ADVANCES IN NEUROLOGY
Volume 89

Advances in Neurology

ADVANCES IN NEUROLOGY
Volume 89

Myoclonus and Paroxysmal Dyskinesias

Editors

Stanley Fahn, M.D.

H. Houston Merritt Professor of Neurology
Department of Neurology
Columbia University and
Columbia-Presbyterian
  Medical Center
The Neurological Institute
New York, New York
USA

Steven J. Frucht, M.D.

Assistant Professor
Department of Neurology
Columbia University and
Columbia-Presbyterian
  Medical Center
The Neurological Institute
New York, New York
USA

Mark Hallett, M.D.

Chief
Human Motor Control Section
National Institute of Neurological
  Disorders and Stroke
National Institutes of Health
Bethesda, Maryland
USA

Daniel D. Truong, M.D

The Parkinson's and Movement
  Disorder Institute
Fountain Valley, California
USA

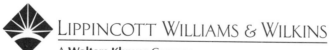

LIPPINCOTT WILLIAMS & WILKINS
A **Wolters Kluwer** Company
Philadelphia · Baltimore · New York · London
Buenos Aires · Hong Kong · Sydney · Tokyo

Acquisitions Editor: Anne M. Sydor
Developmental Editor: Mildred G. Ramos
Production Editor: Thomas J. Foley
Manufacturing Manager: Colin J. Warnock
Compositor: Lippincott Williams & Wilkins Desktop Division
Printer: Maple-Vail Press

Library of Congress Cataloging-in-Publication Data

ISBN: 0-7817-3759-1
ISSN: 0091-3952

Care has been taken to confirm the accuracy of the information presented and to describe generally accepted practices. However, the authors, editors, and publisher are not responsible for errors or omissions or for any consequences from application of the information in this book and make no warranty, expressed or implied, with respect to the currency, completeness, or accuracy of the contents of the publication. Application of this information in a particular situation remains the professional responsibility of the practitioner.

The authors, editors, and publisher have exerted every effort to ensure that drug selection and dosage set forth in this text are in accordance with current recommendations and practice at the time of publication. However, in view of ongoing research, changes in government regulations, and the constant flow of information relating to drug therapy and drug reactions, the reader is urged to check the package insert for each drug for any change in indications and dosage and for added warnings and precautions. This is particularly important when the recommended agent is a new or infrequently employed drug.

Some drugs and medical devices presented in this publication have Food and Drug Administration (FDA) clearance for limited use in restricted research settings. It is the responsibility of the health care provider to ascertain the FDA status of each drug or device planned for use in their clinical practice.

10 9 8 7 6 5 4 3 2 1

Advances in Neurology Series

Contents

Clinical Features of Myoclonus and Myoclonic Syndromes

Neurophysiology of Myoclonus

Genetics of Myoclonus

Pharmacology, Animal Models, and Therapy of Myoclonus

Paroxysmal Disorders and Their Relationship to Epilepsy

Contributing Authors

Charles H. Adler, M.D., Ph.D.
Professor and Chair
Division of Movement Disorders
Department of Neurology
Mayo Clinic Scottsdale
Scottsdale, Arizona,
USA

Sue A. Aicher, Ph.D.
Associate Scientist
Neurological Sciences Institute
Oregon Health & Science University
Beaverton, Oregon
USA

Maria Elisa Alonso, M.D.
Department of Genetics
National Institute of Neurology and Neurosurgery
Mexico City, Mexico

Dong Sheng Bai, M.D.
Chinese Academy of Sciences
Shanghai, China

Robert W. Baloh, M.D.
Professor
Department of Neurology and Surgery
  (Head and Neck)
UCLA Medical School
Director
Neurotology Laboratory
UCLA Medical Center
Los Angeles, California
USA

Thomas G. Beach, M.D.
Director
Laboratory for Neuropathology
Sun Health Research Institute
Sun City, Arizona
USA

Lana Bernstein, M.D.
House Officer
Department of Internal Medicine
Harvard University and Beth Israel Deaconess
  Medical Center
Boston, Massachusetts
USA

Kailash Bhatia, M.D., M.R.C.P.
Senior Lecturer
Department of Clinical Neurology
Institute of Neurology
Consultant Neurologist
Department of Neurology
National Hospital for Neurology
London, United Kingdom

Jaishri Blakeley, M.D.
Intern
Department of Neurology
Parkinson's Disease Center and Movement
  Disorders Clinic
Baylor College of Medicine
Houston, Texas
USA

Eduardo Bonilla, M.D.
Professor
Department of Neurology
Columbia University
New York, New York
USA

Susan B. Bressman, M.D.
Professor
Department of Neurology
Albert Einstein College of Medicine
Bronx, New York
Chairperson
Department of Neurology
Beth Israel Medical Center
Phillips Ambulatory Care Center
New York, New York
USA

Peter Brown, M.D.
Reader in Neurology
Sobell Department of Neurophysiology
Institute of Neurology Queen Square
Honorary Consultant Neurologist
National Hospital of Neurology and Neurosurgery
London, United Kingdom

Paul M. Carvey, Ph.D.
Department of Neurological Sciences
Rush University
Rush-Presbyterian-St. Luke's Medical Center
Chicago, Illinois
USA

Giorgio Casari, M.D.
Human Molecular Genetics Unit
Stem Cell Research Institute
IRCCS San Raffaele Hospital
Milan, Italy

Richard J. Caselli, M.D.
Professor and Chairman
Department of Neurology
Mayo Clinic Scottsdale
Scottsdale, Arizona
USA

John N. Caviness, M.D.
Associate Professor
Department of Neurology
Mayo Medical School
Consultant,
Department of Neurology
Mayo Clinic Scottsdale
Scottsdale, Arizona
USA

Cima Cina, M.Sc.
Research Associate
Department of Pharmacology
Prescient Neuropharma Inc.
Vancouver, British Columbia
Canada

Kristine C. Cowley, Ph.D.
Research Associate
Department of Physiology
Faculty of Medicine
University of Manitoba
Winnipeg, Manitoba
Canada

Meltem Demirkiran, M.D.
Department of Neurology
Çukurova University School of Medicine
Adana, Turkey

Antonio V. Delgado-Escueta, M.D.
Professor
Department of Neurology
University of California
Comprehensive Epilepsy Program
Epilepsy Genetics/Genomics Laboratories
UCLA and VA Greater Los Angeles Healthcare System
West Los Angeles, California
USA

Günther Deuschl, M.D.
Full Professor
Department of Neurology
Department Head
Department of Neurology
Christian-Albrechts-University Kiel
Kiel, Germany

Darryl C. DeVivo, M.D.
Sidney Carter Professor
Departments of Neurology and Pediatrics
Columbia University College of Physicians & Surgeons
New York, New York
USA

Salvatore DiMauro, M.D.
Lucy G. Moses Professor of Neurology
Department of Neurology
Columbia University College of Physicians & Surgeons
New York, New York
USA

Hermann Doose, M.D.
Department of Neuropediatrics
University of Kiel
Kiel, Germany

Stanley Fahn, M.D.
H. Houston Merritt Professor of Neurology
Department of Neurology
Columbia University
Columbia-Presbyterian Medical Center
The Neurological Institute
New York, New York
USA

Chung Yan Fong, M.D.
Division of Neurology
University Department of Medicine
Queen Mary Hospital
Hong Kong, China

Karen P. Frei, M.D.
The Parkinson's and Movement Disorders Institute
Fountain Valley, California
USA

Steven J. Frucht, M.D.
Assistant Professor
Department of Neurology
Columbia University and Columbia-Presbyterian
  Medical Center
The Neurological Institute
New York, New York
USA

Ying-Hui Fu, Ph.D.
Research Associate Professor
Departments of Neurobiology and Anatomy
Howard Hughes Medical Institute
University of Utah
Salt Lake City, Utah
USA

Néstor Gálvez-Jiménez, M.D., F.A.C.P
Associate Professor
Director of Residency Training Program
Head of the Movement and Disorders Section
Department of Neurology
The Cleveland Clinic Florida
Weston, Florida
USA

R. Mark Gardiner, M.D.
Professor
Department of Pediatrics
University College London
Department of Pediatrics
Rayne Institute
London, United Kingdom

Christopher G. Goetz, M.D.
Professor
Department of Neurological Sciences
Rush University
Professor and Associate Chairman
Department of Neurological Sciences
Rush-Presbyterian-St. Luke's Medical Center
Chicago, Illinois
USA

Mark F. Gordon, M.D.
Associate Professor
Department of Neurology
Albert Einstein College of Medicine
Bronx, New York
Attending
Department of Neurology
Long Island Jewish Medical Center
New Hyde Park, New York
USA

Renzo Guerrini, M.D.
Professor of Pediatric Neurology
Neurosciences Unit
Institute of Child Health
The Wolfson Centre
Consultant Pediatric Neurologist
Department of Pediatric Neurology
Great Ormond Street Hospital for Children NHS Trust
London, United Kingdom

Andreas Hahn, M.D.
Department of Neuropediatrics
University of Kiel
Kiel, Germany

Florent Haiss, M.D.
Institute of Anatomy
University of Tübingen
Tübingen, Germany

Mark Hallett, M.D.
Chief
Human Motor Control Section
National Institute of Neurological Disorders and Stroke
National Institutes of Health
Bethesda, Maryland
USA

Ritsuko Hanajima, M.D., Ph.D.
Lecturer
Department of Neurology
University of Tokyo
Tokyo, Japan

Maurice R. Hanson, M.D.
Movement Disorders Program
Department of Neurology
The Cleveland Clinic Florida
Naples, Florida
USA

Melanie J. Hargreave, R.N.
Clinical Research Nurse
Movement Disorders Program
Department of Neurology
The Cleveland Clinic Florida
Naples, Florida
USA

Michio Hirano, M.D.
Assistant Professor
Department of Neurology
Columbia University College of Physicians &
  Surgeons
Assistant Attending
Department of Neurology
New York-Presbyterian Hospital
Columbia Medical Center
New York, New York
USA

Shawn Hochman, Ph.D.
Assistant Professor
Department of Physiology
Emory University School of Medicine
Atlanta, Georgia
USA

Joseph Jankovic, M.D.
Director
Professor of Neurology
Parkinson's Disease Center and Movement
  Disorders Clinic
Senior Attending
Department of Neurology
The Methodist Hospital
Houston, Texas
USA

Joanna C. Jen, M.D., Ph.D.
Assistant Professor
Department of Neurology
UCLA School of Medicine
Los Angeles, California
USA

Anumantha Kanthasamy, Ph.D.
Associate Professor and Director
Parkinson's Research Program
Department of Biomedical Sciences
College of Veterinary Sciences
Iowa State University
Ames, Iowa
USA

Petra Kaufmann, M.D.
Assistant Professor
Department of Neurology
Division of Neuromuscular Disease
Columbia University
Assistant Attending
Department of Neurology
Columbia Presbyterian Medical Center
New York, New York
USA

Michael Kirby, Ph.D.
The Parkinson's and Movement Disorder Institute
Fountain Valley, California
The Parkinson's and Movement Disorder Research
  Laboratory
Long Beach Memorial Research Administration
Long Beach, California
USA

Anthony E. Lang, M.D., F.R.C.P.C.
Jack Clark Chair in Parkinson's Disease Research
Department of Medicine (Neurology)
University of Toronto
Director
Morton and Gloria Shulman Movement Disorders
  Center
Department of Medicine (Neurology)
Toronto Western Hospital
Toronto, Ontario
Canada

Anna-Elina Lehesjoki, M.D., Ph.D.
Professor
Department of Medical Genetics
University of Helsinki
Helsinki, Finland

Ronald P. Lesser, M.D.
Professor
Epilepsy Center
Department of Neurology and Neurosurgery
Johns Hopkins University School of Medicine
Baltimore, Maryland
USA

Sue E. Leurgans, Ph.D.
Professor
Departments of Neurological Sciences and
  Preventive Medicine
Rush Medical College
Chicago, Illinois
USA

Wolfgang Löscher, M.D.
Professor and Chair
Department of Pharmacology
Toxicology and Pharmacy
School of Veterinary Medicine Hanover
Hanover, Germany

Rolando G. Marquez, M.D.
Research Technician
Department of Physiology and Neuroscience
New York University School of Medicine
New York, New York
USA

Rae R. Matsumoto, Ph.D.
Associate Professor
Department of Pharmaceutical Sciences
University of Oklahoma Health Sciences Center
Oklahoma City, Oklahoma
USA

Marco T. Medina, M.D.
California Comprehensive Epilepsy Program
Epilepsy Genetics/Genomics Laboratories
UCLA and VA Greater Los Angeles Healthcare System
West Los Angeles, California
USA
Medical Faculty of Sciences
Honduran Association of Neurologìa
Scientific Unit of Investigation
Autonomous National University of Honduras
Tegucigalpa, Honduras

Berge A. Minassian, M.D. CM
Assistant Professor
Department of Pediatrics (Neurology)
Hospital for Sick Children and University of Toronto
Toronto, Ontario
Canada

Mark E. Molliver, M.D.
Departments of Neurology and Neuroscience
Johns Hopkins University School of Medicine
Baltimore, Maryland
USA

Gholam K. Motamedi, M.D.
Assistant Professor
Department of Neurology
Georgetown University School of Medicine
Director
Epilepsy Monitoring Unit and Epilepsy Surgery Program
Department of Neurology
Georgetown University Hospital
Washington, DC
USA

Bernd A. Neubauer, M.D.
Professor of Pediatrics
Division of Neuropediatrics
Center for Pediatrics and Juvenile Medicine
Justus-Liebig-University
Giessen, Germany

Jose A. Obeso, M.D.
Professor and Consultant
Department of Neurology
Neuroscience Center
Clinica Universitaria and Medical School
University of Navarra
Pamplona, Spain

Elizabeth O'Hearn, M.D.
Assistant Professor
Departments of Neurology and Neuroscience
Johns Hopkins School of Medicine and Johns Hopkins Hospital
Baltimore, Maryland
USA

Shingo Okabe, M.D.
Student of Graduate School of Medicine
Department of Neurology
University of Tokyo
Tokyo, Japan

Laurie Ozelius, M.D.
Molecular Neurogenetics Unit
Massachusetts General Hospital
Charlestown, Massachusetts
USA

Eric J. Pappert, M.D.
Neurology Associates
P.A., Austin, Texas
USA

Lucio Parmeggiani, M.D., Ph.D.
Honorary Consultant Neurophysiologist
Department of Neurophysiology
Institute of Child Health and Great Ormond Street Hospital for Children
The Wolfson Centre
London, United Kingdom

Perla Peirut, M.D.
Department of Neurology
The Cleveland Clinic Florida
Weston, Florida
USA

Dimitris G. Placantonakis, B.S.
Department of Physiology and Neuroscience
New York University School of Medicine
New York, New York
USA

Louis J. Ptáček, M.D.
Associate Investigator
Departments of Neurology and Human Genetics
Howard Hughes Medical Institute
University of Utah
Salt Lake City, Utah
USA

Angelika Richter, D.V.M., Ph.D.
Associate Professor
Department of Pharmacology,
  Toxicology and Pharmacy
School of Veterinary Medicine Hanover
Hanover, Germany

John C. Rothwell, M.D.
Professor of Human Neurophysiology
Sobell Department of Neurophysiology
Institute of Neurology
London, United Kingdom

Mary Sano, M.D.
Assistant Professor of Neuropsychology
Department of Neurology
Columbia University College of Physicians & Surgeons
New York, New York
USA

Rachel Saunders-Pullman, M.D.
Neurologist
The Hyman-Newman Institute for Neurology and
  Neurosurgery
Beth Israel Medical Center
Singer Division
New York, New York
USA

Raphael Schiffmann, M.D.
Acting Chief
Clinical Investigations Section
Developmental and Metabolic Neurology Branch
National Institute of Neurological Disorders and Stroke
Bethesda, Maryland
USA

Brian J. Schmidt, M.D.
Associate Professor
Departments of Medicine and Physiology
University of Manitoba
Consultant Neurologist
Department of Medicine
Health Sciences Centre
Winnipeg, Manitoba
Canada

Peter R. Schofield, Ph.D., D.Sc.
Professor of Medicine
St. Vincent's Hospital
University of New South Wales
Director
Neurobiological Research Program
Garvan Institute of Medical Research
Sydney, Australia

Mohamed Shafiq, M.D.
Clinical Research Fellow
Movement Disorders
Department of Medicine (Neurology)
Toronto Western Hospital
Toronto, Ontario, Canada

Hiroshi Shibasaki, M.D.
Professor
Department of Neurology
Kyoto University Faculty of Medicine
Kyoto University
Shogoin, Sakyo-ku, Kyoto, Japan

Dikoma C. Shungu, M.D.
Assistant Professor
Departments of Neurology and Radiology
Columbia University College of Physicians &
  Surgeons
New York, New York
USA

Jobst Sievers, M.D.
Professor
Department of Anatomy
University of Kiel
Kiel, Germany

Ulrich Stephani, M.D.
Director of Neuropediatric Clinic of the
  University
Department of Neuropediatrics
University of Kiel
Kiel, Germany

Miyabi Tanaka, M.D.
Japan

Kurenai Tanji, M.D., Ph.D.
Fellow in Neuropathology
Department of Pathology
Columbia University College of Physicians &
  Surgeons
Fellow in Neuropathology
Department of Pathology
Columbia Presbyterian Hospital
New York, New York
USA

William T. Thach Jr, M.D.
Professor
Department of Anatomy, Neurobiology, and Neurology
Washington University School of Medicine
St. Louis, Missouri
USA

Philip D. Thompson, M.B.B.S., Ph.D.,
  F.R.A.C.P.
Professor of Neurology
University Department of Medicine
Adelaide University
Director
Department of Neurology
Royal Adelaide Hospital
Adelaide, South Australia

Claudia Trenkwalder, M.D.
Assistant Professor
Department of Neurology
Ludwig-Maximilians-University
Munich, Germany
Assistant Medical Director
Department of Clinical Neurophysiology
University of Goettingen
Goettingen, Germany

Daniel D. Truong, M.D.
The Parkinson's and Movement Disorder Institute
Fountain Valley, California
USA

Shoji Tsuji, M.D.
Department of Neurology
Brain Research Institute
Niigata University, Niigata, Japan

Yoshikazu Ugawa, M.D., Ph.D.
Assistant Professor and Lecturer
Department of Neurology
University of Tokyo
Tokyo, Japan

Toan Q. Vu, M.D.
Department of Neurology
University of Missouri Health Care
Columbia, Missouri
USA

Sarah I. Warsetsky, M.D.
Resident
Departments of Obstetrics and Gynecology
Abington Memorial Hospital
Abington, Pennsylvania
USA

John P. Welsh, M.D.
Associate Scientist
Neurological Sciences Institute
Oregon Health and Sciences University
Beaverton, Oregon
USA

Kristin L. Wetjen, R.N., B.S.N.
Registered Nurse
Department of Neurology
Mayo Clinic Scottsdale
Scottsdale, Arizona
USA

Henrik Wilms, M.D.
Assistant Physician
Clinic for Neurology
Christian-Albrechts-University
Kiel, Germany

Zbigniew K. Wszolek, M.D.
Associate Professor of Neurology
Department of Neurology
Mayo Clinic Jacksonville
Jacksonville, Florida, USA

Kaoru Yuasa, M.D.
Lecturer
Department of Laboratory Medicine
University of Tokyo
Tokyo, Japan

Genevieve S. Yuen, M.D.
Department of Neuroendocrinology
Tri-Institutional M.D. and Ph.D. Program of Weill
  Medical College of Cornell University and
  Rockefeller University
New York, New York
USA

Preface

The clinical features and pathophysiology of myoclonus were last reviewed in a volume published in the *Advances in Neurology* series in 1986. In the past fifteen years we have witnessed tremendous progress in understanding the neurophysiology and genetics of myoclonic disorders. Recent investigations in animal models of myoclonus and in patients with cortical and subcortical myoclonus have yielded important insights that have changed the way neurologists care for these patients. Given these new developments, it seemed an appropriate time to revisit this subject. This book is the result of those efforts.

We chose to include the paroxysmal dyskinesias and related disorders in the treatment of myoclonus because of their shared phenomenology and pathophysiology. To our knowledge, this is the first volume to review these topics. By bringing together these two categories of involuntary movement disorders, we hope to stimulate new ideas for research and treatment.

Each symposium speaker was asked to submit a chapter reviewing recent developments in their field of expertise. In addition, several of the participants who presented posters at the symposium were asked to summarize their work. This book systematically reviews the clinical features, neurophysiology, genetics, and pharmacology of myoclonus. It also reviews the pathophsiology and genetics of paroxysmal movement disorders. We asked contributors to include elements of the commentaries that followed their talks, to emphasize controversies within their field, and to discuss topics that merited further investigation. The result is a volume that we hope will be both comprehensive and stimulating to clinicians and neuroscientists.

Stanley Fahn, M.D.
Steven J. Frucht, M.D.
Mark Hallett, M.D.
Daniel D. Truong, M.D.

Acknowledgments

This book resulted from an international symposium on myoclonus and paroxysmal movement disorders held in October 2000 at the Aberdeen Woods conference center in Atlanta. An international roster of acknowledged experts attended the symposium to review the clinical phenomenology, neurophysiology, genetics, and pharmacology of myoclonus and paroxysmal movement disorders. A series of forty lectures were given, in addition to twenty poster presentations, that reviewed recent research in the field.

The symposium was planned and organized by members of the Myoclonus Study Group. We are indebted to The Myoclonus Research Foundation, The National Institute of Neurological Disorders and Stroke, The Office of Rare Diseases of the National Institutes of Health, UCB Pharma, and the Parkinson's and Movement Disorders Foundation for the financial support for the symposium and publication of the proceedings. Ms. Theodora Mason, of the Myoclonus Research Foundation, handled the logistics of planning such a complicated event with grace and skill. Mr. Norman Seiden supervised all aspects of the planning and execution of the symposium, and was instrumental in its success. His personal dedication to the cause of improving the lives of patients with myoclonus is reflected in this book.

Finally, this symposium was planned as a tribute to the memory of the late C. David Marsden. Professor Marsden's influence is evident throughout this volume, in the seminal work that he published, the investigators that he trained, and in the interest and enthusiasm that he inspired in others. The organizing committee and contributors to this volume dedicate this book to his memory.

ADVANCES IN NEUROLOGY
Volume 89

Myoclonus and Paroxysmal Dyskinesias,
Advances in Neurology, Vol. 89,
edited by S. Fahn, et al.
Published by Lippincott Williams & Wilkins, Philadelphia, 2002.

The Contribution of C. David Marsden to the Study and Treatment of Myoclonus

*Jose A. Obeso, †Kailash Bhatia, and †John C. Rothwell

*Department of Neurology, Neuroscience Center, Clinica Universitaria and Medical School,
University of Navarra, Pamplona, Spain; †Department of Clinical Neurology,
Institute of Neurology and National Hospital for Neurology, London, United Kingdom; and
Sobell Department of Neurophysiology, Institute of Neurology, London, United Kingdom

The first systematic study of a patient with myoclonus was probably Carmichael's case with stimuli-sensitive myoclonic jerks (1). Dawson (2) studied this remarkable patient physiologically in great detail at Queen Square, London, in 1947. He demonstrated that the jerks produced by electrical stimulation of the ulnar nerve were accompanied by large spikes localized over the central area in the electroencephalogram (EEG). The cortical spikes occurred midway between the electrical stimulus and the muscle jerk, and Dawson used, possibly for the first time (3), the term *transcortical reflex* to describe the origin of the myoclonus in this patient. Careful clinical observations (by Dr. Alan Norton) showed that the jerks were mainly provoked by muscle stretch (4), indicating the existence of a transcortical stretch reflex in this patient. The existence of these pathologically enhanced responses gave Dawson the idea of trying to study them in healthy subjects. He first used the technique of photographic superimposition of single EEG sweeps, and then devised the earliest version of an averaging machine for recording the much smaller somatosensory evoked potentials (SEPs) in normal human subjects (4,5).

Professor Carmichael, a fine clinical neurologist who headed the Neurological Research Unit established by the MRC at Queen Square prior to the war, encouraged this conjunction of clinical and basic science research. One of the young scientists attracted to the unit was P. A. Merton, who devoted many years to study reflex muscles responses in humans and originally described the servo theory of muscular control and the silent period (6). With the engineers Hammond and Sutton (7), he described the existence of long latency stretch reflexes in healthy human subjects, but was unsure about whether they were a spinal or cortical phenomenon. In 1968, he met a young (less than 30 years old) C. David Marsden while using the national computer facility at Harwell to calculate power spectra of human tremors, and in the early 1970s they began, together with H. B. Morton, their classic series of experiments that demonstrated the existence of transcortical stretch reflexes in healthy human subjects (8). They observed that the latency to rapid stretching of the flexor pollicis longus (FPL) was approximately twice (around 50 ms) that of the tendon jerk response (Fig. 1). Citing the physiologic anatomy work of Charles Phillips (9), Ed Evarts (10), and others in the monkey that showed direct and rapid connections in motor cortex between sensory inputs and motor outputs, they argued that a similar pathway was operating in humans. This became their transcortical stretch reflex that operated in parallel with the more familiar monosynaptic spinal reflex. At that time (1972), another pa-

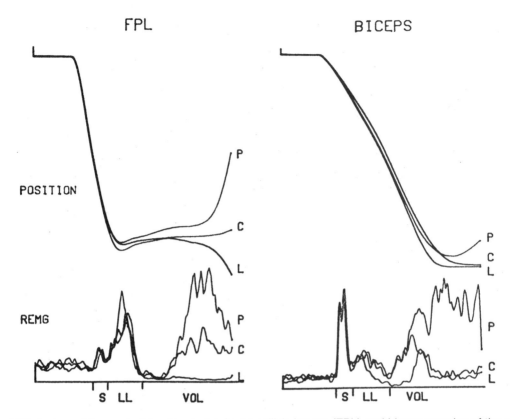

FIG. 1. Long-latency stretch reflex in the flexor pollicis longus (FPL) and biceps muscles of the upper limb. Each trace represents the average of position **(top)** and rectified EMG **(bottom)** in three experimental conditions: *P,* subject tried to resist by pulling against the imposed stretch stimulus; *C,* subject maintained a constant effort; *L,* no opposition to the motor torque was made. The spinal *(S),* the long-latency *(LL),* and the voluntary *(Vol)* component of the EMG responses are labeled. The long-latency stretch reflex has a latency of about 40 ms and is much larger and noticeable in the distal limb muscle FPL than in biceps. (From, Desmedt JE, ed. *Motor Control Mechanisms in Health and Disease.* New York: Raven Press, 1983:510–539.)

tient with stimulus-sensitive myoclonus similar to Carmichael's first case (according with Merton [4] who saw both) was seen in Queen Square. This completed the circle of research that had led from pathology to normal physiology. The patient had giant SEPs and reflex muscles discharges in the upper limb and the "magic" latency of 40 to 50 ms: a clear case of an exaggerated transcortical stretch reflex released by disease.

We believe that the link established in these experiments between physiology and pathology was an important factor in producing

Marsden's drive to understand how the nervous system works. Only in this way could he explain the consequences of disease that he saw in his patients. It was an approach that was followed by Martin Halliday, who also worked in the MRC Unit at Queen Square and who had made the first extensive analysis of the physiology of myoclonus in humans (11).

Marsden was appointed consultant in neurology at King's College Hospital in 1972 and professor of neurology of the Institute of Psychiatry in 1974. Research on the long-latency stretch reflex continued (including one day per week working with Merton and Morton in Queen Square) but his interest in myoclonus per se grew considerably. In particular, Lhermitte's 1971 report (12) of the effect of 5-hydroxytryptophan (5-HTP) in certain forms of myoclonus encouraged his interest in animal models of myoclonus and in pharmacologic trials. For some 12 years (1974 to 1986), Windsor Walk (the site for the animal and physiologic research facilities and Marsden's and his collaborators' offices in the Institute of Psychiatry) became a place where ideas and experimental results were constantly discussed, refined, and finally written up for publication. Marsden (Fig. 2) played a paramount role in all these steps. Admittedly, his international reputation and university commitments had then grown quite considerably, and it became progressively more difficult to find an opening in his busy schedule. Nevertheless, he truly never failed to assist his team in both clinical care and experimental work.

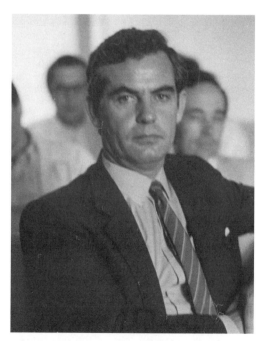

FIG. 2. Photograph of C. David Marsden during a clinical session in the Clinica Universitaria, University of Navarra, Pamplona, 1985.

In 1986, Marsden was appointed to the chair of neurology in Queen Square and also head of the MRC Unit (at this time labeled the Human Movement and Balance Unit). His interest in myoclonus never faded, and he continued to believe, like his predecessor Carmichael, that "it is our goal to make sense of the experiments nature makes in man." Marsden wrote more than 70 papers dealing directly with myoclonus and drove the interest of many basic and clinical neuroscientists into this area (Table 1). We have, somewhat artificially, divided his work for the purpose of this review into clinical, physiologic, and pharmacologic and experimental sections.

CLINICAL STUDIES

Classification

The word "myoclonus" has been abused almost as much as "spasm." Though extensive, the literature on myoclonus does not satisfy, and many reports are ambiguous or lacking in their description of the presentation of the jerks. This was Kinnier Wilson's perception of the state of the art of myoclonus in 1940 (13). Marsden, Hallett, and Fahn (13) made a fundamental contribution to our clinical understanding of myoclonus by providing a nosologic and physiologic classification.

They defined myoclonus as, "muscle jerking, irregular or rhythmic, arising in the central nervous system." They realized that myoclonus could be classified according to clinical presentation, etiology, pathophysiology, and perhaps pharmacologic and biochemical pathology (13). However, the etiologic classification was thought to be more helpful and appropriate for clinical practice. Thus, myoclonus was divided into four main categories: *physiologic myoclonus,* a normal manifestation in healthy people in certain conditions, such as prolonged exercise or during sleep; *essential myoclonus,* where no other neurologic deficit is present and can be sporadic or inherited; *epileptic myoclonus,* where epilepsy dominates the clinical picture and myoclonus was considered as an epileptic manifestation; and *symptomatic my-*

TABLE 1. *Summary of C. David Marsdens' major contributions to myoclonus*

Theme	Publication	Main collaborators
Clinical studies		
Definitions and classification	*Movement Disorders* (book), 1981	Hallett and Fahn
Myoclonic dystonia	*Neurology,* 1983	Obeso, Rothwell, Lang, and Quinn
	Adv Neurol, 1986	
Ramsay-Hunt syndrome	*Mov Disord,* 1989	Obeso and Harding
	Arch Neurol, 1990	
	Brain, 1995	Bhatia and Brown
Myoclonus in CBGD	*Brain,* 1994	Rinne and Thompson
Epilepsia partialis continua	*Brain,* 1985 and 1996	Rothwell, Obeso, and Brown
Long-term evolution of posthypoxic myoclonus	*Mov Disord,* 1997	Brown and Thompson
Physiologic studies		
Cortical and RRM	*J Neurol Neurosurg Psychiatry,* 1977	Adams, Hallett, and Chadwick
	Neurology, 1979	
Spectrum of cortical myoclonus	*Brain,* 1985	Obeso and Rothwell
Physiology of myoclonus in CBGD	*Brain,* 1994	Thompson
Spread of cortical myoclonus	*Brain,* 1991 and 1996	Brown and Rothwell
Hyperekplexia and RRM	*Brain,* 1991	Brown, Rothwell, and Day
	Mov Disord, 1992	Thompson and Obeso
Propriospinal myoclonus	*Brain,* 1991	Brown, Rothwell, and Day
	Mov Disord, 1994	
Pharmacologic and Therapeutic studies		
5-HTP pharmacology and efficacy in postanoxic myoclonus	*Brain,* 1977	Chadwick and Jenner
Polytherapy for severe action myoclonus	*Brain,* 1989	Obeso, Artieda, and Rothwell
Piracetam's efficacy in cortical myoclonus	*Clin Neuropharmacol,* 1988	Obeso and Artieda
	Mov Disord, 1993	Brown
Long-term evolution of chronically treated patients with action myoclonus	*Unpublished*	Bhatia

CBGD, corticobasal-ganglionic degeneration; RRM, reticular reflex myoclonus; 5-HTP, 5-hydroxytryptophan.

oclonus, in the setting of a progressive (i.e., Lafora body disease, G_{M2} gangliosidosis) or static (i.e., anoxia, trauma) encephalopathy. The above definitions and classification were accepted in an experts' meeting organized in 1983 in Arden House (New York State) by S. Fahn (14). The main limitation of this classification was the underlying difficulty with the nosology and pathophysiology of epilepsy and myoclonus. Marsden had a long-standing interest in this theme that was more definitively addressed a few years later (more to follow), when evidence was provided to consider myoclonus of cortical origin as a fragment of epilepsy (15).

The different clinical presentations of myoclonus were further discussed in chapters in a book first published in 1988 and later in 1993 (16). Myoclonus was assessed according the muscles involved, "for this is what one sees when first examining the patient" (16). It was classified as focal/segmental, multifocal, and generalized. An attempt was made to establish a relationship between semiology, physiology, and etiology. For example, focal myoclonus, preferentially involving the limbs distally and sensitive to stimuli, is more likely to have a cortical origin. On the contrary, focal/segmental myoclonus of spontaneous and rhythmic presentation is more likely to have a spinal cord or brainstem origin. Generalized stimuli-sensitive myoclonus is likely to originate in the brainstem (reticular reflex myoclonus).

Myoclonic Dystonia

In 1983, Marsden's group produced a paper entitled "Myoclonic Dystonia" (17) in which it was pointed out that a minority of patients with primary torsion dystonia could, in addition to the typical prolonged, long-lasting spasms in antagonist muscles, exhibit brief myoclonic (less than100 ms) jerks. The condition was sporadic in those cases. The article, however, triggered a good deal of argument at meetings, particularly with colleagues in the United States. This was partially due to semantic problems ("dystonic myoclonus" was a preferred term) but also to differing clinical experience. The matter was hotly debated in a session running late into the night during a dystonia workshop (also organized by S. Fahn in Arden House) in 1986. By then, it had become obvious that the combination of myoclonus and dystonia was specially relevant in patients with a familial form, who exhibited dystonia and/or myoclonus with different degrees of severity without any other major neurologic sign (18). The myoclonus and dystonia of many of such patients are extraordinarily sensitive to alcohol. In an attempt to avoid the semantic and conceptual problems of the combination of myoclonus and dystonia in the same patients, Marsden came up the next morning (in Arden House) with the labeling of "hereditary dystonia with lightning jerks responsive to alcohol." Several families were reported in the next decade, and a marked effort is currently being undertaken to define its genetic basis. The term, however, did not catch on, and myoclonic dystonia (hereditary or alcohol sensitive) is most commonly used (19).

The Ramsay Hunt Syndrome

In the 1987 annual meeting of the American Academy of Neurology held in New York City, Sam Berkovic presented a family with epilepsy, action myoclonus, and ataxia in whom a pathologic diagnosis of adult ceroid lipofuscinosis (Kufs disease) had been made. Analysis of the Montreal Institute series of patients with this combination led Berkovic and Anderman to believe that patients with the typical triad of the so-called Ramsay Hunt syndrome could all be diagnosed if properly investigated for different conditions, which included mitochondrial encephalopathy (myoclonic epilepsy with ragged red fiber myopathy), Lafora body disease, Kufs disease, sialidosis, or progressive myoclonic epilepsy (PME). Berkovic suggested in his oral communication that "this was the right time and place [Ramsay Hunt had made his career in New York] to bury the Ramsay Hunt syndrome as a clinical entity." Marsden and Obeso, who were present in the room, pointed out several reasons to disagree with the attempt to abolish the use of Ramsay Hunt syndrome in clinical practice and indicated that "the burial was far too premature." This set off another polemic, vividly recorded in three review articles published in *Movement Disorders* in 1989 (20–22) where the position and arguments of both groups were discussed in detail and complemented by Anita Harding's own views. This in turn led to a meeting (organized by Andermann and Roger in Marseille in 1989) where the matter was resolved by agreeing that action myoclonus can combine, in the setting of a slowly progressive disease with no recognized etiology, ataxia (progressive myoclonic ataxia [PMA]), epilepsy (PME), or both, with different degrees of severity (23). Thus, the clinical presentation may vary enormously, even within the same family. The gene mutation for PME was found a few years later (24), but it still remains to be established if the same mutation is responsible also for the myoclonic-ataxic predominant forms. In addition, a group of cases studied at Queen Square had celiac disease with action myoclonus of cortical origin and ataxia (25), stressing the plurietiologic origin of PMA and PME and perhaps the value of still maintaining the label of Ramsay Hunt as a clinical syndrome with multiple etiologies. The problem with the term Ramsay Hunt syndrome is that it has been used in the literature in different ways and is still confusing; thus, the tendency is to abandon its use.

Jerky Limbs and Corticobasal Degeneration

Patients with a jerky limb always represent a clinical diagnostic and management challenge. Marsden was particularly interested in this problem, especially because of the relationship between cortical myoclonus and epilepsy. This led his team to document how most cases of epilepsia partialis continua (EPC) had the physiologic characteristics of cortical myoclonus (15,26,27). Among such patients with jerky limbs, there were a few whose disease was of unknown etiology (JM was the initial case) and had many clinical features of cortical myoclonus and EPC, but in whom the SEPs were not "giant," nor was there a cortical wave preceding the action myoclonus. It was also noticed that apparently spontaneous and repetitive myoclonus, producing the clinical impression of EPC (15), was actually the result of bursts of muscle activity triggered by extreme sensitivity to peripheral stimulation. JM's autopsy revealed the pathology of corticobasal ganglionic degeneration (CBGD) (the initial report, however, was that of Parkinson disease!), and this quickly led to the identification of other cases and the detailed clinical and physiologic description of CBGD (28, 29). It is now recognized that a common presentation of CBGD consists of a unilateral "clumsy," stiff, and/or jerky hand. The jerks are stimulus sensitive and aggravated by action and occur so frequently that they may be confused with tremor. The physiologic data also distinguish the jerks of CBGD from other forms of cortical myoclonus. It was postulated that the reflex myoclonus present in patients with CBGD is mediated by direct somatosensory input to the motor cortex, bypassing the usual relay in the somatosensory cortex, thus explaining the lack of giant SEPs (29).

PHYSIOLOGIC AND PHARMACOLOGIC STUDIES

Perhaps the most original and important contribution of Marsden to myoclonus was to combine the pathophysiologic and pharmacologic analysis of myoclonus. Both aspects are treated together in this section.

Cortical and Reticular Reflex Myoclonus

Before 1975, there was only one report by Halliday (11) about the physiology of myoclonus in a large series of patients. However, advances in computing, together with increased understanding of the basic physiology in healthy subjects, soon led to an increase in interest in the field. Hallett and Marsden in London and Shibasaki in Tokyo started independently to apply the technique of EEG back averaging to analyze the cortical activity preceding spontaneous or action-induced muscle jerks. Previously, the only way to demonstrate such activity was by examining the paper readout of a standard EEG record and noting whether there was a spike in the EEG that preceded muscle jerks. Using back averaging, a computer could identify the muscle jerks and then average the EEG activity that preceded them. With this technique they found that they could identify patients with cortical myoclonus who had no obvious spiking on routine EEG.

In addition, Hallett, Chadwick, and Marsden went on to distinguish the new entities of reticular reflex myoclonus (RRM) and cortical reflex myoclonus (CRM) (30,31). Patients with CRM exhibited large SEPs and a cortical spike, time-locked and preceding the action jerks, and the order of recruitment of the generalized jerks followed a rostrocaudal order (30). On the contrary, patients with RRM had no cortical activity related with the jerks, and the recruitment order was best explained by a discharge spreading up the brainstem and down the spinal cord (31). One particular patient (EA), studied (and reported) in great detail over a long period by Marsden and several of his pupils, exhibited both pathophysiologic types of myoclonus. This combination turned out to be rare in patients with postanoxic myoclonus (32) but critically important at the time to understand some pharmacologic differences. Thus, patients with RRM were shown to respond dramatically to treatment with 5-HTP and/or clonazepam, whereas those with CRM improved much less (33). These findings provided a scientific basis for the treatment of action and reflex myoclonus. At the same time, Shibasaki and collaborators in Japan produced evidence for similar physiologic findings in patients with cortical myoclonus and PME, lipidosis, and Lafora body disease (34–36). Shibasaki's work also suggested that the "giant" SEPs seen in patients with reflex myoclonus could have a subtly different cortical origin to the discharge preceding spontaneous and action myoclonus (35). The former was located in postcentral areas, whereas the latter could be more anterior. It

became noticeable that myoclonus of cortical origin was the most common pathophysiologic type in patients with chronic myoclonic encephalopathies (13,36).

Cortical Myoclonus and Epilepsy: Treatments

The clinical and physiologic characteristics of cortical myoclonus were expanded in a series of articles produced by Marsden's group over the next two decades. The spectrum of cortical myoclonus was explained by the fact that increased cortical excitability (Fig. 3) could lead to a combination of reflex jerks and focal and action myoclonus, sometimes progressing to jacksonian seizures or even generalized grand mal epilepsy (15). This provided evidence for considering cortical myoclonus as a fragment of epilepsy, an idea that Marsden

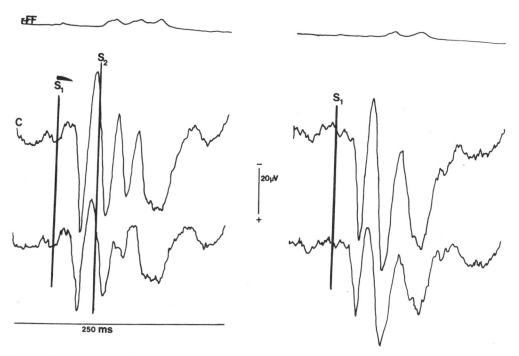

FIG. 3. Giant cortical SEPs and associated reflex discharges recorded from finger flexor muscles *(FF)* of the right forearm. Single stimulation (right) of the median nerve produced a large, double cortical potential, each of the cortical spike preceding the rectified EMG response with an interval of 20 ms. A second electrical stimulus (delivered 40 ms after the first one) induced a third cortical spike and another EMG response with a similar interval. Each trace is the average of 64 responses. (See reference 15 for further details.)

promoted for many years (13). The cortical mechanisms involved in multifocal myoclonus were explored also in great detail (37,38). Importantly, it was recognized that what clinically may look as generalized action myoclonus was in fact the result of the focal cortical discharge spreading to recruit adjacent motor regions and crossing, through the corpus callosum, to excite the contralateral cortex (37). Physiologic studies with transcranial magnetic brain stimulation suggested that this was a consequence of an imbalance in the normal levels of excitation and inhibition in the motor areas of cortex, with obvious parallels to models of cortical epileptic foci (38).

The epileptic nature of cortical myoclonus was further stressed by some initial pharmacologic observations made in patient EA who had a combination of CRM and RRM and occasional generalized seizures By 1980, patient EA's RRM was fairly well controlled with clonazepam, but she was still severely disabled by multifocal spontaneous, reflex, and action myoclonus of cortical origin. She was admitted to Golla Ward in the Maudsley Hospital for evaluation of newer serotoninergic drugs, including the dopamine agonist lisuride (which also has some serotoninergic effect), and the clonazepam daily dose was reduced. Intravenous administration of lisuride improved the CRM of patient EA (39), but as a consequence of the low dose of clonazepam, spontaneous and action myoclonus became increasingly worse and evolved into generalized seizures. Dawson in 1946 had also described how a worsening of spontaneous and action myoclonus could culminate, after a few hours or days, in a grand mal seizure. The normal dose of clonazepam was resumed, but in order to obtain good control of the myoclonus and seizures, Marsden decided to add first valproic acid and subsequently primidone. With that triple therapy, EA's jerks were virtually abolished, her motor performance was normal, and she has not had a seizure again in the past 15 years. As a result of this striking observation, polytherapy, with those three typical antiepileptic drugs and piracetam, was shown a few years later to be the most effica-

cious treatment of cortical myoclonus of any etiology (40). Piracetam in particular was found to be effective against myoclonus of cortical origin only (41,42). Marsden studied and treated a large number of patients with myoclonus in Queen Square. Many of these patients are still being followed up by one of us (K. Bhatia) and other clinicians. Interestingly, the best treatment in those patients with severe action myoclonus even today is triple therapy with piracetam, clonazepam, and valproate. A detailed report of this long-term experience will be published in the near future.

Negative Myoclonus

Marsden's interest in physiologic mechanisms led him to speculate about the cortical origin of negative myoclonus (43). In their original description of postanoxic myoclonus, Lance and Adams pointed out that myoclonic jerks induced by action were caused by an initial brisk muscle contraction, followed by a longer period of electromyography (EMG) silence (44). They noted that the silence, particularly in postural muscles, could be more disabling than the actual muscle jerk and that it was accompanied by a slow wave in the EEG activity over central areas (45,46). Such a combination of muscle excitation followed by silence was also a characteristic of the muscle jerks produced by single pulse transcranial electrical, and later magnetic, stimulation of the human motor cortex, which was explored by Marsden, Merton, and Morton in the 1980s. Marsden noted the resemblance between the clinical phenomenon of "asterixis" and the postural lapses evoked by cortical stimulation (47). He therefore postulated the existence of a type of myoclonus (negative) where the cortical discharge gives rise to muscular silence rather than to active contractions. Negative myoclonus is now well recognized clinically, and its cortical origin has been shown by several groups (48–50).

Startle and Hyperekplexia

The syndrome of hyperekplexia or pathologic startle was also a subject of great interest for Marsden and collaborators, primarily because of a suspected similarity with RRM. However, the initial interest was probably triggered by the case of KP, a 21-year-old woman who, after a minor head injury during a party, woke up with generalized jerks induced by sensory stimulation. Marsden thought she had a new pathophysiologic form of myoclonus because visual threat, sudden sound, or tapping a limb produced a generalized "jump" frequently followed by a salvo of multifocal jerks lasting several seconds. Physiologic studies showed that the latency of the jerks was variable, ranging between 90 and 175 ms, and the order of recruitment was also quite variable and without any specific somatotopic order. It became apparent that certain maneuvers could stop the jerks. Altogether, two of us (JCR and JAO) became convinced the jerks were psychogenic. It took quite an effort to bring Marsden to the physiology laboratory to test our hypothesis because he refused in the majority of cases (at that time) to accept the possibility of a psychogenic origin for any movement disorder. Finally, he reached the same conclusion and cured the patient just by letting her know what the presumed diagnosis was. A few similar patients were encountered later and reported together in 1992 (51). The physiology of startle and hyperekplexia was studied in detail by Brown and colleagues (52,53) in the MRC Unit. In a series of patients with hyperekplexia, they found that the earliest EMG response recorded after the blink triggered by unexpected sound or tapping the face was in the sternocleidomastoid muscles. EMG activity in the masseter and trunk was recorded following the sternocleidomastoid, and limb muscles were recruited much later, like in the normal startle reflex (52). This pattern of muscle activation was compatible with a brainstem origin but differed from that described in RRM by having a much slower descending spinal conduction velocity (30,53). It was suggested that hyperekplexia is the pathologic expression of the normal startle response. It differs from RRM, although both originate in the lower brainstem. In addition, tonic spasms triggered by sensory stimuli may be present in patients with hyperekplexia (53). The pathophysiologic mechanisms of the latter have not been equally well defined but they seem closer to startle epilepsy (54,55).

Propriospinal Myoclonus

This is the latest pathophysiologic type of myoclonus defined by Marsden's school. Patients exhibit nonrhythmic, repetitive myoclonus of the axial musculature, causing flexion of the neck, trunk, and knees (56). The jerks can occur spontaneously or during action or can be induced by tapping. Physiologic studies showed that the order of recruitment and the latencies of the muscles involved in the jerks were compatible with an origin at midthoracic spinal level and spread slowly up and down the cord (56). Typical of Marsden's approach to the study of myoclonus was the effort devoted to understanding the normal physiologic counterpart to propriospinal myoclonus, which shares many characteristics with the long propriospinal pathways documented in animals.

EXPERIMENTAL MODELS OF MYOCLONUS

A good animal model of myoclonus has been very difficult to find. Only recently (see chapter 30) has a fairly good model of posthypoxic myoclonus has been developed in the rat. Jenner and Marsden explored several models of myoclonus, including 5-HTP in the guinea pig and urea and dichlorodiphenyltrichloroethane (DDT) in the rat (57–59). Strenuous attempts to find the physiologic and biochemical counterpart of posthypoxic myoclonus in humans were undertaken in Windsor Walk in the early 1980s, but none of these models became useful for routine studies. Even today, perhaps the best and only animal model of cortical myoclonus is the photosensitive *Papio papio* (60), which indeed shares many physiologic features with photic cortical myoclonus in humans (61). Such a model was routinely used by Meldrum, also working in the neurology department of the

Institute of Psychiatry, for the study of mechanisms of epilepsy. One extremely interesting but largely ignored model at that time was the injection of bicuculline in the caudate of the rat (62). This approach produced focal, repetitive spontaneous jerking of the contralateral limb. In 1980, Nigel Leigh (who followed Marsden in the chair of neurology at the Institute of Psychiatry) spent about one year in Windsor Walk as part of his training and performed detailed experiments with the bicuculline model. The jerks were associated with rhythmic cortical discharges (Fig. 4) and represented a fairly good model of EPC. Nigel Leigh's careful analysis of the injection sites and trajectories suggested, however, that bicuculline was primarily acting at the cortex rather than at the level of the caudate. This

triggered an interesting polemic (with Meldrum) but no definitive conclusion was reached, and the data were never published. After moving to Queen Square, Marsden abandoned the research in animal models of myoclonus and concentrated on the human studies summarized in this chapter.

Conclusions

Marsden made a large number of contributions to the understanding and treatment of myoclonus. He always emphasized the importance of translating new concepts in normal physiology to the pathology seen in patients with myoclonus and vice versa. Indeed, one reason why Marsden, Merton, and Morton finally persuaded the scientific community to

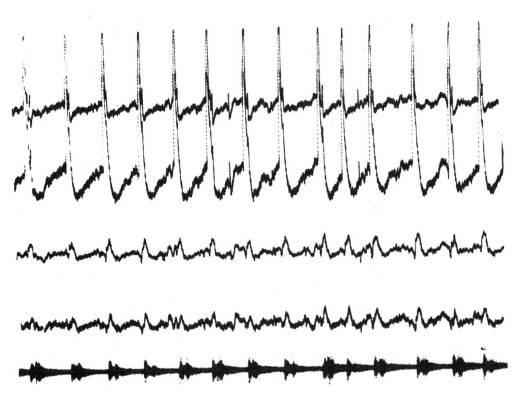

FIG. 4. The picture shows continuously recorded activity over 10 seconds of cortical **(upper two traces)** and striatal **(middle two traces)** extracellular neuronal activity and EMG activity in the right forelimb **(bottom trace)** following bicuculline administration in the left motor cortex of the rat. Rhythmic spike activity at about 1.5 Hz in the left cortex **(second trace from above)** is seen preceding each myoclonic jerk in the contralateral limbs. (N. Leigh, J. C. Rothwell, J. A. Obeso, P. Jenner, and C. D. Marsden, London, 1980, *unpublished observations.*)

accept the idea of transcortical stretch reflexes was their clear demonstration in patients with cortical myoclonus. Marsden always tried to decipher the intimate mechanisms underlying the origin of neurologic manifestations and diseases. He clearly succeeded in this endeavor with myoclonus and other movement disorders. Moreover, his drive to resolve both scientific and clinical challenges was deeply engraved into a whole generation of basal ganglia and movement disorders specialists. We hope his work and spirit will continue to inspire many in the years to come.

ACKNOWLEDGMENT

Ms. Maria Puy Obanos corrected and prepared the article for publication. Most of the studies undertaken by the first author with C. D. Marsden were undertaken with the help of J. C. Rothwell and Brian Day in London and J. Artieda in Pamplona. A large number of the papers published by the author with C. D. Marsden were written in Pamplona thanks to a traveling grant of the University of Navarra and under the inspiration of the product of this region (see reference 20).

REFERENCES

1. Carmichael EA. Myoclonus. *Proc R Soc Med* 1947; 40:553–554.
2. Dawson GD. Investigations on a patient subject to myoclonic seizures after sensory stimulation. J Neurol Neurosurg *Psychiatry* 1947;10:141–162.
3. Dawson GD. Discussion of a case of myoclonus. *Proc R Soc Med* 1947;40:553.
4. Merton PA. Neurophysiology on man. *J Neurol Neurosurg Psychiatry* 1981;44:861–870.
5. Dawson GD. A summation technique for detecting small signals in a large irregular background. *J Physiol* 1951;115:2–3.
6. Merton P. A. Speculations on the servo-control of movement. In: Malcolm JL, Gray JAB, eds. *The spinal cord.* CIBA Foundation Symposium. London: Churchill Livingstone, 1953.
7. Hammond PH, Merton PA, Sutton GG. Nervous gradation of muscular contraction. *Br Med Bull* 1956;12: 14–218.
8. Marsden CD, Merton PA, Morton HB. Servo action in human voluntary movement. *Nature* 1972;238:140–143.
9. Phillips CG. Motor apparatus of the baboon's hand. *Proc R Soc* 1969;B173:141–174.
10. Evarts EV. Relations of pyramidal tract activity to force exerted during voluntary movement. *J Neurophysiol* 1968;31:14–27.
11. Halliday AM. The electrophysiological study of myoclonus in man. *Brain* 1967;40:241–284.
12. Lhermitte F, Peterfalvi M, Marteau R, et al. Analyse pharmacologique d'un cas de myoclonus d'intention et d'action postanoxique. *Rev Neurol* 1971;124:21–31.
13. Marsden CD, Hallett M, Fahn S. The nosology and pathophysiology of myoclonus. In: Marsden CD, Fahn S, eds. *Movement Disorders.* London: Butterworth Scientific, 1981:196–248.
14. Fahn S, Marsden CD, Van Woert MH. Definition and classification of myoclonus. *Adv Neurol* 1986; 43:1–5.
15. Obeso JA, Rothwell JC, Marsden CD. The spectrum of cortical myoclonus. *Brain* 1985;108:193–224.
16. Obeso JA, Artieda J, Marsden CD. Different clinical presentations of myoclonus. In: Jankovic J, Tolosa E, eds. *Parkinson's disease and other movement disorders.* Baltimore: Urban and Schwarzenberg, 1993:315–328. (First published in 1988.)
17. Obeso JA, Rothwell JC, Lang AM, et al. Myoclonic dystonia. *Neurology* 1983;33:825–830.
18. Quinn NP, Rothwell JC, Thompson PD, et al. Hereditary myoclonic myocloni, hereditary torsion myocloni and hereditary essential myoclonus: an area of confusion. *Adv Neurol* 1988;50:391–401.
19. Durr A, Tassin J, Vidailhet M, et al. D2 dopamine receptor gene in myoclonic myocloni and essential myoclonus. *Ann Neurol* 2000;48:127–8.
20. Marsden CD, Obeso JA. The Ramsay Hunt syndrome is a useful entity. *Mov Disord* 1989;4:6–12.
21. Andermann F, Berkovic S, Carpenter S, et al. The Ramsay Hunt syndrome is no longer a useful diagnostic category. *Mov Disord* 1989;4:13–17.
22. Harding AE. Ramsay Hunt syndrome, Unverricht-Lundborg disease or what? *Mov Disord* 1989;4:18–19.
23. Marseille Consensus Group. Classification of progressive myoclonus epilepsies and related disorders. *Ann Neurol* 1990;28:113–115.
24. Pennacchio LA, Lehesjoki AE, Stone NE, et al. Mutations in the gene encoding cystatin B in progressive myoclonus epilepsy (EPM). *Science* 1996;271:1731–1734.
25. Bhatia KP, Brown P, Gregory R, et al. Progressive myoclonic ataxia associated with myoclonic disease. The myoclonus is of cortical origin but the pathology is in the cerebellum. *Brain* 1995;118:1087–1093.
26. Cowan JM, Rothwell JC, Wise RJ, et al. Electrophysiological and positron emission studies in a patient with cortical myoclonus, epilepsia partialis continua and motor epilepsy. *J Neurol Neurosurg Psychiatry* 1986;49: 796–807.
27. Cockerell OC, Rothwell JC, Thompson PD, et al. Clinical and physiological features of epilepsia partialis continua. Cases ascertained in the UK. *Brain* 1996;119: 393–407.
28. Rinne JO, Lee MS, Thompson PD, et al. Corticobasal degeneration. A clinical study of 36 cases. *Brain* 1994; 117:1183–1196.
29. Thompson PD, Day BL, Rothwell JC, et al. The myoclonus in corticobasal degeneration. Evidence for two forms of cortical reflex myoclonus. *Brain* 1994;117: 1197–1207.
30. Hallett M, Chadwick D, Marsden CD. Cortical reflex myoclonus. *Neurology* 1979;29:1107–1125.
31. Hallett M, Chadwick D, Adam J, et al. Reticular reflex

myoclonus: a physiological type of human post-anoxic myoclonus. *J Neurol Neurosurg Psychiatry* 1977;40: 253–264.

32. Brown P, Thompson PD, Rothwell JC, et al. A case of postanoxic encephalopathy with cortical action and brainstem reticular reflex myoclonus. *Mov Disord* 1991; 6:139–144.

33. Chadwick D, Hallett M, Harris R, et al. Clinical, biochemical and physiological features distinguishing myoclonus responsive to 5-hydrosytryptophan, tryptophan with a monoamine oxidase inhibitor and clonazepam. *Brain* 1977;100:455–487.

34. Shibasaki H, Koroiwa Y. Electroencephalographic correlates of myoclonus. *Electroencephogr Clin Neurophysiol* 1975;39:455–463.

35. Shibasaki H, Yamashita Y, Kuroiwa Y. Electroencephalographic studies of myoclonus: myoclonus-related cortical spikes and high amplitude somatosensory evoked potentials. *Brain* 1978;101:447–460.

36. Shibasaki H, Kakigi R, Ikeda A. Scalp topography of giant SEP and pre-myoclonus spike in cortical reflex myoclonus. *Electroencephalogr Clin Neurophysiol* 1991; 81:31–37.

37. Shibasaki H, Yamashita Y, Neshige R, et al. Pathogenesis of giant somatosensory evoked potentials in progressive myoclonic epilepsy. *Brain* 1985;108:225–240.

38. Brown P, Day BL, Rothwell JC, et al. Intrahemispheric and interhemispheric spread of cerebral cortical myoclonic activity and its relevance to epilepsy. *Brain* 1991;114:2333–2351.

39. Brown P, Ridding MC, Werhahn KJ, et al. Abnormalities of the balance between inhibition and excitation in the motor cortex of patients with cortical myoclonus. *Brain* 1996;119:309–317.

40. Obeso JA, Rothwell JC, Quinn NP, et al. Lisuride in the treatment of myoclonus. *Adv Neurol* 1986;43:191–196.

41. Obeso JA, Artieda J, Rothwell JC, et al. The treatment of severe action myoclonus. *Brain* 1989;112:765–777.

42. Obeso JA, Artieda J, Quinn N, et al. Piracetam in the treatment of different types of myoclonus. *Clin Neuropharmacol* 1988;11:529–536.

43. Brown P, Steigert MJ, Thompson PD, et al. Effectiveness of piracetam in cortical myoclonus. *Mov Disord* 1993;8:63–68.

44. Lance JW, Adams RD. The syndrome of intention or action myoclonus as a sequel to hypoxic encephalopathy. *Brain* 1963;86:111–136.

45. Shibasaki H, Ikeda A, Nagamine T, et al. Cortical reflex negative myoclonus. *Brain* 1994;117:477–486.

46. Obeso JA, Artieda J, Burleigh AL. Clinical aspects of negative myoclonus. *Adv Neurol* 1995;67:1–8.

47. Marsden CD, Merton PA, Morton HB. Direct electrical stimulation of corticospinal pathways through the intact scalp in human subjects. In: Desmedt JE, ed. *Motor control mechanisms in health and disease.* New York: Raven Press, 1983:387–391.

48. Shibasaki H. Pathophysiology of negative myoclonus and asterixis. *Adv Neurol* 1995; 67:199–211.

49. Toro C, Hallett M, Rothwell JC, et al. Physiology of negative myoclonus. *Adv Neurol* 1995;67:211–218.

50. Artieda J, Muruzabal J, Larumbe R, et al. Cortical mechanisms mediating asterixis. *Mov Disord* 1992;7: 209–216.

51. Thompson PD, Colebatch JG, Brown P, et al. Voluntary stimulus-sensitive jerks and jumps mimicking myoclonus or pathological startle syndrome. *Mov Disord* 1992;7:257–262.

52. Brown P, Rothwell JC, Thompson PD, et al. New observations on the normal auditory reflex in man. *Brain* 1991;114:1891–1902.

53. Brown P, Rothwell JC, Thompson PD, et al. The hyperekplexias and their relationship to the normal startle reflex. *Brain* 1991;114:1903–1928.

54. Bancaud J, Talairach J, Bonis A. Physiopatogenie des epilepsies-sursaut: a propos d'une epilepsie de l'aire motrice supplementaire. *Rev Neurol* 1967;117:441–453.

55. Brown P. Physiology of the startle phenomena. *Adv Neurol* 1996;67:273–328.

56. Brown P, Thompson PD, Rothwell JC, et al. Axial myoclonus of propriospinal origin. *Brain* 1991;114: 197–214.

57. Chadwick D, Hallett M, Jenner P, et al. 5-hydroxytryptophan-induced myoclonus in guinea pigs: a physiological and pharmacological investigation. *J Neurol Sci* 1978;35:157.

58. Muscatt S, Rothwell JC, Obeso JA, et al. Urea-induced stimulus-sensitive myoclonus in the rat. *Adv Neurol* 1986;43:553–563.

59. Pratt JA, Rothwell J, Jenner P, et al. Myoclonus in the rat induced by p,p'-DDT and the role of altered monoamines function. *Neuropharmacology* 1985;24:193–204.

60. Naquet R, Meldrum BS. Myoclonus induced by intermittent light stimulation in the baboon: neurophysiological and neuropharmacological approaches. *Adv Neurol* 1986;43:611–628.

61. Artieda J, Obeso JA. The pathophysiology and pharmacology of photic cortical reflex myoclonus. *Ann Neurol* 1993;34:175–184.

62. Tarsy D, Pyckock CJ, Meldrum BS, et al. Focal contralateral myoclonus produced inhibition of GABA action in the caudate nucleus of rats. *Brain* 1978;101: 143–162.

Myoclonus and Paroxysmal Dyskinesias,
Advances in Neurology, Vol. 89,
edited by S. Fahn, et al.
Lippincott Williams & Wilkins, Philadelphia © 2002.

1

Overview, History, and Classification of Myoclonus

Stanley Fahn

Department of Neurology, Columbia University, Columbia-Presbyterian Medical Center
Neurological Institute, New York, New York

Myoclonic jerks are defined as sudden, brief, shock–like involuntary movements caused by muscular contractions (positive myoclonus) or inhibitions (negative myoclonus) (1). The duration of the jerk is less than 100 ms., usually less than 50 ms. Because of its short duration, myoclonus is a movement disorder in which electrophysiologic investigation can be enormously helpful to the clinician. Because myoclonic jerks are usually between 10 and 50 ms. in duration and rarely longer than 100 ms., electrical recordings can distinguish myoclonus from other movements. Furthermore, because an individual cannot easily voluntarily produce jerks of durations less than 50 ms., finding these short duration contractions or finding the electrical inhibitions of negative myoclonus on electromyogram (EMG) recordings can help distinguish myoclonic jerks from volitional movements or those due to psychogenic factors. Surface recordings are sufficient for determining the duration of the contraction, so penetrating the skin with needles is not necessary. Applying and recording simultaneous EMG surface electrodes can also determine whether the jerks are synchronous or not. Synchronization is a common feature of myoclonic jerks, and if present could distinguish between myoclonus and other types of abnormal movements and rule out psychogenicity. Finally, another advantage of polyEMG recordings is that they can localize the anatomic origin and de-termine the pathway by which myoclonus spreads in the body, i.e., distinguishing spread via the propriospinal pathway or via the corticospinal tract.

Quantifying the severity of myoclonus would be of enormous benefit for following patients with myoclonic jerks. It would help determine the natural history, the effect of medications, and especially help in evaluating the effectiveness of new therapeutic agents in clinical trials. One attempt to develop a myoclonus rating scale was published by Truong and Fahn (2), with a more user-friendly modification being recently developed, validated, and published in this volume.

The differential diagnosis of myoclonus would be similarly rapid and brief contractions of simple tics. These would be difficult to distinguish from myoclonus, but if complex tics are also present in these patients, the rapid simple tics can be readily recognized because "of the company they keep." Choreic movements are not as rapid as myoclonus, but there could be overlap in speed and duration. Choreic movements tend to flow from point to point on the body and are not repetitively synchronous in other body parts. Excessive startle or hyperekplexia is related to myoclonus in that the speed is fast, but always triggered by startle. Although myoclonus can be triggered by sensory stimuli, they are usually also present with either active voluntary movements (i.e., action myoclonus) or when the body part is at rest (rest myoclonus). Action myoclonus is usually more debilitating than rest myoclonus.

The frequency of myoclonus in the general population has been determined by an epidemiologic study conducted at the Mayo Clinic (3). A prevalence of 8.6 cases per 100,000 and an incidence of 1.3 per 100,000 per year were found. Symptomatic myoclonus was the most common, and within this category, dementing illnesses were the most frequent. A listing of myoclonic syndromes can be found in Marsden et al. (4), Fahn et al. (1), and Caviness (5).

HISTORICAL ASPECTS

The term myoclonus was derived from the longer term *paramyoklonus multiplex* that was first used in a case report by Professor Nikolaus Friedreich in Heidelberg in 1881 (6). Friedreich coined this new term to describe multifocal jerks occurring over the body of a 50-year-old man for 5 years. Friedreich wanted to distinguish the jerks from the clonic contractions of epilepsy and used a combination of terms: *clonus,* quick movements (*klonus* in German); *myo,* muscle; *para,* symmetric; and *multiplex,* multiple sites. Hence, paramyoklonus multiplex. The term caught on and was used, sometimes inaccurately, to describe similar patients in the succeeding years, ultimately being shortened to myoclonus.

However, even before Friedreich's use of this new terminology, similar shock–like movements had been recognized, first considered as part of epilepsy and later as distinct from epilepsy and with the use of other newly minted names. For example, the term *electric chorea* was coined by Dubini (7) 35 years before Friedreich. Dubini reported 38 cases of an acute febrile illness with spasms involving the neck and back; 90% died. It would appear that this affliction was probably an infection, such as meningitis or encephalitis, and the rapid jerks were probably myoclonus. The term *electric chorea* was used several times since then, but for labeling other rapid movements that in retrospect do not seem to be myoclonus. Henoch in 1861 (again before Friedreich) (8) described chronic multifocal jerks in 30 otherwise normal children. The jerks were repetitive, about 3 to 6 per minute, and involved the neck and shoulders predominantly. Most likely these jerks were tics, but Hennig (8) called them electric chorea. In 1880, Bergeron (8), as reported by his pupil Berland, used the term to describe self-limited twitches in children; again, most probably these were tics. Because "electric chorea" had been used to represent different types of rapid movements, Marsden, Hallett, and Fahn (4) recommended that it would be best to "avoid the term electric chorea."

Lowenfeld (9) was the first to use the term *myoclonus* by shortening paramyoklonus multiplex. This was followed by Seeligmüller (10) in his description of a patient who likely had tics. Although the patient was 24 years old, the movements began at age 5 years and also involved vocalizations. When Unverricht reviewed the literature in 1891 (11), he found 40 cases of paramyoclonus multiplex, but rejected 80% as other causes of movement disorders. Lindenmulder (12) described the first family with essential myoclonus.

Several cases thought to be those of myoclonus were probably something else, and different names were used. Kny (13) used the term *myoclonus fibrillaris multiplex,* and the patients probably had fasciculations of amyotrophic lateral sclerosis (ALS). Morvan (14) may have been witnessing myoclonus when he used the term *fibrillary chorea* to describe five patients with acute febrile illness with muscle twitching leading to coma and death. Also thought to be fibrillary chorea were probably examples of myokymia (15), which might have been examples of Isaac's syndrome. Another uncertain syndrome, given the name convulsive tremor because of its paroxysmal nature, was nevertheless thought by Hammond (16) to be similar to Friedreich's case of paramyoclonus multiplex.

Various myoclonic syndromes began to be described. Myoclonic epilepsy was reported by Unverricht (11,17). Following Lundborg's review of myoclonus (18), the syndrome of nondementing familial myoclonic epilepsy was called Unverricht-Lundborg disease. Lundborg described ten families and also classified myoclonus into essential and symptomatic categories. Lafora and Glueck (19) added to this syndrome with their description of myoclonic epilepsy with dementia; amyloid bodies were seen throughout the nervous system at autopsy. Six cases of action myoclonus with cerebellar ataxia were reported by Ramsay Hunt (20) who used the term *dyssynergia cerebellaris myoclonica.* Four also had epilepsy, and two had Friedreich's ataxia. The so-called Ramsay Hunt syndrome is now called progressive myoclonic ataxia (21). A mitochondrial disorder causing myoclonus and epilepsy with ragged red fibers on muscle pathology was described by Fukuhara et al. (22).

Rhythmic myoclonus limited to a body segment was first described to the palatal region (23–25). Later, other segments were described with rhythmic segmental myoclonus (26,27).

A landmark paper was that of Lance and Adams (28), who reported four cases with posthypoxic action myoclonus, characterized predominantly by myoclonus that was most prominent as an active limb reached for a target (intention myoclonus). Action myoclonus had previously been described by Ramsay Hunt (20) and by Wohlfahrt and Hook (29). Nevertheless, the posthypoxic cases were dramatic and reintroduced the phenomenon. Another feature described by Lance and Adams was that sometimes the myoclonic jerks were associated with inhibitions of muscle contractions, so-called negative myoclonus, rather than always with a contraction. Besides the descriptive nature of this paper, highlighting posthypoxic myoclonus was what led to therapeutic trials for myoclonus, including the first effective agent, 5-hydroxytryptophan (30), and then subsequently clonazepam (31), and valproate (32).

The phenomenon of myoclonic jerks as one is falling to sleep is physiologic and is known as hypnic jerks, first reported by De Lisi in 1932 (33). This should not be confused with another phenomenon that occurs during sleep, referred to as nocturnal myoclonus by Symonds (34), but more accurately labeled as periodic movements in sleep by Coleman et al. (35) when polysomnography became available.

Although the recognition of brief inhibitory pauses as negative myoclonus could be attributed to Lance and Adams (28), earlier electrical studies of asterixis (flapping of the limbs) showed these sudden jerks to be due to transient inhibition of the muscles that maintain posture of those extremities (36). Today, asterixis is probably the most common form of negative myoclonus; it is commonly seen accompanying various metabolic encephalopathies (37). Unilateral asterixis has been described with focal brain lesions of the contralateral medial frontal cortex, parietal cortex, internal capsule, and ventrolateral thalamus (38).

CLASSIFICATION

Myoclonus can be classified by clinical appearance, anatomic origin of the jerks based on electrophysiologic characteristics, and by etiology (Table 1.1). Clinically, one should determine if the jerks occur when the affected body part is at rest, engaged in volitional activity, or stimulated by sensory input (reflex myoclonus). Often, action myoclonus is worse when the affected limb is attempting to reach a precise target and is then referred to as intention myoclonus. Action or intention myoclonus is particularly encountered after cerebral hypoxia and with certain degenerative disorders, such as Unverricht-Lundborg disease and the progressive myoclonic ataxias. Usually action myoclonus is more disabling than rest myoclonus. When sudden stimuli such as sound, light, visual threat, or movement triggers the jerks, they are known as reflex myoclonus.

Another clinical distinction that is made is the temporal pattern of the myoclonic jerks. Myoclonus can be irregular (arrhythmic), rhythmic (such as palatal myoclonus and

TABLE 1.1. Classifications of myoclonus

Clinical	Anatomic	Etiology
Relation to action	Cortical	Physiologic myoclonus
At rest	Focal	Essential myoclonus
With action	Multifocal	Epileptic myoclonus
Reflex induced	Generalized	Symptomatic myoclonus
Body part	Epilepsia partialis continua	Storage diseases
Focal	Thalamic	Cerebellar degenerations
Segmental	Brainstem	Basal ganglia degenerations
Multifocal	Reticular	Dementias
Generalized	Startle	Viral encephalopathies
Temporal pattern	Palatal	Metabolic encephalopathies
Irregular	Ocular	Toxic encephalopathies
Oscillatory	Spinal	Hypoxia
Rhythmic	Segmental	Focal damage
	Propriospinal	
	Peripheral	

other segmental myoclonias), or oscillatory, in which the jerks occur as a burst of oscillations and then fade. Rhythmic myoclonus is typically due to a structural lesion of the brainstem or spinal cord (hence, present as a segmental myoclonus), but not all cases of segmental myoclonus are rhythmic. Myoclonic jerks occurring in different body parts are often synchronized, a feature that may be specific for myoclonus.

The last clinical feature to note is the bodily location of the myoclonus. Similarly to classifying other movement disorders, such as dystonia, it is useful to determine if the myoclonus is focal (limited to one region of the body), segmental and axial, multifocal, or generalized.

Anatomically, myoclonus can arise from the cerebral cortex, thalamus, brainstem, cerebellum, spinal cord, and from peripheral sites (nerves, roots, or plexi). Cortical reflex myoclonus usually presents as a focal myoclonus and is triggered by active or passive muscle movements of the affected body part. It is associated with high-amplitude somatosensory evoked potentials and with cortical spikes observed by computerized back averaging, timelocked to the stimulus. Epilepsia partialis continua can sometimes be considered a form of continuous myoclonus arising from the cerebral cortex. Brainstem (reticular) reflex myoclonus is more often generalized or spreads along the body away from the source in a

timed-related sequential fashion. Spinal myoclonus can remain at a specific dermatomal or segmental axial location and be rhythmic, or it can spread along propriospinal pathway to involve several segments. Peripheral myoclonus remains in the distribution of the irritated peripheral nerve or roots.

The etiology of myoclonus is enormous, but can conveniently be classified into four distinct groupings: physiologic, essential, epileptic, and symptomatic. Physiologic myoclonias are the muscle jerks that occur in normal people; in this category are hypnic jerks (sleep jerks) and hiccups. Essential myoclonus is the entity or entities of multifocal myoclonus that occurs without any other neurologic deficit except tremor and mild dystonia and without any known neurodegeneration. The terms *myoclonic dystonia* and *myoclonus-dystonia* may represent disorders that are part of the essential myoclonus spectrum. Essential myoclonus is often familial, and genetic studies are being carried out in such families. Epileptic myoclonias are conditions in which epilepsy is the primary disorder, and myoclonic jerks are present as part of the clinical picture. The most common category of myoclonus is symptomatic myoclonus. Many of these myoclonias are from neurodegenerative diseases, but infections, hypoxia, and trauma are also common.

In Caviness's epidemiologic survey of myoclonus syndromes mentioned earlier, symptomatic myoclonus was the most common, and within this category, dementing illnesses were the most frequent. A listing of myoclonic syndromes can be found in Marsden et al. (4), Fahn et al. (1), and Caviness (5).

REFERENCES

1. Fahn S, Marsden CD, Van Woert MH. Definition and clinical classification of myoclonus. *Adv Neurol* 1986; 43:1–5.
2. Truong DD, Fahn S. Therapeutic trial with glycine in myoclonus. *Mov Disord* 1988;3:222–232.
3. Caviness JN, Alving LI, Maraganore DM, et al. The incidence and prevalence of myoclonus in Olmsted County, Minnesota. *Mayo Clin Proc* 1999;74:565–569.
4. Marsden CD, Hallett M, Fahn S: The nosology and pathophysiology of myoclonus. In: Marsden CD, Fahn S, eds. *Movement Disorders*. London, Butterworth Scientific, 1982:196–248.
5. Caviness JN. Myoclonus. *Mayo Clin Proc* 1996;71: 679–688.
6. Friedreich N. Neuropathologische Beobachtung beim paramyoklonus multiplex. *Virchow's Arch Pathol Anat Physiol Klin Med* 1881; 86:421–434.
7. Dubini A. Primi cenni sulla corea electria. *Annals of the University of Medicine (Milano)*. 1846;117:1–5. Quoted by Marsden, Hallett, and Fahn (4).
8. Wilson SAK. *Neurology* Baltimore: Williams & Wilkins, 1940.
9. Lowenfeld 1883. Quoted by Seeligmüller (10).
10. Seeligmüller A. Ein Fall von Paramyoklonus multiplex (Friedreich) (Myoclonia congenital). *Dtsch Med Wochenschr* 1886;12:405–408.
11. Unverricht H. *Die Myoclonie*. Leipzig und Wien: Franz Deuticke. 1891:128.
12. Lindenmulder FG: Familial myoclonus occurring in three successive generations. *J Nerv Ment Dis* 1933;77: 489–491.
13. Kny E. Über ein dem Paramyoclonus multiplex (Friedreich) nahestehendes Krankheitsbild. *Archives für Psychiatrie und Nervenkrankheiten* 1888;19:577–590.
14. Morvan AM. De la chorée fibrillaire. *Gazette hebdomadaire de Medecine et de Chirurgie* 1890;27:173–176, 187–189, 200–202.
15. Schultze F. Beiträge zur Muskelpathologie. I. Myokymie (Muskelwogen) besonders an den Unterextremitaten. *Dtsch Z Nervenheilk* 1895;6:65–70.
16. Hammond WA. On convulsive tremor. *N Y J Med* 1867; 5:185–198.
17. Unverricht H. Über familiäre Myoklonie. *Dtsch Z Nervenheilk* 1895;7:32–67.
18. Lundborg H. Die progressive Myoklonus-Epilepsie. *Uppsala:Almqvist and Wiksell*, 1903.
19. Lafora G, Glueck B. Beitrag zur Histopathologie der Myokonischen Epilepsie. *Z Neurol Psychiatr* 1911;6: 1–16.
20. Hunt JR. Dyssynergia cerebellaris myoclonica—primary atrophy of the dentate system: a contribution to the pathology and symptomatology of the cerebellum. *Brain* 1921;44:490–538.
21. Marsden CD, Harding AE, Obeso JA, et al. Progressive myoclonic ataxia (the Ramsay Hunt syndrome). *Arch Neurol* 1990;47:1121–1125.
22. Fukuhara N, Tokiguchi S, Shirakawa K, et al. Myoclonus epilepsy associated with ragged red fibers (mitochondrial abnormalities): disease entity or a syndrome? *J Neurol Sci* 1980;47:117–133.
23. Spencer HR. Pharyngeal and laryngeal "nystagmus." *Lancet* 1886;2:702.
24. Klien H. Zur Pathologie der kontinuierlichen rhythmischen Krämpfe der Schlingmuscckulatur. *Neurol Zentralbl* 1907;26:245–254.
25. Guillain G, Mollaret P. Deux cas de myoclonies synchrones et rythmées vélo-pharyngo-laryngo-oculo-diaphragmatiques. Le problème anatomique et physiopathologique de ce syndrom. *Rev Neurol* 1931;2: 545–566.
26. Patrikios MJ. Sur un cas d'automatisme moteur particulier des members supérieurs après traumatisme de la moelle cervicale. *Rev Neurol* 1938;69:179–188.
27. Garcin R, Rondot P, Guiot G. Rhythmic myoclonus of the right arm as the presenting symptom of a cervical cord tumour. *Brain* 1968;91:75–84.
28. Lance JW, Adams RD. The syndrome of intention or action myoclonus as a sequel to hypoxic encephalopathy. *Brain* 1963;86:111–136.
29. Wohlfahrt G, Hook O. A clinical analysis of myoclonic epilepsy (Unverricht-Lundborg), myoclonic cerebellar dyssynergia (Hunt) and hepatolenticular degeneration (Wilson). *Acta Psychiatr Neurol Scand* 1951;26: 219–245.
30. Lhermitte F, Marteau R, Degos C-F. Analyse pharmacologique d'un cas de myoclonus d'intention et d'action post-anoxiques. *Rev Neurol (Paris)* 1972;126:107–114.
31. Boudouresques J, Roger J, Khalil R, et al. A propos de 2 observations de syndrome de Lance et Adams. Effet therapeutique du RO-05-4023. *Rev Neurol (Paris)* 1971;125:306–309.
32. Fahn S. Posthypoxic action myoclonus: review of the literature and report of two new cases with response to valproate and estrogen. *Adv Neurol* 1979:26:49–84.
33. De Lisi L. Su di un fenomeno motorio costante del sonno normale: le mioclonie ipniche fisiologiche. *Riv Pat Nerv Ment* 1932;39:481–496.
34. Symonds CP. Nocturnal myoclonus. *J Neurol Neurosurg Psychiatry* 1953;16:166–171.
35. Coleman RM, Pollak CP, Weitzman ED. Periodic movements in sleep (nocturnal myoclonus): relation to sleep disorders. *Ann Neurol* 1980;8:416–421.
36. Leavitt S, Tyler HR. Studies in asterixis. *Arch Neurol* 1964;10:360–368.
37. Young RR, Shahani BT. Asterixis: one type of negative myoclonus. *Adv Neurol* 1986;43:137–156.
38. Obeso JA, Artieda J, Burleigh A. Clinical aspects of negative myoclonus. *Adv Neurol* 1995;67:1–7.

Myoclonus and Paroxysmal Dyskinesias,
Advances in Neurology, Vol. 89,
edited by S. Fahn, et al.
Lippincott Williams & Wilkins, Philadelphia © 2002.

2

Epidemiology of Myoclonus

John N. Caviness

Department of Neurology, Mayo Clinic Scottsdale, Scottsdale, Arizona

A considerable body of literature describes myoclonus of various etiologies (1). Much effort has also been made to study its pathophysiology through electrophysiologic analysis (2). However, most studies have been based on random clinical ascertainment of cases. Studying myoclonus from an epidemiologic perspective presents a few challenges. Disparate diagnostic entities can variably produce myoclonus, and many of these disorders are rare. There are additional problems associated with ascertainment of myoclonus as a symptom (or sign), since it can either be the main clinical problem or be relatively unnoticed as a relatively minor syndrome component. When small and occurring in a repetitive fashion during muscle activation, myoclonus can be confused with tremor. Despite these problems, it is still important to study the incidence and prevalence of myoclonus. Epidemiology offers a way to study the public health impact of any clinical entity. This information also helps the clinician organize a rational differential diagnosis and can provide clues as to how myoclonus is generated.

Information about the general occurrence of myoclonus has been obtained from the literature through (a) large clinical series, (b) epidemiologic studies of specific diagnoses that commonly produce myoclonus, and (c) epidemiologic study of myoclonus from any cause in a defined population. Random ascertainment, referral bias, and undefined populations are obvious problems with large clinical series. Epidemiologic studies of specific diagnoses are often "point in time" studies and therefore underestimate the accumulative risk of having myoclonus in that particular disorder. We studied the incidence and prevalence of myoclonus in the defined population of Olmsted County, Minnesota (3). Although there are also problems with ascertainment in a defined population, the data represent a more valid epidemiologic perspective on the occurrence of myoclonus in the general population than the aforementioned methods.

LARGE CLINICAL SERIES

In the past 40 years, very few clinical series have been reported as being inclusive for all possible causes of myoclonus. There is no epidemiologic information that can be reliably obtained from large clinical series, because of the problems mentioned previously. Nevertheless, various classification schemes have been presented over the years based on clinical series. Such case collections, when compared with more controlled studies, show an obviously skewed perspective.

Aigner and Mulder described 94 myoclonus cases in 1960 from the Mayo Clinic (4). Seventy-five percent of cases were younger than 20 years old. Most had a pure seizure disorder without other neurologic problems. Approximately 25% had a syndrome consistent with progressive myoclonic epilepsy. A minority had a syndrome consistent with essential myoclonus. Very few had onset of myoclonus after age 50, and none exhibited myoclonus as a result of a late-onset neurodegenerative syndrome.

Swanson et al. reported 67 myoclonus cases seen at Johns Hopkins University (5). In this series, central nervous system infections and toxic/metabolic disturbances were the common causes of myoclonus. No cases of essential myoclonus were reported and progressive myoclonic epilepsy comprised less than 10% of this series. There were just a few cases that may have had a late-onset neurodegenerative syndrome.

Epidemiologic Studies of Specific Diagnoses

The incidence of idiopathic progressive myoclonic epilepsy (Unverricht-Lundborg, EPM1) in Finland is 5 in 100,000 births (6). This is undoubtedly a much larger number than has been seen in other countries. Creutzfeldt-Jakob disease is believed to have an incidence of 0.05 to 0.1 cases per 100,000 person-years (7). Myoclonus is a clinical hallmark of Creutzfeld-Jakob disease, but it does not occur in every case.

Only a few epidemiologic studies of specific diagnoses have reported on the occurrence of myoclonus in the cases being studied. Alzheimer's disease is a prime example. In Alzheimer's disease, cross-sectional studies underestimate the occurrence of myoclonus. Studies in which patients were followed up until death have shown a 40% to 50% accumulative risk of developing myoclonus. One study found an incidence of 1,150 myoclonus cases per 100,000 person/years in a population of persons with Alzheimer's disease (8).

The Clinical Epidemiology of Myoclonus in Olmsted County, Minnesota

Our study (3) was retrospective and restricted to pathologic and persistent myoclonus. Case ascertainment was done through a medical records linkage system. We identified all subjects whose records contained documentation of myoclonus or of diseases known to exhibit myoclonus. A neurologist reviewed the records of all potential patients, and only those records with clearly documented myoclonus were accepted. Population denominators were derived from U.S. census data.

Twenty-one cases were accepted out of the 714 individuals who were identified through the medical records linkage system. Twelve cases were incident from 1976 to 1990, 6 cases were both incident from 1976 to 1990 and prevalent on January 1, 1990, and 3 cases were used as being prevalent only. The average annual incidence rate of pathologic and persistent myoclonus for 1976 through 1990 was 1.3 cases per 100,000 person-years. The lifetime prevalence of myoclonus, as of January 1, 1990, was 8.6 cases per 100,000 population.

When evaluating the 21 cases as a simple clinical series, there were 12 men and 9 women, and most research subjects were aged 60 years or older. A more accurate view is obtained from analyzing the cases from an epidemiologic perspective. The age- and sex-specific average annual incidence rates are plotted in Figure 2.1, and the age- and sex-specific prevalence is plotted in Figure 2.2. These graphs show that the incidence and prevalence of myoclonus increase with age and are generally greater for men than for women. This is in stark contrast to the earlier large clinical series where most cases had a younger age of onset. This is probably because of the random ascertainment as well as a decreased appreciation of myoclonus in disorders with later age of onset in those series.

The average annual incidence rate of 1.3 cases per 100,000 person-years is compared in Table 2.1 to those obtained for other movement disorders in the same database (9–12). The value for myoclonus is actually larger than that for Huntington's disease. It is about half the incidence for idiopathic dystonia and only about eight times less common than idiopathic Parkinson's disease. When comparing the amount of literature that is devoted to these other movement disorders with that of myoclonus, one could argue that myoclonus should be studied more extensively, considering its relative incidence.

In our study, we used the proposed clinical classification for myoclonus of Marsden and

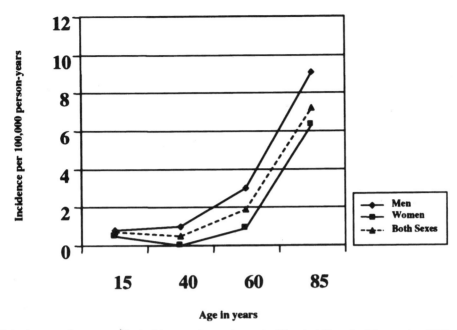

FIG. 2.1. Age- and sex-specific incidence of myoclonus in Olmsted County, Minnesota, 1976–1990.

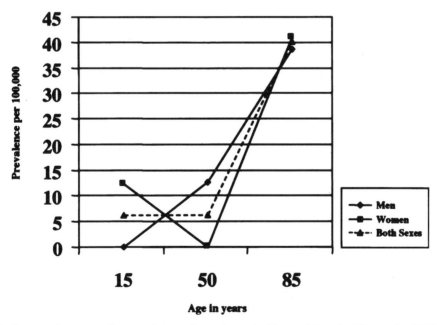

FIG. 2.2. Age- and sex-specific prevalence of myoclonus in Olmsted County, Minnesota, 1976–1990.

TABLE 2.1. Incidence values compared among various movement disorders

Neurological disorder (reference)	Incidence value per 100,000 person-years
Myoclonus	1.3
Huntington's disease (9)	0.3
Idiopathic dystonia (10)	2.6
Parkinson's disease (11)	10.8
Essential tremor (12)	23.7

Fahn (13). Their scheme consists of three major categories of pathologic myoclonus: essential, epileptic, and symptomatic. Our study found that symptomatic myoclonus (72%) was the most common etiologic category, followed by epileptic myoclonus (17%) and essential myoclonus (11%). Within the symptomatic group, posthypoxic syndrome, Alzheimer's disease, and Creutzfeldt-Jakob disease accounted for most of the cases. This is quite different from the large clinical series in the past, where dementing illnesses that affect older individuals and chronic neurodegenerative diseases are uncommon. The difficulties with performing a retrospective epidemiologic study of a symptom are outlined elsewhere (3). One particular problem with our study was the small number of cases. This is the reason why more unusual, but nevertheless important, causes of myoclonus did not appear among the 21 cases.

The myoclonus associated with Alzheimer's disease and Creutzfeldt-Jakob disease was not as disabling to those patients as compared with the patients with posthypoxic myoclonus. For those with Alzheimer's disease and Creutzfeldt-Jakob disease, dementia was the clinically more important symptom. The myoclonus was the most prominent symptom in the juvenile myoclonic epilepsy patients, and the response to treatment was good and superior to that seen in the posthypoxic myoclonus patients. The posthypoxic patients had myoclonus as a prominent cause of their disability, and the treatment response was poor.

SUMMARY

All studies that attempt to evaluate the general occurrence of myoclonus have various biases. Even so, myoclonus has been demonstrated to be an important cause of abnormal movement control when compared to other movement disorders. Clearly, posthypoxia etiology, neurodegenerative disease, and epilepsy syndromes are important individual causes of myoclonus. The epidemiology of myoclonus is worthy of further study in other defined populations.

REFERENCES

1. Caviness JN. Myoclonus: a clinical review. *Mayo Clin Proc* 1996;71:679–688.
2. Shibasaki H. Electrophysiological studies of myoclonus. AAEM Minimonograph no. 30. *Muscle Nerve* 2000;23:321–335.
3. Caviness JN, Alving LI, Maraganore DM, et al. The incidence and prevalence of myoclonus in Olmsted County. *Mayo Clin Proc* 1999;74:565–569.
4. Aigner BR, Mulder DW. Myoclonus: clinical significance and an approach to classification. *Arch Neurol* 1960;2:600–615.
5. Swanson PD, Luttrell CN, Magladery JW. Myoclonus—A report of 67 cases and review of the literature. *Medicine* 1962;339–356.
6. Norio R, Koskiniemi M. Progressive myoclonus epilepsy: genetic and nosological aspects with special reference to 107 Finnish patients. *Clin Genet* 1979;15:382–398.
7. Will RG. Epidemiology of Creutzfeldt-Jakob disease. *Br Med Bull* 1993;49:960–970.
8. Chen JY, Stern Y, Sano M, et al. Cumulative risks of developing extrapyramidal signs, psychosis, or myoclonus in the course of Alzheimer's disease. *Arch Neurol* 1991;48:1141–1143.
9. Kokmen E, Ozekmekci FS, Beard CM, et al. Incidence and prevalence of Huntington's disease in Olmsted County, Minnesota (1950 through 1989). *Arch Neurol* 1994;51:696–698.
10. Nutt JG, Muenter MD, Aronson A, et al. Epidemiology of focal and generalized dystonia in Rochester, Minnesota. *Adv Neurol* 1988;50:361-5.
11. Bower JH, Maraganore DM, McDonnell SK, et al. Incidence and distribution of parkinsonism in Olmsted County, Minnesota, 1976–1990. *Neurology* 1999;12; 52(6):1214-20.
12. Rajput AH, Offord KP, Beard CM, et al. Essential tremor in Rochester, Minnesota: a 45-year study. *J Neurol Neurosurg Psychiatry* 1984;47:466–470.
13. Marsden CD, Marsden CD, Hallett M, et al. The nosology and pathophysiology of myoclonus. In: Marsden CD, Fahn S, eds. *Movement disorders*. London: Butterworths, 1982:196–248.

*Myoclonus and Paroxysmal Dyskinesias,
Advances in Neurology,* Vol. 89,
edited by S. Fahn, et al.
Lippincott Williams & Wilkins, Philadelphia © 2002.

3

Myoclonus in Lewy Body Disorders

*John N. Caviness, *Charles H. Adler, †Thomas G. Beach, *Kristin L. Wetjen,
and *Richard J. Caselli

*Department of Neurology, Mayo Clinic Scottsdale, Scottsdale, Arizona; and †Department of
Neuropathology, Sun Health Research Institute, Sun City, Arizona*

Hyperkinetic movement disorders are common in parkinsonian syndromes. Tremor, at rest and/or during muscle activation, is present in many cases of idiopathic Parkinson's disease (PD) as well as other parkinsonian syndromes (1). Myoclonus is much less common than tremor in parkinsonian syndromes, and the presence of myoclonus usually suggests a less common cause of parkinsonism than idiopathic PD (2). The association of myoclonus and parkinsonism has been observed in multiple system atrophy (MSA), corticobasal degeneration, diffuse Lewy body disease, drug-induced syndromes, postencephalitic parkinsonism, idiopathic PD, and less commonly in other conditions (3–9). However, it cannot be assumed that the myoclonus pathophysiology is identical across these different parkinsonian syndromes. Moreover, different types of myoclonus in the same syndrome may occur.

Electrophysiologic studies of myoclonus in parkinsonism have provided some insight about its mechanism and source. Myoclonus in MSA has been reported to be typical of "cortical reflex myoclonus," with enlarged somatosensory evoked potentials (SEPs), exaggerated long latency electromyographic (EMG) responses (LLRs) to median nerve stimulation, and back-averaged electroencephalographic (EEG) transients (10). In addition, a photic cortical reflex myoclonus and a brainstem source for myoclonus have been described electrophysiologically in MSA

(11,12). In corticobasal degeneration, enhanced EMG facilitation to cutaneous digital stimulation has been found. Despite the lack of back-averaged EEG transients, the overall findings were interpreted as support for a cortical origin of the myoclonus (7,8). In PD with stimulus-sensitive myoclonus and dementia, Chen et al. (9) reported that there was increased EMG facilitation to cutaneous stimulation. In contrast, this facilitation was not found in their normal subjects or PD patients without myoclonus and dementia. In neither group of PD patients was the presence of time-locked EEG transients mentioned, and the source of facilitation was uncertain.

We recently reported the electrophysiologic analysis of a cortical origin myoclonus in two patients with a sporadic, levodopa-responsive parkinsonism that closely resembled clinical PD (13). Since that time, patient 2 of that report has died and at autopsy, showed idiopathic Lewy body PD. In addition, we have also described cortical myoclonus in the familial Lewy body disorder that was described by Muenter (14). In order to further define the occurrence of small-amplitude cortical myoclonus in the spectrum of Lewy body disorders and its clinical and electrophysiologic associations, we studied small-amplitude myoclonus in ten patients with PD and two patients diagnosed as having dementia with Lewy bodies (DLB). We also present the brain autopsy findings of our previously reported case.

METHODS

Clinical Assessment

Ten PD patients who demonstrated small-amplitude, multidirectional jerking of the fingers and wrist were recruited from our movement disorders clinic. All PD patients had a chronic, progressive, asymmetric syndrome of bradykinesia and rigidity, with or without rest tremor, without evidence of another disorder. According to U.K. brain bank guidelines, these criteria should have a 93% chance of fulfilling the pathologic criteria for PD (15,16). Two patients with DLB who demonstrated small-amplitude, multidirectional jerking of the fingers and wrist were also recruited. DLB was diagnosed using the consensus criteria, and both patients had a history of visual hallucinations (17).

All subjects had the motor scale of the Unified Parkinson's Disease Rating Scale (UPDRS) and a Folstein Mini-Mental State Exam (MMSE) recorded while in the "on" state.

Electrophysiology

Combined EEG/EMG recordings, using the Neuroscan (C) system (Neuroscan, Inc., El Paso, Texas), acquired data at a rate of 2500 Hz with a band pass of 1 to 500 Hz (24 dB/octave). Bilateral upper extremity bipolar surface Ag/AgCl EMG electrodes were placed on deltoid, biceps, triceps, wrist flexors, wrist extensors, abductor pollicis brevis (APB), first dorsal interosseus, and abductor digiti minimi (ADQ). Modified 10–20 system Ag/AgCl EEG electrode positions were used with a Fz reference. Recordings were made at rest and during arm movement. EEG/EMG back averaging was done off-line, with cursor placement at the onset of myoclonic EMG activity. The data for back averaging were collected while the muscles were activated by holding the arms outstretched, wrists slightly extended, and the fingers spread apart. Recordings were made in the "on" state.

A GRASS SS8800 stimulator (Grass Instruments Co., Quincy, Massachusetts) was used to obtain cortical SEPs and LLRs bilaterally. For the SEP, two trials of 1000 epochs were recorded with 0.2 ms stimulation at 1.5 Hz of the median nerve at the wrist with sufficient intensity to produce a minimal APB twitch. The attempted elicitation of LLRs was performed by 0.2 ms stimulation to the median nerve at the wrist (sufficient intensity to produce minimal APB twitch) as well as digital stimulation of the index finger at 2 to 3 times the sensory threshold. For the elicitation of LLRs, 20 trials were collected at 5- to 10-second intervals for each type of stimulation with the muscles relaxed. For the SEPs and the LLRs, the same bilateral upper extremity surface EMG electrodes were used as that discussed for the EEG/EMG polygraphy.

RESULTS

Parkinson's Disease

Clinical Assessment. The ten PD subjects consisted of eight men and two women. The average age was 70.4 years (range, 63 to 77). The motor UPDRS average was 22.4 (range, 7 to 29). Hoehn and Yahr staging ranged from 1.5 to 3.0 with a mean of 2.4. At the time of clinical assessment and electrophysiologic testing, 7 of 10 subjects were on antiparkinsonian therapy. The average MMSE was 28.0 (26 to 30).

The myoclonus in those subjects occurred as distally predominant bilateral upper extremity action myoclonus of the wrist and fingers. The myoclonus was only rarely present at rest. Reflex myoclonus could not be demonstrated to touch, stretch, or tendon reflexes. The amplitude was often greater on one side, but this was not always the same side as the more prominent parkinsonian signs. No relationship to antiparkinsonian therapy of any type was appreciated, and three subjects were not on therapy.

Electrophysiology. Myoclonic EMG discharges were seen only rarely during rest. Surface EMG during muscle activation showed both rhythmic trains and sporadic brief (<100 ms) discharges consistent with myoclonus. The discharges occurred primarily in wrist and hand muscles, and less-frequent discharges occurred proximally. A multifocal distribution was seen without bilateral synchronous discharges.

All PD patients showed a focal, short latency, back-averaged EEG transient prior to the myoclonic EMG discharge. In all cases, the transient had a triphasic positive-negative-positive configuration over the sensorimotor cortex contralateral to the myoclonic EMG discharge. The maximum amplitude of the transients was always posterior to the central sulcus in parietal electrodes. Referencing the back-averaged transient to Fz, A1, and A2 or an averaged reference always showed the CP3/4 electrode as having maximum amplitude. SEPs (N20-P25, P25-N33) were not enlarged. Enhanced LLRs following median nerve or digital nerve stimulation at rest were not seen. The grand average for eight of the PD cases (all those done with using right arm activation) is shown in Figure 3.1. At CP3, the transient had the maximal positive-negative amplitude of 8.3 mV (Fz reference). The time

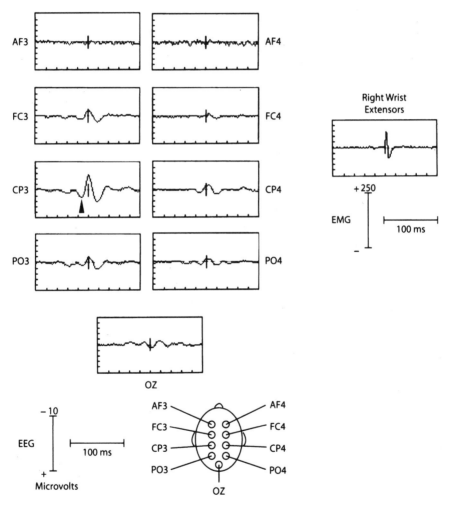

FIG. 3.1. Grand average for eight Parkinson disease subjects (100 epochs each, 800 epochs total). Back-averaging of the myoclonic discharge for the right wrist extensors shows a triphasic positive-negative-positive focal electroencephalogram (EEG) transient over the contralateral sensorimotor region. The *arrow* shows the peak positivity of the initial phase for the CP3 electrode. At CP3, the transient had the maximal positive-negative amplitude of 8.3 mV. The time interval from this peak positivity to the onset of back-averaged electromyogram activity was 27 ms. The EEG electrode positions are shown in the small head-shaped figure. The time and amplitude scales are shown in the reference window.

interval from this peak positivity to the onset of back-averaged EMG activity was 27 ms.

Dementia with Lewy Bodies

Clinical Assessment. The two DLB cases were 76 and 68 years old. They had MMSE scores of 15 and 21, motor UPDRS scores of 29 and 33, and both had a Hoehn and Yahr stage of 2.5. Both of the DLB cases were on antiparkinsonian therapy. The clinical characteristics of the myoclonus in the DLB subjects were nearly identical as those for the PD subjects, except possibly for an increased myoclonus activation at rest.

Electrophysiology. Occasional myoclonic EMG discharges were seen during rest. Surface EMG during muscle activation showed

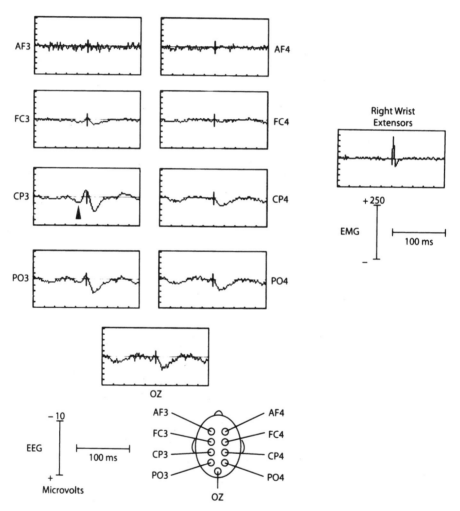

FIG. 3.2. Grand average for the two dementia with Lewy body disease subjects (100 epochs each, 200 epochs total). Back-averaging of the myoclonic discharge for the right wrist extensors shows a triphasic positive-negative-positive focal electroencephalogram (EEG) transient over the contralateral sensorimotor region. The *arrow* shows the peak positivity of the initial phase for the CP3 electrode. At CP3, the transient had the maximal positive-negative amplitude of 4.8 mV. The time interval from this peak positivity to the onset of back-averaged rectified electromyogram activity was 30 ms. The EEG electrode positions are shown in the small head-shaped figure. The time and amplitude scales are shown in the reference window.

both rhythmic trains and sporadic brief (<100 ms) discharges consistent with myoclonus. The discharges occurred primarily in wrist and hand muscles, and less-frequent discharges occurred proximally. A multifocal distribution was seen without bilateral synchronous discharges.

Both DLB patients showed a focal, short latency, back-averaged EEG transient prior to the myoclonic EMG discharge. In all cases, the transient had a triphasic positive-negative-positive configuration with maximum amplitude posterior to the central sulcus in parietal electrodes contralateral to the myoclonic EMG discharge. SEPs (N20-P25, P25-N33) were not enlarged. Enhanced LLRs following median nerve or digital nerve stimulation at rest were not seen. The grand average of the back-averaged EEG transients for the two DLB cases is shown in Figure 3.2. At CP3, the transient had the maximal positive-negative amplitude of 4.8 mV. The time interval from this peak positivity to the onset of back-averaged EMG activity was 30 ms.

BRAIN PATHOLOGY FROM PREVIOUSLY DESCRIBED REPORT (CASE 2)

Gross examination of the brain was unremarkable except for marked depigmentation of the substantia nigra (13). On microscopic appearance, the neocortical areas showed occasional Lewy bodies in the middle temporal gyrus, inferior parietal lobule, and cingulate gyrus, and there were rare Lewy bodies in the pre- and postcentral gyri. The amygdala and entorhinal cortex showed mild gliosis and scattered Lewy bodies. A few neurons in the hypothalamus contained Lewy bodies. The substantia nigra and locus ceruleus are severely depleted of pigmented neurons, and there were Lewy bodies in several remaining neurons in each area. There were sparse to moderate densities of cored plaques in neocortical areas, with similar densities of diffuse plaques, and neurofibrillary tangles were rare. Neurofibrillary tangles were present at high densities in the hippocampus and entorhinal

cortex. The nucleus basalis of Meynert showed a few neurofibrillary tangles but was otherwise unremarkable. Sections of the cerebellum showed patchy Purkinje cell loss in the hemispheric cortex. The dentate nucleus and superior vermis of the cerebellum, medulla, and cervical spinal cord were unremarkable. The findings showed pathologically confirmed PD. The Alzheimer type changes corresponded to "intermediate likelihood" of Alzheimer's disease by the Reagan/National Institute on Aging (NIA) criteria.

DISCUSSION

The observations of the present report confirm and extend our previous clinical and electrophysiologic findings (13). Because the ten patients of the present report included a range of progression, we verified that the small-amplitude myoclonus occurred at early as well as at later stages of the disease. We also obtained support for the notion that the myoclonus was not necessarily associated with dementia. Although subjective complaints of decreased memory were seen in our ten PD patients, none was demented and all had MMSE scores of 26 or greater. These patients will need to be followed in order to determine whether the presence of cortical myoclonus heralds cognitive decline. With regard to the electrophysiologic findings, all patients showed a focal, short latency, back-averaged EEG transient prior to the contralateral myoclonic EMG discharge. The transient always had a maximum amplitude posterior to the central sulcus in CP3/4 electrodes contralateral to the myoclonic EMG discharge. This suggests that the transient may arise from the sensory areas of the sensorimotor cortex rather than from regions anterior to the central sulcus. Inadvertently or due to head shape variation, the CP3/4 electrode in some instances could have had a more anterior location with respect to the cortical area underneath it. However, the parietal waves N20 and P25 of the SEP also always had a maximum in the CP3/4 electrodes. Even though this provides some evidence for parietal localization of this wave, better mapping, as could be done with magnetoencephalography with magnetic resonance imaging coregistration would be more definitive.

The evidence presented here suggests that cortical myoclonus can occur across the spectrum of Lewy body disorders. Our two DLB subjects, as expected, had MMSE scores that were well below those seen in our PD cases. However, even from these two cases, it was evident that the clinical and electrophysiologic characteristics of the action myoclonus were very similar to the PD cases. One possible clinical difference seen in our patients was an increased prominence of myoclonus at rest when compared to the PD cases. The myoclonus seen in PD and DLB also showed many properties in common with the myoclonus that we have reported previously in individuals with hereditary diffuse Lewy body disease (14). For comparison purposes,

the back-averaged EEG transient from our previously reported hereditary case is shown in Figure 3.3.

The combined clinical and electrophysiologic characteristics of the myoclonus in Lewy body patients are different from those seen in other parkinsonian syndromes or other instances of similarly appearing small distal jerks. Such syndromes include MSA, corticobasal degeneration, cortical tremor, minipolymyoclonus, levodopa-induced myoclonus, and asterixis. Our patients did not have enlarged cortical SEPs or enhanced LLRs, which differentiates them from having "typical" cortical reflex myoclonus (18). Hence, this myoclonus has different electrophysiologic characteristics from that seen in any type of myoclonus described in MSA (10–12). The presence of a time-locked EEG transient distinguishes the myoclonus in our patients from that seen in corticobasal degen-

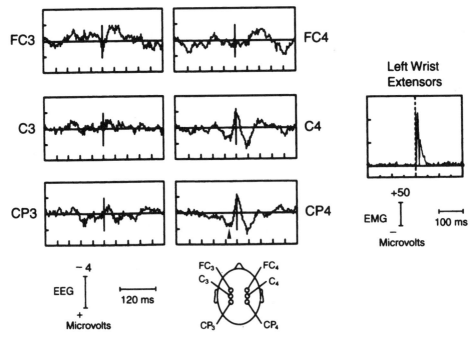

FIG. 3.3. Back-averaged cortical transient for a case of hereditary Lewy body disease from our previously reported case (14). The triphasic positive-negative-positive focal EEG transient over the right sensorimotor cortex preceded the averaged left wrist extensor myoclonic discharge. The peak positive-negative amplitude occurred at the CP4 electrode. The *arrow* denotes the point of the pretrigger positive peak that occurred at 30 ms.

eration (7). The clinical appearance of the small-amplitude distal limb myoclonus is somewhat reminiscent of the movements seen in cortical tremor or minipolymyoclonus (5,19). However, the electrophysiologic findings in cortical tremor are like those found in "typical" cortical reflex myoclonus, which these patients did not demonstrate. The cortical correlate described in minipolymyoclonus by Wilkins and Hallett had a bifrontal negativity, quite unlike that found in our patients (5,19). The electrophysiologic findings for the myoclonus in Alzheimer disease can be variable, but negative potentials followed by the myoclonus at longer latencies than reported here have been found (20). The clinical characteristics of the myoclonus in our patients were unlike those in levodopa-induced myoclonus, as the latter usually occurs from rest, often during sleep or drowsiness, and is sensitive to levodopa dosage (3). Finally, the movements seen in our patients in no way resembled the postural lapses of asterixis.

The specific pathologic correlate of the myoclonus across the spectrum of Lewy body disorders is not clear. Recently, case 2 from our previous report died and had a brain autopsy. This patient had a thirteen-year history of PD with fluctuations followed by a gradual deterioration of mental function with hallucinations over a two-year period. The myoclonus began before clinical evidence of mental decline. As mentioned earlier, there were widespread Lewy bodies and some Alzheimer type pathology. Individuals with DLB show diffusely distributed Lewy bodies and variable but significantly present Alzheimer's disease pathology. Pathologic findings from the Muenter kindred have shown neuronal loss in the substantia nigra and locus ceruleus as well as widespread Lewy bodies (21). In this kindred, the Lewy bodies exist in the substantia nigra, limbic areas, and occasionally in neocortical areas over the convexity. Alzheimer changes are not typically found. Thus, cortical Lewy bodies are a prominent finding in Lewy body disorders that may show myoclonus, but what pathology specifically correlates with the presence of the myoclonus is unknown. It is also unclear what role, if any,

Alzheimer type pathology may play in the generation of myoclonus in Lewy body disorders. Clearly, much more study is needed on the pathologic correlation of myoclonus in Lewy body disorders. Furthermore, neurochemical abnormalities may well play a role as well.

In summary, the myoclonus that we have described in PD, DLB, and hereditary Lewy body cases has been found to have similar clinical and electrophysiologic characteristics. This suggests that there may be unifying causative mechanisms underlying the myoclonus in Lewy body disorders. One possible mechanism for the cortical myoclonus production would be the lack of inhibitory influences and/or excessive excitation of sensorimotor cortex produced by the neurodegeneration occurring locally. On the other hand, neurochemical abnormalities and/or abnormal remote input from other areas may be playing a prominent role. More direct evidence is needed to elucidate this mechanism.

REFERENCES

1. Deuschl G, Bain P, Brin M, et al. Consensus statement of the Movement Disorder Society on Tremor. *Mov Disord* 1998;Suppl 3:2–23.
2. Caviness JN. Myoclonus. *Mayo Clin Proc* 1996;71: 679–688.
3. Klawans HL, Goetz C, Bergen D. Levodopa-induced myoclonus. *Arch Neurol* 1975;32:331–334.
4. Burkhardt CR, Filley CM, Kleinschmidt-DeMasters BK, et al. Diffuse Lewy body disease and progressive dementia. *Neurology* 1988;38:1520–1528.
5. De Wilkins, Hallett M, Erba G. Primary generalised epileptic myoclonus: a frequent manifestation of minipolymyoclonus of central origin. *J Neurol Neurosurg Psychiatry*1985;48:506–516.
6. Wenning GK, Shlomo YB, Magalhaes M, et al. Clinical features and natural history of multiple system atrophy. An analysis of 100 cases. *Brain* 1994;117:835–845.
7. Thompson PD, Day BL, Rothwell JC, et al. The myoclonus in corticobasal degeneration: evidence for two forms of cortical reflex myoclonus. *Brain* 1994;117: 1197–1207.
8. Klawans HL, Tanner CM, McDermott J. Myoclonus and parkinsonism. *Clin Neuropharmacol* 1986;9(2):202–205.
9. Chen R, Ashby P, Lang AE. Stimulus-sensitive myoclonus in akinetic-rigid syndromes. *Brain* 1992;115: 1875–1888.
10. Obeso JA, Rothwell JC, Marsden CD. The spectrum of cortical myoclonus. *Brain* 1985;108:193–224.
11. Artieda J, Obeso JA. The pathophysiology and pharmacology of photic cortical reflex myoclonus. *Ann Neurol* 1993;34:175–184.

12. Clouston PD, Lim CL, Fung V, et al. Brainstem myoclonus in a patient with non-dopa-responsive parkinsonism. *Mov Disord* 1996;11:404–410.
13. Caviness JN, Adler CH, Newman S, et al. Cortical myoclonus in Levodopa-responsive parkinsonism. *Mov Disord*1998;13:540–544.
14. Caviness JN, Gwinn-Hardy KA, Adler CH, et al. Electrophysiological observations in hereditary parkinsonism-dementia with Lewy body pathology. *Mov Disord* 2000;15:140–145.
15. Hughes AJ, Ben-Shlomo Y, Daniel SE, et al. What features improve the accuracy of clinical diagnosis in Parkinson's disease: a clinicopathologic study. *Neurology* 1992;42:1142–1146.
16. Hughes AJ, Daniel SE, Blankson S, et al. A clinicopathologic study of 100 cases of Parkinson's disease. *Arch Neurol* 1993;50:140–148.
17. McKeith IG, Galsko D, Kosaka K, et al. Consensus guidelines for the clinical and pathological diagnosis of dementia with Lewy bodies (DLB): report of the consortium on DLB international workshop. *Neurology* 1996;47:1113–1124.
18. Shibasaki H. Electrophysiologic studies of myoclonus. AAEE Minimonograph no. 30. *Muscle Nerve*1988;11:899–907.
19. Ikeda A, Kakigi R, Funai N, et al. Cortical tremor: a variant of cortical reflex myoclonus. *Neurology* 1990;40:1561–1565.
20. Thompson PD, Shibasaki H. Myoclonus in corticobasal degeneration and other neurodegenerations. *Adv Neurol* 2000;82:69–81.
21. Muenter MD, Forno LS, Hornykiewicz, et al. Hereditary form of parkinsonism-dementia. *Ann Neurol* 1998;43:768–781.

Myoclonus and Paroxysmal Dyskinesias,
Advances in Neurology, Vol. 89,
edited by S. Fahn, et al.
Lippincott Williams & Wilkins, Philadelphia © 2002.

4

Neurodegenerative Causes of Myoclonus

Philip D. Thompson

*University Department of Medicine and Department of Neurology, Royal Adelaide Hospital and
University of Adelaide, Adelaide, South Australia*

Myoclonus is a common finding in neurodegenerative diseases and in some conditions may be a prominent clinical feature. Table 4.1 summarizes those neurodegenerative conditions in which myoclonus may be prominent and of diagnostic significance.

INHERITED METABOLIC ENCEPHALOPATHIES

Myoclonus is a common feature of the neurodegenerative syndrome that accompanies the inherited metabolic diseases of childhood and adolescence. These conditions frequently present with progressive neurologic degeneration and seizures, dementia, and loss of motor skills. These features may be more prominent than myoclonus.

The myoclonus in these syndromes is classified clinically as focal or multifocal action and stimulus-sensitive reflex myoclonus and has been well characterized in numerous reports. These descriptions have formed the basis of the classical accounts of the physiology of cortical reflex myoclonus (1). Reflex myoclonus occurs in response to cutaneous and muscle afferent stimulation. Both action and reflex myoclonus consists of repetitive trains of short duration (25 to 50 ms) hypersynchronous electromyographic (EMG) discharges simultaneously in antagonist muscle pairs. The electroencephalogram (EEG) is often abnormal with spike and wave discharges. Jerk locked averaging of the EEG reveals positive cortical spike or sharp waves preceding myoclonus and cortical

spread of myoclonic spike discharges in the EEG. Cortical somatosensory evoked potentials (SEPs) are enlarged and often referred to as "giant" with a P25-N33 complex of greater than 10 microvolt (2). The latency of reflex myoclonus in hand muscles is of the order of 50 to 60 ms after stimulation of the median (or ulnar) nerve at the wrist.

The common causes of these syndromes of cortical myoclonus often with epilepsy, dementia, and ataxia have traditionally been referred to as "progressive myoclonic epilepsy." In those cases where myoclonus and ataxia are more prominent than epilepsy, the alternative designation "progressive myoclonic ataxia" has been suggested to emphasize this subtle clinical difference. Table 4.1 lists the commoner causes of this syndrome. Increasingly recognized as a cause of progressive myoclonic ataxia is the mitochondrial disease myoclonus epilepsy with ragged red fibers (MERRF).

CEREBELLAR DEGENERATIONS

Cortical reflex myoclonus and a syndrome of progressive myoclonic ataxia are also seen in some spinocerebellar degenerations. Primary (spino)cerebellar degenerations, celiac disease, and postanoxic encephalopathy with action myoclonus are the commonest causes, in addition to late presentations of the inherited metabolic encephalopathies. Even with detailed investigations it has been estimated that up to 40% of progressive myoclonic ataxic syndromes in adult life remain undiagnosed (3).

TABLE 4.1. *Myoclonus in neurodegenerative conditions*

Myoclonus with cognitive decline
Alzheimer disease
Creutzfeldt-Jakob disease
Paraneoplastic encephalopathy

Myoclonus with akinetic-rigid syndromes
Corticobasal degeneration
Multiple system atrophy
Huntington disease
Dentato-rubro-pallido-luysian atrophy

Progressive myoclonus with epilepsy or ataxia
Spinocerebellar degenerations
Myoclonus epilepsy with ragged red fibers
Lafora body disease
Ceroid lipofuscinosis
Unverricht-Lundborg disease (Baltic myoclonus)
Sialidosis
Celiac disease

CORTICOBASAL DEGENERATION

Myoclonus is present in one-third of cases at presentation and develops in a further 20% over the following two years. A jerky limb tremor may evolve into myoclonus as the disease progresses (4). Accordingly, myoclonus is observed in approximately 50% of patients with corticobasal degeneration during the course of the illness (5).

Myoclonus is frequently superimposed on a rigid dystonic posture of the limb, typically the hand and fingers, but it may also be seen in the feet and toes. Movement of the affected limb is followed by repetitive trains of action myoclonus. Apraxia of the limb may further contribute to clumsy limb movement. On examination, stimulus-sensitive reflex myoclonus is elicited by cutaneous stimulation and tendon taps.

The EMG patterns of hypersynchronous discharges in both action and stimulus-sensitive reflex myoclonus are similar to that described in cortical reflex myoclonus (6). However, several physiologic features serve to distinguish the myoclonus of corticobasal degeneration from "typical" cortical reflex myoclonus. There are no time-locked cortical spike or sharp wave discharges in the EEG preceding myoclonus in most cases, and the EEG shows only nonspecific changes (7). Cortical activity preceding myoclonus has been detected on back-averaged magnetoencephalography, but it was not evident on EEG (8).

The parietal components of the SEP (N20-P25-N35) may consist of a broad notched positive wave rather than the normal "W" shape waveform, and in the majority of cases, the wave is not enlarged. In contrast, prefrontal components (P22-N30) are relatively preserved. Enlargement of the P25-N33 component of the cortical SEP, typical of cortical reflex myoclonus, is rare (case 7 in reference 7).

Reflex myoclonus is elicited by a variety of cutaneous stimuli. Electrical stimulation of peripheral sensory nerves elicits reflex myoclonus at intensities near or even below sensory perceptual threshold even in patients with cortical sensory loss (7,9). Reflex myoclonus following stimulation of mixed nerves may be recruited below the threshold for the direct M response, indicating activation of large-diameter sensory afferents. A distinctive feature of the reflex myoclonus in corticobasal degeneration is the short latency of the reflex myoclonus (4,5,7,9,10). C reflexes occur at latencies of the order of 40 ms in hand muscles (after stimulation of the ulnar and median nerves at the wrist) and 80 ms in foot muscles after stimulation at the ankle.

ALZHEIMER DISEASE

Myoclonus is observed during the later stages of sporadic Alzheimer disease and is recognized as a prominent and early clinical feature in the inherited forms of Alzheimer disease, particularly in chromosome-14 linked pedigrees with mutations in the presenilin-1 gene, when myoclonus may be accompanied by seizures.

Physiologic studies of myoclonus in Alzheimer disease indicate both cortical and subcortical origins. The physiologic features of typical cortical reflex myoclonus include enlarged cortical SEPs, stimulus sensitivity with C reflexes (at variable latencies of 36 to

75 ms), and positive cortical sharp wave potentials back-averaged preceding myoclonus (by 25 to 40 ms), with intracortical spread. In other cases, broad negative cortical waves preceded myoclonus by 50 to 180 ms, with normal cortical SEPs, suggesting a subcortical origin (11,12).

CREUTZFELDT-JAKOB DISEASE

Generalized or multifocal and occasionally rhythmic myoclonus may appear in the course of Creutzfeldt-Jakob disease. Generalized myoclonus, typically in response to a loud noise, is a characteristic finding. Normal background rhythms in the EEG are replaced by slower waveforms with variable amplitude, distribution, and morphology. Periodic discharges comprising bilaterally synchronous sharp waves (duration 200 to 400 ms) repeating at a frequency of 0.5 to 1 Hz are a characteristic finding. Dementia, myoclonus, and periodic EEG discharges occurred in 53% of 209 consecutive cases of experimentally transmitted Creutzfeldt-Jakob disease (13).

The relationship between the periodic discharges and myoclonus is variable. Jerk locked averaging revealed the periodic discharges to be widely distributed and predominantly contralateral, and a negative potential preceding myoclonus by 60 ms suggested a subcortical origin (14). Cortical reflex and photic reflex myoclonus may also be seen (15).

MULTIPLE SYSTEM ATROPHY

Approximately 30% of patients with multiple system atrophy exhibit myoclonus (16). Typical cortical reflex myoclonus in the olivopontocerebellar form of multiple system atrophy is well recognized (17) and characterized by stimulus-sensitive reflex myoclonus with enlargement of the P25-N33 component of the cortical SEP (18). Photic cortical reflex myoclonus with generalized muscle jerks following flash stimulation may occur in both the olivopontocerebellar and striatonigral forms of multiple system atrophy (19). Myoclonus of brainstem origin has been described in the striatonigral of multiple system atrophy (20).

HUNTINGTON DISEASE

Myoclonus in Huntington disease is rare but recognized in young-onset akinetic rigid forms when it is often accompanied by seizures. The myoclonus is stimulus sensitive and induced by action (21). Physiologic evidence of a cortical origin was presented in three patients from two families in whom back-averaged cortical spike discharges on EEG preceded multifocal myoclonus with intracortical spread and photic reflex myoclonus. As in typical cortical reflex myoclonus, rapid intracortical spread produced the clinical picture of generalized multifocal myoclonus. Reflex myoclonus in hand muscles following peripheral nerve stimulation had a latency of around 40 ms, similar to corticobasal degeneration (and unlike typical cortical myoclonus). Cortical SEPs were of small amplitude, consistent with previous descriptions of the SEP in Huntington disease (21), but borderline enlargement of the P1-N2 component accompanying reflex myoclonus in hand muscles, 40 ms after stimulation of the median nerve at the wrist, has also been described (22).

DENTATO-RUBRO-PALLIDO-LUYSIAN ATROPHY

Myoclonus is distinctive feature of some families with the myoclonus-epilepsy phenotype of this condition, which are mainly described in Japan. Physiologic studies have not defined the nature of myoclonus.

ACKNOWLEDGMENT

I wish to acknowledge the inspiration of David Marsden in the study of movement disorders in general but particularly for his contribution to the clinical evaluation, investigation, and classification of myoclonus. With Pat Merton, he enthusiastically pursued the physiologic basis of cortical myoclonus and the role of long latency cortical reflexes, arguing that myoclonus was a pathologic aberration of this reflex system and that these reflexes traversed the cortex. This fascination with the interplay between neurologic "accidents of nature" and normal physiology gave great color and clarity to his scientific and clinical teaching and writing.

REFERENCES

1. Dawson GD. The relation between the electroencephalogram and muscle action potentials in certain convulsive states. *J Neurol Neurosurg Psychiatry* 1946; 33339:5–22.
2. Shibasaki H, Yamashita Y, Neshigi R, et al. Pathogenesis of giant somatosensory evoked potentials in progressive myoclonic epilepsy. *Brain* 1985;108:225–240.
3. Marsden CD, Harding AE, Obeso JA, et al. Progressive myoclonic ataxia (the Ramsay Hunt syndrome). *Arch Neurol* 1990 47:1121–1125.
4. Brunt ERP, van Weerden TW, Pruim J, et al. Unique myoclonic pattern in corticobasal degeneration. *Mov Disord* 1995;10:132–142.
5. Rinne JO, Lee MS, Thompson PD, et al. Corticobasal degeneration: a clinical study of 36 cases. *Brain* 1994; 117:1183–1196.
6. Hallett M, Chadwick D, Marsden CD. Cortical reflex myoclonus. *Neurology* 1979;29:1107–1125.
7. Thompson PD, Day BL, Rothwell JC, et al. The myoclonus in corticobasal degeneration: evidence for two forms of cortical reflex myoclonus. *Brain* 1994;117: 1197–1207.
8. Mima T, Nagamini T, Ikeda A, et al. Pathogenesis of cortical myoclonus studied by magnetoencephalography. *Ann Neurol* 1998;43:598–607.
9. Chen R, Ashby P, Lang AE. Stimulus sensitive my-

oclonus in akinetic rigid syndromes. *Brain* 1992;115: 1875–1888.
10. Carella F, Scaioli V, Franceschetti S, et al. Focal reflex myoclonus in corticobasal degeneration. *Funct Neurol* 1991;6:165–170.
11. Wilkins DE, Hallett M, Berardelli A, et al. Physiologic analysis of the myoclonus of Alzheimer's disease. *Neurology* 1984;34:898–903.
12. Ugawa Y, Kohara N, Hirasawa H, et al. Myoclonus in Alzheimer's disease. *J Neurol* 1987;235:90–94.
13. Brown P. Transmissible human spongiform encephalopathy (infectious cerebral amyloidosis): Creutzfeldt-Jakob disease, Gerstmann-Straussler-Schinker syndrome, and Kuru. In: Calne D, ed. *Neurodegeneration*. Philadelphia: WB Saunders, 1994:839–876.
14. Shibasaki H, Motomura M, Yamashita Y, et al. Periodic synchronous discharge and myoclonus in Creutzfeldt-Jakob disease: diagnostic application of jerk-locked averaging method. *Ann Neurol* 1981;9:150–156.
15. Shibasaki H, Neshige R. Photic cortical reflex myoclonus. *Ann Neurol* 1987;22:252–287.
16. Wenning GK, Quinn NP. Multiple system atrophy. In: Quinn NP, ed. *Parkinsonism*. London: Bailliere Tindall, 1997:187–204.
17. Obeso JA, Rothwell JC, Marsden CD. The spectrum of cortical myoclonus. *Brain* 1985;108:193–224.
18. Rodriguez ME, Artieda J, Zubieta JL, et al. Reflex myoclonus in olivopontocerebellar atrophy. *J Neurol Neurosurg Psychiatry* 1994;57:316–319.
19. Artieda J, Obeso JA. The pathophysiology and pharmacology of photic cortical reflex myoclonus. *Ann Neurol* 1993;34:175–184.
20. Clouston PD, Lim CL, Fung V, et al. Brainstem myoclonus in a patient with non-Dopa responsive parkinsonism. *Mov Disord* 1996;4:404–410.
21. Thompson PD, Bhatia KP, Brown P, et al. Cortical myoclonus in Huntington's disease. *Mov Disord* 1994;9: 633–641.
22. Carella F, Scaioli V, Ciano C, et al. Adult onset myoclonic Huntington's disease. *Mov Disord* 1993;8: 201–205.

*Myoclonus and Paroxysmal Dyskinesias,
Advances in Neurology,* Vol. 89,
edited by S. Fahn, et al.
Lippincott Williams & Wilkins, Philadelphia © 2002.

5

Myoclonus in Pallido-Ponto-Nigral Degeneration

*John N. Caviness and †Zbigniew K. Wszolek

*Department of Neurology, Mayo Clinic Scottsdale, Scottsdale, Arizona; and †Department of
Neurology, Mayo Clinic Jacksonville, Jacksonville, Florida*

Many families have now been described under the group of disorders known as frontotemporal dementias linked to chromosome 17 (FTDP-17). These disorders are associated with tau protein gene mutations. Pallido-ponto-nigral degeneration (PPND) is one example of an FTDP-17 syndrome (1). The major clinical features include progressive parkinsonism, dystonia unrelated to medications, dementia, ocular motility abnormalities, pyramidal tract dysfunction, frontal lobe release signs, perseverative vocalizations, eyelid opening and closing apraxia, and bladder incontinence. The average age of disease onset is 43, ranging from 32 to 58 years, and the average survival time is 8.6 years. The onset of the disease is insidious, with half of the patients presenting with parkinsonism and half with personality changes and cognitive impairments. The course is exceptionally aggressive, and four stages of disease progression, each lasting about 2 years, can be delineated (2). Affected patients show poor or no response to levodopa and other dopaminergic agents. Routine laboratory tests are normal. Magnetic resonance imaging findings include cerebral atrophy involving predominantly the frontal, parietal, and temporal lobes. There is also narrowing of the substantia nigra pars compacta and atrophy of the pontine tegmentum (3). Positron emission tomography studies with [^{18}F]-6-fluorodopa have consistently revealed significantly reduced striatal uptake in affected individuals (1,2,4,5). Neuropathologic examinations demonstrated neuronal loss and gliosis in the substantia nigra, globus pallidus, and mesencephalic-pontine tegmentum (thus the name of disorder: pallido-ponto-nigral degeneration) (1,2). However, the other brain structures including amygdala, putamen, and cerebral cortex are also involved in the degenerative process (1,2). There are no Lewy bodies, neurofibrillary tangles, senile plaques, or amyloid deposits (6). Ballooned neurons in the cerebral cortex and neuronal and glial tau inclusions are encountered (6,7). Molecular genetic investigations revealed linkage to *wld* locus on chromosome 17 (8) and the presence of the N279K mutation in the tau gene (9).

Myoclonus has been previously reported in stage II or III of this disorder. Preliminary clinical neurophysiologic studies, including electroencephalography (EEG), EEG background frequency analysis, electromyographic (EMG) recordings, EMG multichannel surface studies, and evoked potential determinations have been performed on certain affected family members (10). Generalized slowing of EEG frequencies that paralleled clinical progression was found. Surface EMG studies on three subjects showed muscle activation tremorlike discharges, and in one patient (stage II), there seemed to be myoclonic EMG discharges. In order to further define the myoclonus in PPND clinically and electrophysiologically, we performed studies on five affected individuals and six at-risk individuals.

METHODS

Clinical Assessment

Each subject was examined for myoclonus and assigned a clinical stage of PPND as previously described (2). A neurologic examination, including a Unified Parkinson's Disease Rating Scale (UPDRS) and a Mini-Mental State Exam (MMSE), was performed.

Electrophysiologic Assessment

Combined EEG/EMG recordings, using the Neuroscan (C) system (Neuroscan, Inc, El Paso, Texas), acquired data at a rate of 2,500 Hz with a band pass of 1 to 500 Hz (24 dB/octave). Bilateral upper-extremity bipolar surface Ag/AgCl EMG electrodes were placed on deltoid, biceps, triceps, wrist flexors, wrist extensors, abductor pollicis brevis (APB), first dorsal interosseus, and abductor digiti minimi. Modified 10 to 20 system Ag/AgCl EEG electrode positions were used with an averaged ear reference. Recordings were made at rest and during arm movement. EEG/EMG back averaging was done off-line, with cursor placement at the onset of myoclonic EMG activity. The data for back averaging were collected while the muscles were activated by holding the arms outstretched, wrists slightly extended, and the fingers spread apart.

A GRASS SS8800 stimulator (Grass Instruments Co, Quincy, Massachusetts) was used to obtain cortical somatosensory evoked potentials (SEPs) and long latency reflexes (LLRs) bilaterally in some subjects. For the SEPs, two trials of 1,000 epochs were recorded with 0.2 ms stimulation at 1.5 Hz of the median nerve at the wrist with sufficient intensity to produce a minimal APB twitch. The attempted elicitation of LLRs was performed by 0.2 ms stimulation to the median nerve at the wrist (sufficient intensity to produce minimal APB twitch) as well as digital

stimulation of the index finger at 2 to 3 times the sensory threshold. For the elicitation of LLRs, 20 trials were collected at 5- to 10-second intervals for each type of stimulation with the muscles relaxed. For the SEPs and the LLRs, the same bilateral upper-extremity surface EMG electrodes were used as those mentioned earlier for the EEG/EMG polygraphy.

RESULTS

Three of the five affected individuals had small-amplitude multifocal action myoclonus of the upper extremities. Myoclonus was not present at rest. Reflex myoclonus could not be demonstrated to touch, stretch, or tendon reflexes. The surface EMG showed short-duration (less than 100 ms) discharges occurring in mostly in an agonist-only pattern and less commonly with synchronous discharges in multiple muscles. Figure 5.1 shows the EMG polygraphy while the arms were outstretched in one of the affected individuals with myoclonus. No gross EEG correlate was seen. For all three affected individuals, back averaging of these myoclonic discharges in two or more muscles failed to show an EEG transient preceding the myoclonus. The other two affected individuals showed no myoclonus. One of these individuals had SEPs that were not enlarged and unremarkable LLRs.

Five of the six at-risk individuals showed no myoclonus. Two of these individuals had unremarkable SEPs and no LLRs. One of the at-risk individuals showed small- to moderate-amplitude multifocal action myoclonus of the upper extremities. Myoclonus was not present at rest. Reflex myoclonus could not be demonstrated to touch, stretch, or tendon reflexes. During the arms-outstretched maneuver, there was a smooth continuous surface EMG pattern that was commonly interrupted by trains of short duration (less than 100 ms) discharges occurring primarily in wrist extensors with spread into more distal muscles. No gross EEG correlate was seen. Back averaging showed a focal EEG positive-negative transient preceding the myoclonic EMG discharge (Fig. 5.2). The latency from the posi-

FMY

Florida Gulf Coast University

10501 FGCU Blvd. S.

Ft. Myers, FL 33965-6501

Route to:

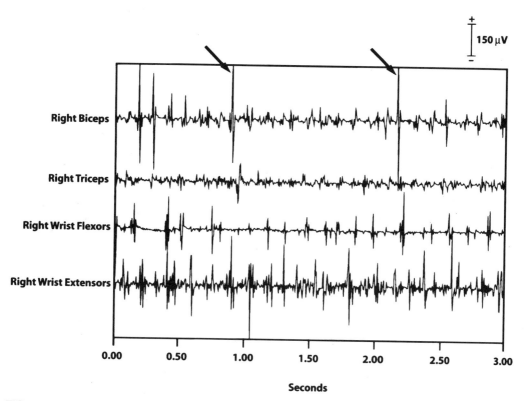

FIG. 5.1. Electromyographic (EMG) polygraphy while the arms were outstretched in one of the affected individuals with myoclonus. *Arrows* show some of the most prominent myoclonic EMG discharges.

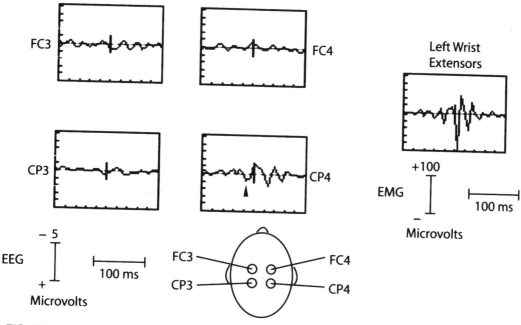

FIG. 5.2. Back-averaging of left wrist extensor muscle group shows a focal electroencephalogram positive-negative transient preceding the myoclonic electromyographic discharge. The *arrow* shows the positive phase of the premyoclonic transient at the CP4 electrode. The latency from the positive peak to the back-averaged myoclonic discharge was 11 ms, and the peak-to-peak positive-negative amplitude was 3.5 mV

tive peak to the back-averaged myoclonic discharge was 11 ms, and the peak-to-peak positive-negative amplitude was 3.5 mV.

DISCUSSION

The affected individuals tested in this study variably showed myoclonus in the upper extremities. When present, the myoclonus was small, subtle, and action induced, without detectable activation with rest or stimuli. For the affected individuals, clinical progression was more advanced for the myoclonus cases than for those without myoclonus. This may simply suggest that the appearance of myoclonus is a marker for progressive pathology in this syndrome. However, the presence of the myoclonus in the at-risk individual contradicts this notion. One possibility is that the timing of the myoclonus in the clinical progression signifies and/or correlates with different definable phenotypes within PPND, thus differentiating a "late myoclonus" phenotype versus a "early myoclonus" phenotype. If so, myoclonus and its electrophysiologic confirmation could be used to study phenotypic variability within the specific genotype of the N279K tau mutation. An alternative explanation would be that the myoclonus physiology evolves through the various clinical stages and may in some cases be seen very early (presymptomatic), then disappears, but then reappears at a later clinical stage. Some combination of these explanations may be more correct. One of the authors (ZKW) has personally examined 19 affected PPND cases, and myoclonus does not always occur. Since phenotypic variability is a very important concept in neurodegenerative disease, it would be useful to study this issue further.

The exact physiology of the myoclonus in PPND is unclear and may be heterogeneous. The finding of the cortical transient back-averaged to the myoclonus in one of the at-risk individuals suggests a cortical origin for the myoclonus within the sensorimotor cortex. However, multiple attempts at back-averaging a cortical correlate in the affected individuals showed no transient. SEPs and LLRs were not obtained for any of the subjects that demonstrated myoclonus, but these studies in other PPND patients have been normal. Although more data are needed, it is probable that the myoclonus physiology in this syndrome is diverse, and the clinical-electrophysiologic phenotype differs from the classical "typical" cortical reflex myoclonus (11).

Pathologically, there are abundant ballooned neurons in neocortical and subcortical regions as well as tau-rich inclusions in the cytoplasm of neurons and oligodendroglia morphologically similar to those seen in corticobasal degeneration, but in a distribution pattern resembling progressive supranuclear palsy. Thus, the abnormalities in PPND, like other tau mutation disorders, are diffuse. This makes it difficult to define a specific neuropathologic substrate for a given type of myoclonus in this syndrome at this time. Pathologic and neurochemical studies will need to be correlated with clinical-electrophysiologic phenotypes to further elucidate symptom production in PPND.

Myoclonus is well established to occur in PPND, but it has not been mentioned prominently in other FTDP-17 syndromes (12). Recently, three additional kindreds with N279K mutation have been reported, including two Japanese families and one French family (13–15). Myoclonus was not reported as part of the clinical phenotype, but systematic studies to look for subtle features were not performed. Among the sporadic disorders that are considered to be "tauopathies," corticobasal degeneration is the one entity that commonly demonstrates myoclonus. It is interesting to note that, similar to the affected PPND individuals studied here, the myoclonus in corticobasal degeneration shows no cortical correlate and usually a SEP that is not enlarged (16). Corticobasal degeneration patients can show enhanced long latency EMG reflexes, and it would be important to study the PPND subjects for the same long latency EMG reflex characteristics.

In summary, myoclonus variably occurs in individuals affected with the N279K tau mutation that causes PPND. The clinical-electrophysiologic characteristics of this myoclonus do not match exactly with those seen in other myoclonic disorders. The physiology of the myoclonus may change over the course of the disorder, reflecting progressive cortical pathology and possibly changes in other brain regions as well. Further study of the myoclonus in PPND will be valuable for the study of sporadic tau disorders, phenotypic variability in neurodegenerative disease, and myoclonus physiology in general.

REFERENCES

1. Wszolek ZK, Pfeiffer RF, Bhatt MH, et al. Rapidly progressive autosomal dominant parkinsonism and dementia with pallido-ponto-nigral degeneration. *Ann Neurol* 1992;32:312–320.
2. Wszolek ZK, Pfeiffer RF. Rapidly progressive autosomal dominant parkinsonism and dementia with pallido-ponto-nigral degeneration. In: Stern MB, Koller WC, eds. *Parkinsonian syndromes*. New York: Marcel Dekker Inc, 1993:297–312.
3. Cordes M, Wszolek ZK, Calne DB, et al. Magnetic resonance imaging studies in rapidly progressive autosomal dominant parkinsonism and dementia with pallido-ponto-nigral degeneration. *Neurodegeneration* 1992;1:217–224.
4. Cordes M, Wszolek ZK, Pfeiffer RF, et al. Examination of the presynaptic dopaminergic system using positron emission tomography in a family with autosomal dominant parkinsonism and dementia due to pallido-ponto-nigral degeneration (PPND). Radiologica Diagnostica 1993;34:141–145.
5. Kishore A, Wszolek ZK, Snow BJ, et al. Presynaptic nigrostriatal function in genetically tested asymptomatic relatives from pallido-ponto-nigral degeneration family. *Neurology* 1996;47:1588–1590.
6. Yamada T, McGeer EG, Schelper RL, et al. Histological

7. and biochemical pathology in a family with autosomal dominant parkinsonism and dementia. *Neurol Psychiatry Brain Res* 1993;2:26–35.
7. Reed LA, Schmidt ML, Wszolek ZK, et al. The neuropathology of a chromosome 17-linked autosomal dominant parkinsonism and dementia (pallido-ponto-nigral degeneration). *J Neuropathol Exp Neurol* 1998;57:588–601.
8. Wijker M, Wszolek ZK, Wolters EC, et al. Localization of the gene for rapidly progressive autosomal dominant parkinsonism and dementia with pallido-ponto-nigral degeneration to chromosome 17q21. *Hum Mol Genet* 1996;5:151–154.
9. Clark LN, Poorkaj P, Wszolek Z, et al. Pathogenic implications of mutations in the tau gene in pallido-ponto-nigral degeneration and related neurodegenerative disorders linked to chromosome 17. *Proc Natl Acad Sci USA* 1998;95:13103–13107.
10. Wszolek ZK, Lagerlund TD, Steg RE, et al. Clinical neurophysiologic findings in patients with rapidly progressive familial parkinsonism and dementia with pallido-ponto-nigral degeneration. *Electroencephalogr Clin Neurophysiol* 1998;107:213–222.
11. Caviness JN, Kurth M. Cortical myoclonus in Huntington's disease associated with an enlarged somatosensory evoked potential. *Mov Disord* 1997;12:1046–1051.
12. Reed LA, Wszolek ZK, Hutton M. Phenotypic correlations in FTDP-17. *Neurobiol Aging (in press)*. 2001;22(1):89-107.
13. Delisle M-B, Murrel JR, Richardson R, et al. A mutation at codon 279 (N279K) in exon 10 of the tau gene causes a tauopathy with dementia and supranuclear palsy. *Acta Neuropathol* 1999;98:62–77.
14. Yasuda M, Kawamata T, Komure O, et al. A mutation in the microtubule-assocciated protein tau in pallido-nigro-luysian degeneration. *Neurology* 1999;53:864–868.
15. Arima K, Kowalska A, Hasegawa M, et al. Two brothers with frontotemporal dementia and parkinsonism with an N279K mutation of the tau gene. *Neurology* 2000;54:1787–1795.
16. Thompson PD, Shibasaki H. Myoclonus in corticobasal degeneration and other neurodegenerations. *Adv Neurol* 2000;82:69–81.

Myoclonus and Paroxysmal Dyskinesias,
Advances in Neurology, Vol. 89,
edited by S. Fahn, et al.
Published by Lippincott Williams & Wilkins, Philadelphia, 2002.

6

Myoclonus in Gaucher Disease

*Karen P. Frei and †Raphael Schiffmann

*The Parkinson's and Movement Disorders Institute, Fountain Valley, California; and
†Developmental and Metabolic Neurology Branch, National Institute of Neurological Disorders
and Stroke, Bethesda, Maryland

Gaucher disease is the most common lysosomal storage disease resulting from a deficiency of the enzyme glucocerebrosidase (1). It is transmitted through autosomal recessive inheritance, and the gene has been localized to chromosome 1q21. This enzyme deficiency leads to an accumulation of glucocerebroside within macrophages producing Gaucher cells (GC). Clinically, the disorder can be divided into three subtypes; type 1, the nonneuronopathic form; type 2, the acute neuronopathic form; and type 3, the chronic neuronopathic form. The onset of type 2 Gaucher disease is usually within the first six months of life, presenting with hepatosplenomegaly and horizontal supranuclear gaze palsy. Dysphagia, dysarthria, and laryngeal spasms ensue. Myoclonus and seizures may occur. Bilateral sixth nerve palsies, retroflexion of the head, and spasticity develop as the disease progresses. Death is usually by 4 years of age. Patients with type 3 Gaucher disease have nonneurologic manifestations of varying severity. Disease onset can occur from early childhood through adulthood (2,3). Horizontal supranuclear gaze palsy appears to be a universal finding (4). Most patients remain neurologically stable for many years with enzyme replacement therapy (5). Myoclonus and seizures may occur midway through the disease in some patients with type 3 Gaucher disease, or they may be the presenting symptom. In those patients, myoclonic ataxia and spasticity as well as de-

mentia tend to occur as the disease progresses (6). The ocular abnormality often progresses to a complete extraocular palsy. The myoclonus tends to be progressive and refractory to treatment. It often interferes with daily activities and can prevent ambulation. Death usually results from complications of either the systemic or the neurologic disease manifestations. Treatment of disease with enzyme replacement has not resulted in regression of myoclonus or other neurologic manifestations (5,7). In this chapter, we describe the myoclonus that is seen in neuronopathic Gaucher disease as reported in the literature and discuss possible mechanisms responsible for the myoclonus.

MATERIALS AND METHODS

Twelve patient reports of neuronopathic Gaucher's disease were reviewed from the literature dating from 1978 to the present. There were three type 2 patients of the acute infantile variety (8,9) and seven type 3 chronic neuronopathic patients (3,6,9–12,). The remaining two patients were of intermediate severity between types 2 and 3 with onset in infancy, a slightly slower progression, and death by 36 months of age (transitional type) (10,12,13).

RESULTS

A summary of the clinical descriptions from the twelve case reports is presented in Table 6.1.

TABLE 6.1. *Summary of Gaucher cases*

Author, date	Type	Age at onset	Splenectomy	Myoclonus	Seizures	Age at death	EEG
Grover et al.,[a] 1978	Transitional	10 mo	No	Unspecified	Yes	32 mo	Multifocal Spike wave
Wenger et al., 1983	3	4 yr	No	Progressive Segmental to continuous	Akinetic Myoclonic	12.5 yr	Multifocal Spike wave
Nishimura and Barranger,[a] 1980	3	7 yr	Yes	Multifocal Progressive Action Stimulus sensitive	Generalized Myoclonic	NR	3–7 Hz spike wave Photomyoclonus
	3	9 yr	Yes	Multifocal Progressive	Generalized	16 yr	3–5 Hz slow and spike wave Photomyoclonus
Kaga et al., 1982	2	3 mo	No	Unspecified	Myoclonic Generalized	16 mo	—
Winkelman et al.,[a] 1983	3	18 yr	No	Progressive Continuous Stimulus sensitive	Generalized	43 yr	—
	3	29 yr	No	Stimulus sensitive Heralded seizure	Generalized	NR	—
Kaye et al., 1986	2	5 mo	No	Unspecified	Yes	16 mo	—
	2	7 mo	No	Unspecified	Yes	14 mo	—
	3	6 mo	No	None	None	6.7 yr	Mild slow Photo-convulsive
Conradi et al., 1991	Transitional	10 mo	Yes	Progressive Stimulus sensitive	Myoclonic	32 mo	2–3 Hz spike wave Myoclonus assoc.
Verghese et al., 2000	3	18 mo	No	Multifocal Action Progressive Negative Stimulus sensitive Continuous	Myoclonic	6 yr	Normal

NR, not reported; EEG, electroencephalogram.
[a]Patients are related.

Myoclonus

Myoclonus and seizures developed in all but one patient who had oculomotor apraxia only. Electroencephalography (EEG) of this patient included a photoconvulsive response, and therefore the possibility of ongoing subclinical seizure activity exists. Four type 3 patients had myoclonic seizures in addition to myoclonus and generalized seizures.

The myoclonus was described as progressive, stimulus sensitive, and generally refractory to medication. The myoclonus was not described in detail in the three type 2 patients and one of the transitional patients. It was progressive in one of the infantile-onset patients and in all six of the type 3 patients. In general, the myoclonus would begin as jerks involving the extremities and progress to include stimulus sensitivity toward noise, touch, or movement with action myoclonus and then proceed to become continual, involving the extremities, face, and in one case the neck and trunk, often interfering with ambulation or feeding. Two type 3 patients had photomyoclonus. Negative myoclonus was seen in one of the type 3 patients.

The development of seizures usually preceded the onset of myoclonus. Occasionally, a generalized seizure may herald the new onset of myoclonic epilepsy. The time lapse between seizure onset and development of myoclonus was mentioned in four type 3 patients. One patient had the onset of myoclonus occurring four years after the onset of generalized seizures at age 10 (6). A second patient had a gradual development of myoclonus and myoclonic seizures within months following the initial onset of generalized seizures at age 14 (6). Two siblings with type 3 had the onset of myoclonus occur 5 and 12 years after the onset of seizures at age 29 and 38 years, respectively (3). In both of these patients, myoclonus would often progress in amplitude, leading to the onset of a generalized seizure. Myoclonus was reported to begin between 7 and 14 months of age in the three type 2 cases. The two transitional patients reported myoclonus occurring at 16 months of age. Myoclonus was noted to begin at 3 years, 4 years, 14 years in two patients, 34 years, and 50 years of age in six of the type 3 patients.

The EEG results in seven patients were reported. One type 2 patient had high voltage with diffuse spike and wave activity. One transitional patient had multifocal spike and waveform activity (10). Another transitional patient had three EEGs performed during the course of the disease. The first EEG at 9 months was normal, the second at 10 months revealed 3.5-Hz polyspike and wave activity, and the third at 13 months showed 2- to 3-Hz spike and wave activity with associated myoclonus (13). One type 3 patient with stimulus-sensitive and negative myoclonus had a normal EEG without spike correlation with the myoclonus (11). One revealed mild slowing and two had generalized 3- to 7-Hz spike and wave activity with photomyoclonus (6,9).

Somatosensory evoked potentials (SEPs) were not reported in any of the twelve patients. Brainstem auditory evoked responses were evaluated in one of the type 2 patients. Waveforms I, II, and III were prolonged in the right side at 6 months of age, and two months later the latencies were prolonged further and wave III was lost on the right side. The left side revealed near normal latencies for waves I, II, and III also with absence of the subsequent waves, but without significant change between the studies.

Neuropathology

Neuropathology was reported in all three of the type 2 patients, in both of the transitional patients and in four of the type 3 patients. A summary of the neuropathology can be found in Table 6.2. The amount of neuropathology was varied and did not appear to correlate with disease severity. Perivascular GCs were seen in the brain in seven of the nine patients reported. The majority of the perivascular clusters of GCs were found in the white matter, and cerebral cortex, thalamus, and basal ganglia were also involved. One of the type 2 patients reported perivascular GCs in the pons.

Gaucher cells were also seen intraparenchymally predominantly in the occipital region. In two of the type 2 patients there was a gradient in the density of GCs from the frontal to the occipital region, and the occipital region had the greatest amount of these storage cells. One of the transitional patients had intraparenchymal accumulations of GCs most prominent in the occipital and temporolateral cortex. In these regions a band of cells was seen in lamina IV of the cortex (13). Intraparenchymal accumulations of GCs were also seen in the cerebellum. One type 3 patient had a single cluster of GCs in the occipital lobe (11). GCs were not reported in four patients.

Signs of neuronal degeneration were reported in six of the nine patients. The pons appeared to be the site mainly affected with mild neuronal cell loss seen in two type 2 patients, in one transitional patient, and in two type 3 patients (3,9,10,12,13). The cortex showed neuronal cell loss in two cases, and astrocytosis and astrogliosis were seen in a band corresponding to lamina IV of the cortex in a transitional patient with the same distribution of GCs (13). Neuronal cell loss was seen in the substantia nigra in three cases (3,8,13). A single patient with type 3 Gaucher disease had selective fiber (myelin and axonal) loss in the superior cerebellar peduncle and not in the cerebellar white

TABLE 6.2. *Summary of neuropathology*

Author, date	Type	Perivascular Gaucher cells	Intraparenchymal Gaucher cells	Neuronal degeneration	Purkinje cell loss	Dentate cell loss	Olive involvement
Grover et al., 1978	Infantile onset	+[a]	+[a]	—	—	—	—
Wenger et al., 1983	3	None	None	Pons—mild Cortex—irregular	Severe	Severe	—
Kaga et al., 1982	2	Cerebrum	None	Cortex Ammon's horn	None	Mild	None
Winkelman et al., 1983	3	White matter Thalamus Basal ganglia Subaracnoid space Around cerebellum	None	Brainstem nuclei Oculomotor nucleus Red nucleus Superior colliculus SN Reticular formation	None	Severe	Inferior olive—moderate
Kaye et al., 1986	2	White matter Cerebral cortex Thalamus SN	Gradient from Cerebral cortex Thalamus—mild SN	Pons frontal to occipital	—	None	—
	2	White matter Cerebral cortex Thalamus Thalamus SN	Gradient from frontal to occipital Cerebral cortex SN	—	—	—	—
	3	Thalamus	None	None	—	—	—
Conradi et al., 1991	Infantile onset	White matter Gray matter	Lamina IV Occipital and temporolateral cortex	SN Pons	Mild	Severe	None
Verghese et al., 2000	3	None	1 cluster occipital lobe	Superior cerebellar peduncle	Severe	—	—

SN, substantia nigra.

[a]Gaucher cells present in brain; not specified whether perivascular or intraparenchymal.

matter, which is indicative of involvement of the dentatorubrothalamic pathway (11).

The cerebellum appeared to be involved, with reports of Purkinje cell loss and/or dentate nucleus cell loss in five patients. Purkinje cell loss was found to be severe in two type 3 patients and mild in one of the transitional patients (11–13). Dentate nucleus cell loss appeared to be severe in all four cases reported: one type 2, one transitional, and two type 3 patients (3,11–13).

DISCUSSION

The myoclonus seen in neuronopathic Gaucher disease appears to be progressive, starting with intermittent, spontaneous multifocal jerks of the extremities and progressing to a near continual state resulting in significant disability, even interfering with ambulation. It is stimulus sensitive and occurs with action. Negative myoclonus may also occur (11,14,15). Many of these patients have associated seizures. Thus, by clinical description the myoclonus may be considered progressive myoclonic epilepsy (PME) and therefore of the cortical type. Associated EEG findings with myoclonus and photic myoclonus lend support to the cortical nature of the myoclonus seen in Gaucher disease. As such, it is similar to the myoclonus seen in other genetic/metabolic diseases, such as neuronal ceroid lipofuscinosis and sialidosis (16,17).

The cortical origin of the myoclonus is demonstrated by the presence, in type 3 Gaucher patients with PME, of a large-amplitude SEP (giant potential) that is time locked to the electromyographic correlate of the myoclonus (18). Patients with type 3 Gaucher disease who do not exhibit myoclonus have an increased amplitude of the SEP compared to age-matched controls. This amplitude inversely correlates with the intelligence quotient of the patients (18). These findings suggest that a defect in cortical inhibition underlies the neurologic manifestation of this form of Gaucher disease.

The presence of negative myoclonus, a loss of postural tone as seen in asterixis, is compatible with the classification of cortical myoclonus, which can be composed of both positive and negative myoclonus (19). Similar mechanisms are postulated for both types. Paroxysmal activation of motor regions, either of primary motor cortex or of inhibitory motor cortical areas, are thought to produce positive or negative myoclonus (20).

A single patient with reticular reflex myoclonus, which is thought to originate from the brainstem, was reported (11). The subcortical origin that was proposed was based on the clinical description of the myoclonus and the lack of EEG correlate. This is not inconsistent with the classification of cortical myoclonus, and both cortical and reticular reflex myoclonus may coexist (16).

Other than EEG spikes correlating with myoclonus, multifocal spike and wave discharges, diffuse slowing of the background, and photomyoclonus were found in six of the seven EEGs reported. This is consistent with previous reports of EEGs in neuronopathic Gaucher disease. However, the rapid 6 to 10 per second spike and sharp waves seen in the posterior brain region of type 3 patients were not specified (21). Photomyoclonus has been seen in other metabolic disorders such as neuronal ceroid lipofuscinosis and Lafora disease. Photomyoclonus is a form of stimulus sensitive myoclonus triggered by light flashes. The

myoclonus appears to originate from abnormal cortical activity in the premotor and motor cortex following a normal cortical potential from the occipital cortex (22). The flash frequency resulting in a myoclonic response may be a distinguishing factor between these disorders with Gaucher disease most responsive to light flashes at 6 to 10 Hz (17).

Brainstem auditory evoked responses (BAERs) have been studied in type 2 Gaucher disease patients. Generally, it is thought that the BAER is a noninvasive method for assessing brainstem function. Brainstem abnormalities are prominent in type 2 Gaucher disease; therefore, these patients would appear to be good candidates to monitor disease progression with BAER. Wave I arises from the eighth cranial nerve, wave II from the cochlear nucleus or from the auditory nerve, wave III from the superolivary complex, and waves IV through VII from the midpontine and more rostral regions (23). Abnormalities in BAER have been reported for type 2 Gaucher disease, primarily with absence of waveforms beyond wave III. Three cases of type 2 have revealed only waves I and II and a small wave III that disappeared with disease progression (8,23,24). Absences of waves III through VII have been seen in other disorders such as asphyxia, Pelizaeus-Merzbacher disease, metachromatic leukodystrophy, brainstem tumors, and adrenoleukodystrophy (25). However, the neuropathology of these patients did not correlate with the abnormality seen on BAER. It ranged from the preservation of the nuclei and tracts of the brainstem (8) to neuronal cell loss and gliosis of the cochlear nerve, superior olivary complex, and cochlear nucleus (24), with almost complete neuronal loss in the vestibular and cuneate nuclei (23). BAER may be able to detect abnormalities of the brainstem prior to pathologic changes.

The neuropathology reported in these patients mainly point to presence of GCs and neuronal cell loss and neuronophagia. Gaucher cells appear to be present both perivascularly and intraparenchymally predominantly in the cortex, white matter, and thalamus and inconsistently in the basal ganglia. An increase in GCs was reported to occur in the occipital and temporal cortex in both types 2 and 3 (9,11,13). This has been reported in the nor-bottnian form of Gaucher disease as well, considered a variant of type 3 Gaucher disease (26). The accumulation of GCs in the occipital lobe may represent accumulation of storage material and an increase in glucocerebroside has been found to coincide with this (9). It is interesting to speculate that disruption of the occipital cortex may contribute to the pathogenesis of the photomyoclonus seen in many of the type 3 patients.

The presence of GC accumulation in lamina IV is intriguing (13), and other studies have found abnormalities in the cortical laminar structure as well. Verity and Montasir (27) found focal neuronal aggregation in lamina IV of the occipital cortex in a type 2 infant. Conradi et al. (13) found neuronal loss in layers III and V, forming stripes through the cortex. Cortical lamina IV receives thalamocortical fibers that are specific afferents from thalamic nuclei (28). The predominant cell type of lamina IV is spiny stellate cells that are excitatory and are thought to have burst generator properties. Epileptiform events appear to begin where these types of neurons are located (29). Similar mechanisms responsible for hypersynchronous activities, such as a myoclonic burst or epileptic discharge, are common (30). Thus, a shared mechanism is postulated to produce both myoclonus and epilepsy, which coexist in progressive myoclonic epilepsy. It is possible that neuronal abnormalities in cortical lamina IV produce the heightened excitability of the cortex needed to produce cortical myoclonus. Spread of the spontaneous discharge may result in motor seizures (31). Reutens et al. (32) found using transcranial magnetic stimulation that progressive myoclonic epilepsy is spread via transcortical pathways, lending support to this theory.

Neuronal cell loss in the cerebellum appeared to be the most consistent finding among the patients reviewed. Involvement of the Purkinje cells and/or the dentate nucleus was most common (3,8,10–13,24). The cere-bellum has also been found to be the site of the greatest glucocerebroside accumulation (26). This was also seen in a patient with sap-C deficiency, a sphingolipid activator protein also involved in the breakdown of glucosylce-ramide, which produces Gaucher disease (33). Pathology of the cerebellum seems to be a consistent finding in many patients with action myoclonus, including Lafora body disease, progressive myoclonic ataxia, and posthypoxic myoclonus (16,34). Purkinje cell output inhibits the deep cerebellar nuclei, which have an excitatory action on the brainstem reticular formation. Thus, a reduction in Purkinje cells would theoretically produce a heightened excitability to sensory input. However, this is likely not a primary cause of myoclonus since cerebellar abnormalities are not correlated with disease severity (16).

Based on this information, it appears likely that Gaucher disease produces progressive myoclonic epilepsy through some form of disturbance of the sensorimotor cortex, thus producing a hyperexcitable state. Since cortical hyperexcitability is present in type 3 Gaucher patients who do not have overt myoclonus (18), the presence of myoclonus represents one end of the clinical spectrum in neurono-pathic Gaucher disease. This cortical inhibitory defect may be caused by accumulation of glucocerebroside or by production of a neurotoxin, which leads to an alteration of neuronal function. Neuronal cell cultures treated with a glucocerebrosidase inhibitor have been found to show an increased sensitivity toward glutamate and other metabolic inhibitors, suggesting compromised neuronal function. A release of calcium appears to be related to this increased sensitivity, resulting in cell death (35). The addition of glucocere-brosidase to the cultured cells prevents neuronal cell death. However, treatment of patients with neuronopathic Gaucher disease does not reverse neurologic symptoms (5,7). Thus the problem may be the inability of the enzyme to cross the blood–brain barrier.

Psychosine (glucosylsphingosine) is another possible neurotoxin that has been found in the brains of neuronopathic Gaucher patients (26,36). Psychosine was found in greater amounts in the cerebellum than in the cerebrum in patients with type 2 Gaucher disease and its concentration in the brain may correlate with both the clinical course and the neuropathologic abnormality. Glucosylpsychosine is degraded by glucocerebrosidase and may act as a detergent; as such, it is toxic to neurons (37).

CONCLUSIONS

We hypothesize that the combination of hypersensitivity to glutamate or other metabolic toxins such as psychosine of glucocerebrosidase-deficient neurons is responsible for the initial cortical neuronal dysfunction that generates the cortical myoclonus seen in neuronopathic Gaucher disease. Somehow this function causes dysfunction of burst generator cells in cortical lamina III and V in sensory cortex and layer IV in the visual cortex, which results in spontaneous myoclonus. As the disease progresses, increased neuronal dysfunction or toxicity allows the transcortical spread of the myoclonic discharges, resulting in progressive myoclonic epilepsy. As a result of the progressive myoclonus, the dentate nucleus and Purkinje cells of the cerebellum become affected. This hypothesis is incomplete and leaves many details to be resolved before the physiology behind the development of PME in neuronopathic Gaucher disease is defined and appropriate treatment can be given for this condition.

REFERENCES

1. Brady RO, Kanfer JN, Bradley RM, et al. Demonstration of a deficiency of glucocerebroside-cleaving enzyme in Gaucher's disease. *J Clin Invest* 1966;45:1112–1115.
2. King JO. Progressive myoclonic epilepsy due to Gaucher's disease in an adult. *J Neurol Neurosurg Psychiatry* 1975;38:849–854.
3. Winkelman MD, Banker BQ, Victor M, et al. Non-infantile neuronopathic Gaucher's disease: a clinicopathologic study. *Neurology* 1983;33:994–1008.
4. Patterson MC, Horowitz M, Abel RB, et al. Isolated horizontal supranuclear gaze palsy as a marker of severe systemic involvement in Gaucher's disease. *Neurology* 1993;43:1993–1997.
5. Altarescu G, Hill S, Wiggs E, et al. The efficacy of enzyme replacement therapy in patients with chronic neuronopathic Gaucher disease. *J Pediatr* 2001;138(4):539-547
6. Nishimura R, Omos-Lau N, Ajmone-Marsan C, et al. Electroencephalographic findings in Gaucher disease. *Neurology* 1980;152–159.
7. Schiffmann R, Heyes MP, Aerts JM, et al. Prospective study of neurological responses to treatment with macrophage-targeted glucocerebrosidase in patients with type 3 Gaucher's disease. *Ann Neurol* 1997;42:613–621.
8. Kaga M, Azuma C, Imamura T, et al. Auditory brainstem response (ABR) in infantile Gaucher's disease. *Neuropediatrics* 1982;13:207–210.
9. Kaye EM, Ullman MD, Wilson ER, et al. Type 2 and Type 3 Gaucher disease: a morphological and biochemical study. *Ann Neurol* 1986;20:223–230.
10. Grover WD, Tucker SH, Wenger DA. Clinical variation in 2 related children with neuronopathic Gaucher disease. *Ann Neurol* 1978;3:281–283.
11. Verghese J, Goldberg RF, Desnick RJ, et al. Myoclonus from selective dentate nucleus degeneration in Type 3 Gaucher disease. *Arch Neurol* 2000;57:389–395.
12. Wenger DA, Roth S, Kudoh T, et al. Biochemical studies in a patient with subacute neuronopathic Gaucher disease without visceral glucosylceramide storage. *Pediatr Res* 1983;17:344–348.
13. Conradi N, Kyllerman M, Mansson JE, et al. Late-infantile Gaucher Disease in a child with myoclonus and bulbar signs: neuropathological and neurochemical findings. *Acta Neuropathol* 1991;82:152–157.
14. Tripp JH, Lake BD, Young E, et al. Juvenile Gaucher's disease with horizontal gaze palsy in three siblings. *J Neurol Neurosurg Psychiatry* 1977;40:470–478.
15. Yamanouchi H, Arima M. Negative myoclonus. *Nippon Rinsho* 1993;51:2995–2999.
16. Lance JW. Action myoclonus, Ramsay Hunt syndrome and other cerebellar myoclonic syndromes. *Adv Neurol* 1986;43:33–55.
17. Rapin I. Myoclonus in neuronal storage and Lafora diseases. *Adv Neurol* 1986;43:65–85.
18. Garvey MA, Toro C, Goldstein S, et al. Somatosensory evoked potentials as a marker of disease burden in type 3 Gaucher disease. *Neurology* 2001:13;56(3):391-394.
19. Shibasaki H. Pathophysiology of negative myoclonus and asterixis. *Adv Neurol* 1995;67:199–209.
20. Toro C, Hallett M, Rothwell JC, et al. Physiology of negative myoclonus. *Adv Neurol* 1995;67: 211–217.
21. Nishimura RN, Barranger JA. Neurologic complications of Gaucher's disease, Type 3. *Arch Neurol* 1980; 37:92–93.
22. Artieda J, Obeso JA. The pathophysiology and pharmacology of photic cortical reflex myoclonus. *Ann Neurol* 1993;34:175–184.
23. Lacey DJ, Terplan K. Correlating auditory evoked and brainstem histologic abnormalities in infantile Gaucher's disease. *Neurology* 1984;34:539–541.
24. Kaga M, Ono M, Yakumaru K, et al. Brainstem pathology of infantile Gaucher's disease with only wave I and II or auditory brainstem response. *J Laryngol Otol* 1998;112:1069–1073.
25. Kaga M, Murakami T, Naitoh H, et al. Studies on pediatric patients with absent auditory brainstem response (ABR) later components. *Brain Dev* 1990;12:380–384.
26. Conradi NG, Sourander P, Nilsson O, et al. Neuro-

pathology of the Norbottnian type of Gaucher disease. *Acta Neuropathol* 1984;65:99–109.

27. Verity MA, Montasir M. Infantile Gaucher's disease: neuropathology, acid hydrolase activities and negative staining observations. *Neuropadiatrie* 1977;8(1):89–100.
28. Carpenter MB. *Core text of neuroanatomy,* 3rd ed. Baltimore: Williams & Wilkins, 1985:351–352.
29. Block CH. The neocortex: structure and function. In: Wyllie E, ed. *The treatment of epilepsy.* Philadelphia: Lea & Febiger, 1993:12–13.
30. Tassinari CA, Rubboli G, Shibasaki H. Neurophysiology of positive and negative myoclonus. *Electroencephalogr Clin Neurophysiol* 1998;107(3):181–195.
31. Vignal JP, Biraben A, Chauvel PY, et al. Reflex partial seizures of sensorimotor cortex (including cortical reflex myoclonus and startle epilepsy). *Adv Neurol* 1998;75:207–224.
32. Reutens DC, Puce A, Berkovic SF. Cortical hyperexcitability in progressive myoclonus epilepsy: a study with transcranial magnetic stimulation. *Neurology* 1993;43:186–192.
33. Pampols T, Pineda M, Giros ML, et al. Neuronopathic juvenile glucosylceramidosis due to sap-C deficiency: clinical course, neuropathy and brain lipid composition in this Gaucher disease variant. *Acta Neuropathol* 1999;97:91–97.
34. Brown P. Myoclonus. *Curr Opin Neurol* 1996;9:314–316.
35. Pelled D, Shogomori H, Futerman AH. The increased sensitivity of neurons with elevated glucocerebroside to neurotoxic agents can be reversed by imiglucerase. *J Inherit Metab Dis* 2000;23:175–184.
36. Nilsson O, Svennerholm L. Accumulation of glucosylceramide and glucosylsphingosine (Psychosine) in cerebrum and cerebellum in infantile and juvenile Gaucher disease. *J Neurochem* 1982;39:709–718.
37. Suzuki K. Twenty-five years of the "psychosine hypothesis": a personal perspective of its history and present status. *Neurochem Res* 1998;23(3):251–259.

Myoclonus and Paroxysmal Dyskinesias,
Advances in Neurology, Vol. 89,
edited by S. Fahn, et al.
Lippincott Williams & Wilkins, Philadelphia © 2002.

7

Toxin and Drug-Induced Myoclonus

Mark F. Gordon

Department of Neurology, Long Island Jewish Medical Center, New Hyde Park, New York

The term *myoclonus* literally means "a quick muscle movement." It describes a sudden, brief shocklike involuntary movement caused by muscle contractions (positive myoclonus) or sudden brief lapses of muscle contraction in active postural muscles (negative myoclonus, or asterixis). The myoclonus can be focal, multifocal, or generalized. Lesions at many levels of the central nervous system (CNS), including cerebral cortex, brainstem, and spinal cord, as well as lesions of the peripheral nervous system (PNS), including spinal roots or peripheral nerve, may trigger myoclonus.

Various toxins and medications may induce myoclonus in people. Animal models for substance-induced myoclonus may suggest some of the mechanisms for the toxic effects in humans.

The diagnosis of a toxin- or medication-induced myoclonus is often a diagnosis of exclusion. Bleecker (1) proposed the following diagnostic criteria for neurotoxic disease: (a) verified exposure; (b) appropriate temporal association between the exposure and symptoms; (c) objective evidence of the underlying pathology by neurologic examination, neuropsychologic examination, electroencephalography (EEG), electromyography (EMG), evoked potentials, computerized axial tomography, magnetic resonance imaging, positron emission tomography, and single-photon emission computed tomography; (d) exclusion of another chronic disease; (e) exclusion of a primary psychiatric disease; and (f) exclusion of a genetic etiology.

Myoclonus may present as part of a more complex neurologic syndrome related to various toxins or medications. Typically, the myoclonic jerks are generalized or multifocal, asymmetric, and nonrhythmic. They are commonly stimulus sensitive or induced by voluntary movement. Exceptions include metrizamide (2), other water-soluble contrast agents (3), and diclofenac (4), which characteristically cause segmental myoclonus. Generally, the myoclonic jerking occurs with encephalopathy, altered mental status, or even coma. Other neurologic signs, such as ataxia, headache, and seizures, may be present with certain intoxications. The various agents, their clinical findings, and treatments are summarized in Table 7.1.

Asterixis, considered a form of negative myoclonus (6), is a gross, brief, arrhythmic involuntary lapse of posture at a joint. This postural lapse occurs only during the tonic contraction. Adams and Foley (7) reported asterixis in patients with hepatic encephalopathy. Asterixis has since been seen in various metabolic and toxic encephalopathies (8). Asterixis may also be seen in the recovery phase of general anesthesia, with sedative or anticonvulsant drug administration, and in normal drowsy individuals (8,9). Asterixis is commonly described in the wrist flexors and extensors, but muscles of the face, neck flexors, and hip extensors are also involved. When the amplitude of the asterixis is very low, it may resemble a tremor. EMG recording of the asterixis shows brief (50 to 200 ms)

TABLE 7.1. *Medication- and toxin-associated myoclonus*

Agent	Myoclonus description	Other neurologic signs	Treatment	References
Aluminum	—	Dementia, seizures	Change dialysate, chelation	16
Amantadine	Multifocal or generalized, spontaneous or action induced; especially with renal impairment	Encephalopathy, delirium	Stop drug	95–97
Anesthetics (etomidate)	Generalized, stimulus sensitive	Tremor, dystonia, abnormal eye movements	Transient	73–77
Anesthetics (enflurane)	Generalized	Often in patients with seizures	Transient	79,80
Antibiotics (penicillin, cephalosporins, imipenem, quinolones)	Nonrhythmic, asymmetric, stimulus sensitive	Seizures, psychosis, delirium	Stop drug	164–174
Antihelminthics (piperazine)	Generalized, asymmetric, nonrhythmic	Confusion, somnolence, headache, ataxia, seizures, coma, death	Stop drug, administer anticonvulsants	176
Antihistamines	Multifocal, asymmetric, stimulus sensitive	—	Stop drug	114
Baking soda	Multifocal, nonrhythmic or generalized	Metabolic alkalosis, paresthesias	Stop agent	
Benzodiazepine withdrawal	Often facial, nocturnal	—	—	186,187
Bismuth	Multifocal or generalized, asymmetric, stimulus sensitive, action induced	Encephalopathy, ataxia, seizures, coma, death	Stop drug; chelation with British anti-Lewisite (BAL)	12,31,32
Bromocriptine	Generalized, arrhythmic, spontaneous, with action (such as walking), and increased by auditory and tactile stimuli	Dyskinesias	Lower or stop drug	93–94
Buspirone	Generalized, nonrhythmic	Dystonia	Stop drug	152
Calcium-channel antagonists (especially CNS-selective)	Sometimes irregular, symmetric, occasionally dystonic	Dystonia, parkinsonism	Stop drug	99–102
Cannabinoids	Asymmetric, multifocal, action induced, stimulus sensitive	Behavioral changes	Stop exposure	185
Carbamazepine	Myoclonus or asterixis	Tic-like movements, ataxia, nystagmus	Stop drug	116,118
Carbon monoxide	Rare	Delayed onset; other movement disorders are parkinsonism, dystonia, chorea	Stop exposure	65
Carvedilol	Intermittent, arrhythmic, multifocal, generalized	—	Stop drug	180
Chloralose	Spontaneous, stimulus sensitive, sometimes generalized	Agitation, stupor, coma	Stop exposure; diazepam, propofol	84,85
Chlorambucil	Multifocal	Confusion, hallucinations, agitation, seizures, ataxia	Stop drug	88,89
Cimetidine	—	Encephalopathy, psychosis, seizures	Stop drug	178
Cocaine	Generalized, action-induced	Opsoclonus, dystonia, chorea, tics, and exacerbations of underlying tic disorders	Transient	144,181

TABLE 7.1. *Continued.*

Agent	Myoclonus description	Other neurologic signs	Treatment	References
Contrast medium—ionic—diatrizoate meglumine—inadvertent intrathecal use during myelography	Ascending myoclonic spasms	Seizures, rhabdomyolysis	Elevate head, remove CSF, administer anticonvulsants, diuresis, sedation, neuromuscular blockade	192
Contrast media—water-soluble (iothalamate meglumine, iocarmate meglumine, angiografin, myelografin, metrizamide)	Segmental (generally limited to the legs), rhythmic, stimulus sensitive	Seizures	Transient, diazepam	2,3, 188–191
Cyclic antidepressants	Face, limbs or generalized, often action induced, during wakefulness or sleep	Choreoathetosis, tremor, delirium, stupor, coma, seizures, respiratory depression, pupillary dilatation, dry mucous membranes, tachycardia, hypotension, urinary retention	Stop drug; clonazepam	140–143
Dichloroethane	—	Ataxia, somnolence	Transient	60
Diclofenac	Segmental, generalized	Encephalopathy	Stop drug	4,154
Dopamine-receptor blockers (antipsychotics and antiemetics)	Multifocal, action-induced myoclonus, affecting the limbs and face; asterixis	Tremor, parkinsonism, dystonia, orofacial dyskinesia, neuroleptic malignant syndrome	Stop drug	102–108, 194
Gabapentin	Focal and multifocal myoclonus, asterixis	—	Stop drug	122,123
Ifosfamide (chloroacetaldehyde)	Multifocal, asymmetric, stimulus sensitive	Sedation, coma, seizure, ataxia, dystonia, chorea, cranial nerve palsies	Transient	86,87
Lamotrigine	Erratic; patients had intractable cryptogenic generalized epilepsy with mild preexisting jerks	—	Stop drug	124
Levodopa	Single, multifocal, or hemi; commonly in trunk and limbs	Dyskinesias	Lower the drug; methysergide may help	91,92
Lithium	Generalized, spontaneous, stimulus sensitive	Postural tremor, somnolence, delirium, stupor, coma, fasciculations, hypertonia, hyperreflexia, parkinsonism, chorea, ataxia, nystagmus	Stop drug	112,113
Mercury, organic	Generalized, action induced	Encephalopathy, tremor, ataxia	Chelation therapy	24
Methaqualone	Generalized or asymmetric, stimulus sensitive	Hypertonia, hyperreflexia, stupor, coma, generalized seizures, withdrawal	Supportive	182
Methyl bromide	Multifocal, action induced, stimulus induced	Encephalopathy, psychosis, dyarthria, ataxia, tremor, coma, death	Stop exposure	35–38
Methyl chloride	Stimulus sensitive	Encephalopathy, stuttering, ataxia	Stop exposure	42,43

continued

TABLE 7.1. *Continued.*

Agent	Myoclonus description	Other neurologic signs	Treatment	References
Methylenedioxymeth-amphetamine (MDMA)	Myoclonus	Perceptual changes, anxiety, tremor, diaphoresis, salivation, blurred vision, mydriasis, nystagmus, ataxia, tachycardia, hypertension, nausea, "flashbacks"; serotonin syndrome	Stop exposure; rapid cooling; forced diuresis	144
Methyl ethyl ketone	Multifocal	Coma, metabolic acidosis, peripheral neuropathy	Stop exposure; correct acidosis	15
Monoamine oxidase inhibitor	Spontaneous; during wakefulness and sleep	Delirium, psychosis, serotonin syndrome, hypertensive crisis	Stop drug, lorazepam	149,150
Opioids (morphine, fentanyl, hydrocodone, meperidine)	Intoxication or withdrawal states; myoclonus, hiccups	Choreoathetosis, ataxia	Stop drug; benzo-diazepines (for the intoxication or withdrawal); naloxone (for the intoxication only)	144, 155–163
Organochlorine insecticides (convulsant and nonconvulsant cyclodienes, DDT)	Rest, postural, action induced, stimulus induced	Anxiety, psychosis, paresthesias, headache, tremor, seizure, ataxia, weakness, dizziness	Stop exposure, lavage, cholestyramine, propranolol	47,49,51, 53
Oven cleaner	Irregular, dystonic, stimulus sensitive	Anorexia, fatigue	Stop exposure, transient	61
Phenobarbitone	Asterixis of hands	Nystagmus, ataxia	Stop drug	116
Phenytoin	Myoclonus, asterixis	Chorea, ballism, dystonia, tremor	Stop exposure	116,117
Primidone	Asterixis of hands	Nystagmus, ataxia	Stop drug	116
Serotonin reuptake inhibitors	Spontaneous, action, reflex, and stimulus sensitive, nonrhythmic, multifocal	Chorea, dystonia, stereotypies	Stop exposure	132–134
Strychnine	Generalized, stimulus sensitive	Delirium	Stop exposure	68
Tetraethyl lead	Generalized, action induced, stimulus sensitive	Hallucinations, ataxia, irritability	Stop drug; chelation	59
Tetanus from *Clostridium tetani*	Generalized, stimulus sensitive (auditory and tactile stimuli)	Trismus (lockjaw), generalized stiffness, rigidity, opisthotonus, spasms, laryngeal obstruction	Stop exposure, antitoxin, anti-biotics, mecha-nical ventilation, sedatives, mus-cle relaxants	67,68
Thallium	—	Neuropathy, dysarthria, dysphagia	Gastric lavage, oral Prussian blue, diuresis, hemodialysis, hemoperfusion	29
Toluene	Segmental, reflex and stimulus-sensitive spinal	*Acute:* fatigue, headache, incoordination, confusion, weakness, loss of consciousness; *chronic:* cognitive impairment, pyramidal signs, gait and limb ataxia, dysarthria, opsoclonus, ocular flutter, ocular dysmetria, nystagmus, diminished olfaction, sensorineural hearing loss, postural tremor	Stop exposure	62–64

TABLE 7.1. *Continued.*

Agent	Myoclonus description	Other neurologic signs	Treatment	References
L-Tryptophan (eosinophilia-myalgia syndrome)	Myoclonus (late feature); unclear if related to contaminants or to L-tryptophan itself	Eosinophilia, myalgias, peripheral neuropathy, myopathy, cognitive impairment (especially memory), tremors, and myokymia	? Steroids	153
Valproate	Asterixis	Tremors	Stop drug	119–121

CNS, central nervous system; CSF, cerebrospinal fluid; DDT, dichlorodiphenyltrichloroethane.

silent periods that correlate with the lapses in posture. These silent periods and jerks are not bilaterally synchronous, except in the face. Asterixis is typically bilateral or generalized; however, unilateral asterixis (6,10) or even bilateral asterixis (11) caused by focal lesions may be observed.

Toxic agents and systemic metabolic disturbances are among the most common causes of "curable" myoclonus. The list of poisonous substances (12) and drugs (13) that can cause myoclonus is long and expanding. It may be difficult to differentiate these etiologies from others, such as neurodegenerative or infectious. For instance, a patient with myoclonic encephalopathy in whom Creutzfeldt-Jakob disease was suspected was identified to have bismuth subsalicylate poisoning from an over-the-counter remedy for gastrointestinal complaints (14). Poisoning by methyl ethyl ketone in a printer was identified as a curable cause of alcohol-sensitive progressive myoclonic encephalopathy (15). Withdrawal from the source of the poison led to a gradual recovery, though the patient required treatment with clonazepam and propranolol as well.

NEUROTOXIC COMPOUNDS

Neurotoxic compounds may be generally classified as gases, metals, organic solvents, pesticides, and others (1) (Table 7.2).

Toxin-Induced Myoclonus

The myoclonus in toxic encephalopathies is typically triggered by an external stimulus and aggravated by action. Toxin-induced causes of myoclonus include bismuth, heavy metals, methyl bromide, dichlorodiphenyl-trichloroethane (DDT), gasoline sniffing, toxic oil syndrome, chloralose, and methyl ethyl ketone.

TABLE 7.2. *Classification of neurotoxic compounds*

Gases	Metals	Organic solvents	Pesticides	Others
Carbon monoxide, ethylene oxide, formaldehyde, hydrogen sulfide, nitrous oxide, methyl chloride	Alkyltins, aluminum, arsenic, lead, manganese, mercury, thallium	Acetone, carbon disulfide, ethyl benzene, methanol, methyl chloroform, methl n-butyl ketone, methylene chloride, n-hexane, styrene, toluene, trichlorothylene, xylene, mixture of solvents	Aldrin, carbamates, chlordane, chlordecone, 2,4-dichlorphenoxy acetic acid, 2,4,5-trichlorophenoxy acetic acid, lindane, methyl bromide, organophosphate compounds, pyrethroids	Acrylamide, β-dimethylamino-proprionitrile

Aluminum

Aluminum is used as an electrical insulation and for high-temperature applications such as the bricks, mufflers, industrial and household utensils, paints, deodorants, oral antacid, and antidiarrhea agents. With few exceptions, aluminum does not typically affect brain function in individuals with normal kidney function. Occupational exposure to Al-containing materials is sometimes associated with pulmonary disease and certain malignancies; however, it is rarely linked to neurologic disease. Acute and chronic encephalopathic states from Al overload occur in adults and children with impaired kidney function who are treated with oral phosphate-binding agents that contain Al and/or Al-containing dialysates. Chelation and removal of aluminum can reverse the course of this otherwise progressive and fatal neurotoxic disorder. In uremic patients, acute neurotoxicity with plasma Al levels greater than 500 mg per mL may (a) manifest as grand mal seizures during dialysis with heavily Al-contaminated solutions, (b) appear within days of treatment with deferoxamine chelation therapy due to displacement of sequestered Al from bone and other compartments, or (c) present after weeks or months of oral administration of a combination of citrate and Al compounds. Onset of aluminum toxicity is sudden in adults, with agitation, confusion, seizures, myoclonic jerking, coma, and death within days to weeks (16). Children may have a more insidious onset, with intellectual impairment, seizures, and regression of verbal and motor skills (17).

Chronic Al neurotoxicity in uremic patients is commonly associated with fractures, osteomalacia, and microcytic anemia. Dialysis encephalopathy is seen in patients with Al plasma levels of 100 to 200 mg per mL after years of parenteral Al exposure from Al-contaminated dialysate. Patients insidiously develop a speech disorder (stuttering and stammering), personality changes, disorientation, seizures, and visual and auditory hallucinations. Dementia appears gradually, first as disturbed concentration, lack of attention, and disorientation, then memory deterioration, and then confusion and possibly paranoia and suicidal ideation. Asterixis and myoclonus occur. About 7 to 9 months after onset, the patient may become mute, globally demented, and die (16). Histologic examination of the brains of patients who died with dialysis encephalopathy reveals mild spongiform pathology in the cerebral cortex and nonspecific neuronal changes (18). The gray-matter aluminum levels in patients with dialysis encephalopathy are about three times higher than in dialysis patients without neurologic disease (19).

Aluminum levels in plasma are used to monitor dialysis patients and other subjects at risk for iatrogenic aluminum toxicity. Al levels less than 10 mg per mL are considered normal; 60 mg per mL suggests the possibility of an increased body Al burden; greater than 100 mg per mL indicates a potential toxicity and a need for increased monitoring; greater than 200 mg per mL is often associated with overt Al toxicity, and greater than 500 mg per mL indicates acute Al intoxication. Prevention of aluminum toxicity in renal patients has been achieved through use of dialysis fluids containing low Al concentrations, calcium-based instead of Al-based phosphate binders, regular plasma aluminum monitoring, and if indicated, once-weekly intramuscular administration of deferoxamine prior to dialysis, with removal of the chelate during dialysis.

Occupational exposure to aluminum, such as in smelting, may be associated with neuropsychologic impairment and less commonly with motor impairment (20). There are isolated reports of individuals who developed neurologic disease consistent with aluminum toxicity. A metal worker developed jerking movements, impaired coordination, and seizures (21). Another Al-factory worker inhaled Al dust and developed focal epilepsy (repeated episodes of clonic jerking of the left arm and leg), increased tendon reflexes, extensor plantar reflexes, and dementia (22). He ultimately developed generalized seizures, coma, and died. A postmortem analysis of lungs and brain revealed Al concentrations 20 times normal. Lungs showed histologic evidence of fibrosis.

Aluminum smelter-pot-room workers may develop incoordination, tremor, ataxia, cognitive deficits, and spastic paraparesis. It is unclear, however, whether this syndrome is related to chronic aluminum toxicity; exposure to various chemicals such as particulate alumina, fluorides, hydrogen sulfide, sulfur oxides, carbon monoxide, carbon dioxide, cyanide, lithium, and polycyclic aromatic hydrocarbons; chronic alcohol intake; or neurologic disease, such as multiple sclerosis (23).

Mercury

Organic mercurials can cause myoclonus, often generalized or action induced, as well as tremor, ataxia, and encephalopathy (24). The organic mercurials are still responsible for poisoning epidemics (for example, the methyl mercury in contaminated fish). Inorganic elemental mercury intoxication, which causes tremor and intention myoclonus, has rarely been seen since it was ascribed to be Mad Hatter syndrome (25). Sporadic cases of acute mercury exposure are still reported (26). Chronic low-level exposure, such as in dentists (27), may be a concern.

Arsenic

The heavy metal arsenic targets the gastrointestinal tract, skin, bone marrow, kidneys, and peripheral nervous system. After an acute arsenic intoxication and less commonly with chronic intoxication, patients may subacutely develop peripheral neuropathy with numbness and tingling in the legs, hyperalgesia, and spontaneous pain. Patients may uncommonly develop CNS impairment, including memory and learning impairment, diminished concentration, agitation, emotional lability, and fluctuating mental states. Myoclonus is not reported.

Lead

Intoxication with the metal lead can cause impaired growth (in children), anemia, nephropathy, neuropathy, and encephalopathy. Myoclonus is not reported.

Manganese

The metal manganese can cause an extrapyramidal dysfunction. After a chronic exposure to manganese dust, miners may gradually develop asthenia, restlessness, lumbago, muscle stiffness or cramping, apathy, anorexia, somnolence, and disturbed sexual function. Psychomotor excitement may be the presenting symptom, characterized by compulsive acts, delusions, and hallucinations. This general or psychiatric initial phase is followed in a few months by the appearance of progressive extrapyramidal symptoms, including hypokinesia, fixed gaze, masked face, monotonous speech, incoordination, micrographia, tremor, dystonia, abnormal gait, and postural instability (28). A rest tremor is unusual. Tremors of the hands (with posture), tongue, and lips are common. Myoclonus is not typically described.

Thallium

Thallium is a rare but ubiquitous element in the Earth's crust. It is present in the dust of zinc and lead smelters. Its major use is as a rodenticide and insecticide. Generally, thallium toxicity involves combined neurologic, gastrointestinal, and hair abnormalities. Acute intoxication is followed by a sensory neuropathy with pain and paresthesias in the lower limbs, followed by sensory abnormality in the fingers. Distal weakness occurs as part of a motor neuropathy. In more advanced cases, proximal weakness produces dysarthria, dysphagia, and respiratory difficulties. Other problems may develop, including emotional lability, anxiety, sleep disorders, headache, tremor, myoclonus, ataxia, choreoathetosis, and cranial nerve involvement. (29). Alopecia, the hallmark of thallium poisoning, begins at 2 weeks and is complete by 1 month. Cardiotoxicity including tachycardia, irregular pulse, and angina may occur.

Chronic thallium intoxication presents with abdominal pain, insomnia, and weight loss. Abnormal movements, such as myoclonus, polyneuritis, inappropriate behavior, depression, fever, hypertension, cardiac disturbances, and hair loss may be seen.

Thallium-induced neuropathologic findings include ganglion cell changes in the cortex and brainstem, edema of the white matter, mild involvement of the spinal cord, and segmental myelin degeneration of the peripheral nerves. Treatment involves gastric lavage, oral Prussian blue, forced diuresis, and in more severe cases, hemodialysis and charcoal hemoperfusion.

Bismuth

Burns et al. (30) described five patients from Australia with an encephalopathy characterized by confusion, ataxia, tremor, and intense myoclonic jerking. Each had undergone a colostomy for carcinoma of the colon and had received treatment with oral bismuth subgallate to improve stool consistency and odor for a period of 6 months to 6 years. No cause for the encephalopathy was found. All patients improved when the bismuth intake was stopped. Burns et al. suggested that bismuth subgallate could produce a toxic encephalopathy.

At the same time, bismuth encephalopathy was recognized in France. Buge et al. (31) reported six cases with a similar clinical presentation to the Australian cases and found elevated plasma levels of bismuth. Those six patients had received bismuth subnitrate, and none had had a gastrointestinal operation. Bismuth was implicated as the cause of the encephalopathy.

Between 1973 and 1977, approximately 50 cases were diagnosed in Australia (32) and more than 1,000 cases were detected in France, where 72 deaths were recorded (33,34).

In bismuth encephalopathy there is a prodromal phase lasting weeks or months, characterized by depression, irritability, or apathy. This is followed by a rapid deterioration with confusion and hallucinations, myoclonic jerking, truncal ataxia, and dysarthria. Generalized convulsions, stupor, and coma may develop. Recovery occurs if bismuth intake is stopped early in the course. In severe cases,

chelation therapy using dimercaprol (BAL) may promote a more rapid recovery.

The myoclonus in bismuth encephalopathy is mainly present with action, but it is also very sensitive to external stimuli. The jerks may occur spontaneously. They may be multifocal or generalized. (12)

In bismuth encephalopathy, the somatosensory evoked response (SEP) was enlarged bilaterally, and the EEG showed spike-and-wave activity preceding the myoclonus (35). In one patient who survived 5 years with a stupor and intense myoclonus, the pathology showed bilateral necrosis of the inferior colliculi, gliosis of the upper brainstem reticular formation, and moderate gliosis and degeneration of the cerebellar Purkinje cells.

Methyl Bromide

Methyl bromide, a fumigant, can cause multifocal and action-induced myoclonus with encephalopathy, psychosis, dysarthria, ataxia, and intention tremor (35–37). A permanent severe intention myoclonus has been described after accidental exposure during fumigation of a house; however, posthypoxic intention myoclonus due to a status epilepticus could not be excluded (38). In humans, acute exposure produces mucosal irritation, followed in several hours by malaise, nausea, emesis, headache, dizziness, gastrointestinal, and pulmonary symptoms. A latent period of several hours may occur that is followed by visual symptoms, dysarthria, ataxia, myalgias, numbness, paresis, confusion, delirium, psychosis, tremors, myoclonus, seizures, and death. The few postmortem neuropathologic studies have followed acute, high-dose exposures and have shown cerebral edema, petechial hemorrhage, cell loss in the cerebral and cerebellar cortex, changes in the dentate and various brainstem nuclei, and lesions in the inferior colliculi and mammillary bodies, microscopically similar to those seen in Wernicke encephalopathy (39,40). Chronic human exposure to methyl bromide may resemble acute toxicity with a mixture of peripheral neuropathy, pyramidal and cerebellar dysfunction, and neuropsychiatric disturbance.

Methyl Chloride

Methyl chloride is used as an aerosol propellant, solvent, and extractant. Chronic MeCl intoxication in six workers produced diplopia, ataxia, memory difficulties, stuttering, dizziness, and confusion (41). Myoclonus and seizures may be elicited by light manipulation (42,43). The mechanism for the MeCl neurotoxicity is unknown.

Methyl Ethyl Ketone

Methyl ethyl ketone (MEK) or 2-butanone is a volatile hydrocarbon solvent used in paint, glue, paint removers, printing ink, rubber cement, and resins. Orti-Pareja et al. (15) described a 27-year-old graphics worker with occupational exposure to MEK who developed dizziness, asthenia, anorexia, weight loss, postural and action tremor in the hands, face, tongue, and voice, multifocal myoclonic jerks in the limbs, ocular flutter, and ataxic gait. EEG showed a normal background activity with occasional bursts of θ waves at 6 to 7 Hz and generalized spikes. The ataxia, myoclonus, and tremor showed a dramatic, but transient, improvement after intake of 20 g ethanol. The syndrome resolved after one month of therapy with clonazepam and propranolol and cessation of the exposure to MEK. The clonazepam and propranolol were then withdrawn without reappearance of the signs after a 10-month follow-up. MEK can produce ataxia, tremor, encephalopathy, and coma (44). Chronic exposure to the solvent MEK and other related compounds, such as methyl-*n*-butyl ketone or *n*-hexane may cause a peripheral neuropathy (45).

Organochlorine Insecticides

Chlorinated Cyclodienes

Chlorinated cyclodiene insecticides (CCIs) are a class of organochlorine insecticide (46). The CCIs are classified as either *nonconvul-* *sant* caged cyclodienes (mirex, chlordecone) or *convulsant* CCIs (chlordane, aldrin, dieldrin, endrin).

Chlordecone (Kepone) is an organochlorine ant and roach pesticide. Due to its toxicity, in 1974, the U.S. Environmental Protection Agency prohibited its sale or use. From March 1974 to July 1975, in 133 chlordecone-production workers, 64 % with a mean blood chlordecone level of 2.53 ppm developed nervousness, tremor, ataxia, weight loss, pleuritic and joint pain, liver function test abnormalities, and oligospermia (47). A tremor of low amplitude and irregular directions was common. This tremor occurred primarily upon action or posture maintenance; however, it was sometimes present at rest. The tremor stopped in sleep and increased with anxiety or fatigue. Some patients developed blurred vision and chaotic eye movements resembling opsoclonus, some developed startle myoclonus, disorientation, confusion, and auditory and visual hallucinations. Chlordecone has multiple mechanisms, including inhibition of adenosine triphosphatase in the brain, heart, and liver, inhibition of brain mitochondrial oxidative phosphorylation, inhibition of calcium uptake, and alteration of dopamine and γ-aminobutyric acid (GABA) activities. Cholestyramine significantly increased fetal excretion of the pesticide (48). Propranolol in doses up to 200 mg per day lessened the tremor in some patients.

The convulsant CCIs produce a reversible seizure disorder in humans and animals by interfering with the function of GABA, the major inhibitory neurotransmitter in the vertebrate and insect CNS. These insecticides were used widely in North America in the 1940s to the 1960s. However, the environmental persistence of many organochlorine insecticides, coupled with their potential for bioconcentration and biomagnification in various chains, caused avian and other species to accumulate body burdens that were linked to disrupted reproductive success. The use of organochlorine insecticides is banned in North America and Europe; however, extensive use continues in less-developed parts of the world. Poisoning with these insecticides has been associated with ingestion of contaminated seed grain or flour, occupational exposures during manufacture or application of CCIs, homicide, and suicide. In humans, intoxication produces myoclonus, convulsions, headache, nausea, vomiting, malaise, dizziness, and muscle weakness. Circumoral numbness, anorexia, nausea, fatigue, and myoclonic jerks were reported in a woman exposed to chlordane for 1 to 4 weeks (49). Convulsions induced by chlordane are accompanied by confusion, incoordination, excitability, and, in some cases, coma (50). Symptoms of intoxication, including myoclonic jerking, irritability, and memory loss were reported for up to 1 year following 6 to 12 months of oral exposure to grain containing aldrin and lindane (51).

Blood or serum levels are used to monitor exposure to most of the CCIs. Exposure to endrin is determined from urinary metabolites, since this CCI has a very short biologic half-life in the blood. Characteristic EEG findings of CCIs are bilateral, synchronous θ wave activity, and occasional bilateral, synchronous spike-and-wave complexes (52).

Treatment of organochlorine insecticide intoxication is symptomatic. Contaminated skin is washed with soap and water and eyes are flushed with water for at least 10 minutes. Treatment for ingestion includes gastric lavage, avoiding aspiration into the lungs, followed by intragastric administration of 3 to 4 tablespoons of activated charcoal and 30 g of magnesium or sodium sulfate in 30% solution. Fats, oils, and milk should be avoided because these promote absorption of organochlorine insecticides from the intestinal tract. Convulsions are treated with a single, or if needed, repeated intravenous application of an anticonvulsant benzodiazepine, such as diazepam.

Dichlorodiphenyltrichloroethane and Chlorinated Cyclodiene Insecticides

DDT and CCIs have been used to control typhus, malaria, dengue fever, and filariasis. DDT and its metabolite, DDE, are highly lipophilic compounds that accumulate in adipose tissue for prolonged periods of time. DDT is found in other tissues, including the brain. In humans, dermal and respiratory absorption are low, but oral doses are well absorbed. DDT interferes with sodium ion conductance across excitable membranes, prolongs the duration of the recovery phase of the action potential, increases the excitability of the nerve to stimulation, and thereby induces repetitive axonal discharges to stimuli that normally elicit a single response.

Clinical features of DDT poisoning begin 0.5 to 6 hours after the exposure and include hyperesthesias of the mouth, tongue, and lower face (typically the initial feature), then disequilibrium, paresthesias and tremors of the limbs, confusion, malaise, headache, fatigue, and delayed emesis. Recovery occurs over several days in severe poisoning when convulsions have occurred. Residual weakness and ataxia of the hands have been reported 5 weeks after the ingestion (53). Chronic exposure to DDT causes weight loss, anorexia, mild anemia, muscle weakness, tremors, anxiety, excitability, fear, myoclonic jerks, and generalized seizures. EEG may reveal sharp waves, excessive θ waves, spike-and-sharp complexes, and low-voltage, rhythmic spikes (54). There is no specific treatment for DDT poisoning. Animal studies suggest that sedatives (such as diazepam), ionic calcium, and glucose may be useful (53).

Organophosphate

The organophosphate compounds (55), the largest group of pesticides, induce cholinergic toxicity by inhibition of acetylcholinesterase at nerve endings and the subsequent accumulation of acetylcholine at cholinergic synapses. The symptoms and signs of acute organophosphate poisoning can be grouped into muscarinic (largely parasympathetic), nicotinic (sympathetic and motor), and CNS effects. Muscarinic features include lacrimation, miosis, salivation, sweating, increased bronchial secretions, bronchoconstriction, dyspnea, pulmonary edema, nausea, emesis, abdominal cramping, diarrhea, bradycardia, hypotension, arrhythmias, and urinary frequency and incontinence. Nicotinic features include muscle weakness, twitching, and cramps, fasciculations, pallor, hyperglycemia, tachyarrhythmias, and hypertension. CNS effects include anxiety, confusion, irritability, blurred vision, seizures, tremors, opsoclonus, respiratory depression, and coma. The time between exposure and onset of symptoms varies with the particular organophosphate, route, and degree of exposure: within a few minutes after massive ingestion, or delayed several hours with slowly absorbed organophosphates. Patients generally recover from the major cholinergic signs within a few days to a few weeks. Therapy includes decontamination, induction of vomiting, gastric lavage, administration of atropine (to counteract the muscarinic effects) and pralidoxime (to reduce the acetylcholine levels by restoring the acetylcholinesterase activity).

Toxic Cooking Oil

In 1981 in Spain there was an epidemic of an "atypical pneumonia" with neurologic symptoms, such as muscle pain, spasms, and weakness, and decreased vision. Generalized severe muscle wasting, absent tendon jerks, and patchy sensory loss were the most common neurologic findings on the examination. Myoclonus, a late complication in 2% to 3% of cases, was typically spontaneous, multifocal and often asymmetric, repetitive, and semirhythmic (56). Epidemiologic studies implicated edible rapeseed oil, which had been contaminated with anilines and propanediols (57,58). The latency period between the exposure and the onset of the illness was 4 to 10 days.

Gasoline Sniffing

Gasoline sniffing may cause an acute encephalopathy due to intake of tetraethyl lead. Visual hallucinations, ataxia, insomnia, irritability, and myoclonic jerking characterize this syndrome. The myoclonus is usually generalized, increased by action, and provoked by external stimuli. The encephalopathy may become permanent after repeated exposure to the toxin (59).

Dichloroethane

Accidental ingestion of the dry cleaning agent dichloroethane has produced myoclonus and somnolence (60). The myoclonic movements typically resolve within days, but the ataxia may persist.

Oven Cleaners

Oven cleaners may also produce a myoclonic encephalopathy. Peatfield and Boothman reported a previously well 46-year-old woman who, after prolonged cleaning of her oven with Sanmex spray, developed progressive nausea, anorexia, fatigue, involuntary, irregular, jerking movements (described as myoclonus with a dystonic component) involving the chest, neck, and upper abdomen. The movements occurred spontaneously and also were triggered by auditory stimuli. She received valproate and the movements abated over 2 days. EEG showed a normal α rhythm. Simultaneous surface EMG recordings showed myoclonic jerks, mostly lasting 90 to 130 ms, that were not accompanied by any EEG change. The authors suspected that the butane in the cleaner triggered the myoclonus, but they were unable to confirm this (61).

Toluene

Toluene is a volatile, aromatic hydrocarbon used in the production of adhesives, glues, lacquer, paints, rubbers, and thinners. It may be abused by inhalation. Acute effects of toluene intoxication are dose dependent and include fatigue, headache, incoordination, confusion, weakness, and loss of consciousness. Chronic toluene abuse produces the following neurologic abnormalities: cognitive (inattention, diminished memory, visuospatial function, and complex cognition), pyramidal (spastic paraparesis, hyperactive deep tendon reflexes, clonus, and Babinski signs), cerebellar (gait and limb ataxia, dysarthria), cranial nerve and brainstem (opsoclonus, ocular flutter, ocular dysmetria, nystagmus, diminished olfaction, and sensorineural hearing loss), and postural tremor (62,63).

Sugiyama-Oishi et al. (64) reported a 48-year-old male painter with stimulus-sensitive spinal myoclonus from chronic toluene (paint thinner) intoxication. He had occasional episodes of headache, nausea, and dizziness from acute thinner intoxication and a chronic hand tremor and memory disturbance. Neurologic examination revealed bilateral postural tremor of his hands and rhythmic reflex myoclonic jerking in his right arm (elicited by tapping the brachioradialis muscle tendon). Surface EMG revealed repetitive grouping discharges beginning about 100 ms after the tendon tap and lasting about 30 to 50 ms. A long loop reflex (C-reflex) and giant SEPs were not observed in his right arm, and EEG showed no spike. Urinary excretion of N-benzoylglycine, a metabolite of toluene, was increased (1.17 g per L). His myoclonic jerks were considered to be stimulus-sensitive spinal myoclonus, because they were induced segmentally and because cortical hyperexcitability was not seen.

Carbon Monoxide

Carbon monoxide poisoning may cause a delayed-onset movement disorder, but only rarely myoclonus. Of 242 patients with CO poisoning examined between 1986 and 1996, delayed movement disorders were diagnosed in 32 (13.2%); 23 (71.9%) had parkinsonism; 5, dystonia; 3, chorea; and 1 myoclonus. All were associated with delayed CO encephalopathy. The median latency between CO poisoning and the onset of movement disorders was 4 weeks for parkinsonism, 51 weeks for dystonia, 4 weeks for chorea, and 8 weeks for myoclonus. Dystonia was notable for the longest latency to onset after the CO poisoning. There were variable findings on computed tomography in the delayed-onset movement disorders after CO poisoning (65).

Strychnine

Strychnine, a naturally occurring toxic alkaloid first isolated from *Strychnos ignatti,* has been used as a poison to control vermin since the sixteenth century. It is used as an experimental tool to study glycine receptors in the brain and spinal cord and as a convulsant agent to model epileptiform activity. Strychnine poisoning is generally by ingestion of rodenticide compounds. It produces anxiety, restlessness, hyperreflexia, myoclonus, particularly of the head and neck, convulsions (triggered by external stimuli, such as loud noises or sudden movements), and respiratory paralysis (66). Urgent management includes maintenance of breathing; prevention of convulsions (with intravenous diazepam, pentobarbital, or phenobarbital); gastric lavage with activated charcoal (to reduce toxin absorption); neuromuscular blockade and artificial respiration when convulsions are uncontrollable; and treatment in a dark, quiet room (which reduces the external stimuli that trigger the seizures). Once convulsions are controlled, treatment focuses on the severe lactic acidosis, rhabdomyolysis, and hyperthermia that result from the convulsions. Strychnine produces neuronal excitation by blocking the inhibitory neurotransmitter glycine.

Tetanus Toxin

Tetanus toxin, derived from *Clostridium tetani,* presents locally with trismus (lockjaw) and headache or, more commonly, with a generalized stiffness, rigidity, opisthotonus, and spasms, which can lead to laryngeal obstruction (67). The spasms may represent a stimulus-sensitive myoclonus (68), induced by auditory and tactile stimuli. The spasms are excruciatingly painful and may be uncontrollable, leading to respiratory arrest and death. Spasms are most prominent in the first 2 weeks; autonomic disturbance usually starts some days after spasms and reaches a peak during the second week of the disease. Rigidity may last beyond the duration of both spasms and autonomic disturbance. Treatment of tetanus includes penicillin or metronidazole antibiotic, mechanical ventilation, muscle relaxants, and sedatives.

Endogenous Toxins from Metabolic Derangements

Endogenous toxins from metabolic abnormalities, such as uremia (69,70), hepatic coma (68), hypercapnia (68), and hypoglycemia (71), may induce myoclonus. Metabolic alkalosis may cause paresthesias, muscle twitching, and rarely myoclonus and may be partially due to decreased serum levels of ionized calcium. Razavi (72) reported a patient who developed a metabolic alkalosis, paresthesias, facial twitching, prolonged QT interval, and positive Trousseau sign compatible with hypocalcemia from excessive ingestion of baking soda. These metabolic derangements usually produce multifocal, arrhythmic myoclonic jerks affecting predominantly the face and proximal musculature. Later in the illness, patients can demonstrate generalized myoclonus.

In metabolic encephalopathy with myoclonus, the EEG reveals paroxysms of slow-wave and spike-and-slow-wave activity not temporally related to the myoclonic jerks (70). The myoclonus typically resolves as the encephalopathy is corrected. No specific pharmacologic interventions are generally recommended for the myoclonus related to metabolic derangements.

DRUG-INDUCED MYOCLONUS

Multiple drugs may induce multifocal spontaneous and action myoclonus. Klawans et al. published a review in 1986 (13). These drugs include insoluble bismuth salts, anesthetics, chloralose, antineoplastics, levodopa and other antiparkinsonian agents, dopamine receptor blockers (such as antipsychotics and antiemetics), lithium, anticonvulsant drugs overdoses (phenytoin, carbamazepine, valproate, gabapentin, lamotrigine), antidepressants (serotonin reuptake inhibitors, cyclic antidepressants, and monoamine oxidase inhibitors [MAOIs]), diclofenac, opiates (morphine, meperidine, hydrocodone, fentanyl), antibiotics (penicillin, cephalosporins, imipenem, quinolones), antihelminthic (piperazine), antiviral (acyclovir), antihistamines, cimetidine, β-agonists and β-blockers, cocaine, methaqualone, cannabinoid compounds, benzodiazepine withdrawal, and contrast media.

Anesthetics

Various anesthetic agents may cause myoclonus. *Etomidate*, an ultrashort-acting, non-barbiturate hypnotic, commonly causes involuntary muscle movements that are myoclonic in 74%, averting movements in 7%, tonic movements in 10%, and eye movements in 9% (73). Tremor and dystonia have also been observed (74). Etomidate produces a transient, generalized, and stimulus-sensitive dose-related myoclonus (75–77).

Islander and Vinge (78) reported two patients who developed delayed neuroexcitatory symptoms after an uneventful anesthesia. The first patient developed muscle hypertonicity, jerky movements, and unconsciousness after an uneventful anesthesia with propofol, and later the same thing happened after anesthesia with thiopentone. The second patient developed similar symptoms after an uneventful anesthesia with propofol, but she did not fully recover. The authors commented that in these two patients the causal relationship between propofol and the neuroexcitatory symptoms was uncertain.

Prolonged maintenance of deep anesthesia with the gaseous agent *enflurane* may rarely cause myoclonus, generally in patients with seizure disorders (79,80). The myoclonus is generalized and resolves spontaneously within days. The myoclonus is associated with periodic spike-dome complexes alternating with electrical silence on EEG.

Spinal anesthesia may rarely cause myoclonus. Fox et al. (81) reported a patient with transient, bilateral, lower-extremity myoclonus during the recovery phase after spinal anesthesia. The myoclonus responded partially to diazepam and cleared in 24 hours.

γ-Hydroxybutyrate

Oxybate, or γ-hydroxybutyrate (GHB), a metabolite of the inhibitory neurotransmitter GABA, is present in the brain in one-thousandth of the concentration of GABA. Formerly used as an anesthetic, it is still used in Europe for the treatment of narcolepsy, alcohol dependence, and opiate dependence (82). Its sale was banned in the United States in 1990. More recently, it has been used recreationally and for intended sexual assault. Toxic effects of the street form of GHB include rapid onset of drowsiness, nausea, vomiting, bradycardia, hypothermia, myoclonic seizures, and short-duration coma (82,83).

Chloralose

Moene et al. (84) described six patients intoxicated with the rodenticide chloralose who developed an intense spontaneous and stimulus-sensitive myoclonus that worsened to generalized myoclonic status. Most patients were agitated, stuporous, or comatose during the jerking. The myoclonus was asynchronous with spike-wave activity on the EEG. Chloralose increases activity of cortical neurons while selectively depressing the ascending reticular formation. Diazepam generally controls the myoclonus. Propofol was used successfully in a patient whose myoclonic jerks did not respond to high dose diazepam (85).

Antineoplastics

Some antineoplastics may induce myoclonus.

Ifosfamide, an analog of cyclophosphamide, is an oxazaphosphorine alkylating agent used to treat various pediatric and adult tumors, including lung cancer, sarcoma, gynecologic malignancies, germ cell tumors, and lymphomas. Side effects include sedation, coma, seizures, ataxia, cranial nerve palsies, and rarely myoclonus. Anderson and Tandon (86) reported a 61-year-old man treated with ifosfamide for adenocarcinoma of the lung and abdominal lymphoma who developed confusion, myoclonus, blepharospasm, torticollis, opistho-

tonus, and chorea. Intravenous diphenhydramine abolished the extrapyramidal abnormality. The metabolite chloracetaldehyde may be the cause of the CNS toxicity. The chloracetaldehyde is found in a tenfold higher concentration after metabolism of ifosfamide compared to cyclophosphamide, which dose not have CNS toxicity. Chloracetaldehyde is chemically similar to acetaldehyde, a neurotoxic metabolite of ethanol. Aldehyde dehydrogenase degrades both chloracetaldehyde and acetaldehyde (87).

Chlorambucil is a slow-acting nitrogen mustard treatment for chronic lymphocytic leukemia and malignant lymphomas. Chlorambucil may produce multifocal myoclonus, sometimes with seizures, confusion, hallucinations, agitation, and ataxia. These problems may be seen in patients receiving therapeutic doses or an overdose or having impaired renal function (88,89). The EEG shows paroxysms of high-amplitude spike-wave activity not temporally related to the myoclonus. The movement abnormality and the EEG resolve after stopping the drug.

The antineoplastic *prednimustine* may rarely induce myoclonus (90).

Antiparkinsonian Drugs

Myoclonus is an infrequent complication of Parkinson disease (PD) drug therapy. *Levodopa* can induce myoclonus and asterixis (91). The trunk and limbs are most commonly affected. Facial muscle involvement is unusual. Levodopa can induce myoclonus during sleep (nocturnal myoclonus) as well as during fatigue, dozing, or even wakefulness. These movements are generally single, abrupt jerks of the limbs, often occurring bilaterally and symmetrically, or occasionally in an arm and leg on the same side simultaneously (92). The myoclonus abates with drug cessation. Methysergide, a serotonin-specific antagonist, eliminates the levodopa-induced myoclonus without worsening the levodopa-induced dyskinesias.

The dopamine agonist *bromocriptine* may also induce myoclonus (93,94). A 33-year-old mentally retarded man with anoxic birth injury and a progressive generalized dystonia received increasing doses of bromocriptine (without concomitant drugs). His dystonia improved; however, he developed a generalized, arrhythmic myoclonus affecting primarily the proximal arms and axial muscles. The myoclonus occurred spontaneously, with action (such as walking), and was increased by auditory and tactile stimuli. The myoclonus improved with discontinuation of the bromocriptine; however, the dystonia worsened (94).

Amantadine hydrochloride was initially used as an antiviral agent in the prophylaxis of influenza A; however, it is now mainly used to treat PD patients. Amantadine is a dopamine-reuptake inhibitor, a dopamine agonist, and also an N-methyl-D-aspartate (NMDA) receptor agonist. Amantadine may rarely produce myoclonus with a delirium (95). It was implicated as the cause of myoclonus of the larynx, pharynx, and face in a PD patient on concomitant levodopa (96). The myoclonus improved with stopping the amantadine. Matsunaga et al. (97) described three patients with confusion and cortical myoclonus induced by amantadine. The myoclonus was multifocal and asymmetric in all limbs and neck, tongue, and face. Two of the three patients had high plasma amantadine levels and renal impairment. It can accumulate to toxic levels in patients with renal impairment because about 90% of the oral dose is excreted in the urine, and little is removed by hemodialysis (98).

Dopamine Antagonists

Drugs that antagonize the striatal dopamine receptors frequently produce various movement disorders, such as acute dystonic reactions, acute akathisia, parkinsonism, neuroleptic malignant syndrome, and tardive syndromes (dyskinesias) such as buccolingual masticatory syndrome, stereotypies, tardive dystonia, tardive tourettism, tardive tremor, tardive myoclonus, and tardive akathisia. Possible causative agents include neuroleptics to treat psychotic disorders such

as schizophrenia; the benzamides (i.e., metoclopramide, sulpiride, cleopride, veralipride) to treat nausea, emesis, gastrointestinal upset, and menopausal hot flashes; and calcium channel blockers (i.e., flunarizine, cinnarizine, nifedipine, verapamil, diltiazem, especially those that are CNS selective) to treat vertigo, migraine, and cardiovascular disorders. Isolated cases have been reported with verapamil (99), diltiazem (100), and nifedipine (101,102). The myoclonus induced by the calcium channel antagonists occurs predominantly in the limbs both at rest and with intention. It is often irregular and symmetric and sometimes dystonic. The myoclonus is typically dose related and subsides with withdrawal of the offending drug.

Myoclonus is the predominant feature in a small number of cases of tardive dyskinesia (103). This publication reported prominent postural myoclonus in the arms in 32 of 133 psychiatric patients who had received neuroleptic treatment for at least 3 months. In addition to myoclonus, the patients showed other drug-induced movement disorders, such as tremor, parkinsonism, and orofacial dyskinesias. In 6 of the 32 cases EMG was performed, and typical positive myoclonic discharges 30- to 40-ms long were detected. In a follow-up paper (104), the myoclonus correlated with the dose of the neuroleptic.

Little and Jankovic (105) reported a 46-year-old psychotic woman on chronic antipsychotic treatment who developed tardive myoclonus within 5 months after stopping the neuroleptic. The movement disorder was characterized by 1- to 2-Hz neck jerks accompanied by synchronous contractions of the platysma, frontalis, and sternocleidomastoid muscles. The myoclonus persisted for 7 months and ceased after restitution of the neuroleptic.

The atypical antipsychotic clozapine can cause a dose-related increase in major motor seizures as well as myoclonus (106). Knoll (107) reported a 40-year-old man with chronic schizophrenia who developed oropharyngeal myoclonus after 1 month of therapy with clozapine while on concurrent sertraline. The myoclonus resolved with a reduction of the dose. Since the myoclonus was time linked with changes in the dose of clozapine, Knoll postulated that the clozapine triggered the myoclonus; however, he also considered the possibilities that sertraline itself may have directly induced the myoclonus or that sertraline may have indirectly induced the myoclonus by increasing the clozapine levels. Sajatovic and Meltzer (108) reported clozapine-induced myoclonus or generalized seizures in 11 (7.4%) of 148 patients with schizophrenia or schizoaffective disorder who were treated with clozapine monotherapy.

Myoclonus has been associated with neuroleptic malignant syndrome (NMS) induced by haloperidol (109).

Lithium

Lithium commonly produces a fine hand tremor (8 to 10 Hz), especially in patients who are receiving concomitant neuroleptics and antidepressants (110,111). Acute lithium intoxication typically produces neurologic symptoms (112). Initial symptoms are apathy and sluggishness, followed by delirium, stupor, or coma. Frequent neurologic manifestations include coarse tremor, fasciculations, myoclonus (generalized, spontaneous, and stimulus sensitive), and muscle twitching. Less common are muscular hypertonicity, hyperreflexia, parkinsonism, choreoathetoid dyskinesia, dysarthria, ataxia, downbeat nystagmus, gaze palsy, and generalized seizures. The estimated rate of persistent neurologic sequelae following acute intoxication is 10% (113). The mechanism of lithium's neurotoxic effects is unclear. Lithium influences the cholinergic and aminergic transmitter systems, GABA and peptidergic processes, and the second messenger (phosphoinositide) system.

Antihistamines

Antihistamines can cause dyskinesias that are clinically similar to classic tardive dyskinesia.

Overdosages of antihistamines alone (114) or in combination with pseudoephedrine and paracetamol (114) have been associated with multifocal, asymmetric myoclonus.

Anticonvulsants

Phenytoin is the antiepileptic drug most frequently associated with the development of movement disorders. It has been reported to induce orofacial chorea, ballism, dystonia, tremor, asterixis, and myoclonus (116,117). In the review of the literature by Harrison et al. (117), 77 cases were reported until 1993; however, phenytoin-related myoclonus is only rarely described. Some patients developed the involuntary movements even at phenytoin levels within the therapeutic range. Some 68% of the patients who developed movement disorders were taking other antiepileptic drugs in combination with phenytoin. Young and Shahani (8) reported that phenytoin exacerbated unilateral asterixis secondary to thalamic lesion.

Carbamezepine (CBZ) may rarely induce myoclonus or asterixis, even at serum levels in the therapeutic range. Wendland (118) reported an 11-year-old boy with benign occipital epilepsy who developed nonepileptic myoclonus and ticlike movements after 2 weeks of CBZ therapy (15 mg per kg per day). Drug withdrawal produced a resolution of the involuntary movements within several days, and drug rechallenge produced myoclonus. The myoclonus occurred with CBZ serum levels in the therapeutic range. Chadwick et al. (116) described a 66-year-old woman with trigeminal neuralgia who developed asterixis of her outstretched hands, nystagmus, and ataxia on CBZ with serum levels in the therapeutic range. Lowering the CBZ dose lessened the movement disorder, but her tic worsened.

Primidone and *phenobarbitone* may also induce a syndrome of asterixis of outstretched hands, nystagmus, and gait ataxia that improves with withdrawal of the anticonvulsants (116).

In about 10% of patients, *valproate* may cause a dose-related tremor that resembles essential tremor syndrome (119). Asterixis (negative myoclonus) due to valproate is occasionally reported (120,121).

Asconape et al. (122) reported that in a retrospective review of clinic charts of 104 consecutive patients started on *gabapentin* (GBP) for the treatment of epilepsy, 13 patients experienced myoclonus. All patients had refractory epilepsy and were taking other antiepileptic drugs. Six patients had a severe chronic static encephalopathy, and 5 patients had no medical diagnosis other than seizures. Ten patients developed multifocal myoclonus. Three patients developed focal myoclonus, contralateral to their epileptic focus. Two patients had an exacerbation of preexisting myoclonus. An EEG performed during myoclonus on 3 patients showed no correlate. The myoclonus persisted as long as the GBP was maintained, whereas stopping GBP resulted in rapid cessation of the myoclonus. In all cases, the myoclonus was subtle and did not significantly interfere with daily activities. Jacob et al. (123) reported a patient with postherpetic neuralgia who developed asterixis while being treated with GBP.

Janszky et al. (124) described disabling "erratic" myoclonus in two patients with mental retardation who were receiving *lamotrigine* therapy for childhood-onset intractable cryptogenic generalized epilepsy. A combination of lamotrigine and valproate produced excellent benefit; however, after 2 to 3 years of therapy, both patients developed disabling myoclonic jerks. The dosage of lamotrigine was the same before and at the onset of myoclonus; however, when the severe myoclonus started, both patients had a serum lamotrigine level (16.5 and 17.7 mg per L) higher than prior levels. Disabling myoclonus was also present during lamotrigine monotherapy with 15 mg per L serum level. Lamotrigine may worsen myoclonus in generalized epilepsies, possibly correlating with serum drug levels.

Serotonergic Drugs

In both certain animal models and people, substances that increase CNS serotonin can produce a myoclonic syndrome. Klawans et al. (125) reported the production of myoclonus in intact guinea pigs after the subcutaneous injection of 5-hydroxytryptophan (5-HTP), the immediate precursor of serotonin. In guinea pigs, intraperitoneal 5-HTP induced a myoclonic phenomenon linked to serotonin-receptor stimulation that is dependent on brainstem and spinal cord centers (126).

The *serotonin syndrome* is characterized by a triad of mental status changes, autonomic dysfunction, and neuromuscular abnormalities. Features include restlessness, agitation, delirium, incoordination, tremor, myoclonus, ataxia, seizures, muscular, hypertonia, hyperreflexia, shivering, diaphoresis, tachycardia, hypertension, and hyperpyrexia. This state may progress to coma and death from cardiovascular collapse, hyperpyrexia, and other systemic complications (127). The serotonin syndrome arises from an increase in the biologic activity of serotonin (127,128). The syndrome is mediated by 5-HT_{1A} receptors located in the brainstem (128).

Any drug or combination of drugs that increases serotonergic transmission can precipitate the *serotonin syndrome*. As described by Sternbach (127) and LoCurto (128), mechanisms of the serotonin syndrome and examples of related drugs include the following:

- *Inhibition of serotonin reuptake:* selective serotonin reuptake inhibitors (SSRIs), the tricyclic antidepressants (especially clomipramine because of all the tricyclic antidepressants, it most potently blocks the serotonin reuptake), amphetamine, cocaine, dextromethorphan, meperidine, methylenedioxymethamphetamine (MDMA or ecstasy), and venlafaxine
- *Increased substrate supply:* the serotonin precursor L-tryptophan
- *Inhibition of serotonin metabolism:* moclobemide and MAOIs
- *Combination of drugs:* MAOIs and meperidine (which is particularly risky)
- *Increased serotonin release:* amphetamine, cocaine, fenfluramine, reserpine, and MDMA

- *Direct receptor antagonism:* buspirone, lysergic acid diethylamide, and sumatriptan
- *Dopamine agonism:* amantadine, bromocriptine, bupropion, and levodopa

Nayuda and Scheftner (129) reported a paranoid schizophrenic patient with chronic neuroleptic intake who developed a withdrawal syndrome (with myoclonus, agitation, nightmares, nausea, and piloerection) after olanzapine discontinuation. Symptoms improved with reinstitution of the drug. The authors suspected a serotonin syndrome and speculated that sudden cessation of serotonin-receptor blockade may produce a rebound phenomenon in postsynaptic receptors, which have been sensitized or increased in number by the 6-month blockade.

Myoclonus, the most common neurologic sign in serotonin syndrome, is seen in 58% of cases (130). The presence of myoclonus helps distinguish the serotonin syndrome from NMS, although it is often not possible to distinguish the two on clinical grounds alone. Unlike NMS, the serotonin syndrome often resolves within 24 hours. Frequently, patients with serotonin syndrome require only supportive care, but in more critically ill patients, intubation and mechanical ventilation may be required. Mortality is high (11%), and patients should be managed in an intensive care unit. Gastric decontamination (such as gastric lavage and activated charcoal) may be considered, especially with a recent (less than 1 hour) ingestion of a life-threatening agent, such as a MAOI. Propranolol, diphenhydramine, chlorpromazine, diazepam, lorazepam, and methysergide have been used to treat serotonin syndrome. Cyproheptadine, a histamine-1 receptor blocker with 5-HT$_{1A}$ antagonist properties, reversed clinical signs within hours (131).

The serotonin reuptake inhibitor (SRI) class of antidepressants has been associated with the development of movement disorders. Fluoxetine has been reported to produce a myoclonus or more complex movement disorders combining myoclonus, chorea, dystonia, and stereotypies (132,133). Lauterbach (132)

reported a patient with presumed Pick disease who developed an intermittent rhythmic myoclonus while taking chronic haloperidol and fluoxetine, followed by a resolution of the myoclonus after stopping the fluoxetine (yet continuing the haloperidol). Later, after stopping the haloperidol and rechallenge with fluoxetine or trazodone, the myoclonus reappeared. The authors postulated that the myoclonus was related to activation of the serotonin 5-HT$_{1A}$ receptors (possibly supersensitive in Pick disease) or to a dopamine-deficient state.

Ghika-Schmid et al. (134) reported the first patient with myoclonus induced by fluoxetine in a patient without underlying brain disease. The myoclonus developed spontaneous, action (i.e., gait), reflex, and induced (by proprioceptive, luminous, and auditory stimulation) nonrhythmic involuntary transient myoclonic jerks of head, arms, and legs. On EEG no correlation was found between the movement and electrical cortical activity. The myoclonus resolved within 2 days of stopping the fluoxetine. The authors postulated that the involvement of the face as well as the limbs and the absence of EEG correlation suggested a reticular reflex myoclonus. Since the introduction of fluoxetine in the market, 184 cases of myoclonus have been reported (133). Among the SSRIs, fluoxetine has the most prolonged action and has plasma levels of an active metabolite for up to 5 weeks.

One of the liver cytochrome P-450 enzymes (CYP2D6) is mainly responsible for the elimination of some of the SSRIs and the tricyclic antidepressant drugs (135). Since fluoxetine is a potent inhibitor of this enzyme (136), it may potentially increase the toxicity of tricyclic drugs if prescribed concomitantly. Concomitant treatment with other drugs that inhibit CYP2D6, such as neuroleptics and dextropropoxyphene, may inhibit the metabolism of the antidepressant and increase the risk of myoclonus and seizures (137).

Cyclic antidepressants, classified as tricyclic and tetracyclic (such as clomipramine, imipramine, desipramine, amitriptyline, doxepin, trazodone, nortriptyline, and maprotiline), block the reuptake of serotonin and norepinephrine and also block the 5-HT$_2$ sero-tonergic, α_1-adrenergic, muscarinic, and H$_1$ and H$_2$-histaminic receptors. These drugs induce dyskinesias either secondary to an acute intoxication or after a chronic administration (138,139). Both the anticholinergic and serotonin reuptake-inhibiting properties of the cyclic antidepressants may be related to the development of the abnormal movements (138,140).

The most common movement disorders associated with acute exposure to cyclic antidepressants are myoclonus, choreoathetosis, and tremor (140,141). Other features of intoxication include delirium, stupor or coma, generalized seizures, respiratory depression, pupillary dilatation, dry mucous membranes, tachycardia, hypotension, and urinary retention.

Myoclonus is a common side effect of therapeutic doses of cyclic antidepressants, occurring in about 40% of patients (140,142). The myoclonus occurred within 1 month of therapy in 81% and within 2 weeks in 46% of patients. The myoclonus usually involves the face or limbs and occurs both during wakefulness and sleep. In most, the myoclonus is mild and infrequent; however, up to 10% of patients experience prominent myoclonic jerks that force a change in the therapy. The myoclonus is typically dose related and usually disappears with drug withdrawal. In patients who are unable to tolerate the withdrawal and in whom no antidepressant is better tolerated, clonazepam may be tried for the myoclonus. The tricyclic-induced myoclonus is associated with an increase in the cortical SEP amplitudes, suggesting cortical excitation or disinhibition, possibly due to the potentiation of serotonin (142).

Myers et al. (143) described a 49-year-old woman with depression who developed severe "nocturnal cataclysms of myoclonus" attributed to clomipramine. A sleep EEG showed myoclonus, but no seizures. The myoclonus improved with clonazepam.

MDMA is a popular mood-altering recreational drug known as ecstasy or Adam. Available in powders or pills, it is usually taken orally, and infrequently intranasally or parenterally. MDMA produces perceptual changes including vivid color enhancement, illusions, hallucinations (visual, tactile, auditory, olfactory, or gustatory), anxiety, tremor, myoclonus, muscle tightness, jaw clenching, diaphoresis, profuse salivation, blurred vision, mydriasis, nystagmus, ataxia, tachycardia, hypertension, and nausea. Effects usually disappear within 24 hours, but users have reported jaw tightness, blurred vision, fatigue, nausea, anxiety, depression, or insomnia lasting days or even weeks. Flashbacks have occurred (144). Ingestion of extremely high doses of MDMA may produce a life-threatening hyperpyrexia, tachycardia, muscle rigidity, tachyarrhythmia, rhabdomyolysis, disseminated intravascular coagulation, seizures, panic, and delirium. This syndrome resembles heatstroke. The most important management is rapid cooling plus a forced diuresis to enhance myoglobin clearance and prevent acute renal failure. Persistent deficits in visual and verbal memory may occur (145).

Acute effects of MDMA are due to increases in extracellular serotonin and dopamine. It releases serotonin, blocks its reuptake, and inhibits tryptophan hydroxylase in serotonergic nerve terminals in the CNS. Thus, acute MDMA toxicity enhances the serotonin and may produce a serotonin syndrome, including myoclonus. Repeated high doses cause depletion of serotonin-uptake sites and destruction of serotonergic nerve terminals, especially in the rostral brain (i.e., frontal cortex, hippocampus, and striatum) (146). MDMA is biotransformed by multiple chemical pathways. It is converted to the catecholamine, dihydroxymethamphetamine (DHMA), by CYP2D6. This enzyme's polymorphic distribution in humans may produce genetically determined differences in neurotoxicity (147,148).

Monoamine Oxidase Inhibitors

Myoclonus is the most common neurotoxic effect of MAOIs at therapeutic doses, which is usually up to 90 mg per day of phenelzine and 60 mg per day of tranylcypromine. The patients often describe the myoclonus as "twitchiness" (149). Phenelzine at 45 mg per day after 44 days of therapy was implicated in producing myoclonus (mainly of the legs) and episodic delirium and psychosis in a 55-year-old woman with agoraphobia and anxiety. Withdrawal of the phenelzine and initiation of lorazepam produced resolution of the symptoms after 7 days (150). MAOI-induced myoclonus occurs mostly during rest, sleep onset and sleep, and less often during wakefulness (149).

The MAOI drugs may produce a hypertensive crisis in association with foods containing tyramine. The MAOI hypertensive crisis is a hyperadrenergic reaction that can occur when patients taking MAOIs consume foods containing tyramine (such as aged cheeses, aged meats, concentrated yeast extracts, sauerkraut, broad bean pods, tap beer, and excessive alcohol) (151). Symptoms include hypertension, headache, diaphoresis, mydriasis, excitation, and cardiac arrhythmia. The syndrome occurs when tyramine, no longer capable of being deaminated by hepatic MAO after its intestinal absorption, triggers the widespread release of norepinephrine from presynaptic stores. The MAOI drugs may also induce the serotonin syndrome (see earlier discussion). Both the hypertensive reaction and the serotonin syndrome may occur for up to 3 weeks after MAOI discontinuation, because MAO enzyme levels recover slowly from their inhibition or depletion.

Buspirone

A myoclonic syndrome with dystonia and akathisia was observed after only two 5-mg doses of buspirone, a serotonin agonist with 5-HT$_{1A}$ receptor activity (152). Symptoms subsided after the withdrawal of buspirone and administration of clonazepam. The case suggests that buspirone may induce myoclonus, but the patient had multiple medical problems that could have contributed to or caused the myoclonus.

Eosinophilia-Myalgia Syndrome

In the 1980s, a syndrome called *eosinophilia-myalgia syndrome* (EMS), character-

ized by eosinophilia and incapacitating myalgias, was recognized in some patients after the intake of L-tryptophan-containing products (generally for insomnia, premenstrual syndrome, and depression). It remains unclear whether EMS reflects contaminants, such as (phenylamino) alanine and 1,1'-(ethylenebis)-tryptophan, in certain batches of L-tryptophan or whether the illness can be triggered by L-tryptophan itself.

Kaufman et al. (153) described tremors, myoclonus, and myokymia as late sequelae in some patients with EMS. Peripheral neuropathy, myopathy, and neurocognitive symptoms (especially memory disturbances) may occur.

Analgesics

Myoclonus has been described after the administration of various types of analgesics, including nonsteroidal antiinflammatory agents and opiates.

Diclofenac

Myoclonus of the legs occurred in a 34-year-old woman who was receiving the nonsteroidal antiinflammatory agent diclofenac, 150 mg per day for 4.5 months for spondyloarthritis. The myoclonus resolved 2 days after the drug was stopped (4). Another patient with renal insufficiency developed encephalopathy and myoclonus from diclofenac (154).

Opioids

Numerous cases of myoclonus and rare cases of hiccups have been reported after opioid administration (155). A wide variety of opiates (hydrocodone, meperidine, norpethidine, fentanyl, morphine, diamorphine, hydromorphone, sufentanil) and routes of administration (oral, intramuscular, intravenous, intrathecal) have been implicated, but high doses, the presence of other agents (antipsychotics, antiemetics, nonsteroidal antiinflammatory agents, and antidepressants), and comorbid medical conditions may pose special risks. Opiate-induced myoclonus is often generalized. Opiate-induced myoclonus usually responds to either naloxone or benzodiazepines.

Myoclonus is a rare side effect in patients receiving the opiate agonist *morphine* by oral, intravenous, epidural, and intrathecal routes (156–158). The myoclonus is often dose related and may be managed with a benzodiazepine, such as midazolam or diazepam, or by stopping the morphine (156–158).

Meperidine, a synthetic opiate structurally unlike morphine, produces morphinelike effects. Symptoms of meperidine intoxication are similar to those of morphine and heroin, but constipation and urine retention are less pronounced. The meperidine metabolite normeperidine causes CNS excitation with tremor, muscle twitches, agitation, delirium, hallucinations, myoclonus, and seizures (159,160). Normeperidine's usual half-life of 15 to 20 hours is greatly prolonged in patients with renal failure, sickle cell disease, and cancer. When meperidine is combined with a MAOI, excitatory symptoms are exacerbated and fatal respiratory depression has been reported (161).

Lauterbach (155) described a patient with hiccups, intermittently accompanied by apparent focal rhythmic diaphragmatic myoclonus, after *hydrocodone* administration. A 55-year-old man developed myoclonus after receiving the synthetic opioid *fentanyl* (162). Additionally, Lane et al. (163) reported choreoathetoid movements, ataxia, and myoclonus in five children after fentanyl infusions for sedation during mechanical ventilation. The more usual manifestations of opioid withdrawal, such as tremor, irritability, and insomnia, were also noted, but autonomic manifestations of opioid withdrawal were absent. No treatment was instituted, and all patients made a complete recovery without neurologic sequelae.

In adults, the signs and symptoms of *opiate withdrawal* are disagreeable but rarely dangerous. Opiate withdrawal does not typically produce seizures, hallucinations, or delirium. The withdrawal causes irritability, anxiety, weakness, lacrimation, excess sweating, and yawning, then achiness, mydriasis, tachycardia, piloerection, anorexia, nausea, diarrhea,

abdominal cramps, fever, sweating alternating with chills, cough with clear sputum, and muscle spasms of the back and limbs (144). In contrast to adults, newborns of opiate-dependent mothers develop potentially fatal withdrawal signs, including myoclonus and seizures (which can be difficult to distinguish from nonepileptic jitteriness) (144). Opiate withdrawal myoclonus may be stimulus sensitive, associated with D_2-antagonist coadministration, and responsive to benzodiazepines and unresponsive to naloxone (155).

Antibiotics

Antibiotics such as penicillin, carbenicillin, ticarcillin, and the cephalosporins may rarely produce a nonrhythmic, asymmetric, stimulus-sensitive myoclonus with seizures and hallucinations. The myoclonus resolves when the drug is withdrawn. Patients receiving high-dose continuous infusions, those with renal dysfunction, or those with impaired blood–brain barriers are most vulnerable (164–169). Recently, Fishbain et al. (170) reported a 74-year-old woman with renal failure, coronary artery disease, peripheral vascular disease, and bacteremia treated with cefepime, a cephalosporin, who developed unresponsiveness and multifocal face and arm more so than leg arrhythmic and asynchronous twitching.

Penicillin impedes the GABA inhibitory neurotransmission by blocking the chloride channel associated with the $GABA_A$ receptor and increasing membrane excitability. Cephalosporins may have similar mechanism.

Myoclonus is a rare side effect of imipenem, a carbapenem antibiotic. In a series of 2,516 patients treated with imipenem, seizures were reported in 26 (1.5%), and only 1 patient developed myoclonus, accompanied by confusion (171). Frucht and Eidelberg (172) reported imipenem as the possible agent causing myoclonus in a patient with advanced ovarian adenocarcinoma. The myoclonus primarily affected the arms and was present at rest, increased with action, and improved after stopping the drug.

Quinolone antibiotics, such as ciprofloxacin, may produce numerous neurologic side effects including agitation, confusion, insomnia, delirium, psychosis, myoclonus, and seizures. Patients who have renal failure and concomitant use of theophylline increase the risk of drug toxicity (173,174).

Antihelminthic Agents

Piperazine compounds, used as antihelminthic agents, may produce generalized, asymmetric, nonrhythmic, myoclonus with somnolence, incoordination, ataxia, headache, confusion, and sometimes seizures, coma, and death. Symptoms are more common in brain-damaged persons or in those with renal failure. (175,176).

Acyclovir

Acyclovir, a synthetic purine nucleoside analog, is used in the treatment of herpes simplex and varicella-zoster virus infections. Acyclovir blocks replication by inhibiting viral DNA synthesis. Acyclovir is eliminated by the kidneys. A rare reversible encephalopathy occurs in less than 1% of patients treated with conventional doses. Disorientation and confusion develop initially, followed by a florid delirium with hallucinations, dysarthria, restlessness, and tremor, and in severe cases, myoclonus and seizures. Patients with renal insufficiency and bone marrow transplantation recipients are predisposed to this encephalopathy. Symptoms usually improve with stopping the drug (177).

Cimetidine

Cimetidine, a histamine H_2-receptor antagonist, is used to treat gastric and duodenal ulcers. Cimetidine can cause a dose-related acute encephalopathy, especially in patients with hepatic or renal dysfunction or in the elderly. The encephalopathy includes confusion and mild disorientation, occasionally progressive cognitive impairment, and rarely toxic psychosis with hallucinations, myoclonus,

and abnormal electroencephalograms (178). The encephalopathy gradually abates after drug withdrawal.

β-Agonists and β-Blockers

The selective β_2 agonist *salbutamol* has been implicated in myoclonus. Micheli et al. (179) described three patients whose onset and remission of myoclonus were closely correlated with high-dose salbutamol intake and withdrawal, although concomitant factors (hypoxia, subdural hematoma, and malignancy, seen in one patient each) may have been contributory. Surprisingly, myoclonus was also attributed to carvedilol, a nonselective β-adrenergic antagonist with α_1 blocking activity, used for the treatment of congestive heart failure (CHF) and hypertension. Fernandez and Friedman (180) described an 81-year-old man with ischemic cardiomyopathy, recurrent CHF, paroxysmal atrial fibrillation, and recent cardiac pacer placement who developed intermittent, arrhythmic, and multifocal myoclonic jerks of the face, trunk, and limbs after an increased dose of carvedilol. The myoclonus was present at rest and persisted unchanged by posture or action. It resolved after drug cessation.

Cocaine

Opsoclonus and myoclonus have rarely been reported following cocaine use (181). Other movement disorders, such as acute dystonia, chorea, tics, and exacerbations of underlying tic disorders (such as Tourette syndrome) are more commonly associated with cocaine use (144).

Methaqualone

Methaqualone, a sedative-hypnotic, causes sedation by an unknown mechanism. Toxic doses of methaqualone may produce generalized or asymmetric, stimulus-sensitive myoclonus with increased resting tone and hyperreflexia, generally accompanied by stupor or coma, and sometimes by generalized seizures

(182). The toxicity of methaqualone may be increased by diphenhydramine (183). Treatment of methaqualone overdose is supportive and includes hemoperfusion through activated charcoal or cation exchange resins. Methaqualone use can lead to physical dependence, and withdrawal symptoms follow abstinence. Methaqualone became a popular recreational drug in the 1970s and was withdrawn from the United States market in the 1980s. A similar syndrome was reported with chronic use of the sedative-hypnotic bromisovalum (184).

Cannabinoid Compounds

The hemp plant, *Cannabis sativa*, contains numerous cannabinoid compounds (cannabinols) with different pharmacologic properties. Marijuana is made from the cut tops and leaves of the whole plants. Cannabinoids indirectly affect a number of CNS transmitter systems, including the dopaminergic "reward circuit" from the midbrain ventral tegmental area to the nucleus accumbens and the medial prefrontal cortex. Marijuana may produce asymmetric, multifocal, action-induced, or stimulus-sensitive myoclonus in some patients without previous brain injury (185).

Withdrawal from benzodiazepines may produce myoclonus, but this is rarely a prominent part of the syndrome. Myoclonic jerks are generally nocturnal, are often limited to the facial muscles, and resolve within days to weeks (186,187).

Contrast Agents

Various water-soluble radiographic contrast agents, such as iothalamate meglumine (3), iocarmate meglumine (188), Angiografin (189), myelografin (190), and metrizamide (2,191), have caused segmental myoclonus, generally limited to the legs, often rhythmic and stimulus sensitive, without accompanying EEG changes. Movements are diminished after diazepam and resolve spontaneously within hours or days.

Myelography is generally performed safely using nonionic water-soluble radiographic contrast media. However, inadvertent introduction of ionic contrast media into the thecal space can produce myoclonic spasms, convulsions, rhabdomyolysis, or death. Killefer and Kaufman (192) reported an inadvertent use of *diatrizoate meglumine*, an ionic contrast agent, instead of the nonionic contrast agent during intraoperative myelography. The patient developed ascending myoclonic spasms, resulting in rhabdomyolysis. Treatment included elevation of the head, removal of cerebrospinal fluid, administration of anticonvulsants, diuresis, sedation, and neuromuscular blockade. The patient recovered without sequelae.

CONCLUSION

Numerous toxins and drugs affecting various neurotransmitters, such as opiate, serotonin, dopamine, and GABA, can induce myoclonus in people. Similarly, heterogeneity is noted in animal models of myoclonus. There are multiple mechanisms for the production of myoclonus, but a unifying one has not yet been identified. Various anatomic sites and transmitters in the CNS may underlie the myoclonus. The drugs and toxins induce various distributions (focal, segmental, multifocal, or generalized) and patterns (rest, spontaneous, action, stimulus induced, and rhythmicity) of myoclonus. Many substances that induce myoclonus also induce seizures; however, the correlation is imperfect, and myoclonus is often reported in the absence of definable epileptiform activity on the EEG, suggesting that in some cases, the pathogenesis of the myoclonus and seizures may be different.

Further study of myoclonus induced by drugs and toxins may reveal clues to the etiology and pathophysiology of various forms of myoclonus and may potentially lead to improved prevention and therapy.

REFERENCES

1. Bleecker ML. Clinical presentation of selected neurotoxic compounds. In: Bleecker ML, Hansen JA, eds. *Occupational neurology and clinical neurotoxicology.* Baltimore: Williams & Wilkins, 1994:209–233.

2. Junck L, Marshall WM. Neurotoxicity of radiologic contrast agents. *Ann Neurol* 1983;13:469.
3. Praestholm J, Lester J. Water-soluble contrast lumbar myelography with meglumine iothalamate (conray). *Br J Radiol* 1970;43:303.
4. Alcalay M, Thomas P, Reboux JF, et al. Myoclonus during a treatment with diclofenac. *Semin Hop Paris* 1979;55:679–680.
5. Pappert EJ, Goetz CG. Treatment of myoclonus. In: Kurlan R, ed. *Treatment of movement disorders.* Philadelphia: JB Lippincott Co, 1995:289–290.
6. Shahani BT, Young RR. Asterixis: a disorder of the neural mechanisms underlying sustained muscle contraction. In: Shahani M, ed. *The motor system: neurophysiology and muscle mechanisms.* Amsterdam: Elsevier, 1976:301.
7. Adams RD, Foley JM. The neurological changes in the more common types of severe liver disease. *Trans Am Neurol Assoc* 1949;74:217.
8. Young RR, Shahani BT. Asterixis: one type of negative myoclonus. *Adv Neurol* 1986;43:137–156.
9. Young RR, Shahani BT. Anticonvulsant asterixis. *Electroencephalogr Clin Neurophysiol* 1973;34:760a.
10. Yagnik P, Dhopesh V. Unilateral asterixis. *Arch Neurol* 1981;38:601.
11. Degos J-D, Verroust J, Bouchareine A, et al. Asterixis in focal brain lesions. *Arch Neurol* 1979;36:705.
12. Obeso JA, Viteri C, Martinez Lage JM, et al. Toxic myoclonus. *Adv Neurol* 1986; 43:225–230.
13. Klawans HL, Carvey PM, Tanner CM, et al. Drug-induced myoclonus. *Adv Neurol* 1986;43:251–264.
14. Gordon MF, Abrams RI, Rubin DB, et al. Bismuth subsalicylate toxicity as a cause of prolonged encephalopathy with myoclonus. *Mov Disord* 1995;10:220–222.
15. Orti-Pareja M, Jimenez-Jimenez FJ, Miquel J, et al. Reversible myoclonus, tremor, and ataxia in a patient exposed to methyl ethyl ketone. *Neurology* 1996;46:272.
16. Alfrey AC. Dialysis encephalopathy. In: Yasui M, Strong MJ, Ota K, et al, eds. *Mineral and metal neurotoxicity.* Boca Raton: CRC Press, 1997:127.
17. Sedman AB, Wilkening GN, Warady BA, et al. Encephalopathy in childhood secondary to aluminum toxicity. *J Pediatr* 1984;105:836.
18. Burks JS, Alfrey AC, Huddlestone J, et al. A fatal encephalopathy in chronic hemodialysis patients. *Lancet* 1976;1:764.
19. Sideman S, Manor D. The dialysis dementia syndrome and aluminum intoxication. *Nephron* 1982;31:1.
20. Spencer PS. Aluminum and its compounds. In: Spencer PS, Schaumberg HH, Ludolph AC, eds. *Experimental and clinical neurotoxicology,* 2nd ed. New York: Oxford University Press, 2000:142–151.
21. Spofforth J. Case of aluminium poisoning. *Lancet* 1921;1:1301.
22. McLaughlin AIG, Kazantos G, King E, et al. Pulmonary fibrosis and encephalopathy associated with inhalation of aluminum dust. *Br J Indust Med* 1962; 19:253.
23. White DM, Longstreth WT, Rosenstock L, et al. Neurologic syndrome in 25 workers from an aluminum smelting plant. *Arch Intern Med* 1992;152:1443.
24. Snyder RD. The involuntary movements of chronic mercury poisoning. *Arch Neurol* 1972;26:379.
25. Neal PA, Jones RR. Chronic mercurialism in the hatter's fur-cutting industry. *JAMA* 1938;110:337–343.
26. Roullet E, Nizou R, Jedynak P, et al. Myoclonies d'intention et d'action revelatrices d'une intoxication professionnelle par le mercure. *Rev Neurol* 1984;140:55–58.
27. Shapiro IM, Cornbluth DR, Summer AJ. Neurophysiological and neuropsychological functions in mercury-exposed dentists. *Lancet* 1982;2:1147–1150.
28. Mena I. Manganese poisoning. In: Vinken PJ, Bruyn GW, eds. *Handbook of clinical neurology,* vol. 36. Amsterdam: Elsevier/North Holland, 1979:217.
29. Manzo L, Blum K, Sabboni E. Neurotoxicity of selected metals. In: Blum K, Manzo L, eds. *Neurotoxicology.* New York: Marcel Dekker, 1985:385–404.
30. Burns R, Thomas DW, Barron VJ. Reversible encephalopathy possibly associated with subgallate ingestion. *Br Med J* 1974;1:220–223.
31. Buge A, Rancurel G, Poisoon M, et al. Vingt observations d'encephalopathies aigues avec myoclonies au cours de traitements oraux par les sels de bismuth. *Ann Med Interne (Paris)* 1974;125:877.
32. Australian Drug Evaluation Committee. Adverse effects of bismuth subgallate: a further report from the Australian Evaluation Committee. *Med J Aust* 1974;2:664.
33. Le Quesne PM. Toxic substances and the nervous system: the role of clinical observation. *J Neurol Neurosurg Psychiatry* 1981;44:1–8.
34. Martin-Bouyer G. Intoxication par le sals de bismuth administer par vioe orale. *Gastroenterol Clin Biol* 1975;2:349–356.
35. Goulon M, Nouailhat F, Escourelle R, et al. Intoxication par le bromure de methyle. *Rev Neurol* 1975;131:445.
36. Rondot P, Said G, Ferrey G. Les hyperkinesias volitionnelles. Etudes electrologiques: classification. *Rev Neurol* 1972;126:415.
37. Moses H, Klawans HL. Bromide intoxication. In: Vinken PJ, Bruyn GW, eds. *Intoxications of the nervous system, part I, vol 36. Handbook of Clinical Neurology.* Amsterdam 1979:291–318.
38. Prockop LD, Smith AO. Seizures and action myoclonus after occupational exposure to methyl bromide. *J Fla Med Assoc* 1986;73:690–692.
39. Hauw JJ, Escourolle R, Baulac M, et al. Postmortem studies on posthypoxic and post-methyl bromide intoxication: case reports. *Adv Neurol* 1986;4:201.
40. Squier MV, Thompson J, Rajgopalan B. Case report: neuropathology of methyl bromide intoxication. *Neuropathol Appl Neurobiol* 1992;18:579.
41. Scharnweber HC, Spears GN, Cowles SR. Chronic methyl chloride intoxication in six industrial workers. *J Occup Med* 1974;16:112–113.
42. Hartman TL, Wacker W, Roll RM. Methyl chloride intoxication. *N Engl J Med* 1955;253:552.
43. McNally WD. Eight cases of methyl chloride intoxication with three deaths. *J Ind Hyg Toxicol* 1946;28:94.
44. Ropelman PG, Kalfayan PY. Severe metabolic acidosis after ingestion of butanone. *Br Med J* 1983;286:21.
45. Altenkirch H, Mager J, Stoltenburg G, et al. Toxic polyneuropathies after sniffing a glue thinner. *J Neurol* 1977;214:137.
46. Spencer PS, Schaumburg HH. Chlorinated cyclodienes. In: Spencer PS, Schaumburg HH, Ludolph AC, eds. *Experimental and clinical neurotoxicology, 2nd ed.* New York: Oxford University Press, 2000:364–370.
47. Cannon SB, Veazey JM Jr, Jackson RS, et al. Epidemic

Kepone poisoning in chemical workers. *Am J Epidemiol* 1978;17:529.

48. Cohn WJ, Boylan JJ, Blanke RV, et al. Treatment of chlordecone (Kepone) toxicity with cholestyramine. *N Engl J Med* 1978;298:243.

49. Garrettson LK, Guzelian PS, Blanke RV. Subacute chlordane poisoning. *J Toxicol Clin Toxicol* 1985;22:565.

50. Olanoff LS, Bristow WJ, Colcolough J, et al. Acute chlordane intoxication. *J Toxicol Clin Toxicol* 1983;20:291.

51. Gupta PK. Neurotoxicity of chronic chlorinated hydrocarbon insecticide poisoning: a clinical and electroencephalographic study in man. *Indian J Med Res* 1975;63:601.

52. Joy RM. Chlorinated hydrocarbon insecticides. In: Ecobichon DF, Joy RM, eds. *Pesticides and neurological diseases.* Boca Raton: CRC Press, Florida, 1982:91.

53. Smith AG. Chlorinated hydrocarbon insecticides. In: Hayes WJ Jr, Laws ER Jr, eds. *Handbook of pesticide pathology, Vol. 2: classes of pesticides.* San Diego: Academic Press, 1991:731.

54. Mayersdorf A, Israeli R. Toxic effects of chlorinated hydrocarbon insecticides on the human encephalogram. *Arch Environ Health* 1974;28:159.

55. Lotti M. Organophosphorus compounds. In: Spencer PS, Schaumberg HH, Ludolph AC, eds. *Experimental and clinical neurotoxicology,* 2nd ed. New York. Oxford University Press, 2000:897–925.

56. Leiva C, Fernandez Gonzalez F, De Blas G, et al. Abnormal movements in the Spanish toxic oil syndrome. *J Neurol* 1985;232:242.

57. Hill RH Jr, Schurtz HH, Posada de la Paz M, et al. Possible etiologic agents for toxic oil syndrome: fatty acid esters of 3-(N-phenylamino)-1,2-propanediol. *Arch Environ Contam Toxicol* 1995;28:259.

58. Posada de la Paz M, Philen RM, Schurz H, et al. Epidemiological evidence for a new class of compounds associated with the toxic oil syndrome. *Epidemiology* 1999;10:130.

59. Hansen KS, Sharp FR. Gasoline sniffing, lead poisoning, and myoclonus. *JAMA* 1978;240:1375–1376.

60. Dorndorf W, Kresse K, Christain W, et al. Dichloroethane poisoning with myoclonic syndrome, seizures, and irreversible cerebral defects. *Arch Psychiatr Nervenkr* 1975;220:373–379.

61. Peatfield RC, Boothman BR. Transient myoclonus after exposure to oven cleaner. *Mov Disord* 1991;6(1):90-1.

62. Hormes JT, Filley CM, Rosenberg NL. Neurologic sequelae of chronic solvent vapor abuse. *Neurology* 1986;36: 698–700.

63. Lazar RB, Ho SU, Melen O, et al. Multifocal central nervous system damage caused by toluene abuse. *Neurology* 1983;33:1337–1340.

64. Sugiyama-Oishi A, Arakawa K, Araki E, et al. A case of chronic toluene intoxication presenting stimulus-sensitive segmental spinal myoclonus [Japanese]. *No To Shinkei* 2000;52:399–403.

65. Choi IS, Cheon HY. Delayed movement disorders after carbon monoxide poisoning. *Eur Neurol* 1999;42:141–144.

66. Smith BA. Strychnine poisoning. *J Emerg Med* 1990;8:321.

67. Farrar, JJ, Yen LM, Cook T, et al. Tetanus. *J Neurol Neurosurg Psychiatry* 2000;69:292–301.

68. Swanson PD, Luttrell CN, Magladery JW. Myoclonus: a report of 67 cases and a review of the literature. *Medicine (Baltimore)* 1962;41:339.

69. Raskin NH, Fishman RA. Neurologic disorders in renal failure. *N Engl J Med* 1976;294:143.

70. Chadwick D, French AT. Uraemic myoclonus: an example or reticular reflex myoclonus? *J Neurol Neurosurg Psychiatry* 1979;42:52.

71. Nicoli F, Bartolomei F, Swiader L, et al. Diffuse, segmental, asynchronous myoclonus, manifestations of severe hypoglycemia [letter]. *Presse Med* 1991;20:1783.

72. Razavi B. Baking soda toxicity. *Am J Med* 2000;108: 756–757.

73. Prof Info Amidate, 1995.

74. Reddy RV, Moorthy SS, Dierdorf SF, et al. Excitatory effects and electroencephalographic correlation of etomidate, thiopental, methoxital, and propofol. *Anesth Analg* 1993;77:1008–1011.

75. Dubois DJ, Bastenier GJ, Genicot C, et al. A comparative study of etomidate and methohexital as induction agents for analgesia anesthesia. *Acta Anaesthesiol Belg Suppl* 1976;27:187.

76. Gooding JM, Corssen G. Etomidate: an ultrashort-acting non-barbiturate agent for anesthesia induction. *Anesth Analg* 1976;55:286.

77. Famenco CE, Odugbesan CO. Further experience with etomidate. *Can Anaesth Soc J* 1978;25:130–132.

78. Islander G, Vinge E. Severe neuroexcitatory symptoms after anaesthesia - with focus on propofol anaesthesia [report]. *Acta Anaesthesiol Scand* 2000;44:144–149.

79. Ng AT. Prolonged myoclonic contractions after enflurane anesthesia. *Can Anaesth Soc J* 1980;27:502–503.

80. Hudson R, Ethans CT. Alfathesin and enflurane: synergistic central nervous system excitation? *Can Anaesth Soc J* 1981;28:55–56.

81. Fox EJ, Villanueva R, Scutta HS. Myoclonus following spinal anesthesia. *Neurology* 1979;29:379–380.

82. Kam PC, Yoong FF. Gamma-hydroxybutyric acid: an emerging recreational drug. *Anaesthesia* 1998;53:1195.

83. Anon. Adverse events associated with ingestion of gamma-butyrolactone. Minnesota, New Mexico, and Texas, 1998–1999. *MMWR Morb Mortal Wkly Rep* 1999;48:137.

84. Moene Y, Cuche M, Trillet M, et al. Problemes diagnostiques poses par l'intoxication aigue a chloralose (a propos de 6 cas). *J Med Lyon* 1969;12:1483–1493.

85. Quinio P, Bouche O, Rossignol B, et al. Propofol in the management of myoclonus syndrome induced by chloralose poisoning [correspondence]. *Anesthesiology* 1995;83:875.

86. Anderson NR, Tandon DS. Ifosfamide extrapyramidal neurotoxicity. *Cancer* 1981;68:72.

87. Pratt CB, Green AA, Horowitz ME. Central nervous system toxicity following the treatment of pediatric patients with isosfamide/mesna. *J Clin Oncol* 1986;4:1253.

88. Ammenti A, Reitter B, Muller-Wiefel DE. Chlorambucil neurotoxicity: report of two cases. *Helv Paediatr Acta* 1980;35:281–287.

89. Byrne TN, Moseley TA, Finer MA. Myoclonic seizures following chlorambucil overdose. *Ann Neurol* 1981;9:191.

90. Martin M, Diaz-Rubio E, Casado A, et al. Prednimustine-induced myoclonus: a report of three cases. *Acta Oncol* 1994;33:81–82.

91. Glantz R, Weiner WJ, Goetz CG, et al. Drug-induced asterixis in Parkinson's disease. *Neurology* 1982;32: 553–555.

92. Klawans HL, Goetz C, Bergen D. Levodopa induced myoclonus. *Arch Neurol* 1975;32:331–334.

93. Vardi J, Glaubman H, Rabey JM, et al. Myoclonic attacks induced by L-dopa and bromocriptin in Parkinson patients: a sleep EEG study. *J Neurol* 1978;218:35–42.

94. Buchman AS, Bennett DA, Goetz CG. Bromocriptine-induced myoclonus. *Neurology* 1987;37:885.

95. Lang AE, Blain RDG. Anticholinergics and amantadine in the treatment of Parkinson's disease. In: Calne DB, ed. *Drugs for the treatment of Parkinson's disease.* Berlin: Springer Verlag, 1989:307.

96. Pfeiffer RF. Amantadine-induced "vocal" myoclonus. *Mov Disord* 1996;11:104–105.

97. Matsunaga K, Uozumi T, Qingrui L, et al. Amantadine-induced cortical myoclonus. *Neurology* 2001;56: 279–280.

98. Aoki FY, Sitar DS. Clinical pharmacokinetics of amantadine hydrochloride. *Clin Pharmacokinet* 1988; 14:35–51.

99. Hicks CB, Abraham K. Verapamil and myoclonic dystonia. *Ann Intern Med* 1985;103:154.

100. Jeret JS, Somasundaram M, Asaikar S. Diltiazem-induced myoclonus. *N Y State J Med* 1992;92:447–448.

101. Pedro-Botet ML, Bonal J, Caralps A. Nifedipine and myoclonic disorders. *Nephron* 1989;51:281.

102. De Medina A, Biasini O, Rivera A, et al. Nifedipine and myoclonic dystonia. *Ann Intern Med* 1986;104:125.

103. Tominaga H, Fukuzako H, Izumi K, et al. Tardive myoclonus. *Lancet* 1987; 1:322.

104. Fukuzako H, Tominaga H, Izumi K, et al. Postural myoclonus associated with long-term administration of neuroleptic in schizophrenic patients. *Biol Psychiatry* 1990;27:1116–1126.

105. Little JT, Jankovic J. Tardive myoclonus. *Mov Disord* 2:307–311, 1987.

106. Bak TH, Bauer M, Schaub RT, et al. Myoclonus in patients treated with clozapine: a case series. *J Clin Psychiatry* 1995;56:418–422.

107. Knoll JL. Clozapine-related speech disturbance [letter, comment]. *J Clin Psychiatry* 1997;58:219–220.

108. Sajatovic M, Meltzer HY. Clozapine-induced myoclonus and generalized seizures. *Biol Psychiatry* 1996;39:367–370.

109. Cruz FG, Thiagarajan D, Harney JH. Neuroleptic malignant syndrome after haloperidol therapy. *South Med J* 1983;76:684–686.

110. Lemus CZ, Lieberman JA, Johns CA. Myoclonus during treatment with clozapine and lithium: the role of serotonin. *Hillside J Clin Psychiatry* 1989;11:127–130.

111. Devanand DP, Sackeim HA, Brown RP. Myoclonus during combined tricyclic antidepressant and lithium treatment. *J Clin Psychopharmacol* 1986;8:446–447.

112. Favarel-Garrigues B, Favarel-Garrigues JC, Bourgeois M. Two cases of severe poisoning by lithium carbonate [French]. *Annal Med Psychol* 1972;1:253–257.

113. Hansen HE, Amdisen A. Lithium intoxication. *Q J Med* 1978;47:123.

114. Schipior PG. An unusual case of antihistamine intoxication. *J Pediatr* 1967;71:589–591.

115. Jacquesson M, Saudeau D, Pantin B, et al. Myoclonia induced by a combination of triprolidine, pseudoephedrine and paracetamol. *Nouv Presse Med* 1982; 11:2298–2299.

116. Chadwick J, Reynolds EH, Marsden CD. Anticonvulsant-induced dyskinesias: a comparison with dyskinesias induced by neuroleptics. *J Neurol Neurosurg Psychiatry* 1976;39:1210–1218.

117. Harrison MB, Lyons GR, Landow ER. Phenytoin and dyskinesias: a report of two cases and a review of the literature. *Mov Disord* 1993;8:19–27.

118. Wendland KL. Myoclonus following doses of carbamezepine. *Nervenarzt* 1968;39:231–233.

119. Hyuman N, Dennis PD, Sinclar KG. Tremor due to sodium valproate. *Neurology* 1979;29:1177.

120. Bodensteiner JB, Morris HH, Golden GS. Asterixis associated with sodium valproate. *Neurology* 1981;31: 186.

121. Aguglia U, Gambardella A, Zappia M, et al. Negative myoclonus during valproate-related stupor: neurophysiological evidence of a cortical non-epileptic origin. *Electroencephalogr Clin Neurophysiol* 1995;94: 103–108.

122. Asconape J, Diedrich A, DellaBadia J. Myoclonus associated with the use of gabapentin. *Epilepsia* 2000;41 (4):479-81.

123. Jacob PC, Poovathoor C, Chand RP, et al. Asterixis induced by gabapentin [report]. *Clin Neuropharmacol* 2000;23:53.

124. Janszky J, Rasonyi G, Halasz P, et al. Disabling erratic myoclonus during lamotrigine therapy with high serum level: report of two cases. *Clin Neuropharmacol* 2000;23:86–89.

125. Klawans HL, Goetz C, Weiner WJ. 5-Hydroxytryptophan-induced myoclonus in guinea pigs and the possible role of serotonin in infantile myoclonus. *Neurology* 1973;23:1234–1240.

126. Chadwick D, Hallett M, Jenner P, et al. 5-hydroxytryptophan-induced myoclonus in guinea pigs. *J Neurol Sci* 1978;35:157–165.

127. Sternbach H. The serotonin syndrome. *Am J Psychiatry* 1991;148:705.

128. LoCurto MJ. The serotonin syndrome. *Emerg Med Clin North Am* 1997;15:665–675.

129. Nayudu SK, Scheftner WA. Case report of withdrawal syndrome after olanzapine discontinuation. *J Clin Psychopharmacol* 2000;20:489–490.

130. Mason PJ, Morris VA, Balcezak TJ. Serotonin syndrome: presentation of 2 cases and review of the literature. *Medicine* 2000;79:201–209.

131. Graudins A, Stearman A, Chan B. Treatment of the serotonin syndrome with cyproheptadine. *J Emerg Med* 1998;16:615–-619.

132. Lauterbach EC. Reversible intermittent rhythmic myoclonus with fluoxetine in presumed Pick's disease. *Mov Disord* 1994;9:343–346.

133. Bharucha KJ, Sethi KD. Complex movement disorders induced by fluoxetine. *Mov Disord* 1996;11:324–236.

134. Ghika-Schmid F, Ghika J, Vuadens P, et al. Acute reversible myoclonic encephalopathy associated with fluoxetine therapy. *Mov Disord* 1997;12:622–623.

135. Brosen K, Gram LF. Clinical significance of the sparteine/debrisoquine oxidation polymorphism. *Eur J Clin Pharmacol* 1989;36:537–547.

136. Bergstrom RF. Peyton AL, Lembeger L. Quantification and mechanism of the fluoxetine and tricyclic an-

tidepressant interaction. *Clin Pharmacol Ther* 1992; 51:239–248.

137. Spigset O, Hedenmalm K, Dahl ML, et al. Seizures and myoclonus associated with antidepressant treatment: assessment of potential risk factors, including CYP2D6 and CYP2C19 polymorphisms, and treatment with CYP2D6 inhibitors. *Acta Psychiatr Scand* 1997;96:379–384.

138. Fann WE, Sullivan JL, Richman BW. Dyskinesias associated with tricyclic antidepressants. *Br J Psychiatry* 1976;128:490–493.

139. Kettl P, DePaulo JR Jr. Maprotiline-induced myoclonus. *J Clin Psychopharmacol* 1983;3:264–265.

140. Garvey MJ, Tollefson GD. Occurrence of myoclonus in patients treated with cyclic antidepressants. *Arch Gen Psychiatry* 1987;44:269–272.

141. Noble J, Matthew H. Acute poisoning by tricyclic antidepressants: clinical features and management of 100 patients. *Clin Toxicol* 1969;2:403.

142. Forstl H, Pohlmann-Eden B. Amplitudes of the somatosensory evoked potentials reflect cortical hyperexcitability in antidepressant-induced myoclonus. *Neurology* 1990;40:924–926.

143. Myers BA, Klerman GL, Hartman E. Nocturnal cataclysms with myoclonus: a new side effect of clomipramine. *Am J Psychiatry* 1986;143:1490–1491.

144. Brust JCM. *Neurologic aspects of substance abuse.* Stoneham, Mass., Butterworth-Heinemann, 1993:16, 70.

145. Bolla KI, McCannUD, Ricaurte GA. Memory impairment in abstinent MDMA ("ecstasy") users. *Neurology* 1998;51:1532.

146. Slikker W Jr, Paule MG, Broening HW. Role of serotonergic systems in behavioral toxicity. In: Chang L, Slicker W Jr, eds. *Neurotoxicology: approaches and methods.* New York: Academic Press, 1995:371.

147. Daly AK, Cholerton S, Gregory W, Idle JR. Metabolic polymorphisms. *Pharmacol Ther* 1993;57:129–160.

148. Tucker GT, Lennard MS, Ellis SW, et al. The demethylation of methylenedioxy methamphetamine (ecstasy) by debrisoquine hydroxylase (CYP2D6). *Biochem Pharmacol* 1994;47:1151–1156.

149. Lieberman JA, Kane JM, Reife R. Neuromuscular effects of monoamine oxidase inhibitors. *Adv Neurol* 1986;43:231.

150. White PD. Myoclonus and episodic delirium associated with phenelzine: a case report. *J Clin Psychiatry* 1987;48:340–341.

151. Schulman KI, Walker SE, MacKenzie S, et al. Dietary restriction, tyramine, and the use of monoamine oxidase inhibitors. *J Clin Psychopharmacol* 1989;9:397.

152. Ritchie EC, Bridenbaugh RH, Jabbori B. Acute generalized myoclonus following buspirone administration. *J Clin Psychiatry* 1988;49:242–243.

153. Kaufman LD, Kaufman MA, Krupp LB. Movement disorders in eosinophilia-myalgia syndrome: tremor, myoclonus, and myokymia. *J Rheumatol* 1995;22: 157–160.

154. Bandelot JB, Mihout B. Myoclonic encephalopathy due to dicofenac. *Nouv Presse Med* 1978;7:1406.

155. Lauterbach EC. Hiccup and apparent myoclonus after hydrocodone: review of the opiate-related hiccup and myoclonus literature. *Clin Neuropharmacol* 1999;22: 87–92.

156. Littrell RA, Kennedy LD, Birmingham WE, et al. Muscle spasms associated with intrathecal morphine therapy: treatment with midazolam. *Clin Pharm* 1992; 11:57–59.

157. de Armendi AJ, Fahey M, Ryan JF. Morphine-induced myoclonic movements in a pediatric pain patient. *Anesth Analg* 1993;77:191–192.

158. De Conno F, Caraceni A, Martini C, et al. Hyperalgesia and myoclonus with intrathecal infusion of high-dose morphine. *Pain* 1991;47:337–339.

159. Hershey LA. Meperidine and central neurotoxicity. *Ann Intern Med* 1983;98:548.

160. Hochman MS. Meperidine-associated myoclonus and seizures in long-term hemodialysis patients. *Ann Neurol* 1983;14:593.

161. Meyer D, Halfin V. Toxicity secondary to meperidine in patients on monoamine oxidase inhibitors: a case report and a critical review. *J Clin Psychopharmacol* 1981;1:319.

162. Stuerenburg HJ, Claassen J, Eggers C, et al. Acute adverse reaction to fentanyl in a 55-year-old man [letter]. *J Neurol Neurosurg Psychiatry* 2000;69:281–282.

163. Lane JC, Tennison MB, Lawless ST, et al. Movement disorder after withdrawal of fentanyl infusion. *J Pediatr* 1991;119:649–651.

164. Bloomer HA, Berten LJ, Maddock RK. Penicillin-induced encephalopathy in uremic patients. *JAMA* 1967; 200:121.

165. Fossieck B, Parker RH. Neurotoxicity during intravenous infusion of penicillin: a review. *J Clin Pharmacol* 1974;14:504.

166. Lerner PI, Smith H, Weinstein L. Penicillin neurotoxicity. *Ann N Y Acad Sci* 1967;145:310.

167. Lothman EW. Intravenous penicillin and myoclonus. *Arch Neurol* 1983;13:221–222.

168. Kallay MC, Tabechian H, Riley GR, et al. Neurotoxicity due to ticarcillin in a patient with renal failure. *Lancet* 1979;1:608–609.

169. Kurtzman NA, Rogers PW, Harter HR. Neurotoxic reaction to penicillin and carbenicillin. *JAMA* 1970;214: 1320–1321.

170. Fishbain JT, Monahan TP, Canonico MM. Cerebral manifestations of cefipime toxicity in a dialysis patient. *Neurology* 2000;55:1756–1757.

171. Calandra GB, Brown KR, Grad LC, et al. Review of adverse experiences and tolerability in the first 2,516 patients treated with imipenem/cilastin. *Am J Med* 1985;78(6A):73–78.

172. Frucht S, Eidelberg D. Imipenem-induced myoclonus. *Mov Disord* 1997;12:621–622.

173. *Physicians' desk reference.* Montvale, NJ: Medical Economics, 2001.

174. Schwartz MT, Calvert JF. Potential neurologic toxicity related to ciprofloxacin. *DICP* 1990;24:138–140.

175. Kompf D, Neundorfer B. Neurotoxic side effects of piperazine in adults. *Arch Psychiatr Nervenkr* 1974; 218:223–233.

176. Schuch P, Stephan U, Jacobi G. Neurotoxic side-effects of piperazines. *Lancet* 1966;1:1218.

177. Schaumburg HH. Acyclovir. In: Spencer PS, Schaumburg HH, Ludolph AC, eds. *Experimental and clinical neurotoxicology,* 2nd ed. New York: Oxford University Press, 2000:135–136.

178. Van Sweden B. Toxic "ictal" confusion in middle age:

treatment with benzodiazepines. *J Neurol Neurosurg Psychiatry*1985;48:472.

179. Micheli F, Cersosimo MG, Scorticati MC, et al. Neurotoxic side effects of piperazine. *Lancet* 1967;1:895.

180. Fernandez HH, Friedman JH. Carvedilol-induced myoclonus [letter]. *Mov Disord* 1999;14:703.

181. Scharf D. Opsoclonus-myoclonus following the intranasal usage of cocaine [letter]. *J Neurol Neurosurg Psychiatry*1989;52:1447.

182. Abboud RT, Freedman MT, Rogers RM, et al. Methaqualone poisoning with muscular hyperactivity necessitating the use of curare. *Chest* 1974;65:204–205.

183. Coleman JR, Barone JA. Abuse potential of methaqualone-diphenhydramine combination. *Am J Hosp Pharm* 1981;38:160.

184. Harenko A. Neurologic findings in chronic bromisovalum poisoning. *Ann Med Interne (Paris)* 1967;56:181–188.

185. Feeney DM, Spiker M, Weiss GK. Marijuana and epilepsy: activation of symptoms by delta-9-THC. In: Cohen S, Stillman RO, eds. *The therapeutic potential of marihuana.* New York: Plenum, 1975:343–362.

186. Melcor CS, Jain VK. Diazepam withdrawal syndrome: its prolonged and changing nature. *Can Med Assoc J* 1982;127:1093–1096.

187. Moore C. Oxazepam withdrawal syndrome. *Med J Aust* 1982;2:220.

188. Bonneau R, Morris JM. Complications of water-soluble contrast lumbar myelography. *Spine* 1978;3:343–345.

189. Loser R, Vogelsang H. Can angiografin be used for lumbar myelography? *Fortsch Geb Rontgenstr Nuklearmed* 1973;116:654–657.

190. Urso S, Barbuti D. Lumbosacral radiculography with a new water-soluble contrast medium: myelografin. *Ital J Orthop Traumatol* 1979;5:321–330.

191. Killebrew K, Whaley RA, Hayward JN. Complications of metrizamide myelography. *Arch Neurol* 1983;40:78–80.

192. Killeffer JA, Kaufman HH. Inadvertent intraoperative myelography with Hypaque: case report and discussion. *Surg Neurol* 1998;49:574.

Myoclonus and Paroxysmal Dyskinesias,
Advances in Neurology, Vol. 89,
edited by S. Fahn, et al.
Lippincott Williams & Wilkins, Philadelphia © 2002.

8

Myoclonus in Parkinsonian Disorders

Mohamed Shafiq and Anthony E. Lang

Department of Medicine (Neurology), Toronto Western Hospital, Toronto, Ontario, Canada

Myoclonus has been observed in association with a variety of parkinsonian disorders including Parkinson's disease (PD), Lewy body dementia (LBD), multiple system atrophy (MSA), corticobasal degeneration (CBD), and postencephalitic parkinsonism (Table 8.1). A wide variety of disorders may, less commonly, combine parkinsonism and myoclonus such as dentato-rubro-pallido-luysian atrophy, Huntington disease, and drug-induced syndromes. The clinical presentation, origin, and pathophysiology of myoclonus can vary across these disorders. This chapter will concentrate on the more common neurologic diseases that usually cause parkinsonism sometimes associated with myoclonus. Many other disorders not included in this review do occasionally manifest this combination, but other features generally predominate (e.g., Alzheimer disease, Creutzfeldt-Jakob disease, frontotemporal dementia, and Huntington disease).

TABLE 8.1. *More common causes of myoclonus and parkinsonism*

Myoclonus associated with predominant parkinsonism
Corticobasal degeneration
Multiple system atrophy
Dentato-rubro-pallido-luysian atrophy
Huntington disease
Drug induced
Myoclonus associated with predominant dementia
Alzheimer disease
Lewy body dementia
Creutzfeldt-Jakob disease
Paraneoplastic

ENCEPHALITIS LETHARGICA

Encephalitis lethargica (von Economo disease) occurred in epidemic form between 1917 to 1928. Although mainly of historical interest at the present time, rare sporadic cases are still occasionally seen (1,2). One of the recognized presentations was termed the hyperkinetic or myoclonic form (encephalitis algo-myoclonica) where onset was associated with myoclonic movements (3). Both generalized and focal myoclonus could occur; at times these were rhythmic, involving the face, neck, shoulders, diaphragm, abdomen, arms and legs. Myoclonus of the abdomen producing distinct movements of the umbilicus was considered a pathognomonic sign (4). In some patients, the myoclonus resolved completely, whereas in others it persisted indefinitely. Parkinsonism and myoclonus were the sequelae in some patients with von Economo disease (5).

MYOCLONUS IN PARKINSON DISEASE

Myoclonus in Parkinson Disease Unrelated to Medications

Myoclonus is not a typical feature of idiopathic PD (Table 8.2). Klawans et al. (6) described three patients who presented with mild parkinsonism and prominent myoclonus. Only one of these patients had signs and symptoms suggestive of PD. The remaining two younger patients had an unusual syndrome responsive to adrenocorticotrophic hormone.

TABLE 8.2. *Myoclonus in Parkinson disease*

Untreated PD	Treated PD

Focal myoclonus—rare
Multifocal postural and
    action myoclonus
	L-Dopa induced
	  Toxic
	    Myoclonus +/−
	      asterixis
	  Nontoxic
	    Nocturnal—bilateral
	      and symmetrical
	    Beginning of dose
	    Peak dose
	  Bromocriptine
	  Amantadine

PD, Parkinson disease.

Caviness et al. (7) observed myoclonic movements of the fingers and wrists in two patients with a levodopa responsive parkinsonian syndrome most consistent with PD. Myoclonus was multifocal and asynchronous, brought out by postural maintenance and action, and present in the hand and wrist muscles. The electrophysiologic studies in these patients provided evidence for a cortical origin of the myoclonus. However, somatosensory evoked potentials (SEPs) were not enlarged, and long latency reflexes (LLRs) were not grossly exaggerated, distinguishing this form of cortical myoclonus from those seen in MSA (see below) and Alzheimer disease.

Drug-Induced Myoclonus in Parkinson Disease

The association between myoclonus and PD has been described most often in relation to levodopa intake. In a study of 12 patients who developed myoclonus after taking levodopa for 12 months, abnormal movements consisted of single, abrupt jerks of the extremities (8). These movements were usually bilateral and symmetric, involving the arms and the legs. The jerks were observed during sleep in all 12 patients. The frequency of the jerks varied from as low as 2 per night to up to 30 per night. These movements also occurred during drowsiness and awakening but rarely during activity. The major clinical impact of levodopa-induced myoclonus was to disrupt the drowsiness and sleep of these pa-

tients. Reduction in dose of levodopa resulted in a decrease in the severity and frequency of myoclonus. The addition or withdrawal of anticholinergic agents had no effect on myoclonus. Methysergide was noted to eliminate the levodopa-induced myoclonus in all patients but had no effect on parkinsonism, stressing the role of serotonin in this type of drug-induced myoclonus.

Even more common than this form of drug-induced myoclonus in PD is a "toxic" multifocal myoclonus often associated with asterixis (negative myoclonus) typically evident in patients experiencing psychiatric side effects with or without a toxic confusional state. This complication is more often found in patients with underlying dementia. (see below)

Levodopa is not the only drug to cause myoclonus in patients with PD; other antiparkinsonian medications have also been implicated. Vardi et al. (9) described six patients with PD who developed nocturnal myoclonic attacks after prolonged treatment with levodopa. These attacks were described as abnormal movements occurring during sleep, consisting of repetitive abrupt jerks of the extremities, neck, or body. The frequency varied from 6 to a maximum of 11 attacks per night. Levodopa therapy was interrupted, and after a month of treatment with bromocriptine exclusively, myoclonus persisted as recorded by sleep electroencephalogram (EEG). This suggest that in selected patients, dopamine agonists alone may be capable of inducing certain forms of myoclonus.

Isolated facial muscle involvement is unusual in drug-induced myoclonus. Pfeiffer et al. (10) described a patient with PD treated with amantadine who developed myoclonus primarily involving the laryngeal and pharyngeal muscles triggered by attempts to talk. This resulted in "stuttering" speech characterized by speech arrests and involuntary vocalization. There was "dramatic improvement" in the myoclonus after discontinuation of amantadine. Recently, Matsunaga et al. (11) described generalized, asymmetric, and multifocal myoclonus involving extremities, neck, tongue, and face muscles in three patients treated with amantadine. Two patients had PD, and the third had chronic renal failure and was on hemodialysis. In all cases, myoclonus disappeared rapidly after amantadine was discontinued, even though the dose of levodopa was increased in the two patients with PD.

Levodopa Dose-Related Myoclonus

Luquin et al. (12) studied the nature of levodopa-induced dyskinesias in 168 patients with PD. Six of the patients had spontaneous and action-induced multifocal myoclonus occurring exclusively during the "on" period (i.e., a peak-dose phenomenon). On the other hand, Marconi et al. (13) observed myoclonus occurring in a beginning-of-dose pattern in 10 of 15 patients carefully studied through the course of their response to levodopa.

MYOCLONUS IN LEWY BODY DEMENTIA

Myoclonus is rarely mentioned in available case series and not considered in the clinical diagnostic criteria for LBD. However, as mentioned above, myoclonus (drug related or not) is recognized to occur in patients combining dementia with PD. The role of more widespread Lewy body pathology in the pathogenesis of this feature is uncertain.

In a comparative study of extrapyramidal features in 31 pathologically confirmed cases of LBD and 34 pathologically confirmed cases of PD, myoclonus was found more common in LBD (18.5%, 5 of 27) than PD (0%, 0 of 26). In this study, patients with LBD were ten times more likely than those with PD to have one of the following: myoclonus, absence of rest tremor, no response to levodopa, or no perceived need to treat with levodopa (14).

Burkhardt et al. (15) reported that myoclonus was present in 15% of 34 patients with LBD (4 new, 30 literature). This figure is probably an underestimation of myoclonus in LBD since stimulus-sensitive myoclonus was not assessed (16). Indeed, stimulus-sensitive myoclonus, with exaggerated facilitation of all upper limb muscles at a latency similar to

the normal E2 response (51 to 64.5 ms), may be found in patients combining dementia with PD, probably due to LBD (16). This form of stimulus-sensitive myoclonus may increase further with systemic insults such as concurrent pneumonia.

Finally, rare patients with LBD may be misdiagnosed as having Creutzfeldt-Jakob disease (CJD), in part due to the presence of prominent myoclonus. Haik et al. (17) described ten patients with pathologically proven LBD in whom CJD was suspected initially due to rapid progression. Myoclonus was the most common feature (nine of ten) in these patients (17). Four of five patients with LBD in the series of Burkhardt et al. (see above) were also initially diagnosed as having CJD (15).

MYOCLONUS IN CORTICOBASAL DEGENERATION

Myoclonus is observed in about 55% of patients clinically diagnosed with CBD (18) and is one of the most distinctive features of the disorder (19–21). Given the increasing recognition of other clinical phenotypes associated with the pathology of CBD (22,23), the true prevalence of this feature is uncertain.

Myoclonus is usually focal and predominantly distal and occurs spontaneously, on action and in response to stimuli. Electromyography (EMG) demonstrates brief (25 to 50 ms) hypersynchronous bursts, often in runs of two to four discharges with an interburst interval of 60 to 80 ms. At times, repetitive trains of grouped bursts (each lasting 100 to 500 ms) give the appearance of 2-Hz tremor (24).

It is generally believed that myoclonus of CBD is of cortical origin but has a different set of electrophysiologic characteristics than does typical cortical reflex myoclonus (CRM). Thompson et al. (20) studied the electrophysiologic characteristics of myoclonus in 14 patients with CBD compared to 13 patients with CRM associated with epilepsia partialis continua and progressive myoclonic ataxia (PMA). In contrast to the enlarged cortical SEPs and time-locked cortical discharges of CRM, in 13 of the 14 CBD patients reflex myoclonus was not associated with enlargement of the cortical SEPs, and there were no jerk-locked spikes evident on EEG back-averaging. Reflex myoclonus in hand muscles had a latency of about 40 ms, which is considerably shorter than that found in typical CRM. Prefrontal components of the SEP were relatively preserved, but the later components of parietal SEP were poorly formed. Magnetic stimulation but not electrical stimulation of the brain evoked repetitive bursts of myoclonus, suggesting cortical hyperexcitability. Strong evidence for a cortical origin comes from the use of magnetoencephalography (MEG). Mima et al. (25) reported a cortical origin of myoclonus in one clinically diagnosed CBD patient using this technique. Finally, Manto et al. (26) recorded rhythmic cortical and muscle discharges induced by fatigue in one CBD patient. This was similar to the oscillatory activity found in the sensorimotor cortex in patients with typical CRM (27) and that underlies the normal cortical control of muscle activity by the brain (26).

Combining the evidence for enhanced motor cortical excitability, which is further supported by subsequent studies using transcranial magnetic stimulation (28,29); and the rather short cortical relay times necessary for reflex myoclonus with such short latencies, it was proposed that myoclonus in CBD might be due to enhancement of a direct sensory thalamocortical relay to the precentral motor cortex (20). Such a connection is thought to account for the normal P22. Alternatively, prominent parietal lobe involvement could result in a loss of inhibitory input from the somatosensory to the motor cortex, or thalamic pathology might result in a loss of thalamocortical recurrent inhibition.

It is uncertain whether there are electrophysiologic features that are specific for the pathology of CBD. Certainly, depending on when they are studied over the course of the illness, not all patients with myoclonus and CBD will demonstrate each of the features reported by Thompson et al. (20). For example, we have seen at least one patient whose diagnosis was subsequently confirmed at autopsy in whom reflex latencies were more akin to typical CRM. On the other hand, we have seen patients with a CBD phenotype, later shown to be due to parietal prominent Pick disease (30) and motor neuron disease-inclusion dementia (31), whose reflex myoclonus also did not have the "classical" electrophysiologic features of CBD. If the specificity and sensitivity of the electrophysiologic features were known, then their presence or absence in a patient who clinically appears to have CBD with myoclonus might be helpful in confirming or refuting the diagnosis. Further clinical, electrophysiologic, and pathologic correlation studies will be required to address this issue.

MYOCLONUS IN MULTIPLE SYSTEM ATROPHY

Myoclonus is increasingly recognized as a common manifestation of MSA. The existing literature markedly underestimates its true prevalence. Indeed, this feature was not even mentioned in a review of 203 pathologically proven cases (32). When recognized, it may not be referred to as such; for example, Quinn and Marsden used the term "irregular jerky tremor" (33). Several distinct types of myoclonus have been reported in these patients (Table 8.3). In a study of 100 patients with probable MSA, Wenning et al. (34) reported that myoclonus was present in 37% of those with a parkinsonian phenotype (MSA-P) and 6% of those with a cerebellar predominant form (MSA-C). This, too, is almost certainly an underestimate of the frequency since these patients did not undergo careful electrophysiologic studies.

Stimulus-sensitive myoclonus may be one of the commonest forms of myoclonus found in patients with MSA. In contrast to the impression obtained from the report of Wenning et al. (34), Obeso et al. (35) found that stimulus-sensitive myoclonus occurred more frequently in patients with the olivopontocerebellar form of MSA (MSA-C), although 92% of their patients had bradykinesia and 50% had rigidity. Focal reflex myoclonus was elicited in response to somesthetic stimuli in 23 of their 24 Olivopontocerebellar Atrophy

TABLE 8.3. *Electrophysiologic origin of various clinical forms of myoclonus described in multiple systematrophy*

Clinical features	Origin		References
	Cortical	Brainstem	
Stimulus (somaesthetic)-sensitive myoclonus	+	+	16,36,39,40
Photic-reflex myoclonus	+	−	38
Postural/action myoclonus (including minipolymyoclonus)	+	+	37,39,40
Spontaneous myoclonus	−	+	39
Exaggerated startle response (to sound, tapping the nose, visual stimuli)	−	+	42
Generalized myoclonus in sleep	−	+	39

(OPCA) patients (36). These were comprised of brisk, sometimes multiple jerks of finger flexors and extensors in response to a single stimulus. Fifty-four percent of these patients also had photic reflex myoclonus, and 12.5% each had spontaneous and action-induced myoclonus. Sixteen patients showed a reflex muscle discharge (C wave) recorded from the relaxed forearm muscles after electrical stimulation of the wrist, with a mean latency of 39.9 ms. The SEPs had a normal latency, but the mean amplitudes of the N20/P25 and P25/N33 waves were significantly increased indicating that this was a form of CRM. Chen et al. (16) reported a pathologic exaggeration of the long latency cutaneous reflex or E2 in 3 MSA-P patients with focal reflex myoclonus. The latency of this response was longer (51 to 64.5 ms) than that in the OPCA patients studied by Rodriguez et al., and the SEPs were not enlarged. This suggests that more than one type of somaesthetic stimulus-induced CRM can occur in MSA.

Salazar et al. (37) noted abnormal jerky movements of hands and fingers ("jerky tremor") in 9 of 11 consecutive patients with MSA-P. Electrophysiologic studies confirmed this to be a form of postural and action myoclonus, which they referred to as minipolymyoclonus. Only 3 of these patients had additional reflex myoclonic jerks. SEPs were normal, and no EEG spike time locked to EMG activity on back-averaging technique was noted. However, reflex response latency was 55.3 ± 4.1 ms, compatible with an exaggerated cutaneous reflex or E2, suggesting

that motor cortex hyperexcitability accounts for this minipolymyoclonus.

Another form of myoclonus originating in the cerebral cortex of MSA patients is photic cortical reflex myoclonus (38). Artieda and Obeso found this present in five of six patients with MSA (all six had CRM and two had action myoclonus). Electrophysiologic studies recorded a large (36.9 uV) positive/negative wave maximum in the midfrontal region following visual stimuli (~3.8 ms later) preceding the myoclonus in a time-locked fashion. The myoclonus was markedly responsive to both levodopa and piracetam, as well as, but less so, to 5 hydroxytryptophan.

In contrast to the cortical origin emphasized in the studies discussed above, Clouston et al. (39) reported a patient who presumably had MSA-P with a brainstem origin for the myoclonic jerks. This patient had both spontaneous and somaesthetic reflex jerks (90 to 150 ms) in hands and face while awake as well as frequent more generalized jerks in sleep. There were no giant SEPs or photically induced myoclonus and no preceding EEG activity. The reflex latencies were consistent with a brainstem origin. Although the patient did not demonstrate startle response to auditory stimuli, motor evoked potentials revealed that the central efferent pathway was slow conducting, similar to that involved in a pathologic startle response and unlike the fast conducting pathway involved in the reticular myoclonus that occurs in the setting of anoxic encephalopathy.

Finally, Koffler et al. (40,41) reported both cortical and brainstem hyperexcitability in a patient with pathologically proven MSA-P (striatonigral degeneration) who had marked postural and action myoclonus as well as exaggerated startle response to acoustic, somatosensory, and visual stimuli. Their patient demonstrated the presence of nonhabituating facial and whole body jerks in response to tapping the nose, which the authors attributed to hyperexcitability of the brainstem. We have found that this is an extremely common feature in patients with MSA.

CONCLUSION

The frequency of occurrence, clinical presentation, electrophysiologic characteristics, and pathogenesis of myoclonus can vary across different parkinsonian disorders. Future studies will address the specificity of electrophysiologic subtypes of myoclonus for various pathologies. Further studies are also needed to clarify the genetic, neurochemical, or pathologic basis of different myoclonus phenotypes.

REFERENCES

1. Howard RS, Lees AJ. Encephalitis lethargica. *Brain* 1987;110:19–33.
2. Blunt SB, Lane RJM, Turjanski N, et al. Clinical features and management of two cases of encephalitis lethargica. *Mov Disord* 1997;12:354–359.
3. von Economo C. *Encephalitis lethargica: its sequelae and treatment.* London: Oxford University Press, 1931.
4. Krusz JC, Koller WC, Ziegler DK. Historical review: abnormal movements associated with epidemic encephalitis lethargica. *Mov Disord* 1987;2:137–141.
5. Wilson SAK. Epidemic encephalitis. In: Bruce AN, ed. *Neurology* London: Edward Arnold, 1940:99–144.
6. Klawans HL, Tanner CM, McDermott J. Myoclonus and parkinsonism. *Clin Neuropharmacol* 1986;9:202–205.
7. Caviness JN, Adler CH, Newman S, et al. Cortical myoclonus in levodopa-responsive parkinsonism. *Mov Disord* 1998;13:540–544.
8. Klawans HL, Goetz C, Bergen D. Levodopa-induced myoclonus. *Arch Neurol* 1975;32:331–334.
9. Vardi J, Glaubman H, Rabey JM, et al. Myoclonic attacks induced by L-dopa and bromocriptine in Parkinson patients: a sleep EEG study. *J Neurol* 2001;218:35–42.
10. Pfeiffer RF. Amantadine-induced "vocal" myoclonus. *Mov Disord* 1996;11:104–106.
11. Matsunaga K, Uozumi T, Qingrui L, et al. Amantadine-induced cortical myoclonus. *Neurology* 2001;56:279–280.
12. Luquin MR, Scipioni O, Vaamonde J, et al. Levodopa-induced dyskinesias in Parkinson's disease: clinical and pharmacological classification. *Mov Disord* 1992;7:117–124.
13. Marconi R, Lefebvre-Capprros D, Bonnet AM, et al. Levodopa-induced dyskinesias in Parkinson's disease: phenomenology and pathophysiology. *Mov Disord* 1994;9:2–12.
14. Louis ED, Klatka LA, Liu Y, et al. Comparison of extrapyramidal features in 31 pathologically confirmed cases of diffuse Lewy body disease and 34 pathologically confirmed cases of Parkinson's disease. *Neurology* 1997;48:376–380.
15. Burkhardt CR, Filley CM, Kleinschmidt-DeMasters BK, et al. Diffuse Lewy body disease and progressive dementia. *Neurology* 1988;38:1520–1528.
16. Chen R, Ashby P, Lang AE. Stimulus-sensitive myoclonus in akinetic-rigid syndromes. *Brain* 1992;115:1875–1888.
17. Haik S, Brandel JP, Sazdovitch V, et al. Dementia with Lewy bodies in a neuropathologic series of suspected Creutzfeldt-Jakob disease. *Neurology* 2000;55:1401–1404.
18. Kompoliti K, Goetz C, Boeve BF, et al. Clinical presentation and pharmacological therapy in corticobasal degeneration. *Arch Neurol* 1998;55:957–961.
19. Riley DE, Lang AE, Lewis A, et al. Cortical-basal ganglionic degeneration. *Neurology* 1990;40:1203–1212.
20. Thompson PD, Day BL, Rothwell JC, et al. The myoclonus in corticobasal degeneration: evidence for two forms of cortical reflex myoclonus. *Brain* 1994;117:1197–1207.
21. Thompson PD, Shibasaki H. Myoclonus in corticobasal degeneration and other neurodegenerations. Adv *Neurol* 2000;82:69–81.
22. Bergeron C, Pollanen MS, Weyer L, et al. Unusual clinical presentations of cortical-basal ganglionic degeneration. *Ann Neurol* 1996;40:72–79.
23. Boeve BF, Maraganore DM, Parisi JE, et al. Clinical heterogeneity in patients with pathologically diagnosed cortical-basal ganglionic degeneration. *Mov Disord* 1996;11:351–352.
24. Brunt ERP, van Weerden TW, Pruim J, et al. Unique myoclonic pattern in corticobasal degeneration. *Mov Disord* 1995;10:132–142.
25. Mima T, Nagamine T, Ikeda A, et al. Pathogenesis of cortical myoclonus studied by magnetoencephalography. *Ann Neurol* 1998;43:598–607.
26. Manto MU, Jacquy J, Van Bogaert P, et al. Rhythmic cortical and muscle discharges induced by fatigue in corticobasal degeneration. *Clin Neurophysiol* 2000;111:496–503.
27. Brown P, Marsden CD. Rhythmic cortical and muscle discharge in cortical myoclonus. *Brain* 1996;119:1307–1316.
28. Yokota T, Saito Y, Shimizu Y. Increased corticomotoneuronal excitability after peripheral nerve stimulation in dopa-nonresponsive hemiparkinsonism. *J Neurol Sci* 1995;129:34–39.
29. Lu CS, Ikeda A, Terada K, et al. Electrophysiological studies of early stage corticobasal degeneration. *Mov Disord* 1998;13:140–146.
30. Lang AE, Bergeron C, Pollanen MS, et al. Parietal Pick's disease mimicking cortical-basal ganglionic degeneration. *Neurology* 1994;44:1436–1440.
31. Grimes DA, Bergeron CB, Lang AE. Motor neuron dis-

ease-inclusion dementia presenting as cortical-basal ganglionic degeneration. *Mov Disord* 1999;14:674–680.

32. Wenning GK, Tison F, Ben Shlomo Y, et al. Multiple
system atrophy: a review of 203 pathologically proven
cases. *Mov Disord* 1997;12:133–147.

33. Quinn NP, Marsden CD. The motor disorder of multiple
system atrophy. *J Neurol Neurosurg Psychiatry* 1993;
56:1239–1242.

34. Wenning GK, Ben Shlomo Y, Magalhaes M, et al. Clinical features and natural history of multiple system atrophy: an analysis of 100 cases. *Brain* 1994;117:835–845.

35. Obeso JA, Rodriguez ME, Artieda J, et al. Focal reflex
myoclonus: a useful sign in the differential diagnosis of
parkinsonism. *Ann Neurol* 1989;26:164–165.

36. Rodriguez ME, Artieda J, Obeso JA, et al. Reflex myoclonus in olivopontocerebellar atrophy. *J Neurol Neurosurg Psychiatry* 1994;57:316–319.

37. Salazar G, Valls-Solé J, Martí MJ, et al. Postural and action myoclonus in patients with parkinsonian type multiple system atrophy. *Mov Disord* 2000;15:77–83.

38. Artieda J, Obeso JA. The pathophysiology and pharmacology of photic cortical reflex myoclonus. *Ann Neurol*
1993;34:175–184.

39. Clouston PD, Lim CL, Fung V, et al. Brainstem myoclonus in a patient with non-dopa-responsive parkinsonism. *Mov Disord* 1996;11:404–410.

40. Kofler M, Wenning GK, Poewe W. Cortical and brain
stem hyperexcitability in striatonigral degeneration.
Mov Disord 1998;13:602–607.

41. Kofler M, Wenning GK, Poewe W, et al. Cortical and
brain stem hyperexcitability in a pathologically confirmed case of multiple system atrophy. *Mov Disord*
2000;15:362–363.

42. Tasker RR, Lang AE, Lozano AM. Pallidal and thalamic
surgery for Parkinson's disease. *Exp Neurol* 1997;
144:35–40.

Myoclonus and Paroxysmal Dyskinesias,
Advances in Neurology, Vol. 89,
edited by S. Fahn, et al.
Lippincott Williams & Wilkins, Philadelphia © 2002.

9

The Clinical Challenge of Posthypoxic Myoclonus

Steven J. Frucht

Department of Neurology, Columbia-Presbyterian Medical Center, The Neurological Institute,
New York, New York

In 1960, Dr. James Lance traveled from Australia to the United States to pursue a fellowship at the Massachusetts General Hospital. Interested in movement disorders, he was shown four patients who survived a cardiac arrest only to be afflicted with severe myoclonic jerks and frequent falls. Struck by their similarity to patients with progressive myoclonic epilepsy, he set out to explore the clinical features and neurophysiology of this unusual movement disorder (1). An article entitled "The Syndrome of Intention or Action Myoclonus as a Sequel to Hypoxic Encephalopathy," a classic of the neurologic literature, resulted from these studies (2).

Subsequently known as the Lance-Adams syndrome, intention myoclonus following cardiac arrest has attracted the concerted research effort of only a handful of investigators. This is a pity, because the phenomenology, neurochemistry, and neurophysiology of this syndrome are fascinating. More important, many patients who develop the Lance-Adams syndrome are left with permanent and significant disability. One of the major goals of the Myoclonus Research Foundation, founded nearly 25 years ago by Norman Seiden and Drs. Stanley Fahn and Arnold Gold, was to focus attention and research efforts on this particular problem.

In this chapter, I review what is known about the Lance-Adams syndrome, focusing on phenomenology, natural history, and treat-ment. The neurophysiology of cortical and subcortical myoclonus (both of which may be present in these patients) is considered in chapter 10, and a detailed discussion of the rodent model of posthypoxic myoclonus may be found in chapters 25, 30, and 32.

PHENOMENOLOGY

Little has been added to the original description of the disorder (2). Myoclonus "showed uniform qualities in all patients . . . sometimes single but more often comprising a series of contractions of variable amplitude, which were mostly confined to the active limb but occasionally spread to an adjacent group of muscles or those on the opposite side of the body." Patients were disabled by myoclonic jerks that were specifically triggered by action, or by the attempt to move, "Voluntary movement could be initiated normally but was interrupted by both jerks and pauses, resulting in a chaotic fragmentation of contraction . . . [as seen in] the attempt to perform a finely co-ordinated, willed movement such as conveying food to the mouth, drinking from a glass or reaching for a paper clip in a cup. Here there was a marked difference between performing the task with an empty glass or merely placing the fingers in an empty cup, which brought out only a slight tendency to myoclonus, and taking a full glass of water or retrieving a single paper clip from the cup, which inaugurated a series of violent jerks making effective movement impossible." Patients are especially disabled by this phenomenon, which at times seems cruel: the harder they try to perform a task, the more severe the myoclonus.

In addition to action and intention myoclonus, Lance and Adams recognized that negative myoclonic jerks often left patients severely disabled, "Failure to sustain muscular contraction was even more apparent when the patients attempted to walk, and their tendency to fall appeared to be due to a lapse in contraction of antigravity muscles which might or might not be associated with a visible myoclonic jerk." Negative myoclonus may involve the hamstring and quadriceps muscles, producing a characteristic "bouncing" gait that may be misinterpreted as psychogenic by an untrained observer. Another peculiar tendency of these patients is their susceptibility to startle, "Walking was possible on an even surface at a slow pace, but if the foot should unexpectedly strike the leg of a chair or the toe of the shoe catch on the edge of a carpet, the proximal limb and trunk muscles would suddenly contract and immediately there would follow one or more myoclonic jerks, and possibly a lapse of posture and a fall" (2). Patients afflicted with this problem quickly learn to fear walking alone. The combination of negative myoclonus and exaggerated startle usually confines a patient to a wheelchair.

Although other neurologic deficits may be present, they are usually overshadowed by myoclonus. Dysmetria, mild dysarthria, and ataxia were present in all four of Lance and Adams' patients; however, pyramidal and extrapyramidal deficits were absent. Although patients may appear cognitively normal, formal neuropsychological testing often reveals evidence of subtle disorders of attention, memory, and executive function.

DISEASE COURSE AND NATURAL HISTORY

By 1986, 88 patients with posthypoxic myoclonus had been reported in the literature (3). Thirty-four additional cases were re-

ported between 1986 and 1999, bringing the total to 122 patients with posthypoxic myoclonus reported between 1963 and 1999 (4).

Asthmatic attack, cardiac arrest or infarction, airway obstruction, and drug intoxication are the most common triggers of the syndrome. Anesthesia mishaps such as esophageal intubation have become less common with the practice of end-tidal CO_2 monitoring. Most patients who develop posthypoxic myoclonus are between the ages of 15 and 60. This probably reflects the relative resistance of the young brain to hypoxia and the poor survival of older adults after cardiac arrest.

It is impossible to predict if a patient will develop posthypoxic myoclonus after surviving an arrest. Although many cases may go unreported, it is likely that the disorder is rare. Patients who eventually develop posthypoxic myoclonus usually remain in coma for 4 to 7 days. Seizures and myoclonus are common at this stage, although the medical staff may not recognize myoclonic movements. Family members who observe the patient at the bedside may report that he or she startles easily to sounds or alarms. In those who survive, emerge from coma, and enter the chronic stage of the disorder, at least one-third will have dysarthria and ataxia, and more than two-thirds have difficulty walking. Seizures are frequent but are usually well controlled by antiepileptic medications.

What happens to patients with posthypoxic myoclonus over time? Werhahn et al. (5) followed 14 patients with posthypoxic myoclonus for an average of 3.7 years. In most patients, myoclonus slowly improved over time. Walking, speech, activities of daily living, and global disability all improved. This study confirmed the general impression that unlike most intractable movement disorders, posthypoxic myoclonus is not a progressive condition, and it may even slowly remit.

PHARMACOTHERAPY

Like most forms of myoclonus, the treatment of posthypoxic myoclonus remains empiric. Posthypoxic myoclonus is best thought of as a syndrome rather than a single entity. Patients may have cortical myoclonus, subcortical myoclonus, or both. Similarly, they may have action and intention myoclonus, negative myoclonus with postural lapses, or both. It is impossible to determine solely by examination whether myoclonus is cortical or subcortical, and it can sometimes be difficult to tell if negative myoclonus is present. Unfortunately, most published reports of patients' response to treatments do not include detailed clinical or neurophysiologic assessments. All that can be learned from these cases is whether a patient with posthypoxic myoclonus did or did not respond to the medication. The nature of the response is also at issue, because almost all available reports are descriptive.

Despite these caveats, several lessons emerged from a recent review (4). Clonazepam significantly improved posthypoxic myoclonus in 24 of 47 patients in whom it was prescribed, and valproate was similarly effective in 10 of 22 patients. L-5-Hydroxytryptophan (L-5-HTP) was effective in only 17 of 43 patients, often with intolerable side effects. Piracetam was effective in 3 of 6 patients. Drugs that did not produce significant benefit in even one patient include nitrazepam, primidone, phenobarbital, phenytoin, and tetrabenazine.

In March 2000, the novel antiepileptic agent levetiracetam was released in the United States. Krauss et al. (6) showed that levetiracetam, an analog of piracetam, was effective in two patients with posthypoxic myoclonus. As part of an open-label, add-on pilot study of the tolerability and efficacy of the drug in patients with chronic myoclonus (7), one patient with posthypoxic cortical myoclonus had dramatic benefit, two did not improve, and one could not tolerate it. I have subsequently used levetiracetam in another posthypoxic patient with excellent results, and another patient with cortical myoclonus of different etiology had similar benefit.

TREATMENT RECOMMENDATIONS

Typically, neurologists are called to see patients with posthypoxic myoclonus in the intensive care unit. As patients emerge from coma, myoclonic jerks are probably best managed with clonazepam. This drug has a short half-life, and its sedative properties may be welcome in an encephalopathic agitated patient. When patients recover and enter the chronic stage of the illness, I obtain magnetic resonance imaging of the head and also define the neurophysiology of the myoclonus wherever possible. Enlarged somatosensory evoked potentials suggest cortical myoclonus, but definitive proof requires back-averaged electroencephalography. This technique is not routinely available, and the neurologist must often rely on clinical clues that point to a cortical origin. These include the presence of stimulus-sensitive myoclonus, distal predominance of myoclonus, and very prominent action myoclonus. In contrast, reticular reflex myoclonus tends to involve the proximal limbs and trunk, producing violent flexion jerks, and in my experience it is much less common than cortical myoclonus.

Having established a cortical focus by either physiology or clinical examination, there are several options for treatment. Piracetam is available in Europe and Canada, is well tolerated, and is effective in many patients with cortical myoclonus. Side effects are minimal, although patients must be able to swallow pills because the effective dose ranges from 16.8 to 24 g per day (a liquid formulation is available). Piracetam is not approved for use in the United States. Levetiracetam *is* currently available in the United States and in Europe. It, too, has few side effects, is not metabolized, and is excreted unchanged in the urine. As mentioned before, several patients with cortical myoclonus have benefited dramatically from the drug. The advantage of levetiracetam is that an effective daily dose of 2,000 mg per day can be given in the form of two pills. It is unknown whether piracetam or levetiracetam is more effective in treating cortical myoclonus. Therefore, it seems reasonable to choose either drug for patients with proven or suspected cortical posthypoxic myoclonus. If a patient does not respond to one drug, the other should be tried because there have been anecdotal reports of patients responding to only one agent.

Once treatment with levetiracetam or piracetam has begun, I attempt to wean patients off clonazepam in order to minimize its potential side effects (sedation, depression, personality change, and impotence). For patients who do not obtain adequate relief from these drugs, valproic acid is another option. However, in my opinion, its side-effect profile and its potential effects on hematologic and liver function parameters make this a second-line drug.

Posthypoxic myoclonus patients who are afflicted with reticular reflex myoclonus pose a particular challenge. Clonazepam is often helpful; however, drugs that are effective in cortical myoclonus are generally of little benefit. In these patients, and in patients with cortical myoclonus who do not respond to any of the drugs mentioned before, I consider using 5-HTP. This agent requires pretreatment with carbidopa, and even then nausea and gastrointestinal upset are a major nuisance. The drug can be found in many health food stores, although the purity of the preparation is unknown. In the past, an impurity in one lot of 5-HTP triggered a potentially lethal eosinophilia-myalgia syndrome, raising concern about the source of the agent. At present, few patients take the drug, and ideally it should be used only with an institutional review board–approved protocol that includes written informed consent.

FUTURE WORK

Nearly four decades after the original description, many questions remain unanswered. How rare is posthypoxic myoclonus? What is the mechanism responsible for generating myoclonic jerks? Why do certain patients develop cortical myoclonus and others subcortical myoclonus? Why do some patients with cortical myoclonus respond to medications and others do not? How can the clinical and neurophysiologic features of the syndrome be reconciled with the complex neurochemistry of the serotonin system? The answers to these and other questions await further work. However, the availability of new medications and the interest of basic and clinical investigators in this syndrome offer tangible hope to these patients and their families.

REFERENCES

1. Lance JW, Adams RD. Negative myoclonus in posthypoxic patients: historical note. *Mov Disord* 2001;16:162–163.
2. Lance JW, Adams RD. The syndrome of intention or action myoclonus as a sequel to hypoxic encephalopathy. *Brain* 1963;86:111–136.
3. Fahn S. Posthypoxic action myoclonus: literature review update. *Adv Neurol* 1986;43:157–169.
4. Frucht S, Fahn S. The clinical spectrum of posthypoxic myoclonus. *Mov Disord* 2000;15(S)1:2–7.
5. Werhahn KJ, Brown P, Thompson PD, et al. The clinical features and prognosis of chronic posthypoxic myoclonus. *Mov Disord* 1997;12:216–220.
6. Krauss GL, Bergin A, Kramer RE, et al. Suppression of posthypoxic and post-encephalitic myoclonus with levetiracetam. *Neurology* 2001;56:411–412.
7. Frucht SJ, Louis ED, Chuang C, et al. A pilot tolerability and efficacy study of levetiracetam in patients with chronic myoclonus. *Neurology* 2001;57(6):1112-4.

*Myoclonus and Paroxysmal Dyskinesias,
Advances in Neurology,* Vol. 89,
edited by S. Fahn, et al.
Lippincott Williams & Wilkins, Philadelphia © 2002.

10

Neurophysiology of Cortical Positive Myoclonus

*Yoshikazu Ugawa, *Ritsuko Hanajima, †Shingo Okabe, and ‡Kaoru Yuasa

*Department of Neurology, Division of Neuroscience, †Graduate School of Medicine,
‡Department of Laboratory Medicine, University of Tokyo, Tokyo, Japan*

There are two kinds of myoclonus (a sudden, brief, jerky, shocklike involuntary movement arising from the central nervous system): positive myoclonus and negative myoclonus (1). Jerks are produced by brief electromyographic (EMG) activation in positive myoclonus and by an abrupt cession of ongoing tonic EMG activity in negative myoclonus. This chapter deals with physiologic features of cortical positive myoclonus, and studies of negative myoclonus are described in chapter 12. Cortical positive myoclonus is a myoclonus caused by transient discharges in a certain cortical area. Many studies have already been performed on cortical myoclonus, probably because cortical activities associated with myoclonus can be easily detected with noninvasive methods, such as electroencephalography (EEG) or magnetoencephalography (MEG). The results have been reviewed in several excellent articles (1–11). Most studies have shown hyperexcitability of cortical areas, such as sensorimotor cortex (12–15) or visual cortex (16,17), by studying several characteristics of the cortical activities. In this chapter, we review a few studies that demonstrated sensorimotor cortical hyperexcitability in cortical myoclonus. In addition, we briefly describe our recent study of interhemispheric connection between bilateral hand motor areas in normals and patients with cortical myoclonus.

HYPEREXCITABILITY OF THE MOTOR CORTEX

Cortical discharges responsible for cortical spontaneous myoclonus can sometimes be seen in conventional EEG/EMG polygraphic recordings. However, they often cannot be detected in polygraphs. In such cases, cortical activities associated with myoclonus can be usually detected by the jerk-locked back-averaging method, which was first applied to research on myoclonus by Shibasaki et al. (18,19). This method allows not only the ability to detect a small EEG activity correlating with myoclonus (premyoclonus spike), but also the ability to conduct detailed analyses of the premyoclonus spike. At first sight, the premyoclonus spike was considered to originate from the motor cortex because it causes a muscle contraction. However, scalp topographic study of premyoclonus spikes (20) suggested that it was localized in the postcentral sensory cortex. In a patient with cortical myoclonus, abnormal activity occurred in the postcentral sensory cortex in spontaneous myoclonus as well as in cortical reflex myoclonus (21,22). Resection of this part of the cortex abolished myoclonus in the patient. That case supports the idea that the premyoclonus spike originates from the sensory cortex. Later studies of a myoclonic cortical activity using a dipole source localization of EEG (23) or MEG (12,15,24) revealed that most of premyoclonus cortical spikes originate from the motor cortex, although a part of them come from the sensory cortex. The fact that abnormal discharges spontaneously occur in the motor cortex should indicate hyperexcitability of the motor cortex.

Paired magnetic stimulation of the motor cortex has given us other evidence for motor cortical hyperexcitability in cortical myoclonus. Kujirai et al. (25) first reported that a subthreshold magnetic conditioning stimulus reduced the size of responses to a suprathreshold magnetic test stimulus when the conditioning stimulus preceded the test stimulus by 1 to 5 ms. They concluded that this suppression was produced by an activation of GABA-ergic inhibitory interneurons in the motor cortex by the conditioning stimulus. This idea was confirmed by pharmacologic experiments in humans (26). Since then, this method has been widely used for studying pathophysiologic mechanisms underlying many movement disorders. Cortical myoclonus is one of them (27,28).

Figure 10.1 shows examples of this experiment. Responses in a normal subject are shown on the *left*. Responses to the test stimulus preceded by the conditioning stimulus by 1 to 6 ms (the interstimulus interval [ISI] is 1 to 6 ms) are smaller than the response to the test stimulus given alone (control response, *second row*). A time course of the suppression was depicted as a size ratio of the conditioned response to the control response against an ISI. The mean (±SD) time course for normal subjects (dots in the bottom figure on the *right*) demonstrates that significant suppression occurs at ISIs of 1 to 5 ms. The top figure on the right shows responses in a patient with cortical myoclonus. Conditioned responses at ISIs of 3 and 5 ms were not smaller than the control response, whereas at an ISI of 1 ms suppression was evoked. The mean (±SD) time course for cortical myoclonic patients is shown in the bottom figure on the right. No suppression was seen at ISIs of 3 to 5 ms. This suggests that GABA-ergic inhibitory circuits in the motor cortex are affected in cortical myoclonus (27,28). Brown et al. (27) emphasized that reduced suppression in this experiment was observed in cortical myoclonic patients in whom a cortical activity spreads from an original focus to surrounding areas in the same sensorimotor cortex or to the contralateral sensorimotor cortex ("spreaders," they were called). Another interesting point of this result is that suppression occurred at an ISI of 1 ms in patients with cortical myoclonus. We, and probably other investigators, consider that, in addition to GABA-ergic systems, some other mechanisms must contribute to the suppression at an ISI of 1 ms, but this point will not be discussed here.

HYPEREXCITABILITY OF THE SENSORY CORTEX

It is well known that many patients with cortical myoclonus have prominently enlarged somatosensory evoked potentials (giant SEPs) to peripheral sensory stimuli and reflex muscle contractions at long intervals (long loop reflex [LLR]). The *upper traces* in Figure 10.2 are one example of a giant SEP and a LLR. Median nerve stimulation at the wrist elicited an enlarged SEP at normal la-

FIG. 10.1. Paired magnetic stimulation of the motor cortex. Traces on the left are responses in a normal subject. A conditioning stimulus evoked no responses (subthreshold) (top trace). A test stimulus given alone elicited a response (approximately 0.1 to 0.3 mV) (second trace). The conditioning stimulus reduced the size of responses to the stimulus when it preceded the test stimulus by 1 to 6 ms. This suppression is considered to be an event at the motor cortex and should reflect GABA-ergic inhibitory circuits in the motor cortex. Responses from a cortical myoclonic patient are shown in the upper traces on the right. In contrast to normal subjects, the suppression was not evoked at ISIs of 3 and 5 ms, whereas it was evoked at an ISI of 1 ms. Mean (±SE) time courses of intracortical inhibition are shown in the lower figure on the right. Inhibition at short intervals (1 to 5 ms) was seen in normals, but reduced in patients with cortical myoclonus.

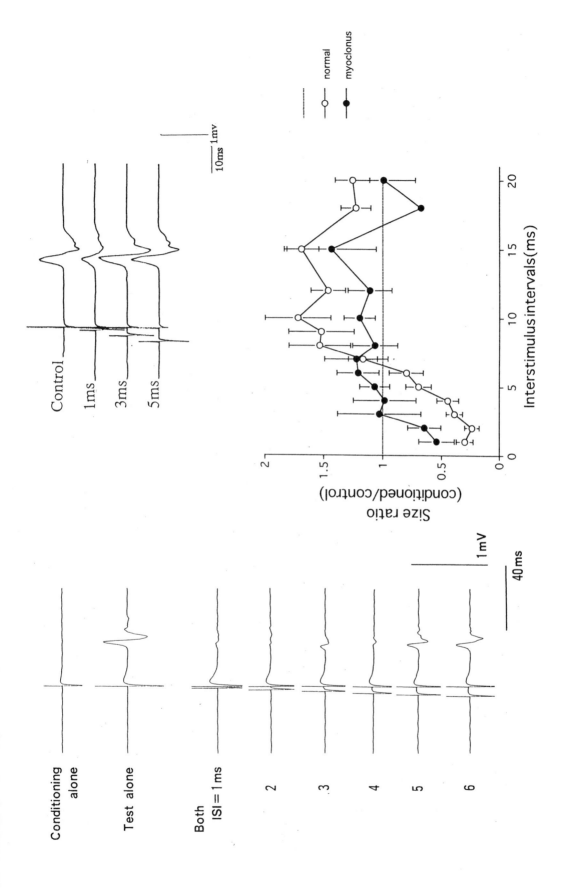

tency. The N20 component was normal in size, whereas later components were abnormally enlarged (P25-P33 amplitude was about 40μV). LLRs were evoked at about 40 ms after the median nerve stimulation. This enhanced SEP suggests hyperexcitability of a certain cortical area, and we usually first consider it to be hyperexcitability of the sensory cortex.

Hallett et al. (29) named this type of myoclonus *cortical reflex myoclonus*. Many studies have since been done to elucidate the pathomechanisms underlying a giant SEP (13,14, 20–22,30–33). Such works have focused on

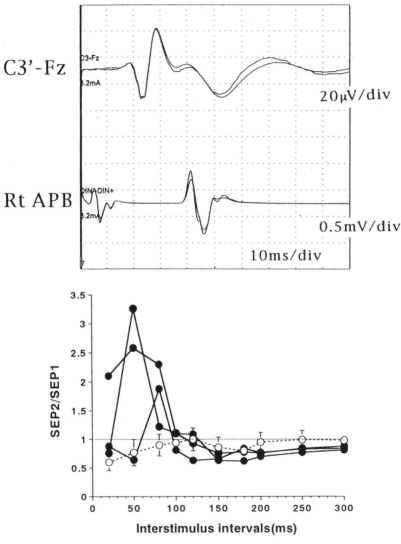

FIG. 10.2. Giant somatosensory evoked potential (SEP) and long loop reflex (LLR). **Upper traces** are a giant SEP and a LLR. A prominently enhanced SEP was evoked by median nerve stimulation at the wrist. Its P25-N33 amplitude was 51.3μV. A LLR was elicited in the APB 37.5 ms after the median nerve stimulation. Time courses of recovery in paired stimulation SEP are shown in the **lower figure**. In normals (○), the SEP to the second stimulus (SEP 2) was significantly smaller than the SEP to the first stimulus (SEP 1) at ISIs shorter than 100 ms, whereas it was markedly enhanced at short ISIs in patients with cortical myoclonus (●).

the difference in generators between a giant SEP and a premyoclonus spike. The question of whether an enhanced component of a giant SEP originates from the sensory cortex or motor cortex has also been one of the topics in this field. Topographic studies of giant SEPs (20,30) suggested that they originate from the sensory cortex. Another report on a giant SEP using an excellent new technique (32) showed that abnormally enhanced activation of the sensory cortex is responsible for giant SEPs. Ikeda et al. (31) found that either a tangential or a radial component, or both of them, was enlarged in a giant SEP. They carefully stated that their study did not answer the question about the source of an enhanced radial component of giant SEP. MEG analyses (13,14) revealed that the generators of enhanced P25 component were in the precentral motor cortex or postcentral sensory cortex. In a patient with cortical reflex myoclonus, subdural electrode recordings demonstrated an enhanced response over the presumed motor cortex (33). Based on all these results, we think that prominently enhanced SEPs are mostly generated by the motor cortex and partly by the sensory cortex. The presence of a giant SEP, therefore, indicates hyperexcitability of the sensory cortex in some patients with cortical reflex myoclonus.

Another line of evidence for hyperexcitability of the sensory cortex again comes from a paired stimulation experiment (2,34, 35), similarly to the paired magnetic stimulation for the motor cortical hyperexcitability. In paired stimulation SEP experiments, an SEP to the second stimulus (SEP 2) was significantly smaller than an SEP to the first stimulus (SEP 1) at ISIs shorter than 100 ms (*circles* in the bottom figure in Figure 10.2). This suppression is considered to be produced by activation of inhibitory interneurons in the sensory cortex. In contrast, the suppression was not observed in some patients with cortical myoclonus or even facilitation was seen (*dots* in the bottom figure of Figure 10.2), which reflect dysfunction of sensory cortical inhibitory interneurons. This dysfunction may cause hyperexcitability of the sensory cortex.

INTERHEMISPHERIC INTERACTION BETWEEN THE MOTOR CORTICES OF BOTH HEMISPHERES

In patients with cortical reflex myoclonus, LLRs are elicited in limb muscles near to the stimulated nerve, and sometimes they are also evoked in contralateral muscles about 10 ms later than the ipsilateral ones. Such bilateral LLRs are shown in the upper traces in Figure 10.3. Stimulation of the right median nerve elicited a giant SEP over the left-hand sensory area at normal latency and a LLR in the right abductor pollicis brevis (APB). Moreover, an enlarged SEP was evoked over the right-hand sensory area (ipsilateral to the stimulated nerve), and a small LLR was evoked in the left APB. Both of these rare responses appeared about 10 ms later than the conventional SEPs and LLRs. This phenomenon has already been described previously (19,36). Pathomechanisms for these responses are supposed to be as follows. An original myoclonic activity elicited by peripheral nerve stimulation (giant SEP) must spread to the sensory cortex of the other hemisphere through the corpus callosum, which produces an enlarged SEP on the other side. This abnormal activity should cause contralateral LLRs.

Focal magnetic stimulation of the motor cortex sometimes elicited ipsilateral later responses as well as contralateral short latency responses in patients with cortical myoclonus. A typical example is shown in Figure 10.3 (lower traces). Focal stimulation over the left motor cortex with a figure-of-8 coil evoked a short latency EMG potential in the right first dorsal interroseous muscle (FDI) with a latency of about 20 ms, and a small response in the left FDI with a latency of about 30 ms. This phenomenon has also been already described by Thompson et al. (37). Transcallosal spreads of an activity produced by magnetic stimulation must be responsible for these ipsilateral responses in cortical myoclonus. Brown et al. (38,39) studied these spreads of a myoclonic activity through the corpus callosum in detail. This idea of transcallosal spreads has inspired us to study interhemi-

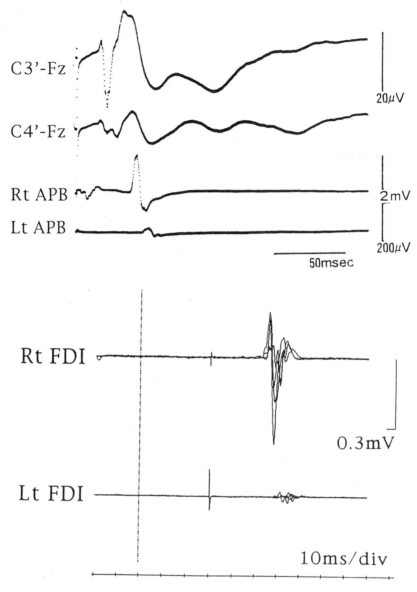

FIG. 10.3. Bilateral LLRs (**upper traces**) and bilateral magnetic cortical responses (**lower traces**) in a patient with cortical myoclonus. Upper traces: SEPs and EMG responses from abductor pollicis brevis (APB) muscles after the right median nerve stimulation. A markedly enhanced SEP was evoked over the left-hand sensory area at normal latency (*top trace*). The latency of a large positive peak was 22 ms. In the right APB, a small M wave was followed by an LLR whose onset latency was 38 ms (*third trace*). Over the right-hand sensory area (*second trace*), a small potential at the same latencies as the SEP on the left was followed by a large positive potential whose latency was 30 ms. Even in the muscle contralateral to the side of stimulation (*left APB*), an LLR was elicited at 47 ms after the stimulation (*bottom trace*). The latency difference between these positive peaks and the onset of responses from a contralateral APB was approximately 16 to 17 ms, which was compatible with cortical latencies of those muscles in cortical stimulation. Latency differences between the two sides were 8 or 9 ms, which were compatible with a transcallosal conduction time. **Lower traces**: Magnetic cortical responses in another patient with cortical myoclonus. Magnetic stimulation over the left-hand motor area elicited responses at 22 ms after the stimulation in the right FDI, and responses at 29 ms in the left FDI. Such ipsilateral responses were never evoked in normal subjects. The difference of onset latencies was again compatible with a transcallosal conduction time.

spheric connection of the hand motor areas of both hemispheres in humans.

Interhemispheric interaction between the motor cortices in humans was first studied by Ferbert et al. (40). They used two stimuli: one was given over one hemisphere, and the other stimulus over the other hemisphere. They found inhibitory interaction through the corpus callosum at ISIs longer than 5 to 6 ms. Later studies on normal subjects (41,42) revealed that the hand motor area has a facilitatory connection with the homotopic area in the contralateral motor cortex, which is surrounded by a larger area of more powerful inhibition (surround inhibition). A point-to-point facilitation surrounded by powerful inhibitory areas is consistent with the effect of callosal stimula-

tion on the motor cortex in animal experiments (43–45). Because the surround effect was so prominent, interhemispheric facilitation was often difficult to observe, or it was seen only when intensities of the conditioning and test stimuli were finely adjusted and they were given strictly over the motor points of both hemispheres (44,45). Under several other conditions, only interhemispheric inhibition was evoked with no facilitation. What occurs in this experiment in patients with cortical myoclonus who should have dysfunction of inhibitory interneurons in the cortex? It is reasonably supposed that interhemispheric facilitation is easily evoked and interhemispheric inhibition is reduced in cortical myoclonus. We show that this is the case in the following paragraph.

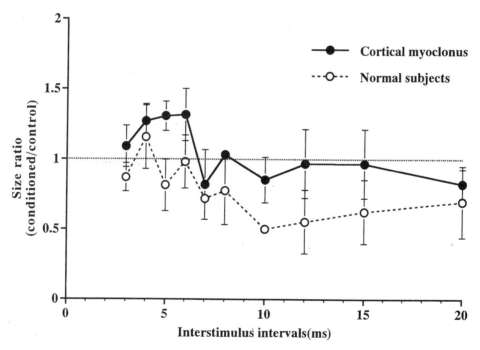

FIG. 10.4. Time courses of effects of a hand motor area stimulation on the excitability of the contralateral hand motor area. In normal subjects (○), suppression was evoked in the contralateral motor cortex at ISIs later than 7 ms with no facilitation at early ISIs. This suppression is considered to be produced by powerful surround inhibition in the motor cortex (42). In contrast, in patients with cortical myoclonus (●), the suppression was not evoked. Moreover, facilitation of the motor cortex was seen at ISIs of approximately 4 to 6 ms. These ISIs taken together with the time required for activation of corticospinal neurones by I3 waves are compatible with the interhemispheric conduction time through the corpus callosum. This facilitation should reflect a homotopic interhemispheric facilitation between bilateral motor cortices. This homotopic facilitatory connection is suppressed by powerful surround inhibition and not apparent in normals. In the patients, it must be released from surround inhibition and could be detected.

EMG responses were recorded from FDIs on both sides. Although we recorded responses from active muscles in the above experiments that revealed interhemispheric facilitation in normals, we used relaxed muscles in this experiment because the patients cannot make constant contraction due to myoclonic jerks. As the test stimulus, we gave a magnetic stimulus that induced posteriorly directed currents in the brain. Its intensity was adjusted to evoke a response with an amplitude of approximately 0.1 to 0.3 mV in the relaxed FDI. As the conditioning stimulus, we used a magnetic stimulus over the motor point of the conditioning motor cortex, which induced medially directed currents in the brain. Its intensity was fixed at just above the active threshold. Under this condition, interhemispheric inhibition at later intervals was evoked, and no facilitation was seen, which is usual in normals. Figure 10.4 shows mean (±SE) time courses of transcallosal effects in normals and patients. Interhemispheric inhibition was evoked at ISIs later than 7 ms in normals. In contrast, in patients with cortical myoclonus, facilitation was seen at ISIs of 4 to 6 ms, and no inhibition was evoked at later intervals (46). These results suggest that in cortical myoclonus, involvement of motor cortical inhibitory interneurons must release the interhemispheric facilitatory connection, which is masked by powerful surround inhibition in normals. This release should explain longer latency EMG responses to focal magnetic stimuli over the ipsilateral motor cortex in cortical myoclonus.

CONCLUSION

Disinhibition or hyperexcitability of the sensorimotor cortex is responsible for cortical myoclonus, irrespective of causes for disinhibition. This disinhibition reflects involvement of cortical inhibitory interneurons. Abnormally enhanced responses of the sensorimotor cortex to transcallosal inputs must produce LLRs in muscles contralateral to the activated peripheral nerve, and they also cause responses to a focal magnetic stimulation in muscles ipsilateral to the side of stimulation.

REFERENCES

1. Tassinari CA, Rubboli G, Shibasaki H. Neurophysiology of positive and negation myoclonus. *Electroencephalogr Clin Neurophysiol* 1998;107:181–195.
2. Shibasaki H, Yamashita Y, Tobimatsu S, et al. Electroencephalographic correlates of myoclonus. *Adv Neurol* 1986;43:357–372.
3. Rothwell JC, Obeso JA, Marsden CD. Electrophysiology of somatosensory reflex myoclonus. *Adv Neurol* 1986;43:385–398.
4. Shibasaki H. Pathophysiology of negative myoclonus and asterixis. *Adv Neurol* 1995;67:199–209.
5. Ugawa Y, Uesaka Y, Terao Y, et al. Pathophysiology of sensorimotor cortex in cortical myoclonus. *Clin Neurosci* 1996;3:198–202.
6. Rothwell JC, Brown P. The spread of myoclonic activity through sensorimotor cortex in cortical reflex myoclonus. *Adv Neurol* 1995;67:143–155.
7. Shibasaki, H. Electrophysiological studies of myoclonus. AAEE minimonograph no. 30. *Muscle Nerve* 1988;11:899–907.
8. Shibasaki H. Myoclonus. *Curr Opin Neurol* 1995;8:331–334.
9. Obseo JA, Rothwell JC, Marsden CD. The spectrum of cortical myoclonus: from focal reflex jerks to spontaneous motor epilepsy. *Brain* 1985;108:193–224.
10. Tassinari CA, Rubboli G, Parmeggiani L, et al. Epileptic negative myoclonus. *Adv Neurol* 1995;67:181–197.
11. Toro C, Hallett M, Rothwell JC, et al. Physiology of negative myoclonus. *Adv Neurol* 1995;67:211–217.
12. Mima T, Nagamine T, Ikeda A, et al. Pathogenesis of cortical myoclonus studied with magnetoencephalography. *Ann Neurol* 1998;43:598–607.
13. Mima T, Nagamine T, Nishitani N, et al. Cortical myoclonus: sensorimotor hyperexcitability. *Neurology* 1998;50:933–942.
14. Uesaka Y, Ugawa Y, Yumoto M, et al. Giant somatosensory evoked magnetic field in patients with myoclonus epilepsy. *Electroencephalogr Clin Neurophysiol* 1993;87:300–305.
15. Uesaka Y, Terao Y, Ugawa Y, et al. Magnetoencephalographic analysis of cortical myoclonic jerks. *Electroencephalogr Clin Neurophysiol* 1996;99:141–148.
16. Shibasaki H, Neshige R. Photic cortical reflex myoclonus. *Ann Neurol* 1987;22:252–257.
17. Yokota T, Tsukagoshi H. Cortical activity-associated negative myoclonus. *J Neurol Sci* 1992;111:77–81.
18. Shibasaki H, Kuroiwa Y. Electroencephalographic correlates of myoclonus. *Electroencephalogr Clin Neurophysiol* 1975;39:455–463.
19. Shibasaki H, Yamashita Y, Kuroiwa Y. Electroencephalographic studies of myoclonus: myoclonus-related cortical spikes and high amplitude somatosensory evoked potentials. *Brain* 1978;101:447–460.
20. Shibasaki H, Yamashita Y, Neshige R, et al. Pathogenesis of giant somatosensory evoked potentials in progressive myoclonus epilepsy. *Brain* 1985;108:225–240.
21. Cowan JM, Rothwell JC, Wise RJ, et al. Electrophysiological and positron emission studies in a patient with cortical myoclonus, epilepsia partials continua and motor epilepsy. *J Neurol Neurosurg Psychiatry* 1986;49:796–807.
22. Rothwell JC, Obeso JA, Marsden CD. On the significance of giant somatosensory evoked potentials in cortical myoclonus. *J Neurosurg Psychiatry* 1984;47:33–42.

23. Celesia GG, Parmeggiani L, Brigell M. Dipole source localization in a case of epilepsia partialis continua without premyoclonic EEG spikes. *Electroencephalogr Clin Neurophysiol* 1994;90:316–319.

24. Hanajima R, Terao Y, Ugawa Y, et al. Magnetoencephalographic analysis of epilepsia partials continua in a patient with RSSE. In: Kimura J, Shibasaki H, eds. *Recent advances in clinical neurophysiology* Amsterdam: Elsevier, 1996;867–871.

25. Kujirai T, Caramia MD, Rothwell JC, et al. Cortico-cortical inhibition in human motor cortex. *J Physiol* 1993; 471:501–520.

26. Ziemann U, Lönnecher S, Steinhoff BJ, et al. Effects of antiepileptic drugs on motor cortex excitability in humans: a transcranial magnetic stimulation study. *Ann Neurol* 1996;40:367–378.

27. Brown P, Ridding MC, Werhahn KJ, et al. Abnormalities of the balance between inhibition and excitation in the motor cortex of patients with cortical myoclonus. *Brain* 1996;119:309–317.

28. Hanajima R, Ugawa Y, Terao Y, et al. Ipsilateral corticocortical inhibition of the motor cortex in various neurological disorders. *J Neurol Sci* 1996;140:109–116.

29. Hallett M, Chadwick D, Marsden CD. Cortical reflex myoclonus. *Neurology* 1979;29:1107–1125.

30. Kakigi R, Shibasaki H. Generator mechanisms of giant somatosensory evoked potentials in cortical reflex myoclonus. *Brain* 1987;110:1359–1373.

31. Ikeda A, Shibasaki H, Nagamine T, et al. Peri-rolandic and frontoparietal components of scalp-recorded giant SEPs in cortical myoclonus. *Electroencephalogr Clin Neurophysiol* 1995;96:300–309.

32. Veleriani M, Restuccia D, DiLazzaro V, et al. The pathophysiology of giant SEPs in cortical myoclonus: a scalp topography and dipole source modelling study. *Electroencephalogr Clin Neurophysiol* 1997;104:122–131.

33. Ashby P, Chen R, Wennberg R, et al. Cortical reflex myoclonus studied with cortical electrodes. *Clin Neurophysiol* 1999;110:1521–1530.

34. Ugawa Y, Genba K, Shimpo T, et al. Somatosensory evoked potential recovery (SEP-R) in myoclonic patients. *Electroencephalogr Clin Neurophysiol* 1991;80: 21–25.

35. Ugawa Y, Genba-Shimizu K, Kanazawa I. Somatosensory evoked potential recovery (SEP-K) in various neurological disorders. *Electroencephalogr Clin Neurophysiol* 1996;100:62–67.

36. Wilkins DF, Hallett M, Berardelli A, et al. Physiologic analysis of the myoclonus of Alzheimer's disease. *Neurology* 1984;34:898–903.

37. Thompson PD, Rothwell JC, Brown P, et al. Transcallosal and intracortical spread of activity following cortical stimulation in a patient with generalized cortical myoclonus [abstract]. *J Physiol* 1993;459: 6P.

38. Brown P, Day BL, Rothwell JC, et al. Intra-hemispheric and inter-hemispheric spread of cerebral cortical myoclonic activity and its relevance to epilepsy. *Brain* 1991;114:2333–2352.

39. Rothwell JC, Brown P. The spread of myoclonic activity through sensorimotor cortex in cortical reflex myoclonus. *Adv Neurol* 1995;67:143–155.

40. Ferbert A, Priori A, Rothwell JC, et al. Inter-hemispheric inhibition of the human motor cortex. *J Physiol* 1992;453:526–546.

41. Ugawa Y, Hanajima R, Kanazawa I. Interhemispheric facilitation of the hand area of the human motor cortex. *Neurosci Lett* 1993;160:153–155.

42. Hanajima R, Ugawa Y, Machii K, et al. Interhemispheric facilitation of the hand motor area in humans. *J Physiol* 2001;531:849-859.

43. Chang HT. Cortical response to activity of callosal neurons. *J Neurophysiol* 1953;16:117–131.

44. Asanuma H, Okamoto K. Unitary study on evoked activity of callosal neurons and its effect on pyramidal tract cell activity on cats. *Jpn J Physiol* 1959;9:437–483.

45. Asanuma H, Okuda O. Effects of transcallosal valleys on pyramidal tract all activity of cat. *J Physiol* 1962;25: 198–208.

46. Hanajima R, Ugawa Y, Okabe S, et al. Interhemispheric interaction between the hand motor areas in patients with cortical myoclonus. *Clin Neurophysiol* 2001;112: 793–799.

Myoclonus and Paroxysmal Dyskinesias,
Advances in Neurology, Vol. 89,
edited by S. Fahn, et al.
Published by Lippincott Williams & Wilkins, Philadelphia, 2002.

11

Neurophysiology of Brainstem Myoclonus

Mark Hallett

Human Motor Control Section, National Institute of Neurological Disorders and Stroke,
National Institutes of Health, Bethesda, Maryland

Myoclonus reflects an exaggerated hyperactivity of the nervous system and may originate at almost any level. Of subcortical sites (but above the spinal cord), myoclonus arising from the reticular formation is the best understood (1). Other sites have been proposed, such as the thalamus (2,3), but detailed physiology is lacking. Three types of brainstem myoclonus are reticular reflex myoclonus, exaggerated startle, and palatal myoclonus (palatal tremor). There is some evidence that the relevant pathophysiology of opsoclonus-myoclonus syndrome is in the brainstem, but this is not yet clear (4). Only reticular reflex myoclonus is covered here.

The notion of myoclonus coming from the brainstem originated with an animal model, myoclonus resulting from the administration of urea (5–7). In the rat, with urea-induced myoclonus, there were no EEG discharges related to myoclonic discharges and no enlarged SEP components. On the other hand, such EEG changes were seen with catechol-induced myoclonus, which is a model of cortical myoclonus. The C reflex in urea-induced myoclonus is not reduced by sensorimotor cortex lesions (6). Moreover, the latency of the C reflex was 10.2 ms, shorter than the C reflex with catechol-induced myoclonus which was 13.4 ms. This is compatible with a subcortical origin for urea-induced myoclonus. Detailed investigations showed that the origin of the myoclonus was in the nucleus reticularis gigantocellularis where paroxys-

mal depolarization shifts (PDSs) were found with intracellular recording (5). It is not certain how urea induces myoclonus, but there is some evidence that it inhibits glycine binding (8); this would give it some similarity to hereditary hyperekplexia (9).

A human correlate of the animal model appears to be what is now called reticular reflex myoclonus. Myoclonus can be divided into two broad categories, epileptic and non-epileptic, depending on its relationship to epilepsy. Reticular reflex myoclonus can be said to be a fragment of a type of generalized epilepsy since the cellular correlate is a PDS. Some authorities argue that epilepsy must have a cortical origin, and, if this argument is accepted, then reticular reflex myoclonus is non-epileptic.

From a clinical point of view, the jerks of reticular reflex myoclonus are usually generalized with predominance that is proximal more than distal and flexor more than extensor. Voluntary action (intention myoclonus) and sensory stimulation (reflex myoclonus) increase the jerking.

Reticular reflex myoclonus was first described in the setting of chronic post-hypoxic myoclonus, the Lance-Adams syndrome (1). Subsequent cases have also been described (10,11). It has also been described in the setting of renal insufficiency (12), not surprising since urea is what precipitates this physiologic type in the rat. One patient with parkinsonism had myoclonus with physiology consistent with brainstem origin (13). Other single cases have been described in the setting of Lyme disease (14), procarbazine therapy for Hodgkin disease (14), and cervical trauma (15).

It is likely that the myoclonus seen in the acute post-hypoxic state is also of brainstem origin. This type of myoclonus occurs very shortly after a hypoxic episode and is characterized by generalized, often massive, body jerks (16, 17). Patients are in a deeply comatose state. The jerks can be associated with seizures. The electroencephalogram (EEG) shows bursts of generalized spike and polyspike activity with the jerks and can often be silent in between (burst suppression pattern) (16,17). The myoclonus can be stimulus sensitive (16,18). While some of these patients survive, most die. The physiology of this state has not been studied in detail, but the my-

oclonus likely arises from a brainstem generator. One reason for postulating this is that the cortex is severely damaged in this state and may not be capable of generating activity. Additionally, generalized jerks are characteristic of a brainstem origin.

With reticular reflex myoclonus, there are brief generalized EMG bursts lasting 10 to 30 ms that are triggered by sensory stimulation such as touch or muscle stretch or by action (Fig. 11.1). The EEG correlates, if present, are generalized spike and wave discharges that are not time locked to the muscle activation (Fig. 11.2). The pattern of EMG activation in cranial nerve muscles, when involved, is with the sternocleidomastoid muscle activated first and the other cranial nerve muscles activated in reverse numerical order.

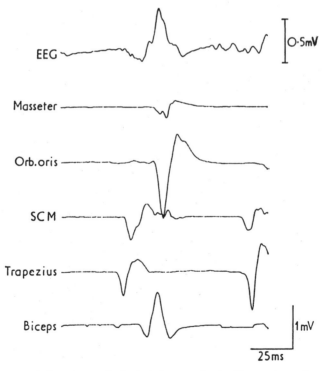

FIG. 11.1. Spontaneous induced myoclonic jerk in a patient with posthypoxic reticular reflex myoclonus. Note that sternocleidomastoid and trapezius precede orbicularis oris which itself precedes masseter. The earliest electromyographic activity precedes the earliest electroencephalographic discharge. (From Hallett M, Chadwick D, Adam J, et al. Reticular reflex myoclonus: a physiological type of human post-hypoxic myoclonus. *J Neurol Neurosurg Psychiatry* 1977;40:253–264, with permission.)

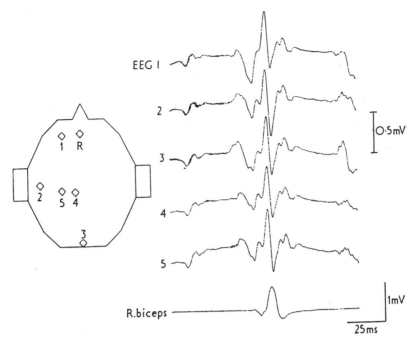

FIG. 11.2. Electroencephalogram (EEG) correlate to a spontaneous jerk in the same patient as in Figure 11.1. Note a widespread spike discharge. This is a single sweep; the EEG spike was not time locked to the electromyogram. (From Hallett M, Chadwick D, Adam J, et al. Reticular reflex myoclonus: a physiological type of human post-hypoxic myoclonus. *J Neurol Neurosurg Psychiatry* 1977;40:253–264, with permission.)

A variant of reticular reflex myoclonus has been called carotid brainstem reflex myoclonus (19). A patient comatose after acute anoxia developed bilaterally synchronous, periodic myoclonic jerks most prominently in the bilateral upper limbs. Although the myoclonus seemed to occur spontaneously, electrophysiologic studies showed that the myoclonic jerks correlated in timing and size with arterial pulses and were suppressed by massage over the carotid sinus. The authors proposed that the myoclonus was a brainstem reflex triggered by the arterial pulses.

Detailed analysis of the relative timing of jerks in different muscles gives information about central nervous system efferent conduction times (1). The latencies of C reflexes after stimulation at different body levels makes it possible to obtain information about the afferent pathways to the brainstem that mediate the myoclonus. Calculations showed a rapid spinal cord efferent conduction time (but slower conduction up the brainstem). The afferent spinal cord conduction time was slow. This pattern of conduction times differs from startle where afferent conduction is fast and efferent conduction is slow (20).

In human investigations and animal studies, reticular reflex myoclonus and cortical reflex myoclonus can coexist (21). In one case of post-hypoxic myoclonus, the action myoclonus was cortical, and the sensory-induced myoclonus was reticular (22).

In two patients with posthypoxic myoclonus who were thought on clinical and electrophysiologic grounds to have reticular reflex myoclonus, thyrotropin-releasing hormone (TRH) enhanced the onset of myoclonus, shortened the latency of the C reflex and increased its amplitude, but produced no change in the SEP (23). These results are consistent with the concept that TRH stimulates medullary reticular neurons, thereby enhancing reticular reflex myoclonus. No such changes are seen in cortical reflex myoclonus. Hence, the TRH test may be helpful as a diagnostic aid.

Treatment of reticular reflex myoclonus may differ from cortical myoclonus. Patients may well respond to clonazepam (12,24,25), and the response can be better than cortical myoclonus. This is also true for the response to 5-hydroxytryptophan (24), but this agent is no longer widely used. On the other hand, only cortical myoclonus seems to respond to piracetam (26,27).

REFERENCES

1. Hallett M, Chadwick D, Adam J, et al. Reticular reflex myoclonus: a physiological type of human post-hypoxic myoclonus. *J Neurol Neurosurg Psychiatry* 1977;40:253-264.
2. Jacob PC, Chand RP. A posttraumatic thalamic lesion associated with contralateral action myoclonus. *Mov Disord* 1999;14:512-514.
3. Gatto EM, Zurru MC, Rugilo C, et al. Focal myoclonus associated with posterior thalamic hematoma. *Mov Disord* 1998;13:182-184.
4. Tsutada T, Izumi T, Murakami T. Correlation of clinical improvement with pontine lesions in opsoclonus-myoclonus syndrome. *Osaka City Med J* 1996;42:53-60.
5. Zuckermann EG, Glaser GH. Urea-induced myoclonic seizures. An experimental study of site of action and mechanism. *Arch Neurol* 1972;27:14-28.
6. Touge T, Takeuchi H, Yamada A, et al. Electrophysiological comparison between catechol- and urea-induced myoclonus models in the rat. *Int J Neurosci* 1993;71:159-171.
7. Muscatt S, Rothwell J, Obeso J, et al. Urea-induced stimulus-sensitive myoclonus in the rat. *Adv Neurol* 1986;43:553-563.
8. Chung E, Yocca F, Van Woert MH. Urea-induced myoclonus: medullary glycine antagonism as mechanism of action. *Life Sci* 1985;36:1051-1058.
9. Floeter MK, Hallett M. Glycine receptors: a startling connection. *Nature Genetics* 1993;5:319-320.
10. Werhahn KJ, Brown P, Thompson PD, et al. The clinical features and prognosis of chronic posthypoxic myoclonus. *Mov Disord* 1997;12:216-220.
11. Hallett M. Physiology of posthypoxic myoclonus. *Mov Disord* 2000;15(Suppl 1):8-13.
12. Chadwick D, French AT. Uraemic myoclonus: an example of reticular reflex myoclonus? *J Neurol Neurosurg Psychiatry* 1979;42:52-55.
13. Clouston PD, Lim CL, Fung V, Yiannikas C, et al. Brainstem myoclonus in a patient with non-dopa-responsive parkinsonism. *Mov Disord* 1996;11:404-410.
14. Rektor I, Kadanka Z, Bednarik J. Reflex reticular myoclonus: relationship to some brainstem pathophysiological mechanisms. *Acta Neurol Scand* 1991;83:221-225.
15. Bettoni L, Bortone E, Dascola I, et al. Transient traumatic reticular myoclonus. Case report. *Funct Neurol* 1990;5:365-370.
16. Van Cott AC, Blatt I, Brenner RP. Stimulus-sensitive seizures in postanoxic coma. *Epilepsia* 1996;37:868-874.
17. Young GB, Gilbert JJ, Zochodne DW. The significance of myoclonic status epilepticus in postanoxic coma. *Neurology* 1990;40:1843-1848.
18. Niedermeyer E, Bauer G, Burnite R, et al. Selective stimulus-sensitive myoclonus in acute cerebral anoxia. A case report. *Arch Neurol* 1977;34:365-368.
19. Hanakawa T, Hashimoto S, Iga K, et al. Carotid brainstem reflex myoclonus after hypoxic brain damage. *J Neurol Neurosurg Psychiatry* 2000;69:672-674.
20. Brown P, Rothwell JC, Thompson PD, et al. The hyperekplexias and their relationship to the normal startle reflex. *Brain* 1991;114:1903-1928.
21. Hallett M. Myoclonus and myoclonic syndromes. In: Engel JJ, Pedley TA, ed. *Epilepsy: A Comprehensive Textbook*. Philadelphia: Lippincott-Raven; 1997:2717-2723.
22. Brown P, Thompson PD, Rothwell JC, et al. A case of postanoxic encephalopathy with cortical action and brainstem reticular reflex myoclonus. *Mov Disord* 1991;6:139-144.
23. Takeuchi H, Touge T, Miki H, et al. Electrophysiological and pharmacological studies of somatosensory reflex myoclonus. *Electromyogr Clin Neurophysiol* 1992;32:143-154.
24. Chadwick D, Hallett M, Harris R, et al. Clinical, biochemical, and physiological features distinguishing myoclonus responsive to 5-hydroxytryptophan, tryptophan with a monoamine oxidase inhibitor, and clonazepam. *Brain* 1977;100:455-487.
25. Witte OW, Niedermeyer E, Arendt G, et al. Post-hypoxic action (intention) myoclonus: a clinico-electroencephalographic study. *J Neurol* 1988;235:214-218.
26. Obeso JA, Artieda J, Quinn N, et al. Piracetam in the treatment of different types of myoclonus. *Clin Neuropharm* 1988;11:529-536.
27. Brown P, Steiger MJ, Thompson PD, et al. Effectiveness of piracetam in cortical myoclonus. *Mov Disord* 1993;8:63-68.

Myoclonus and Paroxysmal Dyskinesias,
Advances in Neurology, Vol. 89,
edited by S. Fahn and S. J. Frucht.
Lippincott Williams & Wilkins, Philadelphia © 2002.

12

Physiology of Negative Myoclonus

Hiroshi Shibasaki

Department of Neurology, Kyoto University,
Shogoin, Sakyo–ku, Kyoto, Japan

The history of negative myoclonus goes back to 1949 when Adams and Foley (1) described quasi-rhythmic involuntary movements of fingers during active maintenance of posture in patients with hepatic encephalopathy. Later they demonstrated a brief lapse of electromyographic (EMG) discharge in association with those movements, and introduced the term *asterixis* (2). In 1976, Shahani and Young (3) coined the term *negative myoclonus*, and later they characterized asterixis as one type of negative myoclonus (4). Tassinari (5) in 1981 introduced the term *epileptic negative myoclonus* (ENM) for negative myoclonus of epileptic nature that can be seen in patients with different types of epilepsy. Since 1994 when the Workshop on Negative Motor Phenomena was held in Atlanta (6), there has been some progress in the understanding of negative myoclonus. This chapter reviews the more recent literature and discusses the possible mechanisms underlying the generation of negative myoclonus.

CLASSIFICATION OF NEGATIVE MYOCLONUS

Obeso et al. (7) classified negative myoclonus into four clinical categories: physiologic negative myoclonus, asterixis, postural lapses, and ENM. Etiologically, negative myoclonus can be classified into at least three groups: (a) ENM; (b) asterixis seen in patients with metabolic or toxic encephalopathy, hepatic encephalopathy in particular; and (c) unilateral asterixis due to focal central nervous system (CNS) lesions. ENM is usually seen in patients with partial epilepsy, and the cerebral cortex, especially the sensorimotor cortex in the wide meaning, is involved in its pathogenesis (5,8,9). Asterixis seen in most cases of metabolic or toxic encephalopathy is considered to be subcortical in its origin, but the cerebral cortex might be also involved in some cases (10,11). The responsible sites for unilateral asterixis are variable, but cases associated with thalamic lesions have been most commonly reported (12).

EPILEPTIC NEGATIVE MYOCLONUS

Electroencephalographic Correlates of Epileptic Negative Myoclonus

In ENM, the EMG silent period is often preceded by an abrupt increase in the EMG discharge. In this chapter, this complex of positive followed by negative myoclonus is called *complex negative myoclonus* in contrast with *pure negative myoclonus*. In the well-known paper on posthypoxic myoclonus published by Lance and Adams (13) in 1963, they paid special attention to the relationship of the initial EMG burst and the following silent period to the electroencephalographic (EEG) spike and the following slow wave, respectively. They noted the comparable duration of the EEG slow wave and the EMG silent period. Furthermore, they found that the H reflexes were elicited during the silent periods, suggesting that the inhibition did not take place at the spinal cord level (13). Oguni et al. (14) reported seven children with partial epilepsy who manifested unilateral brief atonia associated with a single sharp and slow wave complex on the contralateral EEG. They found significant correlation between the amplitude of the EEG sharp activity at the centroparietal region and the intensity of the atonia (14). In other words, the larger the paroxysmal EEG activity, the more prominent was the observed atonia.

Generating Mechanisms of Paroxysmal Electroencephalographic Activity Associated With Epileptic Negative Myoclonus

As for the generator source of the cortical epileptic activity associated with the negative myoclonus, Baumgartner et al. (15) reported a patient presenting with brief repetitive lapses in postural tone of the right upper extremity, the onset of which was preceded by the left frontal EEG spike by 20 to 40 ms. In their case, the EEG spike was estimated to arise from the left premotor cortex. They further showed, by using single photon emission computed tomography superimposed on magnetic resonance imaging, an increased blood flow in the left middle frontal gyrus during the episodes of negative myoclonus of the right upper limb (15). Rubboli et al. (16) also reported an epileptic patient whose interictal EEG spikes were either associated with or without the EMG silent periods. By using the technique of spike averaging, they demonstrated that the EEG spikes associated with the EMG silent period consisted of two peaks, whereas those spikes without the associated EMG silent period had a single peak. The first peak of

the spikes associated with the silent period and the peak without the associated silent period were maximal at the contralateral central region, whereas the second peak of the spikes associated with the silent period was maximal at the contralateral frontal region (Fig. 12.1) (16). These findings suggest that the ENM of upper limb in those cases might be related to an epileptic activity in the contralateral premotor area. Lüders et al. (17) defined the negative motor area as the cortical areas where repetitive electric stimulation at high frequency (50 Hz) causes the inability to continue voluntary phasic movements or sustained muscle contraction without disturbance of consciousness. The question as to whether or not the premotor areas found by Baumgartner et al. (15) and Rubboli et al. (16) correspond to the primary negative motor area as defined by Lüders et al. (17) remains to be clarified.

Postural Lapses

Involvement of axial and leg muscles by ENM is particularly disabling to patients because they tend to fall abruptly (drop attack). In a patient with progressive myoclonus epilepsy who frequently showed complex negative myoclonus while standing, being associated with silent periods in leg EMGs following an abrupt EMG burst (Fig. 12.2), back-averaging of the simultaneously recorded EEG with respect to the onset of the muscle jerk showed a small spike followed by a slow wave maximal at the midline vertex (Cz electrode) (Fig. 12.3). By contrast, back-averaging of the EEG with respect to the onset of the EMG silent period by using the method of Ugawa et al. (18) showed a less-conspicuous sharp activity that was maximal at the frontal region and similarly followed by a central slow wave (Fig. 12.4). In this case, therefore, the EMG silence was more precisely time locked to the EEG slow wave than to the preceding sharp activity (Matsumoto, *unpublished data*).

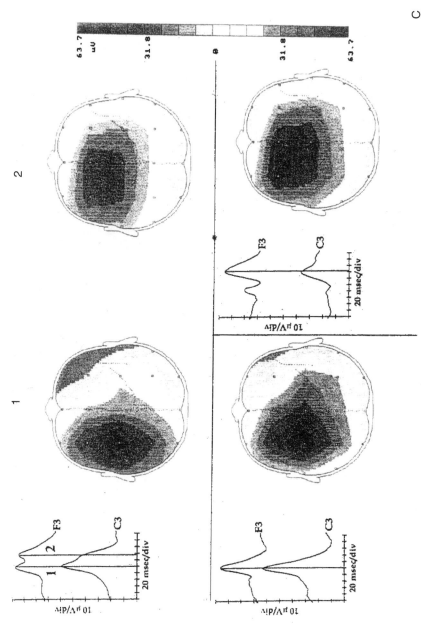

FIG. 12.1. Topography of electroencephalographic spikes associated with (**A**) and without (**B**) negative myoclonus in a patient with epileptic negative myoclonus. Data of peak averaging. The second peak of the spike associated with negative myoclonus (*A-2*) is maximal slightly more anterior to the preceding peak (*A-1*) or to the spike without the associated negative myoclonus (**B**). **C:** data obtained by subtracting (**B**) from (**A**). (From Rubboli G, Parmeggiani L, Tassinari CA. Frontal inhibitory spike component associated with epileptic negative myoclonus. *Electroencephalogr Clin Neurophysiol* 1995;95:201–205, with permission.)

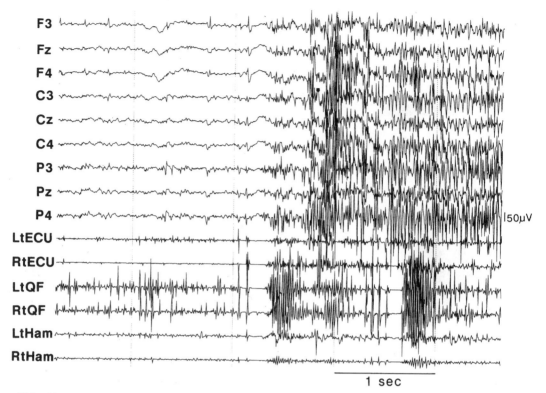

FIG. 12.2. Electroencephalogram/electromyogram (EEG/EMG) polygraph recorded in a patient with progressive myoclonus epilepsy while standing. Note an EMG burst followed by a long clear silent period associated with a spike and wave on the EEG in the middle of the record. (Courtesy of Dr. Riki Matsumoto and Dr. Akio Ikeda.)

Role of the Sensorimotor Cortex

The primary somatosensory and motor cortices seem to be essential for the generation of ENM. Noachtar et al. (19) reported a patient presenting with unilateral ENM due to the contralateral postcentral cortical dysplasia in whom they had an opportunity to record cortical activities from subdurally implanted electrodes. In their case, repetitive spikes from the left postcentral area were consistently followed by an EMG silent period in the right arm, with the time interval of 20 to 30 ms (Fig. 12.5). Furthermore, they found a positive correlation between the size of the EEG spike and the duration of the EMG silent period. In relation to this, Ikeda et al. (20) recently investigated the effect of a single electric shock applied to subdurally implanted electrodes at the perirolandic region in three patients with medically intractable partial epilepsy. In all patients, single pulse stimulation of some parts of the sensorimotor cortex elicited a motor evoked potential (MEP) followed by a silent period lasting 300 ms in the contralateral distal hand muscles. In these cases, the duration of the silent period was proportional to the size of the preceding MEP. It was noteworthy that stimulation of some electrodes, although rare, elicited a pure silent period without any preceding MEP. In the latter case, the stronger stimulus elicited the longer silent period (Fig. 12.6) (20). As regards the primary and supplementary negative motor areas defined by Lüders et al. (17), single pulse stimulation of at least the primary negative motor area produced no silent period in the EMG (20).

PME, Standing

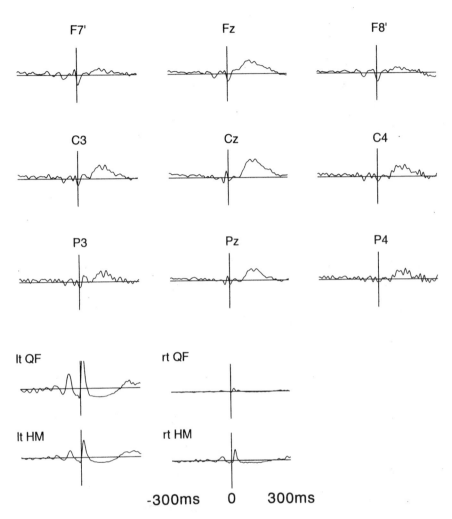

FIG. 12.3. Back-average of electroencephalogram (EEG) with respect to the onset of the electromyogram (EMG) burst of the left quadriceps femoris muscle in the same patient as shown in Figure 12.2. A small EEG spike, maximal at the central vertex (Cz), precedes the EMG onset and is followed by a slow wave. (Courtesy by Dr. Riki Matsumoto and Dr. Akio Ikeda.)

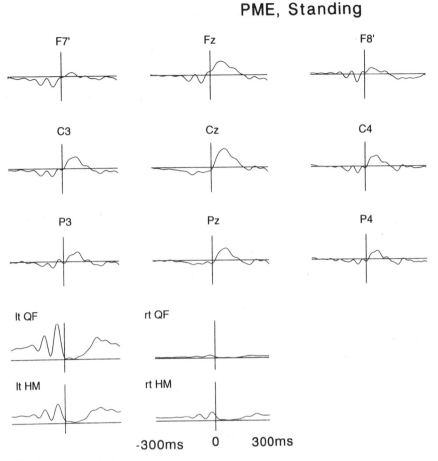

FIG. 12.4. Back-average of electroencephalogram with respect to the onset of the electromyogram silent period recorded from the left quadriceps femoris muscle in the same patient as shown in Figures 12.2 and 12.3. The slow wave starts just at the onset of the silent period and is maximal at Cz. The preceding spike is now less sharp and maximal at the frontal region (F7′, Fz, and F8′). (Courtesy of Dr. Riki Matsumoto and Dr. Akio Ikeda.)

Stimulus Sensitivity

Just like positive myoclonus of cortical origin, ENM can be evoked by somatosensory stimulation (cortical reflex negative myoclonus) (21). In this case, the reflex negative myoclonus is preceded by giant somatosensory evoked potentials (SEPs), and based on the analysis of nonaveraged single data, a significant positive correlation is seen between the amplitude of the giant SEP and the duration of the EMG silent period (21). However, there was no correlation between the duration of the silent period and the size of the preced-

ing C reflex (EMG evoked by the stimuli) (21). Thus, the larger the SEP, the more prominent was the elicited negative myoclonus. The same finding was reported in a patient with Creutzfeldt-Jakob disease who showed negative myoclonus (22). In these patients with cortical reflex negative myoclonus, the recovery function of the SEP, which is studied by paired pulse stimulation with various interstimulus intervals, showed a markedly prolonged recovery, comparable to the duration of the elicited EMG silent period (21,22). This is in strong contrast with the SEP recovery function observed in patients with

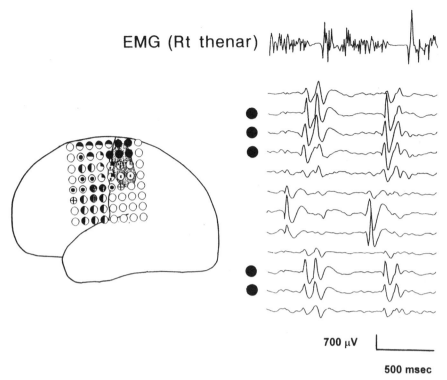

EMG (Rt thenar)

700 μV

500 msec

FIG. 12.5. Subdurally recorded electroencephalogram in association with epileptic negative my-oclonus of the right upper limb in a patient with cortical dysplasia in the left postcentral region. The silent period in the electromyogram of the right thenar muscle is preceded by a cortical spike local-ized to the left postcentral gyrus, including the sensory area corresponding to the right arm. (From Noachtar S, Holthausen H, Lüders HO. Epileptic negative myoclonus: subdural EEG recordings in-dicate a postcentral generator. *Neurology* 1997;49:1534–1537, with permission.)

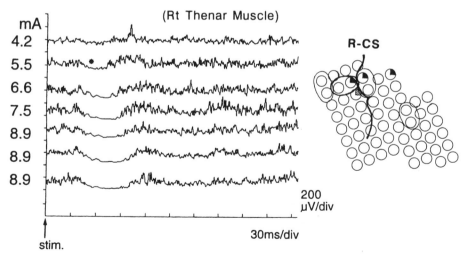

(Rt Thenar Muscle)

mA
4.2
5.5
6.6
7.5
8.9
8.9
8.9

R-CS

200 μV/div

30ms/div

stim.

FIG. 12.6. Pure electromyogram silent period induced in the left abductor pollicis brevis muscle by single pulse electric stimulation of an area of the right postcentral gyrus (identified as the motor area by stimulation study) in a patient with focal motor seizure. Note an increasing duration of the induced silent period with the increasing stimulus intensity. (From Ikeda A, Ohara S, Matsumoto R, et al. Role of primary sensorimotor cortices in generating inhibitory motor response in humans. *Brain* 2000; 123:1710–1721, with permission.)

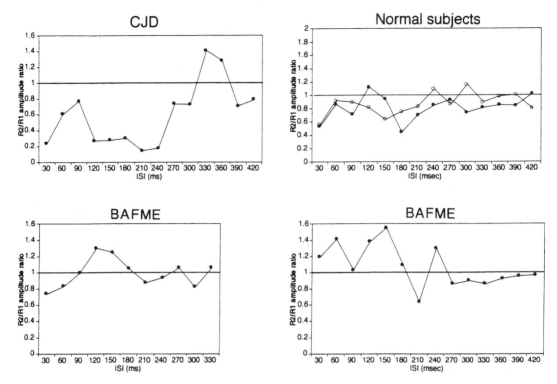

FIG. 12.7. Recovery curve of somatosensory evoked potential (SEP) following electric stimulation of the median nerve in a patient with Creutzfeldt-Jakob disease presenting with negative myoclonus, in comparison with two patients with benign adult familial myoclonic epilepsy and normal subjects. Note a prolonged recovery function of SEP in the patient with negative myoclonus compared to others. (From Matsunaga K, Uozumi T, Akamatsu N, et al. Negative myoclonus in Creutzfeldt-Jakob disease. *Clin Neurophysiol* 2000;111:471–476, with permission.)

cortical reflex positive myoclonus (Fig. 12.7) (21,22). These findings suggest the important role of the primary somatosensory cortex in the generation of reflex negative myoclonus. The cortical reflex negative myoclonus can be also caused by photic stimulation (23).

Excitability of the Motor Cortex

Excitability of the primary motor cortex in ENM was recently studied by Matsunaga et al. (22), by applying transcranial magnetic stimulation (TMS) to the motor cortex in the above-described patient with Creutzfeldt-Jakob disease manifesting negative myoclonus. The MEP threshold was higher as compared to the patients with cortical positive myoclonus, although it was not different from

that of normal subjects. They found a significantly longer silent period following MEP than that seen in patients with cortical positive myoclonus (Fig. 12.8). In normal subjects, TMS of the motor cortex during sustained muscle contraction with increasing stimulus intensity elicits the EMG silent periods of proportionally longer duration (24,25). It is postulated, therefore, that, in patients with ENM, the inhibitory mechanism of the motor cortex is excessively enhanced.

Possible Mechanisms of Epileptic Negative Myoclonus

Taking the currently available information into account, the following hypothesis can be reached for the possible mechanisms underly-

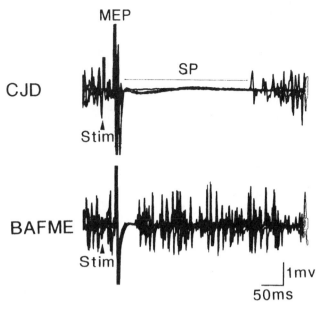

FIG. 12.8. A long silent period of electromyography following motor evoked potential induced in the left abductor pollicis brevis muscle by transcranial magnetic stimulation of the right motor cortex in a patient with Creutzfeldt-Jakob disease presenting with negative myoclonus. Data of a patient with benign adult familial myoclonic epilepsy are shown for control. (From Matsunaga K, Uozumi T, Akamatsu N, et al. Negative myoclonus in Creutzfeldt-Jakob disease. *Clin Neurophysiol* 2000;111: 471–476, with permission.)

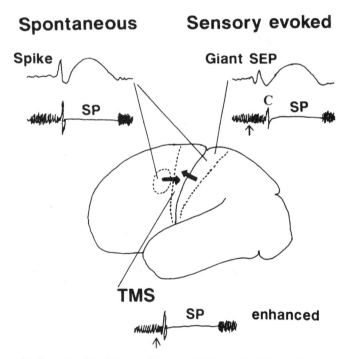

FIG. 12.9. Schematic diagram showing possible mechanisms underlying the generation of epileptic negative myoclonus. The inhibitory function of the primary motor cortex is enhanced as demonstrated by transcranial magnetic stimulation. Inputs into the primary motor cortex from the spontaneous epileptic activity arising either in the premotor area or in the somatosensory cortex, or as the result of sensory stimulation via enhanced excitability of the sensory cortex, might activate the inhibitory system of the motor cortex, producing negative myoclonus of cortical origin.

ing the generation of ENM. In the patients with ENM, the inhibitory activity of the primary motor cortex tends to be abnormally enhanced. Excessive input into the motor cortex as the result of spontaneous epileptic activities arising either from the premotor areas or the postcentral cortex, or as the result of enhanced excitability of the sensory cortex, may activate the inhibitory motor system that is already hyperactive, and suppress the corticospinal tract volley to the anterior horn cells, thus causing the exaggerated EMG silence or negative myoclonus (Fig. 12.9). Stimulus presentation to the motor cortex at various time points during the spontaneous or induced silent period might provide further insight into this mechanism, although the physiologic events taking place under those circumstances have to be clarified at the cellular level in experimental animal models.

ASTERIXIS IN METABOLIC/TOXIC ENCEPHALOPATHY

Typical asterixis or flapping tremor as seen in patients with hepatic encephalopathy is believed to be of subcortical origin, because its EEG correlates cannot be demonstrated even by silent period-locked back-averaging. However, patients with uremic encephalopathy may show myoclonic jerks or asterixis, or both, which fulfill the criteria of cortical reflex myoclonus (10,26,27).

Some anticonvulsants, especially valproic acid (11) and carbamazepine (28), are known to enhance negative myoclonus. Since these drugs are often used for the treatment of progressive myoclonus epilepsy, it creates a confusing situation. In a patient with progressive myoclonus epilepsy, we observed frequent occurrence of muscle jerks but rare occurrence of negative myoclonus when the blood level of valproic acid was 108 μg/mL, and vice versa when its level was up to 148 μg/mL (Ikeda, *unpublished data*). In this case, it is postulated that excessive effect of anticonvulsants, most likely through GABA-ergic inhibition, might suppress facilitatory function of the motor cortex but on the other hand enhance its inhibitory functions.

UNILATERAL ASTERIXIS CAUSED BY FOCAL CENTRAL NERVOUS SYSTEM LESIONS

Unilateral asterixis has been reported in association with focal lesions in various structures such as thalamus, midbrain, and other motor-related areas in the CNS. Tatu et al. (12) recently reported 11 patients with unilateral asterixis caused by isolated vascular lesion in the contralateral thalamus. The anatomic location in their cases suggested ventral lateral or lateral posterior thalamus as the responsible sites.

REFERENCES

1. Adams RD, Foley JM. The neurological changes in the more common types of severe liver disease. *Trans Am Neurol Assoc* 1949;74:217–219.
2. Adams RD, Foley JM. The neurological disorder associated with liver disease. In: Merritt HH, Hare CC, eds. *Metabolic and toxic diseases of the nervous system.* Baltimore: Williams & Wilkins, 1953:198–237.
3. Shahani BT, Young RR. Physiological and pharmacological aids in the differential diagnosis of tremor. *J Neurol Neurosurg Psychiatry* 1976;39:772–783.
4. Young RR, Shahani BT. Asterixis: one type of negative myoclonus. *Adv Neurol* 1986;43:137–156.
5. Tassinari CA. New perspectives in epileptology. In: Japanese Epilepsy Association, ed. *Trends in modern epileptology—proceedings of the International Public Seminar on Epileptology.* Tokyo: Japanese Epilepsy Association, 1981:42–59.
6. Shibasaki H. Pathophysiology of negative myoclonus and asterixis. *Adv Neurol* 1995;67:199–209.
7. Obeso JA, Artieda J, Burleigh A. Clinical aspects of negative myoclonus. *Adv Neurol* 1995;67:1–7.
8. Guerrini R, Dravet C, Genton P, et al. Epileptic negative myoclonus. *Neurology* 1993;43:1078–1083.
9. Tassinari CA, Rubboli G, Shibasaki H. Neurophysiology of positive and negative myoclonus. *Electroencephalogr Clin Neurophysiol* 1998;107:181–195.
10. Artieda J, Muruzabal J, Larumbe R, et al. Cortical mechanisms mediating asterixis. *Mov Disord* 1992;7:209–216.
11. Aguglia U, Gambardella A, Zappia M, et al. Negative myoclonus during valproate-related stupor: neurophysiological evidence of a cortical non-epileptic origin. *Electroencephalogr Clin Neurophysiol* 1995;94:103–108.
12. Tatu L, Moulin T, Martin V, et al. Unilateral pure thalamic asterixis: clinical, electromyographic, and topographic patterns. *Neurology* 2000;54:2339–2342.
13. Lance JW, Adams RD. The syndrome of intention or action myoclonus as a sequel to hypoxic encephalopathy. *Brain* 1963;86:111–136.
14. Oguni H, Sato F, Hayashi K, et al. A study of unilateral brief focal atonia in childhood partial epilepsy. *Epilepsia* 1992;33:75–83.
15. Baumgartner C, Podreka I, Olbrich A, et al. Epileptic negative myoclonus: An EEG-single-photon emission

CT study indicating involvement of premotor cortex. *Neurology* 1996;46:753–758.

16. Rubboli G, Parmeggiani L, Tassinari CA. Frontal inhibitory spike component associated with epileptic negative myoclonus. *Electroencephalogr Clin Neurophysiol* 1995;95:201–205.

17. Lüders HO, Dinner DS, Morris HH, et al. Cortical electrical stimulation in humans: the negative motor areas. *Adv Neurol* 1995;67:115–129.

18. Ugawa Y, Shimpo T, Mannen T. Physiological analysis of asterixis: silent period locked averaging. *J Neurol Neurosurg Psychiatry* 1989;52:89–93.

19. Noachtar S, Holthausen H, Lüders HO. Epileptic negative myoclonus: subdural EEG recordings indicate a postcentral generator. *Neurology* 1997;49:1534–1537.

20. Ikeda A, Ohara S, Matsumoto R, et al. Role of primary sensorimotor cortices in generating inhibitory motor response in humans. *Brain* 2000;123:1710–1721.

21. Shibasaki H, Ikeda A, Nagamine T, et al. Cortical reflex negative myoclonus. *Brain* 1994;117:477–486.

22. Matsunaga K, Uozumi T, Akamatsu N, et al. Negative myoclonus in Creutzfeldt-Jakob disease. *Clin Neurophysiol* 2000;111:471–476.

23. Gambardella A, Aguglia U, Oliveri RL, et al. Photic-induced epileptic negative myoclonus: a case report. *Epilepsia* 1996;37:492–494.

24. Cantello R, Gianelli M, Civardi C, et al. Magnetic brain stimulation: the silent period after the motor evoked potential. *Neurology* 1992;42:1951–1959.

25. Wilson SA, Lockwood RF, Thickbroom GW, et al. The muscle silent period following transcranial magnetic cortical stimulation. *J Neurol Sci* 1993;114:216–222.

26. Shibasaki H, Yamashita Y, Neshige R, et al. Pathogenesis of giant somatosensory evoked potentials in progressive myoclonic epilepsy. *Brain* 1985;108:225–240.

27. Shibasaki H. Electrophysiological studies of myoclonus. AAEM Minimonogram no. 30. *Muscle Nerve* 2000;23:321–335.

28. Nanba Y, Maegaki Y. Epileptic negative myoclonus induced by carbamazepine in a child with BECTS, benign childhood epilepsy with centrotemporal spikes. *Pediatr Neurol* 1999;21:664–667.

Myoclonus and Paroxysmal Dyskinesias,
Advances in Neurology, Vol. 89,
edited by S. Fahn, et al.
Lippincott Williams & Wilkins, Philadelphia © 2002.

13

Palatal Tremor: The Clinical Spectrum and Physiology of a Rhythmic Movement Disorder

Günther Deuschl and Henrik Wilms

Department of Neurology, Christian-Albrechts-University Kiel, Kiel, Germany

Palatal tremor is a disorder characterized by rhythmic movements of the soft palate and sometimes other muscles innervated by cranial or spinal nerves. During the past century palatal tremor has been classified among the myoclonias and was described under various names (palatal myoclonus, oculo-palatal myoclonus, palatal nystagmus, brainstem or palatal myorhythmia). According to a suggestion of C. David Marsden in 1990 (1), it is today classified among the tremors. Palatal tremor is usually considered to indicate a pathology within the Guillain-Mollaret-triangle (2). However, recent findings (3,4) suggest that this conclusion may be true only for the most common form, symptomatic palatal tremor.

ETIOLOGY

Most of the patients with palatal tremor have a defined cause with a localized lesion mostly within the brainstem or the upper cerebellar peduncle. These patients have symptomatic palatal tremor (SPT). The etiologies reported until 1990 have been summarized elsewhere (3). For the purpose of this review, we performed a Medline search with the search categories "palatal tremor" or "palatal myoclonus" for the time period of 1989-2000, and it showed 123 papers. All the case reports that provided enough information to classify them according to the criteria of our earlier paper (3) have been included in Table 13.1. According to

these criteria, almost 100 new cases have been identified. Some etiologies are new; others became a clearer delineation. A unique hereditary syndrome with palatal tremor, ataxia, tetraparesis, and Rosenthal fiber formations has been described (5). Two very similar families have been discussed to be familial leukodystrophies resembling Alexander disease (6,7). Compared to our knowledge in 1990, the syndrome of progressive ataxia and palatal myoclonus is now more clearly described, and we tend to classify this as a separate entity among the neurodegenerative diseases. Rare conditions are cerebrotendinous xanthomatosis (8) and two autopsy-proved cases with progressive supranuclear palsy and (possibly unrelated) palatal tremor (9,10). In this context it is noteworthy, that palatal tremor was not observed in a large group of 203 cases with autopsy-proved multiple systems atrophy (11), and out of 149 patients with presumed olivopontocerebellar atrophy only one patient had SPT (12). Three with Behçets disease (13-15), one case with Krabbe's disease (16), one case with sclerosing leukoencephalopathy in the setting of polycystic lipo membranous osteodysplasia (17), and one case of specific action palatal tremor in a patient with primary intestinal lymphoma (18) have been described. A first case with a proved multiple sclerosis has been found to have SPT (19), but given the high prevalence of multiple sclerosis, this is an exception from the general rule that the disease does not produce palatal

TABLE 13.1. *Etiology of palatal tremor*

Etiology	Number	Reference
Vascular origin		
Hemorrhage	**14**	
Pontine hemorrhage	3	127
Pontine hemorrhage (case 1)	1	128
Pontine hemorrhage (2 cases)	2	75
Pontine hemorrhage (case 2)	1	13
Pontine hemorrhage	1	129
Cerebellar hemorrhage	1	4
Brainstem hemorrhage	1	4
Pontomesencephalic hemorrhage	1	42
Brainstem hemorrhage	1	122
Pontotegmental hemorrhage	1	130
Pontotegmental hemorrhage	1	131
Brainstem AVM	**2**	
—	1	132
—	1	133
Ischemia	**15**	
Dentate/brainstem	1	41
Cases 2, 5, 6, 8	4	106
Cases 1, 2, 5	3	39
Pons	1	134
Case 3, pons	3	73
—	1	128
Cerebellar/corona radiata	1	135
Cerebellar	1	4
Infectious	**5**	
Cases 4, 7	2	106
Basal meningitis	1	136
Cerebellar abscess	1	4
??	1	137
Autoimmune	**4**	
M. Behçet (case 2)	1	13
M. Behçet	1	14
M. Behçet	1	15
Multiple sclerosis	1	19
Degenerative disease		
Progressive ataxia with palatal myoclonus (case 4)	1	39
Progressive ataxia with palatal myoclonus	1	114
Progressive ataxia with palatal myoclonus	1	76
Progressive ataxia with palatal myoclonus	1	4
Progressive ataxia with palatal myoclonus	1	138
Progressive ataxia, spasticity, and palatal tremor	1	139
Spinocerebellar degeneration (case 2)	1	13
Cerebrotendinous xanthomatosis	1	8
Brainstem/cerebellar atrophy (cases 2, 4)	2	73
Krabbe disease	1	16
Brainstem/cerebellar atrophy (2 cases)	2	22
Hereditary palatal myoclonus, ataxia, tetraparesis, and Rosenthal formations	3	5
Hereditary palatal tremor, ataxia, tetraparesis, and Rosenthal formations (presumed Alexander disease)	3	6
Hereditary palatal tremor, ataxia, tetraparesis, and Rosenthal formations (presumed Alexander disease)	2	7
Progressive supranuclear palsy	1	10
Brainstem/cerebellar atrophy	1	140
Polycystic lipomembranous osteodysplasia with sclerosing leukencephalopathy	1	17
Total	**24**	
Trauma		
Case 3	1	39
—	2	66
—	3	91
Removal of a cerebellar tumor	1	141
Total	**7**	
Essential		
—	1	103
—	2	142
—	1	32
—	1	78
—	2	142
—	4	4
—	1	33
—	1	81
—	1	144
—	1	85
—	1	23
—	1	84
—	2	86
—	2	88
—	1	90
Total	**22**	
Others		
Anoxia	1	145
Fluoxetine (reversible palatal tremor)	1	146
Primary intestinal lymphoma	1	18
Celiac disease	1	147
Epilepsia partialis continua	1	46
Epilepsia partialis continua	1	48
Opercular status myoclonic epilepticus	3	49
Total	**22**	
Cases since 1989 (total)	**102**	

An updated list since 1989, listed according to our earlier classification (3).

tremor. Another possible immunologic etiology has been presented in a patient with abnormal serum IgM protein specifically binding to the specific brainstem and cerebellar nuclei (20). A case with palatal tremor and epilepsy showed antibodies to glutamic acid decarboxylase (21) but testing of further patients failed to show these autoantibodies which are usually found in stiff-person syndromes (18,22,23).

For about one-fourth of the patients with palatal tremor, no etiology could be found. These patients have been classified as essential palatal tremor (EPT) (3). They have neither any medical history nor any clinical finding for a brainstem or cerebellar disease except palatal tremor. Their presenting complaint is usually the ear click and earlier investigations have shown, that the tensor veli palatini is producing these clicks (24).

This distinction holds true for the vast majority of patients and has been widely used during the past 10 years. However, some patients had to be left unclassified in the earlier literature, especially when additional symptoms occur (25-27). As an anecdotal observation we have observed two patients (one of them with Mark Hallett, National Institute of Neurologic Disorders and Stroke, Bethesda, Maryland) who exhibited a psychogenic palatal tremor. Both of the patients were aware of true palatal tremor in other patients and both had a clicking sound that did not originate from the tensor but from clapping movements of the soft palate against the tongue. Special motor skills have been described in two subjects that could produce voluntary clicks by activation of the tensor veli palatini (28). This condition is neither involuntary nor a disease and should not be classified among palatal tremors but considered as a specific motor skill of the subjects.

EPIDEMIOLOGY AND MEDICAL HISTORY

Characteristic differences of symptomatic and essential tremor are discussed in other chapters. The sex distribution, the age at onset and the mean age of the two groups are different when looking at a larger series that was reviewed earlier (3). An onset of EPT after 50 years of age is extremely rare. The duration of the disease is not significantly different in the two conditions as much as can be judged from a literature survey (3). Remissions occur in EPT especially when children are affected (29), but they have not been convincingly demonstrated in SPT. SPT is considered a life-long condition once the movement disorder has started, but long-term follow-up studies of patients are not available and most of the cases have been described within a duration of 10 years after the onset of symptoms.

THE SYMPTOMS AND CLINICAL SIGNS OF PALATAL TREMOR

Palatal Hyperkinesias

Palatal tremor is characterized by rhythmic but usually not sinusoidal movements of the soft palate. The movement of the soft palate may be unilateral or bilateral. The palatal movement of SPT is caused by the levator veli palatini muscle whereas the contraction of EPT is caused by the tensor veli palatini muscle (24). The soft palate is supplied by five different muscles, of which the palatoglossus and the palatopharyngeus muscles are depressors of the soft palate. The levator veli palatini muscle lifts the palate in a posterior direction and thereby tightens the free edge of the palate against the upper pharynx. The uvula muscle stiffens the uvula, and the tensor veli palatini lifts the roof of the soft palate because it is connected with the contralateral tensor through a tendon plate. This tendon is turning around the hamulus of the hard palate bilaterally which is serving as a hypomochlion. The tensor veli palatini inserts at the eustachian tube (30). It is interesting to note that the levator muscle is innervated of by the nucleus ambiguus or facial nucleus, but that the tensor muscle is innervated by the trigeminal nucleus (31). Additional muscles may be involved and may cause clinical symptoms. The major complaints of patients, which can be related to the rhythmic hyperkinesias, are summarized in the following paragraphs.

Objective Ear Clicks: The Cardinal Symptom of Essential Palatal Tumor

Ongoing clicks may originate from the ear and they can usually be heard by the examiner sometimes up to a distance of 10 m. Objective measurements within the external acoustic meatus have shown sound pressures between 45 and 80 dB. The click is mostly due to contraction of the tensor veli palatini muscle, which suddenly opens the eustachian tube and thereby causes a sudden breakdown of the surface tension within the tube. For the assessment of these patients, the palate should be inspected. Once the roof of the palate is rhythmically moving it is very likely that the tensor veli palatini is producing the clicks (24,32). Whenever there are clinical doubts, an endoscopic inspection of the upper pharynx with transoral or transnasal endoscopy is recommended. The activation of the tensor veli palatini and the opening of the eustachian tube can be visually inspected with this investigation. In numerous patients, resections of muscles that are commonly not involved have been performed unsuccessfully. Resections of the stapedius muscle have been especially common until now (33) although this muscle almost never produces the click. One otherwise classical EPT case had ear clicks and the authors interpreted this be due to levator activity (33), which rarely inserts at the eustachian tube with some muscle fibers. In their case operative sections of the stapedius and the tensor veli palatini muscles were performed and may have changed the anatomy so much that the levator was indeed tearing at the eustachian tube. The observation is interesting but obviously extremely rare; otherwise, all the patients with SPT having hyperkinesia of the levator would have ear clicks.

Patients with EPT mainly complain about the ear click that seriously affects their ability to concentrate or to sleep. In the older literature, many of the patients with EPT were considered hysteric or psychogenic. Indeed, many patients are extremely distressed by the click:

they quit their jobs, they avoid social activities, and family problems are not uncommon. The psychosocial aspects of this condition have never been formally assessed but our clinical impression is that they are not the primary cause of the clicks but rather a secondary maladaption, as seen in other conditions with a constant acoustic disturbance, such as tinnitus. Further clinical studies are necessary.

Oscillopsia

Involvement of the eye muscles by palatal tremor typically produces a pendular nystagmus. The eyes are involved in SPT but never in EPT. Oscillopsia may develop if the amplitudes of the involuntary eye movements are large enough. We have found that 30% of patients with SPT have pendular nystagmus on clinical examination, but only some of them complain of oscillopsia (3). The eye movements are mostly bilateral. Two types have been identified (34) and may be of localizing value with respect to the abnormal inferior olive (Fig. 13.1). The first shows symmetric bilateral vertical pendular nystagmus (midline form), and the second show a more complicated non-conjugated movement. Usually there are clearly asymmetric jerky nystagmoid eye movements with simultaneous oblique and rotatory components (lateralized form). The vertical component has always a larger amplitude on the side contralateral to the hypertrophied inferior olive. The main component of these ocular oscillations is considered to be similar to the ocular counter-rolling produced by head tilt around an anteroposterior axis lateral to the outer canthus of the eye. The lateralized form is found in patients with unilateral olivary hypertrophy, and the midline form is found in those with bilateral olivary hypertrophy. Unilateral and more complex movements have been rarely described and it is not clear whether these differ from the two types quoted above.

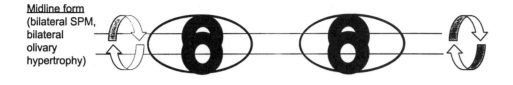

Midline form
(bilateral SPM,
bilateral
olivary
hypertrophy)

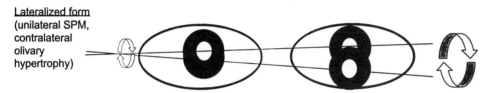

Lateralized form
(unilateral SPM,
contralateral
olivary
hypertrophy)

FIG. 13.1. The two variants of pendular nystagmus seen in SPT.

Tremors or Rhythmic Myoclonias of the Extremities

Less than 10% of patients with SPT exhibit tremors of the head or the extremities. Sometimes the tremor bursts in these cases are found to be time locked with the palatal movements on clinical examination (35-39). This synchrony is the major argument to relate these tremors to the same oscillator as the palatal tremor. These clinical observations are in line with the demonstration of a remote influence of the palatal rhythm on all the motor nuclei contralateral to the hypertrophied inferior olive (4). It is assumed that once this remote effect is strong enough it will produce a rhythmic hyperkinesia time locked with the palatal movements.

However, there are more complex cases exhibiting different rhythms for the palatal and the extremity tremor (37,39,40). The hitherto best-documented case has been published recently: In this patient the rhythm of palatal tremor and extremity hyperkinesia was different and the extremity myoclonus occurred months before the palatal tremor (41). This has been interpreted by the authors, that the same lesion in the brainstem did cause two different hyperkinesias. In another case with pontomesencephalic bleeding, a classical Holmes tremor (or midbrain tremor) with a delay of 9

months developed (as far as can be judged from the description), and 42 and 30 months later palatal tremor developed. Another five cases with SPT and Holmes' tremor have been published (39). At present we interpret these observations in the following way: Lesions within the brainstem/cerebellar region may cause very different movement disorders such as SPT, Holmes tremor, skeletal myoclonus, and others. Thus, it is not surprising that some patients have a second hyperkinesia in addition to SPT following lesions to the brainstem. The critical issue is to look at the time relation between the extremity and palatal tremor bursts and at the clinical history.

Other Rhythmical Symptoms

Rarely, the larynx can be involved thereby producing voice disturbances. In these patients vocal activity is rhythmically modulated, and their speech may be difficult to understand. Even more rarely, and probably unrelated, spasmodic dysphonia has been described in a case of palatal tremor (43). Also very rare in these patients are breathing abnormalities, which are thought to be caused by rhythmical movements of the larynx and pharynx, causing rhythmic modulations of the airflow (44).

The remote influence of palatal tremor on other brainstem and spinal muscles has been reviewed recently (4). We found, that the topographic pattern of the remote effect differs for EPT and SPT. In EPT the tensor veli palatini, moving the soft palate and the pharynx are frequently involved. In SPT, however, besides the pharyngeal and laryngeal muscles, the muscles causing ear click are involved in less than 10% of the cases. These 10% are very old cases that have not been described very thoroughly and thus remain doubtful. Personally, we have never observed a case with SPT and ear clicks.

The most obvious difference is that supranuclear motor centers are rhythmically activated in SPT, but in EPT the movements are restricted to cranial nerve innervated muscles. This will be discussed later.

Further Complaints of the Patients

Usually the major complaints of patients with SPT are not related to the rhythmic hyperkinesia but to the underlying brainstem or cerebellar disease causing the palatal tremor. Hence, the patients often complain about oculomotor disorders, ataxia, or stance or gait disturbances. Various brainstem symptoms are also often present. In sharp contrast, EPT patients do not have any other symptom or clinical sign demonstrating brainstem or cerebellar pathology.

DIFFERENTIAL DIAGNOSIS

Only a few conditions can be confused with palatal tremor. The first are epileptic seizures restricted to the orofacial muscles or even epilepsia partialis continua of these muscles (45,46). Three interesting new case reports appeared meanwhile (47-49), showing such restricted focal epileptic activity; it would be of interest to have video records of the pharynx and larynx to see which muscle groups are involved. In these cases, the sudden onset and atypical frequencies or specific activation characteristics may be important.

The second condition is oculomasticatory myorhythmia (50). This is a very rare disease, which is hitherto described, only in cerebral manifestations of Whipple's disease. The syndrome consists of the triad of (a) slow movements of the masseter and facial muscles, (b) a synchronous vergence nystagmus and usually more complex eye movement abnormalities, and (c) episodes of somnolence lasting hours to days. The slower frequencies and the additional symptoms clearly separate this movement disorder from palatal tremor.

Rarely, tremors of the lips in the setting of the rabbit-syndrome (neuroleptic-induced movement disorder) or in case of chin-tremor (mostly a hereditary action tremor) may be confounded with palatal tremor (51).

The possible confusion of palatal tremor with a variety of different brainstem myoclonias in the setting of cortical or reticular reflex myoclonus has to be mentioned (38,51), but it is never a real diagnostic problem because the myoclonias are usually much more violent and less rhythmic in the latter condition.

PATHOLOGY OF PALATAL TREMOR: OLIVARY HYPERTROPHY IN SYMPTOMATIC PALATAL TREMOR ONLY

It is already known since the earliest descriptions (2,52-56) that patients with palatal tremor usually have a specific abnormality on pathologic examination of the inferior olives called hypertrophic degeneration. This finding was previously described only in patients with SPT, and not a single autopsy of a patient with EPT has been published up to now.

Such olivary hypertrophy can already be seen macroscopically. The area of the inferior olive can be more than twice as large as under normal conditions (57,58). Microscopically, the neurons are enlarged with cytoplasmic vacuolation (59-61). But there is also astrocytic proliferation with typical aggregates of argyrophilic fibers consisting of fibrous astrocytes and interwoven neurites.

Olivary hypertrophy in humans typically develops secondary to a lesion within the cerebellum or brainstem. Initially, the lesion was suggested to lie within the so-called Guillain-Mollaret triangle, which consists of the pathways between the inferior olive, the dentate nucleus and the red nucleus (2). Later it became clear that the olivo-cerebellar projection is never affected in these patients and may even be necessary for the development of the palatal tremor. Detailed studies of Lapresle and Ben Hamida (for review, see reference 36) have shown that the lesion must be situated along the dentato-olivary pathway that originates in the contralateral dentate nucleus and traverses the contralateral superior cerebellar peduncle and the ipsilateral central tegmental tract. The corresponding fibers seem to pass the red nucleus without synapses and terminate within the inferior olive. This projection seems to be somatotopically organized (61,62) which might at least partly explain the differences of muscle involvement among different patients. This fiber tract is presumably a GABA-ergic projection and coincides with a pathway that is already well described in animal models (63,64).

It has been shown in patients that died after a pontine hemorrhage with a variable delay that olivary hypertrophy is a slowly developing process once the typical lesion has occurred (57). The hypertrophy was found to begin about three weeks after the lesion. It has been found retrospectively in a number of stroke patients, that the clinical syndrome of SPT developed after a variable time delay of 2 to 49 months following the cerebral infarction (65). Although it has been reported in trauma patients that the delay between the lesion and the occurrence of the palatal tremor can be much shorter (66), this demonstrates that both phenomena, the hypertrophic degeneration of the inferior olive and the palatal tremor, need time to develop.

There have been several attempts to produce olivary hypertrophy in animals both to study the mechanisms and to eventually produce an animal model for this movement disorder. Olivary hypertrophy can be produced in cats after a brainstem lesion or even after hemicerebellectomy (67-69). In a cat model with hemicerebellar resection, some of the inferior olive (IO) neurons show a similar hypertrophy. They still have an intact mesodiencephalic input and seem

to function similar to normal IO cells (70). Unfortunately, it is unknown whether these animals had any movement disorder. We have recently attempted to confirm this pathogenetic mechanism of olivary hypertrophy in the rat by sectioning the central tegmental tract. Despite the fact that the GABA-ergic dentato-olivary endings of the central tegmental tract were absent in the appropriate inferior olive, a subsequent hypertrophy was not found after 8 months (see chapter 14). We conclude from this, that in the rat either the lesion of the central tegmental tract is not sufficient to produce olivary hypertrophy or olivary hypertrophy cannot be produced in rats at all. Further research is mandatory.

IMAGING OF PATIENTS WITH PALATAL TREMOR

Palatal tremor is mainly a clinical diagnosis. However, a few additional tests can confirm the diagnosis. The most important is magnetic resonance imaging (MRI) of the brainstem with proton density or T2-weighted images showing a hyperintense signal in the region of the inferior olive and additionally an enlargement of the inferior olive. After the first reports of single cases (66,71-77), our study of ten patients with palatal tremor (4) has demonstrated that such MRI abnormalities are typical for SPT.

In contrast, the MRI of patients with EPT was found to be normal in our initial report on four patients with EPT (4). We have meanwhile seen another eight cases that also failed to demonstrate the typical MRI abnormality of SPT. Additionally, more than 20 cases with EPT have been published, some of them reporting the MRI that was always normal and never reported to show olivary hypertrophy (21,23,78-90). Thus, we take for granted that olivary hypertrophy is not a feature of EPT (4).

The abnormal signal of the inferior olive is supporting the diagnosis of SPT. In cases with unilateral palatal tremor, the degeneration of the inferior olive is found always contralateral to the side of the palatal tremor of the m. levator veli palatini muscle. Such imaging studies have uncovered a number of interesting new findings. One single case comparison of MRI and pathology has demonstrated that the abnormal signal on MRI of the inferior olive is indeed equivalent to hypertrophic degeneration according to histologic criteria (76). It is now clear, that the MRI signal in SPT develops within weeks after the insult, which has been demonstrated in two patients with brain trauma (66,91) and in two patients with a brainstem insult (92). According to earlier pathoanatomic studies olivary hypertrophy can change later into an olivary atrophy (57,59) with specific morphologic features (59-61). A recent study has demonstrated atrophy of the cerebellar hemisphere opposite to the abnormal inferior olive (93).

A metananalysis of the MRI scans of nearly 45 published cases came to the conclusion that an increased olivary signal on T2-weighted images appears 1 month after the lesion and persists for at least 3 to 4 years but most likely lifelong (94). Olivary hypertrophy initially develops 6 months after the acute event and resolves by 3 to 4 years (94). It may develop into olivary atrophy, which has been described pathoanatomically (57). Further studies in this field are promising.

THE THERAPY OF PALATAL TREMOR

There is no generally accepted therapy for palatal tremor, neither for the essential nor for the symptomatic form. Because both conditions are very rare, there are no prospective studies; only case reports or open studies in small groups of patients have been published. However, the two conditions have to be separated when it comes to therapy.

Patients with SPT mainly suffer from their additional cerebellar disturbances of movement, which are usually treated by physiotherapy aiming at compensating the typical disabilities. Medical treatment for ataxia is notoriously unsuccessful, and the cerebellar deficits in the setting of palatal tremor are no exception. The rhythmic palatal movement in SPT does not cause discomfort or disability for the patient except when the eyes are involved or when there is an extremity tremor.

Oscillopsia is only rarely treated sufficiently. Single cases with a favorable response to clonazepam have been described (95). Other oral drugs that have been proposed include trihexyphenidyl and valproate. These medications are often not accepted by patients for long-term treatment because of sedative side effects. A relatively new development is the use of botulinum toxin for the treatment of oscillopsia. The toxin can either be injected into the retrobulbar fat tissue or specific muscles can be targeted selectively (96-100). So far no controlled studies are available. In our hands this treatment is helpful for some patients but is not always accepted for long-term use.

For the treatment of tremors carbamazepine was proposed (101), but this is an unusual case that probably corresponds to a myoclonus syndrome of different etiology.

The only complaint of patients with EPT is the ear click. A number of medications have been tried and reported to be successful: valproate (78), trihexyphenidyl (102), and flunarizine (84). Recently sumatriptan has been found to be effective in a few patients (81,85,88), but it was unsuccessful in others (88). The serotonine receptors may thus play a role at least for some patients. As a long-term therapy this drug is not suited for various reasons. Presently the most established therapy is the treatment of the click by injection of botulinum toxin into the tensor veli palatini (32,79, 90,103-105). Low dosages of botulinum toxin (4 to 10 U Botox®) are injected either transpalatally or transnasally under electromyographic guidance. The critical point is to ascertain with endoscopy and electromyography (EMG), through an EMG injection needle isolated until the tip that the needle is definitely placed within the tensor muscle. Spread of botulinum toxin in the soft palate or too-large dosages can otherwise cause severe side effects. Although we have never seen any severe complications in our patients, it must be mentioned that the injection of botulinum toxin into the palatal muscles in rabbits has been introduced as a model for middle ear infections.

PATHOPHYSIOLOGY OF PALATAL TREMOR

The pathophysiology of palatal tremor must be separated for EPT and SPT. Whereas there is almost no relevant information available on EPT, the evidence is steadily growing that SPT is a hyperkinesia due to an olivary oscillator. We will review the relevant findings first and try to integrate clinical, pathophysiologic and experimental findings into our present view.

The Contribution of Functional Imaging

Positron emission tomography can demonstrate the local energy consumption by means of regional glucose uptake. It has been found that in patients with palatal myoclonus there was a statistically significant increase of the glucose consumption in the area of the upper medulla that was interpreted to correspond to the inferior olive (106). Thus, this is the first demonstration of a metabolic "overactivity" of this region. Recently, a patient with essential palatal tremor was described showing hyperactivity of the left inferior olive, the left rubral nucleus, and both dentate nuclei (80). These findings need to be extended in the future and may provide a tool to better understand the differences of EPT and SPT.

Properties of the Oscillator of Palatal Tremor as Revealed with Electrophysiologic Techniques

The persistence of palatal tremor during sleep is unique among the involuntary hyperkinesias (107). In our series of patients with palatal tremor, we found this persistence during sleep in all the cases with SPT. There was a slight but significant decrease of the mean frequency during sleep but the rhythm never stopped. The four patients with EPT showed a cessation of the involuntary hyperkinesia already in early stages of sleep (4). These findings have confirmed earlier clinical observations (for review, see reference 3) and have been strengthened by later case reports. Compared with other tremors, this is almost a unique finding and has led to the proposal that

palatal tremor is due to an autonomous oscillator. Another approach to test the properties of oscillators is to stimulate afferent input in order to change the rhythm of the oscillator. Given a certain rhythm, such a stimulus may prolong or shorten the time until the next tremor burst occurs. This is usually addressed as the resetting property of a central oscillator and has been successfully applied for various tremors (108-110). We have earlier shown that the rhythm of SPT does not change after a masseter and blink reflex stimulus indicating that such weak stimuli are unable to reset the rhythm of SPT (4). A recent study has tested the influence of focal cortical magnetic stimulation on the rhythm of palatal tremor (111). They found that in five patients with SPT, the tremor rhythm can be reset at high stimulus intensities (200% of motor threshold) and that the degree of tremor resetting depends on the stimulus strength.

We conclude that the rhythm of SPT is much more resistant to changes of general activity (like wakefulness, mental activation or sleep stage) than all the other tremors. We do not know which brain structures are involved into the activation or deactivation of the oscillators of tremors, but assuming the IO as the responsible oscillator, it must be mediated through one of its afferent pathways. The main input to the inferior olive comes from the spino-olivary tract and the dorsal column nuclei. Different projections from brainstem structures as the red nucleus, the mesencephalic reticular formation, the superior colliculi, and the pretectum have been described, but there is a significant motor cortex projection (112). At least this latter projection has now been established to be strong enough to reset the rhythm of SPT.

The Distribution of the Rhythmic Activity in Symptomatic Palatal Tremor

The existence of a remote effect of palatal tremor was first demonstrated with an H-reflex technique showing a time-locked enhancement of the soleus H reflex (113). We have demonstrated in our patients by means of averaging of the spontaneous rectified EMG that there is an inhibition of the voluntary EMG of various extremity muscles related to the palatal tremor jerk in the patients with SPT. Moreover, we could show that this effect is restricted to the side contralateral to the abnormal inferior olive. Such an inhibition was not found for patients with EPT. Similar findings in a further patient with symptomatic palatal tremor have been reported (114). Another projection is to the cerebellar or brainstem gaze centers. This is evident through the typical oculomotor abnormality of SPT. The underlying cause for this abnormality is not yet fully clear. Nakada and Kwee (34) proposed that the ocular oscillations in SPT involve vestibulo-ocular reflex adaptation mediated by the flocculus. The distinct clinical features of both conditions are due to either a unilateral or a bilateral activation of the flocculus according to their hypothesis.

Evidence for an Olivocerebellar Malfunction in Symptomatic Palatal Tremor

Despite considerable efforts, the physiologic role of the inferior olive is not yet clear but their involvement in motor control and for motor learning are established (115). The inferior olive is mediating mainly the spinocerebellar input into the cerebellum and is responsible for the fine tuning between cortical movement control and peripheral feedback. Thus it is especially responsible for the delicate timing of muscle activation. Because the only output of the inferior olive is directed to the cerebellum, this comparison is considered to be defective in the case of olivary disturbances. It can be predicted, therefore, that disturbances of movement control in cases of olivary lesions are presenting as cerebellar disturbances, and they may even be indistinguishable from primary cerebellar deficits. Indeed reports from patients with olivary lesions and animal experiments with lesioning of the inferior olive have shown, that the most prominent deficit is ataxia predominantly of the axial type (116). Thus, the search for abnormalities in patients with SPT and olivary hypertrophy should also include the analysis of signs that are typical for cerebellar abnormalities.

Another well-known feature of olivary function is motor learning (117,118). Eyelid conditioning as a classical model of classical condition is impaired after lesioning of the inferior olive, as well as other forms of classical conditioning (119). Recently, Welsh (120) has shown that rats show abnormalities of different forms of motor learning during tremor induced by harmaline. These studies are of special interest for the present question because they could show that abnormalities of learning are related to the malfunction of the IO during harmaline tremor. Similarly, the proposed rhythmic activity of the inferior olive in SPT could lead to functional disturbances of the olivo-cerebellar circuit. Indeed in subjects with SPT a disturbance of motor learning has been demonstrated on the side contralateral to the hypertrophied inferior olive (121).

Two lines of evidence are favoring a disturbance of the olivo-cerebellar circuit in SPT. The first are clinical observations in these patients. Some of them suffer from only small lesions within the pontine area close to the fourth ventricle. Especially small lesions within the central tegmental tract can cause olivary hypertrophy and palatal tremor. This has been shown in earlier pathoanatomic studies (36) and is also found in more recent patients documented with MRI studies (122). For patients who have only a circumscribed lesion of the central tegmental tract, only brainstem abnormalities should be expected. However, there are some cases that have a clear-cut cerebellar symptomatology.

Thus, when considering the question of whether olivary hypertrophy can cause a cerebellar deficit it is most convincing to look to cases with a unilateral olivary hypertrophy and a small lesion of the central tegmental tract. Such a patient has recently been reported to have contralateral ataxia of the extremities and gait and stance ataxia (122).

PATHOPHYSIOLOGIC CONCLUSIONS

Palatal tremor is a rare clinical syndrome but nevertheless it is of special interest for

TABLE 13.2. *Differences of essential and symptomatic palatal tremor*

	Symptomatic palatal tremor	Essential palatal tremor
Etiology	CVD, degenerative disease, encephalitis, MS, trauma, others	Unknown
Age at onset (yr, mean ± SD)	45.1 ± 17.3	24.8 ± 12.9
Sex relation (male:female)	2:1	1:1

CVD, cerebrovascular disease; MS, multiple sclerosis; PT, palatal tremor; SD, standard deviation.

many other movement disorders that are also considered to be generated within the Guillain-Mollaret triangle, such as myoclonias and essential tremor. Fortunately, the study of these pathophysiologic processes is no longer of interest for neurologists but has meanwhile fascinated basic neuroscientists, who have contributed a lot to the understanding and development of new hypotheses for this condition. Our clinical studies have shown, that EPT and SPT differ in many respects (See Table 13.2), which are critical not only for clinical differential diagnosis but show profound differences of the pathophysiology (See Table 13.3). Thus, we propose to clearly keep EPT and SPT separate, and the pathophysiologic considerations for SPT should not be taken over uncritically to the situation of EPT (See Table 13.3).

Symptomatic Palatal Tremor

Earlier attempts have postulated a denervation supersensitivity of IO cells underlying the rhythmic movement (65). Although this would be compatible with the delayed appearance of palatal tremor it is hard to interpret the clock-like rhythmicity of SPT on this basis. It seems much more likely that a physiologic mechanism producing rhythmic discharges is active in this condition. Receptor supersensitivity, which is, for example, assumed for the dyskinesias of Parkinson disease, shows the clinical equivalent of non-rhythmic abnormal movements.

TABLE 13.3. *Criteria separating symptomatic and essential rhythmic palatal tremor*

	Symptomatic palatal tremor	Essential palatal tremor
Etiology	CVD, degenerative disease, encephalitis, MS, trauma	Unknown
Neurologic examination	Mostly brainstem/cerebellar symptoms	Normal (except PT)
Presenting complaint	Mostly unrelated to PT	Ear click
MRI	Abnormal inferior olive	Normal inferior olive
Muscle territory involved	Frequent extrapalatal involvement (especially eyes), rarely ear click	Mostly ear click, never nystagmus or extremity tremors
Activated palatal muscle	Levator veli palatini muscle	Tensor veli palatini muscle
Rhythmically activated brainstem nucleus	Ambiguus or facial nucleus	Trigeminal nucleus
Frequency (mean ± SD per min)	139 ± 51	107 ± 41
Duration of the hyperkinesia	Lifelong	Mostly persistent, remissions may occur
Cessation during sleep	No	Yes
Pathology	Mostly hypertrophic degeneration of the inferior olive; at late stages possibly atrophy of the inferior olive	Unknown, but no evidence for hypertrophic degeneration of the inferior olive

CVD, cerebrovascular disease; MRI, magnetic resonance imaging; MS, multiple sclerosis; PT, palatal tremor; SD, standard deviation.

The release of primitive gill breathing was suggested by Yakolev (123). However, the concept of the release of primitive motor patterns is based on the assumption that the released patterns represent a useful function. Considering the gill breathing as a function of the branchial arch musculature, it is hard to understand why this should include eye movements or even extremity movements. The latter projections can by no means be explained through projections or primitive connections within the brainstem, but they must be conducted through supraspinal projections to the brainstem and spinal cord.

Rhythmic oscillations of single neurons or neuron populations within the central nervous system are, meanwhile, well described for neurons of the inferior olive, thalamic neurons and even spinal motoneurons (64,124). Such a mechanism could account for palatal tremor. The normal action potential is generated by a sudden change in sodium and potassium conductance if the threshold of the cell is reached. In case of the oscillatory mode of these cells, a change of dendritic calcium conductance prolongs the duration of the spike, and a calcium-dependent dendritic change of potassium conductance causes a prolonged afterhyperpolarization. The latter is terminated by a somatic calcium rebound spike, which brings the membrane potential again to the threshold, and the next spike will occur. This can explain why a single cell can oscillate rhythmically.

In case of the inferior olive another feature of the IO cells is explaining why rhythms are synchronized among different cells: They have the capacity of electrotonic coupling mediated by the so-called gap junctions between them (64). If different cells are rhythmically active and time locked at the same frequency, it is more likely that they can mediate their rhythm to the peripheral muscles. It is probably meaningful that the transmission of the gap junctions is known to be regulated by GABA-ergic synapses whose cell bodies are most likely located within the cerebellar nuclei (63). The destruction of such a system could well be responsible for a close coupling of the firing of many IO cells.

Although many questions remain open, presently the most likely interpretation of SPT is that destruction of the dentato-olivary tract causes the cells of the inferior olive to synchronize. The rhythm of the cells is assumed to be dictated by the membrane properties of the cells themselves and is only minimally influenced by changes of physiologic parameters (shown by resistance to external stimulation and sleep). This abnormal rhythmicity is then carried through the inferior cerebellar peduncle to the contralateral cerebellar hemisphere and thus is interfering with physiologic regulations of the oculomotor system (especially the vestibulo-ocular reflex), the cerebello-reticular systems producing the hyperkinesia of brainstem muscles, and the cerebellospinal systems regulating muscle tone.

Essential Palatal Tremor

Much less is known regarding EPT. Until now, no pathologic abnormality has been found for this condition. The negative MRI findings presented here do not exclude morphologic abnormalities, but if they exist they should be different from the one of SPT, which has a clear hyperintense signal of the inferior olive. It is also difficult to assume that EPT is the pure functional analog of SPT since we know that the palatal muscles activated in the two conditions are different, and the rhythmicity is much more likely to be influenced by physiologic conditions like sleep in EPT than SPT. Furthermore, there is no evidence either from our review (3) nor from our electrophysiologic studies (4,125) that patients with EPT do activate a supranuclear motor structure like the oculomotor centers or reticulospinal pathways. Thus, we cannot exclude that EPT is caused by a functional abnormality restricted to one side of the brainstem without any involvement of the contralateral cerebellum (126), especially because there are no other signs of cerebellar abnormality in this condition. In a single case with EPT who could voluntarily suppress the click, an increased activity of the nuclei of the Guillain-Mollaret triangle was demonstrated (80). This interesting finding needs further confirmation. Further investigations are mandatory.

REFERENCES

1. Movement Disorders Society Congress, oral discussion, 1990.
2. Guillain G, Mollaret P, Bertrand I. Sur la lésion responsable du syndrome myoclonique de tronc cérébral. *Rev Neurol (Paris)* 1933;3:666–674.
3. Deuschl G, Mischke G, Schenck E, et al. Symptomatic and essential rhythmic palatal myoclonus. *Brain* 1990; 113:1645–1672.
4. Deuschl G, Toro C, Valls-Sole J, et al. Symptomatic and essential palatal tremor. 1. Clinical, physiological and MRI analysis. *Brain* 1994;117:775–788.
5. Howard RS, Greenwood R, Gawler J, et al. A familial disorder associated with palatal myoclonus, other brainstem signs, tetraparesis, ataxia and Rosenthal fibre formation. *J Neurol Neurosurg Psychiatry* 1993; 56:977–981.
6. Schwankhaus JD, Parisi JE, Gulledge WR, et al. Hereditary adult-onset Alexander's disease with palatal myoclonus, spastic paraparesis, and cerebellar ataxia [see comments]. *Neurology* 1995;45:2266–2271.
7. Deprez M, D'Hooghe M, Misson JP, et al. Infantile and juvenile presentations of Alexander's disease: a report of two cases. [published erratum appears in Acta Neurol Scand 1999 Nov;100(5):354]. *Acta Neurol Scand* 1999;99:158–165.
8. Donaghy M, King RH, McKeran RO, et al. Cerebrotendinous xanthomatosis: clinical, electrophysiological and nerve biopsy findings, and response to treatment with chenodeoxycholic acid. *J Neurol* 1990;237: 216–219.
9. Takeuchi M, Sasaki S, Ito A, et al. [An autopsy case of progressive supranuclear palsy with olivary hypertrophy.] *No To Shinkei* 1991;43:863–867.
10. Suyama N, Kobayashi S, Isino H, et al. Progressive supranuclear palsy with palatal myoclonus. *Acta Neuropathol (Berl)* 1997;94:290–293.
11. Wenning GK, Tison F, Ben SY, et al. Multiple system atrophy: a review of 203 pathologically proven cases. *Mov Disord* 1997;12:133–147.
12. Noda K, Isozaki E, Miyamoto K, et al. [Rhythmical involuntary movement at rest associated with olivoponto-cerebellar atrophy (OPCA). [Japanese.] *Rinsho Shinkeigaku Clinical Neurology* 1993;33:8–14.
13. Yokota T, Atsumi Y, Uchiyama M, et al. Electroencephalographic activity related to palatal myoclonus in REM sleep. *J Neurol* 1990;237:290–294.
14. Iwasaki Y, Kinoshita M, Ikeda K, et al. Palatal myoclonus following Behcet's disease ameliorated by ceruletide, a potent analogue of CCK octapeptide. *J Neurol Sci* 1991;105:12–13.
15. Sakurai N, Koike Y, Kaneoke Y, et al. Sleep apnea and palatal myoclonus in a patient with neuro-Behcet syndrome. *Intern Med* 1993;32:336–339.
16. Yamanouchi H, Kasai H, Sakuragawa N, et al. Palatal myoclonus in Krabbe disease. *Brain Dev* 1991;13: 355–358.
17. Malandrini A, Scarpini C, Palmeri S, et al. Palatal myoclonus and unusual MRI findings in a patient with membranous lipodystrophy. *Brain Dev* 1996;18:59-63.
18. Gambardella A, Zappia A, Valentino P, et al. Action palatal tremor in a patient with primary intestinal lymphoma. *Mov Disord* 1997;12:794–797.
19. Revol A, Vighetto A, Confavreux C, et al. [Oculopalatal myoclonus and multiple sclerosis]. *Rev Neurol (Paris)* 1990;146:518–521.
20. Hitoshi S, Kusunoki S, Chiba A, et al. Cerebellar ataxia and polyneuropathy in a patient with IgM M-protein specific to the Gal(beta 1-3)GalNAc epitope. *J Neurol Sci* 1994;126:219–224.
21. Nemni R, Braghi S, Natali-Sora MG, et al. Autoantibodies to glutamic acid decarboxylase in palatal myoclonus and epilepsy [see comments.] *Ann Neurol* 1994;36:665–667.
22. Davenport C, Foxon R, Todd I, et al. Absence of glutamic acid decarboxylase autoimmunity in symptomatic palatal tremor [letter; comment]. *Ann Neurol* 1995;38:274–275.
23. Vieregge P, Klein C, Gehrking E, et al. The diagnosis of 'essential palatal tremor'. *Neurology* 1997;49:248–249.
24. Deuschl G, Toro C, Hallett M. Symptomatic and essential palatal tremor. 2. Differences of palatal movements. *Mov Disord* 1994;9:676–678.
25. Vali E. Über objektive Ohrgeräusche. *Archiv für Ohrenheilkunde* 1905;66:104–115.
26. Barré JA, Draganesco N, Lieou FJ. Nystagmus giratoire spontané constant bilatéral, myoclonies rythmiques vélo-phryngées, sushyoidiennes et diaphragmatiques. *Revue d'Oto-Neuro-Oculistique* 1926;4:749–757.
27. Lhermitte J, Drouzon J. Un nouveau cas de myoclonies du voile du palais, de la langue, des lèvres et des globes oculaires. Lésions limitées aux noyaux dentelés du pédoncule cérébelleux supérieur et aux olives bulbaires. *Revue Neurologique* 1937;67:390–396.
28. Klein C, Gehrking E, Vieregge P. Voluntary palatal tremor in two siblings. *Mov Disord* 1998;13:545–548.
29. Fox GN, Baer MT. Palatal myoclonus and tinnitus in children. *West J Med* 1991;154:98–102.
30. Hollinshead W. Anatomy for surgeons. Harper and Row: New York, 1982.
31. Strutz J, Hammerich T, Amedee R. The motor innervation of the soft palate. An anatomical study in guinea pigs and monkeys. *Archives of Oto Rhino Laryngology* 1988;245:180–184.
32. Deuschl G, Lohle E, Heinen F, et al. Ear click in palatal tremor: its origin and treatment with botulinum toxin. *Neurology* 1991;41:1677–1679.
33. Jamieson DR, Mann C, O'Reilly B, et al. Ear clicks in palatal tremor caused by activity of the levator veli palatini. *Neurology* 1996;46:1168–1169.
34. Nakada T, Kwee IL. Oculopalatal myoclonus. *Brain* 1986;109:431–441.
35. Holmes G. On certain tremors in organic cerebral lesions. *Brain* 1904;27:327–375.
36. Lapresle J. Rhythmic palatal myoclonus and the dentato-olivary pathway. *J Neurol* 1979;220:223–230.
37. Masucci EF, Kurtzke JF, Saini N. Myorhythmia: a widespread movement disorder. Clinicopathological correlations. *Brain* 1984;107:53–79.
38. Silfverskiöld BP. Rhythmic myoclonias including spinal myoclonus. In: Fahn S, Marsden CD, VanWoert M, eds. *Advances in Neurology* New York: Raven Press, 1986:275–85.
39. Masucci E, Kurtzke J. Palatal myoclonus associated with extremity tremor. *J Neurol* 1989;236:474–477.

40. Hefter H, Logigian E, Witte OW, et al. Oscillatory activity in different motor subsystems in palatal myoclonus. A case report. *Acta Neurol Scand* 1992;86:176–183.

41. Yanagisawa T, Sugihara H, Shibahara K, et al. Natural course of combined limb and palatal tremor caused by cerebellar-brain stem infarction. *Mov Disord* 1999;14: 851–854.

42. Fukui T, Ichikawa H, Sugita K, et al. Intention tremor and olivary enlargement: clinico-radiological study. *Intern Med* 1995;34:1120–1125.

43. Doody RS, Rosenfield DB. Spasmodic dysphonia associated with palatal myoclonus. *Ear Nose Throat J* 1990;69:829–832.

44. Andrews J, Dumont D, Fisher M, et al. Ventilatory dysfunction in palatal myoclonus. *Respiration* 1987;52: 76–80.

45. Thomas JE, Reagan TJ, Klass DW. Epilepsia partialis continua. *Archives of Neurology* 1977;34:266–275.

46. Tatum WO, Sperling MR, Jacobstein JG. Epileptic palatal myoclonus. *Neurology* 1991;41:1305–1306.

47. Emre M. Palatal myoclonus occurring during complex partial status epilepticus. *J Neurol* 1992;239:228–230.

48. Noachtar S, Ebner A, Witte OW, et al. Palatal tremor of cortical origin presenting as epilepsia partialis continua. *Epilepsia* 1995;36:207–209.

49. Thomas P, Borg M, Suisse G, et al. Opercular myoclonic-anarthric status epilepticus. *Epilepsia* 1995; 36:281–289.

50. Schwartz MA, Selhorst JB, Ochs AL, et al. Oculomasticatory myorhythmia: a unique movement disorder occurring in Whipple's disease. *Ann Neurol* 1986;20: 677–683.

51. Dubinsky RM, Hallett M. Palatal myoclonus and facial involvement in other types of myoclonus. *Adv Neurol* 1988;49:263–278.

52. Klien H. Zur Pathologie der kontinuierlichen rhthmischen Krämpfe der Schlingmuskulatur (2 Fälle von Erweichungsherden im Kleinhirn). *Neurologischen Centralblatt* 1907;26:245–246.

53. Lévy G. Un cas de myoclonies rythmiques vélopharyngo-laryngées (nystagmus de voile). Participation de l'hémiface gauche, de l'oeil gauche (nystagmus rotatoire) et du diaphragme - troubles cérébelleux supérieur prédominant à gauche. Zeitschrift für Laryngologie, Rhinologie, Otologie und ihre Grenzgebiete 1925;1:449–455.

54. Guillain G, Mollaret P. Deux cas de myoclonies synchrones et rythmées vélo-pharyngo-laryngo-oculodiaphragmatiques. Le problème antomique et physiopathologique de ce sundrome. *Revue Neurologique* 1931;2:545–566.

55. Grill C, Laurén E. Contribution à l'étude de la pathogénie des myoclonies laryngo-pharyngées. Etude clinique er anatomique. Upsala Läkareförenings Förhandlingar 1932;38:1–34.

56. Lhermitte J, Trelles J-O. L'hypertrophie des olives bulbaires. *Encéphale* 1933;28:588-600.

57. Goto N, Kaneko M. Olivary enlargement: chronological and morphometric analyses. *Acta Neuropathol (Berl)* 1981;54:275–282.

58. Gauthier JC, Blackwood W. Enlargement of the inferior olivary nucleus in association with lesions of the central tegmental tract of dentate nucleus. *Brain* 1961; 84:341–361.

59. Goto N, Kakimi S, Kaneko M. Olivary enlargement:

stage of initial astrocytic changes. *Clin Neuropathol* 1988;7:39–43.

60. Barron KD, Dentinger MP, Koeppen AH. Fine structure of neurons of the hypertrophied human inferior olive. *J Neuropathol Exp Neurol* 1982;41:186–203.

61. Koeppen AH, Barron KD, Dentinger MP. Olivary hypertrophy: histochemical demonstration of hydrolytic enzymes. *Neurology* 1980;30:471–480.

62. Jellinger K. Hypertrophy of the inferior olives. Report on 29 cases. *Z Neurol* 1973;205:153-174.

63. Sotelo C, Gotow T, Wassef M. Localization of glutamic-acid-decarboxylase-immunoreactive axon terminals in the inferior olive of the rat, with special emphasis on anatomical relations between GABAergic synapses and dendrodendritic gap junctions. *J Comp Neurol* 1986;252:32–50.

64. Llinas R, Baker R, Sotelo C. Electrotonic coupling between neurons in cat inferior olive. *J Neurophysiol* 1974;37:560–571.

65. Matsuo F, Ajax ET. Palatal myoclonus and denervation supersensitivity in the central nervous system. *Ann Neurol* 1979;5:72–78.

66. Birbamer G, Buchberger W, Kampfl A, et al. Early detection of post-traumatic olivary hypertrophy by MRI. *J Neurol* 1993;240:407–409.

67. Verhaart WJC, Voogd J. Hypertrophy of the inferior olives in the cat. *Journal of Neuropathology and Experimental Neurology* 1962;21:92–104.

68. Zeeuw CId, Ruigrok TJH, Schalekamp MPA, et al. Ultrastructural study of the cat hypertrophic inferior olive following anterograde tracing, immunocytochemistry and intracellular labelling. *European Journal of Morphology* 1990;28:240–255.

69. Boesten AJ, Voogd J. Hypertrophy of neurons in the inferior olive after cerebellar ablations in the cat. *Neurosci Lett* 1985;61:49–54.

70. Ruigrok TJ, de Zeeuw CI, Voogd J. Hypertrophy of inferior olivary neurons: a degenerative, regenerative or plasticity phenomenon. *Eur J Morphol* 1990;28: 224–239.

71. Sperling MR, Herrmann C, Jr. Syndrome of palatal myoclonus and progressive ataxia: two cases with magnetic resonance imaging. *Neurology* 1985;35: 1212–1214.

72. De Bleecker J, De Reuck J, Van Landegem W, et al. Hypertrophy of the inferior olivary nucleus. A clinicopathological observation. *Acta Neurol Belg* 1988;88: 221–228.

73. Yokota T, Hirashima F, Furukawa T, et al. MRI findings of inferior olives in palatal myoclonus. *J Neurol* 1989;236:115–116.

74. Zarranz JJ, Fontan A, Forcadas I. MR imaging of presumed olivary hypertrophy in palatal myoclonus. *AJNR Am J Neuroradiol* 1990;11:1164.

75. Hirono N, Kameyama M, Kobayashi Y, et al. MR demonstration of a unilateral olivary hypertrophy caused by pontine tegmental hematoma. *Neuroradiology* 1990;32:340–342.

76. Pierot L, Cervera-Pierot P, Delattre JY, et al. Palatal myoclonus and inferior olivary lesions: MRI-pathologic correlation. *J Comput Assist Tomogr* 1992;16:160-163.

77. De Bleecker J, Van Landegem W, Crevits L, et al. Unusual CT and MRI findings in palatal myoclonus. *Acta Neurol Scand* 1992;85:150-153.

78. Borggreve F, Hageman G. A case of idiopathic palatal

myoclonus: treatment with sodium valproate. *Eur Neurol* 1991;31:403-404.

79. Saeed SR, Brookes GB. The use of clostridium botulinum toxin in palatal myoclonus. A preliminary report. *J Laryngol Otol* 1993;107:208-210.

80. Boecker H, Kleinschmidt A, Weindl A, et al. Dysfunctional activation of subcortical nuclei in palatal myoclonus detected by high-resolution MRI. *NMR Biomed* 1994;7:327-329.

81. Scott BL, Evans RW, Jankovic J. Treatment of palatal myoclonus with sumatriptan. *Mov Disord* 1996;11: 748-751.

82. Bauleo S, De Mitri P, Coccagna G. Evolution of segmental myoclonus during sleep: polygraphic study of two cases. *Ital J Neurol Sci* 1996;17:227-232.

83. Saeed SR, Brookes GB. Palatal myoclonus affected by neck posture [letter; comment]. *J Laryngol Otol* 1996; 110:207.

84. Cakmur R, Idiman E, Idiman F, et al. Essential palatal tremor successfully treated with flunarizine. *Eur Neurol* 1997;38:133-134.

85. Jankovic J, Scott BL, Evans RW. Treatment of palatal myoclonus with sumatriptan [letter]. *Mov Disord* 1997;12:818.

86. Bryce GE, Morrison MD. Botulinum toxin treatment of essential palatal myoclonus tinnitus. *J Otolaryngol* 1998;27:213-216.

87. Seidman MD, Arenberg JG, Shirwany NA. Palatal myoclonus as a cause of objective tinnitus: a report of six cases and a review of the literature. *Ear Nose Throat J* 1999;78:292-4, 296-297.

88. Pakiam AS, Lang AE. Essential palatal tremor: evidence of heterogeneity based on clinical features and response to Sumatriptan. *Mov Disord* 1999;14:179-180.

89. Zipfel TE, Kaza SR, Greene JS. Middle-ear myoclonus. J *Laryngol Otol* 2000;114:207-209.

90. Jero J, Salmi T. Palatal myoclonus and clicking tinnitus in a 12-year-old girl—case report. *Acta Otolaryngol Suppl* 2000;543:61-62.

91. Birbamer G, Gerstenbrand F, Kofler M, et al. Posttraumatic segmental myoclonus associated with bilateral olivary hypertrophy. *Acta Neurol Scand* 1993;87: 505-509.

92. Terao S, Sobue G, Takahashi M, et al. [Chronological changes in MR imaging of inferior olivary pseudohypertrophy—report of two cases]. *No To Shinkei* 1994; 46:1184-1189.

93. Kim SJ, Lee JH, Suh DC. Cerebellar MR changes in patients with olivary hypertrophic degeneration. *AJNR Am J Neuroradiol* 1994;15:1715-1719.

94. Goyal M, Versnick E, Tuite P, et al. Hypertrophic olivary degeneration: metaanalysis of the temporal evolution of MR findings. *AJNR Am J Neuroradiol* 2000; 21:1073-1077.

95. Yokota J, Kosaka K, Yoshimoto Y, et al. [Acquired pendular nystagmus after pontine hemorrhage.] *No To Shinkei* 1999;51:1055-1060.

96. Leigh RJ, Tomsak RL, Grant MP, et al. Effectiveness of botulinum toxin administered to abolish acquired nystagmus. *Annals of Neurology* 1992;32:633-642.

97. Leigh RJ, Averbuch HL, Tomsak RL, et al. Treatment of abnormal eye movements that impair vision: strategies based on current concepts of physiology and pharmacology. *Annals of Neurology* 1994;36:129-141.

98. Ruben ST, Lee JP, O'Neil D, et al. The use of botu-

linum toxin for treatment of acquired nystagmus and oscillopsia. *Ophthalmology* 1994;101:783-787.

99. Ruben S, Dunlop IS, Elston J. Retrobulbar botulinum toxin for treatment of oscillopsia. *Australian & New Zealand Journal of Ophthalmology* 1994;22:65-67.

100. Repka MX, Savino PJ, Reinecke RD. Treatment of acquired nystagmus with botulinum neurotoxin A. *Archives of Ophthalmology* 1994;112:1320-1324.

101. Bakheit AM, Behan PO. Palatal myoclonus successfully treated with clonazepam [letter] [see comments]. *J Neurol Neurosurg Psychiatry* 1990;53:806.

102. Jabbari B, Scherokman B, Gunderson CH, et al. Treatment of movement disorders with trihexyphenidyl. *Mov Disord* 1989;4:202-212.

103. Le Pajolec C, Marion MH, Bobin S. [Objective tinnitus and palatal myoclonus. A new therapeutic approach.] *Ann Otolaryngol Chir Cervicofac* 1990;107: 363-365.

104. Deuschl G, Löhle E, Toro C, et al. Botulinumtoxin treatment of palatal tremor (myoclonus). In: Jankovic J, Hallett M, eds. *Therapy with Botulinum Toxin* New York: Marcel Dekker, 1994:567-576.

105. Varney SM, Demetroulakos JL, Fletcher MH, et al. Palatal myoclonus: treatment with Clostridium botulinum toxin injection. *Otolaryngol Head Neck Surg* 1996;114:317-320.

106. Dubinsky RM, Hallett M, Di Chiro G, et al. Increased glucose metabolism in the medulla of patients with palatal myoclonus. *Neurology* 1991;41:557-562.

107. Kayed K, Sjaastad O, Magnussen I, et al. Palatal myoclonus during sleep. *Sleep* 1983;6:130-136.

108. Stein RB, Lee RG, Nichols TR. Modifications of ongoing tremors and locomotion by sensory feedback. *Electroencephalogr Clin Neurophysiol Suppl* 1978;34: 512-519.

109. Britton TC, Thompson PD, Day BL, et al. "Resetting" of postural tremors at the wrist with mechanical stretches in Parkinson's disease, essential tremor, and normal subjects mimicking tremor. *Annals of Neurology* 1992;31:507-514.

110. Britton TC, Thompson PD, Day BL, et al. Modulation of postural wrist tremors by magnetic stimulation of the motor cortex in patients with Parkinson's disease or essential tremor and in normal subjects mimicking tremor. *Ann Neurol* 1993;33:473-479.

111. Chen J, Yu H, Wu Z, et al. Modulation of symptomatic palatal tremor by magnetic stimulation of the motor cortex. *Clin Neurophysiol* 2000;111:1191-1197.

112. Brodal A. Neurological Anatomy in Relation to Clinical Medicine. New York and Oxford: Oxford University Press, 1981.

113. Nagaoka M, Narabayashi H. Palatal myoclonus—its remote influence. *J Neurol Neurosurg Psychiatry* 1984;47:921-926.

114. Elble RJ. Inhibition of forearm EMG by palatal myoclonus. *Mov Disord* 1991;6:324-329.

115. Armstrong DM. Functional significance of connections of the inferior olive. *Physiological Reviews* 1974; 54:358-417.

116. Nashold BS, Slaughter DG. Effects of stimulating or destroying the deep cerebellar regions in man. *J Neurosurg* 1969;31:172-186.

117. Llinas R, Welsh JP. On the cerebellum and motor learning. *Curr Opin Neurobiol* 1993;3:958-965.

118. Raymond JL, Lisberger SG, Mauk MD. The cerebel-

lum: a neuronal learning machine? *Science* 1996;272:
1126-1131.

119. Harvey JA, Romano AG. Harmaline-induced impairment of Pavlovian conditioning in the rabbit. *J Neurosci* 1993;13:1616-1623.

120. Welsh JP. Systemic harmaline blocks associative and motor learning by the actions of the inferior olive. *Eur J Neurosci* 1998;10:3307-3320.

121. Deuschl G, Toro C, Valls-Sole J, et al. Symptomatic and essential palatal tremor. 3. Abnormal motor learning. *J Neurol Neurosurg Psychiatry* 1996;60:520-525.

122. Deuschl G, Jost S, Schumacher M. Symptomatic palatal tremor is associated with signs of cerebellar dysfunction. *J Neurol* 1996;243:553-556.

123. Yakolev PI, Lutrell CN, Bang, F. Discussion of Myoclonus in cats with Newcastle disease virus encephalitis. *Transactions of the American Neurological Association* 1956;81:63-64.

124. Llinas R, Yarom Y. Electrophysiology of mammalian inferior olivary neurones in vitro. Different types of voltage-dependent ionic conductances. *J Physiol (Lond)* 1981;315:549-567.

125. Deuschl G, Jost S, Schumacher M. Symptomatic palatal tremor is associated with signs of cerebellar dysfunction [letter]. *J Neurol* 1996;243:553-556.

126. Kane S, Thach W. Palatal myoclonus and funtion of the inferior olive: are they related? In: Strata P, ed. *The Olivocerebellar System in Motor Control* Berlin: Springer, 1989:427-460.

127. Iwadate Y, Saeki N, Komiya H, et al. [Three cases of involuntary movements following pontine hemorrhage.] *No To Shinkei* 1988;40:869-874.

128. Yokota T, Furukawa T, Tsukagoshi H, et al. [Unilateral palatal myoclonus with peculiar ocular movements—neurotological studies and MRI.] *Rinsho Shinkeigaku* 1989;29:159-163.

129. Chang WN, Lu CS, Chang CS. Oculopalatal myoclonus: report of a case. *J Formos Med Assoc* 1990; 89:487-489.

130. Shepherd GM, Tauboll E, Bakke SJ, et al. Midbrain tremor and hypertrophic olivary degeneration after pontine hemorrhage. *Mov Disord* 1997;12:432-437.

131. Chen SS, Teng MM, Shao KN, et al. Magnetic resonance imaging of unilateral olivary hypertrophy due to pontine tegmental hemorrhage: a case report. *Chung Hua I Hsueh Tsa Chih (Taipei)* 1999;62:648-651.

132. Han SH, Lee WY, Kim JS, et al. MR demonstration of cryptic vascular malformation producing a palatal my-

oclonus—a case report. *J Korean Med Sci* 1989;4: 139-141.

133. Chalk JB, Patterson MC, Pender MP. An intracranial arteriovenous malformation and palatal myoclonus related to pseudoxanthoma elasticum. *Aust N Z J Med* 1989;19:141-143.

134. Yokota T, Tsukagoshi H. Olivary hypertrophy precedes the appearance of palatal myoclonus [letter]. *J Neurol* 1991;238:408.

135. Chua HC, Tan AK, Venketasubramanian N, et al. Palatal myoclonus—a case report. *Ann Acad Med Singapore* 1999;28:593-5.

136. De Bleecker J, Crevits L, De Reuck J. Unilateral ocular involvement in oculo-palatal myoclonus after basal meningitis. *Neuro Opthalm* 1991;11:281-284.

137. Srivastava T, Thussu A. Palatal myoclonus in postinfectious opsoclonus myoclonus syndrome: a case report. *Neurol India* 1999;47:133-135.

138. de la Fuente-Fernandez R. [Hiccup and dysfunction of the inferior olivary complex (see comments)]. *Med Clin (Barc)* 1998;110:22-24.

139. Phanthumchinda K. Syndrome of progressive ataxia and palatal myoclonus: a case report. *J Med Assoc Thai* 1999;82:1154-1157.

140. Kulkarni PK, Muthane UB, Taly AB, et al. Palatal tremor, progressive multiple cranial nerve palsies, and cerebellar ataxia: a case report and review of literature of palatal tremors in neurodegenerative disease. *Mov Disord* 1999;14:689-693.

141. Nishigaya K, Kaneko M, Nagaseki Y, et al. Palatal myoclonus induced by extirpation of a cerebellar astrocytoma. Case report. *J Neurosurg* 1998;88:1107-1110.

142. Yokota T, Hirashima F, Ito Y, et al. Idiopathic palatal myoclonus. *Acta Neurol Scand* 1990;81:239-242.

143. Chang WN, Lu CS, Chee EC, et al. Idiopathic palatal myoclonus: report of two cases. *Chang Keng I Hsueh Tsa Chih* 1992;15:105-109.

144. Tomkinson A, Craven C, Brown MJ. Palatal myoclonus affected by neck position [see comments]. *J Laryngol Otol* 1995;109:61-62.

145. Martinez-Vila E, Martinez-Lage Alvarez P, Luquin MR, et al. Palatal myoclonus and opioid peptides. *Acta Neurol Scand* 1993;88:227-228.

146. Bharucha KJ, Sethi KD. Complex movement disorders induced by fluoxetine [see comments]. *Mov Disord* 1996;11:324-326.

147. Tison F, Arne P, Henry P. Myoclonus and adult coeliac disease. *J Neurol* 1989;236:307-308.

Myoclonus and Paroxysmal Dyskinesias,
Advances in Neurology, Vol. 89,
edited by S. Fahn, et al.
Lippincott Williams & Wilkins, Philadelphia © 2002.

14

Dissection of the Cerebello-Olivary Projection Does Not Induce Neuronal Hypertrophy in the Inferior Olive in the Rat

*Henrik Wilms, †Jobst Sievers, and *Günther Deuschl

*Department of Neurology, Christian-Albrechts-University Kiel, Kiel, Germany; and
†Department of Anatomy, University of Kiel, Kiel, Germany

Symptomatic palatal tremor is characterized by rhythmic activation of the levator veli palatini muscle and often of muscles innervated by various brainstem or spinal motor nuclei at a low frequency between 0.2 and 2 Hz. Affected humans sometimes exhibit a postural and action tremor, which is synchronized to the palatal tremor (1). Almost all cases with symptomatic palatal tremor, however, show a subliminal activation of all the muscles contralateral to the abnormal inferior olive that is synchronous with the jerk of the palatal tremor (2), indicating that rhythmic discharges presumably originating within the inferior olive reach the spinal motoneurons. It is the only human tremor characterized by a morphologic central nervous system alteration known as hypertrophy of the inferior olive, which is caused by either a brainstem or cerebellar lesion and develops with a latency of several months (3,4). In well-documented single cases, development of olivary hypertrophy preceded the occurrence of symptomatic palatal tremor (5,6). In all autopsy cases a lesion of the cerebello-olivary projection from the contralateral cerebellar nuclei to the ipsilateral inferior olive was found. Moreover, classical clinicopathologic correlations have shown that the lesion to produce such olivary hypertrophy can be very limited and restricted to the pontine region (4,7,8). Olivary neurons were characterized by a slight hy-

pertrophy, central chromatolysis, cytoplasmic vacuolization, and gliosis (9–11).

In a comparable animal model in cats, a neuronal "pseudohypertrophy" develops in two subnuclei, the medial accessory olive (MAO) and principal olive (PO) within 8 months after ablation of the **contralateral** hemicerebellum (12–14). An increased number of hypertrophied olivary neurons is seen with longer survival times. Occurrence of olivary pseudohypertrophy after destruction of cerebellar efferents is probably due to the fact that in the normal inferior olive electrotonic coupling between its neurons is reduced by cerebellar GABA-ergic input (15). The destruction of this GABA-ergic pathway on the other hand might enhance this electrotonic coupling (2,16–18) and thus might synchronize the natural tendency of olivary neurons for rhythmical oscillations. From a retrograde tracing study it is known that the cerebello-olivary tract originates within the cerebellar nuclei (17), and in an anterograde tracing study Ruigrok and Voogd (19) showed that these fibers pass the lateral angle of the fourth ventricle and align in the superior cerebellar peduncle as they run rostrally, cross the midline, and project ventrocaudally to the contralateral inferior olive. In the present study we dissected this GABA-ergic projection in rats by a more selective lesion, since a possible induction of olivary hypertrophy in this species might serve as a model for human postural tremor.

MATERIAL AND METHODS

Thirty-four female adult Wistar rats were used in all experiments. The GABA-ergic cerebello-olivary projection was identified in cases from the anterograde tracing study of Ruigrok and Voogd (19). In order to dissect this pathway the animals were placed in a stereotactic frame under deep chloral hydrate anesthesia, and mechanical brainstem lesions were placed either through the lateral margin of the fourth ventricle 5.5 mm rostral to the atlantooccipital membrane (Fig.14.1A) in 12

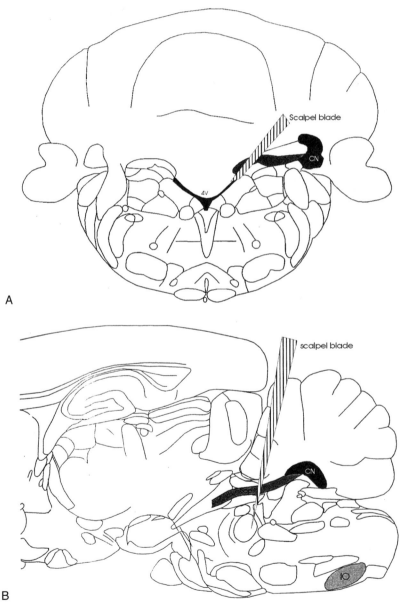

FIG. 14.1. Schematic drawing representing a transversal **(A)** and parasagittal cut **(B)** through cerebellar nuclei *(CN)*, superior cerebellar peduncle *(Scp)*, fourth ventricle *(4V)*, and inferior olive *(IO)* to illustrate the surgical approach.

animals. Alternatively, coronally oriented knife cuts were made at the level of the inferior colliculus (Fig.14.1B) in 22 rats; the coordinates were calculated from the atlas of Paxinos et al. (20). After survival times of 10 to 240 days, the animals were reanesthetized and perfused transcardially with a vascular rinse of 0.9% NaCl followed by 4% buffered paraformaldehyde solution. One hour after termination of the perfusion, the brainstems were dissected out of the cranium, paraffin-embedded, and sectioned coronally at 7 μm. Topography of mesencephalic glial scars was evaluated by immunohistochemistry for glial fibrillary acidic protein (GFAP, 1:1000, rabbit polyclonal, DAKO) or ED1 (marker for monocytes, 1:500, Serotec). Sections through the inferior olive were processed for glutamate decarboxylase (GAD) immunohistochemistry (antiserum kindly provided by Dr. Harvey White, National Institutes of Health, Bethesda, Maryland), since a reduction of staining in the contralateral olive can be expected after successful severance of its GABA-ergic afferents. The GAD antiserum was raised in sheep with a GAD-anti-GAD

complex isolated from rat brain by a primary nonspecific antiserum as immunogen (21,22). Standard immunohistochemical procedures were used, including the use of secondary antibodies coupled to alkaline phosphatase (DAKO, Hamburg; Dianova, Hamburg).

RESULTS

Animals recovered from surgery within 24 hours and showed no motor deficits thereafter. Originating from the cerebellar nuclei, the nucleo-olivary fibers pass the lateral angle of the fourth ventricle very closely aligned in the superior cerebellar peduncle as they run rostrally, cross the midline, and project ventrocaudally to the contralateral inferior olive (19). Both surgical approaches successfully severed this nucleo-olivary projection (Fig. 14.2) in 18 animals: GFAP-positive astrocytes form a glial scar in the lateral angle of the fourth ventricle (Fig. 14.2B; compare to Fig. 14.1A), whereas the coronally orientated scalpel cut (COSC) dissects the fibers as they align in the superior cerebellar peduncle (Fig. 14.2A; compare to Fig.

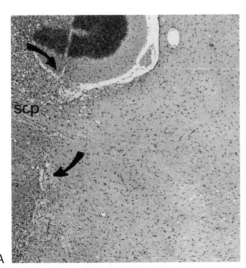
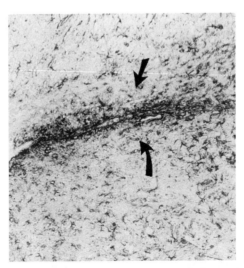

FIG. 14.2. Glial scar in the lateral angle of the fourth ventricle *(4V)* and superior cerebellar peduncle *(scp)* after unilateral mechanical brainstem lesion. Dissection *(arrows)* of the superior cerebellar peduncle *(scp)* (compare to Fig. 14.1B). After a different surgical approach (Fig. 1A), GFAP-positive astrocytes forming a glial scar *(arrows)* involving the lateral angle of the fourth ventricle and superior cerebellar peduncle *(scp)* can be visualized (compare to Fig. 14.1A). Scale corresponds to 600μm in **(A)** and 100μm in **(B)**.

14.2B). Examination of the GAD-immuno-stained sections containing the inferior olive showed that the severance of the nucleo-olivary fibers induced a loss of GABA-ergic boutons within the contralateral medial accessory olive (MAO) (Fig. 14.3A) as compared to the ipsilateral MAO (Fig. 14.3A and B) in one animal after a survival time of 2 months (COSC), and four animals after a survival time of 8 months (one with a lesion through the lateral margin of the fourth ventricle, three animals with COSC). However, no hypertrophy of olivary neurons was found even after 8 months.

DISCUSSION

We have shown that the GABA-ergic nucleo-olivary projection can be selectively destroyed in the rat. Whereas in cats, hypertrophy of olivary neurons may be induced by ablation of the cerebellum (12), this peculiar phenomenon was not observed in our experiments after severance of the cerebellar afferents. This

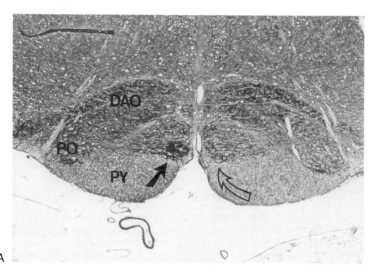

A

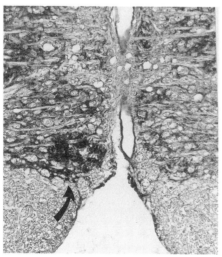

B

FIG. 14.3. Reduced staining of GABA-ergic boutons in the medial accessory olive contralateral to the lesion (*open arrow*) as compared to the ipsilateral side *(filled arrow)* confirms successful severance of the nucleo-olivary projection. Scale bar corresponds to 300μm in **(A)** and 100μm in **(B)**.

species difference regarding olivary reaction might be caused by differences in their afferent connections: though the inferior olive of both cat (23) and rat (24) contains a GABA-ergic innervation, its density may differ resulting in a varying inhibitory influence on the oscillatory property of olivary neurons. Moreover, ultrastructural differences have been observed in olivary neurons with respect to the number and complexity of their glomeruli, which are the morphologic substrate of this coupling (25).

In summary, dissection of the nucleo-olivary projection alone does not induce olivary hypertrophy in the rat after a survival time of 8 months. Our experiments were designed to make a lesion that is as small as possible to dissect primarily the cerebello-olivary GABA-ergic pathway. We conclude that either the rat brain does not show olivary pseudohypertrophy at all or additional hitherto unidentified fiber tracts to the inferior olive have to be lesioned to produce this specific olivary abnormality.

ACKNOWLEDGMENTS

Dr. Ruigrok at Erasmus University in Rotterdam has kindly shown us the original sections from his study in 1990 (19), which enabled us to trace the exact course of the cerebello-olivary tract in the rat. Dr. Harvey White at the National Institutes of Health in Bethesda kindly provided the antiserum for GAD immunohistochemistry. The authors thank Mrs. Rosie Sprang for superior technical assistance. This work was supported by the Deutsche Forschungsgemeinschaft Wi 1762/1-1.

REFERENCES

1. Deuschl G, Mischke G, Schenck E, et al. Symptomatic and essential rhythmic palatal myoclonus. *Brain* 1990;113(Pt 6):1645–1672.
2. Deuschl G, Toro C, Valls-Sole J, et al. Symptomatic and essential palatal tremor. 1: clinical, physiological and MRI analysis. *Brain* 1994;117(Pt 4):775–788.
3. Goto N, Kakimi S, Kaneko M. Olivary enlargement: stage of initial astrocytic changes. *Clin Neuropathol* 1988;7:39–43.
4. Lapresle J, Hamida MB. The dentato-olivary pathway: somatotopic relationship between the dentate nucleus and the contralateral inferior olive. *Arch Neurol* 1970; 22:135–143.
5. Birbamer G, Buchberger W, Kampfl A, et al. Early detection of post-traumatic olivary hypertrophy by MRI. *J Neurol* 1993;240:407–409.
6. Yokota T, Tsukagoshi H. Olivary hypertrophy precedes the appearance of palatal myoclonus [Letter]. *J Neurol* 1991;238:408.
7. Lapresle J, Ben Hamida M. A contribution to the knowledge of the dento-olivary pathway: anatomical study of 2 cases of hypertrophic degeneration of the olivary nucleus following limited softening of the tegmentum mesencephali. *Presse Med* 1968;76:1226–1230.
8. Lapresle J. Rhythmic palatal myoclonus and the dentato-olivary pathway. *J Neurol* 1979;220(4):223–230.
9. Koeppen AH, Barron KD, Dentinger MP. Olivary hypertrophy: histochemical demonstration of hydrolytic enzymes. *Neurology* 1980;30:471–480.
10. Goto N, Kaneko M. Olivary enlargement: chronological and morphometric analyses. *Acta Neuropathol (Berl)* 1981;54:275–282.
11. Yagishita S, Itoh Y, Nakano T. Hypertrophy of the olivary nucleus: an ultrastructural study. *Acta Neuropathol (Berl)* 1986;69:132–138.
12. Verhaart WJC, Voogd J. Hypertrophy of the inferior olives in the cat. *J Neuropathol Exp Neurol* 1962;21:92–104.
13. Voogd J, Boesten AJP. A light- and electron microscopical study of inferior olivary hypertrophy in the cat. *J Anat* 1976;122:712–713.
14. Boesten AJP, Marani E. A light- and electronmicroscopic study of olivary hypertrophy in the cat. *Neurosci Lett* 1979;8:158.
15. Llinas R, Baker R, Sotelo C. Electrotonic coupling between neurons in cat inferior olive. *J Neurophysiol* 1974;37:560–571.
16. Llinas R. Rebound excitation as the physiological basis for tremor: a biophysical study of the oscillatory properties of mammalian central neurons in vitro. In: Findley LJ, Capildeo R, eds. *Movement disorders, Tremor.* London: Macmillan, 1984:339–351.
17. Sotelo C, Gotow T, Wassef M. Localization of glutamic-acid-decarboxylase-immunoreactive axon terminals in the inferior olive of the rat, with special emphasis on anatomical relations between GABA-ergic synapses and dendrodendritic gap junctions. *J Comp Neurol* 1986;252:32–50.
18. de Zeeuw CI, Ruigrok TJ, Schalekamp MP, et al. Ultrastructural study of the cat hypertrophic inferior olive following anterograde tracing, immunocytochemistry, and intracellular labeling. *Eur J Morphol* 1990;28:240–255.
19. Ruigrok TJ, Voogd J. Cerebellar nucleo-olivary projections in the rat: an anterograde tracing study with Phaseolus vulgaris-leucoagglutinin (PHA-L). *J Comp Neurol* 1990;298:315–333.
20. Paxinos G, Watson CR, Emson PC. AChE-stained horizontal sections of the rat brain in stereotaxic coordinates. *J Neurosci Methods* 1980;3:129–149.
21. Oertel WH, Schmechel DE, Tappaz ML, et al. Production of a specific antiserum to rat brain glutamic acid decarboxylase by injection of an antigen-antibody complex. *Neuroscience* 1981;6:2689–2700.
22. Oertel WH, Schmechel DE, Mugnaini E, et al. Immunocytochemical localization of glutamate decar-

boxylase in rat cerebellum with a new antiserum. *Neuroscience* 1981;6:2715–2735.

23. Nelson BJ, Adams JC, Barmack NH, et al. Comparative study of glutamate decarboxylase immunoreactive boutons in the mammalian inferior olive. *J Comp Neurol* 1989;286:514–539.

24. Nelson BJ, Mugnaini E. The rat inferior olive as seen with immunostaining for glutamate decarboxylase. *Anat Embryol* 1988;179:109–127.

25. de Zeeuw CI, Holstege JC, Ruigrok TJ, et al. Ultrastructural study of the GABAergic, cerebellar, and mesodiencephalic innervation of the cat medial accessory olive: anterograde tracing combined with immunocytochemistry. *J Comp Neurol* 1989;284:12–35.

Myoclonus and Paroxysmal Dyskinesias,
Advances in Neurology, Vol. 89,
edited by S. Fahn, et al.
Lippincott Williams & Wilkins, Philadelphia © 2002.

15

Pathophysiology of Spinal Myoclonus

John C. Rothwell

Sobell Department of Neurophysiology, Institute of Neurology, London, United Kingdom

SPINAL MYOCLONUS

Several lines of evidence show that muscle jerks can be produced by the isolated spinal cord. Luttrell et al. (1) showed in the cat that rhythmic myoclonus of the hindquarters could be produced by inoculation of the lumbar spinal cord with Newcastle virus. This persisted after thoracic transection and intradural deafferentation of both hind limbs, suggesting that the generator of the myoclonus was intrinsic to the cord and could discharge even in the absence of peripheral or suprasegmental input. Initially, the muscle jerking in this model was confined to muscles innervated by the lumbar segments. However, in time, jerking spread to the upper body, becoming generalized. This was not due to spread of the virus up the cord since spinal transection abolished jerking above the level of the section. The authors supposed that the jerks were conducted from a lumbar origin to other segments by a spinospinal pathway. A second animal model of spinal myoclonus involves topical application of penicillin to spinal cord segments (2–4). The segmental myoclonus that is produced by this method also persists after spinal transection. The effect of deafferentation was not tested, so it is unclear whether sensory input is necessary to sustain the jerking or whether segmental circuitry alone is sufficient.

In humans, there are also rare cases of patients in whom complete spinal transection is sometimes accompanied by myoclonus in segments below the lesion. L'hermitte described a case in which spinal section was confirmed at post mortem in 1919. More recently, Bussel et al. (5) described a patient in whom rhythmic extension movements of the trunk and lower limbs started 15 months after a traumatic section of the spinal cord, verified by MRI, at the lower cervical cord. In this case, the jerks involved several segments and were probably one of the first physiologically confirmed cases of propriospinal myoclonus (see below). Fouillet et al. (6) described two other cases of tetraplegia with myoclonus of the trunk and legs, but the degree of spinal section was not complete.

There are a variety of possible reasons why the circuitry of the spinal cord should begin to produce jerky muscle contractions. All involve either increased excitability of facilitatory mechanisms or reduced activity of inhibitory mechanisms at the level of interneurons or motoneurons. Most clinical studies suggest that motoneuronal involvement is rare since weakness and denervation potentials are usually absent. Thus in most instances, it is thought that there is some disorder of spinal interneuronal circuits. This could be due to a direct effect of the disease process. Histologic studies of the cord in three cases of presumed viral infection (7,8) showed that the disease had caused preferential loss of small- to medium-sized neurons in the spinal gray matter. Large motoneurons were relatively spared. Alternatively, circuits could be driven abnormally by descending or peripheral inputs. In particular, it is possible that prolonged periods of abnormal input could cause plastic changes in neural circuits that then start to generate myoclonus (9). Deficits in neurotransmitter function are unlikely to cause focal jerking since they are likely to affect all levels of the cord equally. However, they could be responsible for some examples of enhanced spinal reflexes. Stayer and Meinck (10) suggested that a possible disorder of GABA-ergic neurons in the spinal cord of patients with stiff man syndrome was responsible for the jerky spasms provoked by sensory input.

Disordered activity in spinal interneurons is associated not only with myoclonus but also with sustained contraction of muscle. Indeed, spinal interneuronitis is more usually associated with rigidity (11–13) than myoclonus, although some cases are both rigid and jerky (7,14). The essential difference between myoclonus and rigidity is that the activity of motoneurons ceases at the end of a myoclonic jerk, and when it restarts, it does so synchronously and suddenly. Perhaps myoclonus is favored when there remains some strong inhibitory circuit that both terminates a contraction and helps synchronize activation prior to forthcoming jerks. Although a disorder of spinal interneurons is the favored pathology in most cases of spinal myoclonus, there are examples in which motoneurons have been a prime candidate. Histologic evidence was been reported in two cases of segmental spinal myoclonus (15,16). It is thought that injury or infection of motoneurons could cause changes in the distribution of ion channels in the membrane leading to repetitive discharge. If the activity of individual neurons was linked by, for example, Renshaw circuitry, then populations of motoneurons might fire together and cause muscle jerking.

There are several possible causes of spinal myoclonus. These were summarized by Brown (17) and include arteriovenous malformations; intradural tumors that may directly affect spinal circuits; extradural tumors, cysts, or spondylosis that may have indirect effects due to compression of the cord; trauma; multiple sclerosis; amyotrophic lateral sclerosis; and viral infection.

SPINAL SEGMENTAL MYOCLONUS

Segmental myoclonus is a descriptive term that indicates that the distribution of muscle jerking is limited to muscles innervated by one to two contiguous spinal segments. As such, it could be used to describe the muscle jerks that occur in some cases of epilepsia partialis continua or after lesions of peripheral nerve. However, many authors would use the term "focal" to describe such jerks and reserve the term "segmental" for jerks of an implied spinal origin. To avoid any confusion it is probably best to use "spinal segmental myoclonus" to describe jerks with a limited distribution that are thought to have a spinal origin. "Propriospinal myoclonus" can be used to describe jerks of spinal origin that have a wide distribution.

Spinal segmental myoclonus can be rhythmic, as originally emphasized by Halliday (18, 19), or irregular (20,21). In the case of Garcin et al. (22), an astrocytoma of the cervical cord caused regular jerking of the right arm at about 1 Hz (Fig. 15.1), but this became irregular following surgical biopsy. The frequency can vary enormously from patient to patient, sometimes being as rapid as 4 Hz (23), but more usually around 1 Hz. If the jerks are bilateral they are usually synchronous in homologous muscles of the two sides, but occasionally asynchronous jerking has been described (8). Similarly, the jerks are usually synchronous in all muscles of the involved side, although asynchronous activation (24) or alternating activity between antagonists (25) can be observed.

The jerks are often unaffected by mental activity or sleep (19), but several authors have described exacerbation of jerks by action or mental stress or sensory stimulation of distant parts of the body or even by sound, and their disappearance during sleep. In contrast, some forms of propriospinal myoclonus (see below) are only seen during drowsiness (26). In all cases it appears as if external inputs can alter the excitability of spinal circuits involved in the generation of spontaneous jerks.

Spinal segmental myoclonus is often stimulus sensitive (8,25,27), but this is sometimes

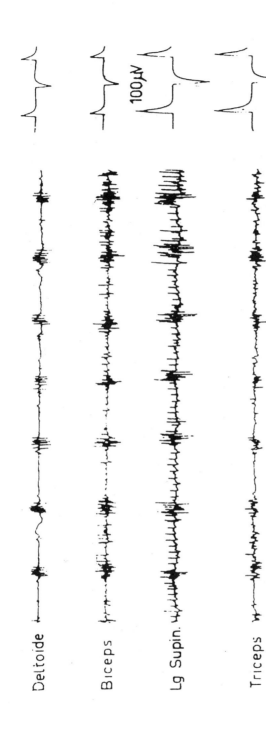

FIG. 15.1. Rythmic spinal segmental myoclonus in a patient with an astrocytoma of the cervical cord. Note the co-contracting regular bursts of electromyographic activity in deltoid, biceps, supinator, and triceps (22).

difficult to observe if the myoclonus is very regular, particularly if there is a refractory period immediately after each spontaneous jerk (28). The latency of the reflex jerks can be variable. Davis et al. (8) reported that stimulation of the right posterior tibial nerve in the popliteal fossa evoked a response in the opposite gastrocnemius at 44 ms, suggestive of a relatively fast crossed spinal reflex. Others have described longer latency responses of 100 ms or more (25,27,28). Such latencies could involve either slow conducting spinal pathways or fast supraspinal pathways. If the sensory field of the reflex is limited to a small area innervated by

affected segments, it may be more likely to be a slow spinal reflex. If responses can be obtained by applying stimuli at distant sites, then a supraspinal origin may be more likely. For example, Sagisaka et al. (28) found that taps to the opposite leg could evoke jerks in a patient with myoclonus of the shoulder. They postulated that this was an enhanced spinobulbospinal reflex (29) revealed because of increased excitability of the affected anterior horn cells.

There have been few investigations of the excitability of spinal reflex pathways in patients with spinal segmental myoclonus. Pathology of the spinal interneurons would be expected to be

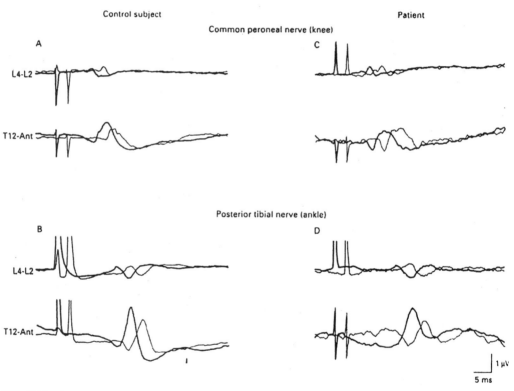

FIG. 15.2. Average sensory evoked potentials recorded from cauda equina (L4-L2) and spinal cord (T12-Ant) in a healthy subject and a patient with spinal segmental myoclonus of the L2-L4 myotomes. The traces show the responses from single *(thick lines)* and paired *(thin lines;* interstimulus interval 3 ms) stimuli applied to the common peroneal *(upper traces)* and posterior tibial *(lower traces)* nerves. Note that the response to the first of the pair of stimuli has been subtracted so that the record shows only the response to the second stimulus of the pair. After stimulation of either nerve, the cauda equina potential has recovered to full amplitude at 3 ms. However, in the healthy subject, the spinal potential is smaller to the paired than the single shock. In the patient, this is true only after stimulation of the posterior tibial nerve, but not after stimulation of the common peroneal nerve (which sends afferents to the affected L2-L4 segments of cord).

associated with changes in, for example, reciprocal inhibition, Renshaw inhibition, and in flexor reflexes. However, in most cases, the presence of continuous jerking makes such studies impossible. DiLazarro et al. (30) managed to record the spinal evoked potentials from a patient with rhythmic myoclonus of muscles innervated by the L2-L4 myotomes (Fig. 15.2). The potentials contain components related to the peripheral nerve volley in the cauda equina as well as to postsynaptic potentials in the dorsal horn. Responses to single nerve stimuli had normal latency and form, but abnormalities were seen in the recovery of excitability using a paired pulse technique. In normal subjects, the peripheral nerve volley produced by the second stimulus of a pair recovers completely at an interstimulus interval of 3 ms, whereas the dorsal horn postsynaptic potential at the same interval is suppressed to about 60% of its control size. In the patient, stimulation of the peroneal nerve, which evokes input to the affected segments of cord, produced facilitation of the dorsal horn response even though the peripheral nerve recovery was normal. The authors concluded that the dorsal horn interneurons were hyperactive in this patient and that this could contribute to the myoclonus.

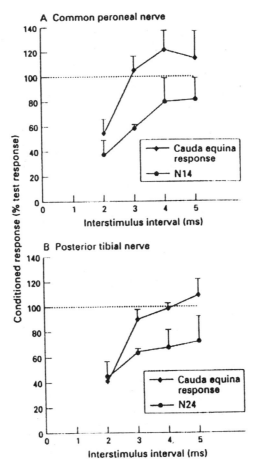

FIG. 15.2. The graphs plot the recovery curve of the cauda equina and spinal dorsal horn potential in 10 healthy subjects. Note that, as in the single traces to the left, that the cauda equina response recovers to full amplitude at an interval of 3 ms, whereas the dorsal horn potential is suppressed (30).

PROPRIOSPINAL MYOCLONUS

Propriospinal myoclonus describes jerking that involves muscles innervated by many different segments of the spinal cord. Myoclonic activity is thought to spread up and down the cord via spinospinal (sometimes called propriospinal) pathways from a more restricted source.

Bussel et al. (5) gave the first electrophysiologic description of this form of spinal myoclonus. They reported a patient with a complete lower cervical cord transection who had rhythmic spontaneous and stimulus-sensitive extension movements of the trunk and legs. The timing of the muscle activation in different muscles remained fixed, but was not measured in detail. Nevertheless, such a pattern would be consistent with spread of activation from a single source. Interestingly, stimulation of peripheral nerve could induce a reflex jerk that provoked a period of alternating flexion/extension of the legs, which the authors thought may have been due to activity in a spinal "pattern generator."

Brown et al. (31) described the detailed electrophysiology of this type of myoclonus in five patients. In all of them the jerks involved flexion of the trunk and sometimes the legs and neck. The jerks were irregular, occurring up to two times per second, and co-contracting in agonist and antagonist muscles. The EMG bursts varied considerably in duration from about 40 ms to 4 s. There was no sign of cortical or reticular involvement in the jerks. In four of the five patients it was possible to identify the order of recruitment of muscles in each jerk from a single spinal generator. The example in Figure 15.3 is typical. This single spontaneous jerk starts in the upper rectus abdominis and then spreads over the next 50 ms to activate more rostral and caudal spinal segments. The speed of conduction suggests a relatively slow spinal conduction velocity of around 5 m per second. In two of the cases, the origin of the myoclonus was thought to be in the lower part of the thoracic cord (as in the patient in Fig. 3). In two others it was thought to be in the cervicothoracic junction. Four of the five patients were stimulus sensitive, with reflex latencies of 100 ms or more. Two of them had shorter latency jerks of around 35 ms in the abdominal recti after taps to the neck or abdomen.

Brown et al. speculated that the activity was conducted from segment to segment through long propriospinal pathways. These are known in cat to be relatively slow conducting (32) and to recruit mainly trunk and proximal limb muscles bilaterally (33,34).

In a later paper, Brown et al. (31) described a further eight patients with truncal jerks, and found that in six of them, each spontaneous jerk consisted of a repetitive series of abdominal contractions at 1 to 7 Hz. The majority of cases had suffered some trauma to the cervical cord prior to the myoclonus, and the authors speculated, like Bussel et al. (5), that cervical damage might have released a "pattern generator" in the lower thoracic cord.

There have been several other reports of patients with propriospinal myoclonus and slow spread of activity from a restricted section of the spinal cord (6,26,35–37). Vetrugno et al. (38) reported a case in which myoclonus was sometimes confined to abdominal muscles as in spinal segmental myoclonus, while at others the jerks seemed to spread slowly (5–15 m per second) up and down the cord to involve muscles in the neck and leg. They postulated that the same generator was involved in both types of jerk and that under conditions of heightened excitability jerks spread away from the area of the primary focus. Schulze-Bonhage et al. (39) described a case with a purely stimulus-sensitive form of propriospinal myoclonus in which stimuli to the back and abdomen could provoke axial jerks at short latency with spread to rostral and caudal segments of the cord.

CONCLUSIONS

Damage to segments of the spinal cord, particularly if it involves loss of or changes in excitability of spinal interneurons, can release activity that produces spontaneous and often rhythmic bursts muscle jerking. The damage may either be direct or it may involve changes in the input to spinal segments

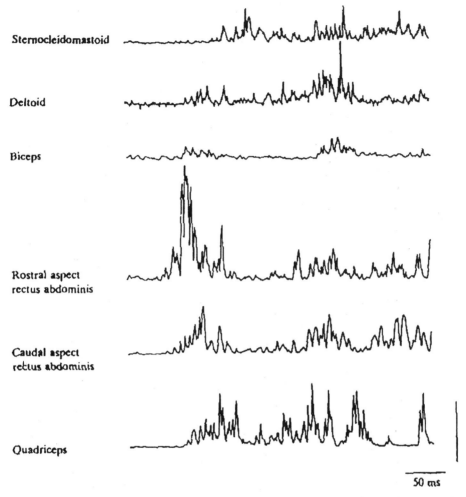

Sternocleidomastoid

Deltoid

Biceps

Rostral aspect
rectus abdominis

Caudal aspect
rectus abdominis

Quadriceps

50 ms

FIG. 15.3. Rectified electromyograms of a single spontaneous jerk in a case of propriospinal myoclonus. Note that the jerk begins with activity in the rostral rectus abdominis and then spreads slowly up and down the cord to other muscles. The vertical calibration is 100 µV for the bottom three channels and 200 µV for the top three channels (40,41).

from other structures both peripheral and supraspinal. The latter could, for example, release intrinsic spinal pattern generators from external control or could provoke plastic reorganization of cord circuits to favor rhythmic discharges.

In some cases, myoclonus remains restricted to the affected segments (spinal segmental myoclonus), but in others it may spread rostrally and caudally (propriospinal myoclonus) to cause jerking in muscles innervated by distant segments. At the present time

it is not clear what distinguishes the pattern of damage that produces myoclonus from that which produces sustained muscle contraction (rigidity). Nor is it clear what factors are involved in facilitating the spread of myoclonus in the propriospinal form.

REFERENCES

1. Luttrell CN, Bang FB, Luxenberg K. Newcastle disease encephalomyelitis in cats. II: physiological studies on rhythmic myoclonus. *Arch Neurol Psychiatry* 1959;81: 285–291.

2. Kao LI, Crill WE. Penicillin-induced segmental my-oclonus. I: motor responses and intracellular recording from motoneurons. *Arch Neurol* 1972;26:156–161.
3. Kao LI, Crill WE. Penicillin-induced segmental my-oclonus. II: membrane properties of cat spinal mo-toneurons. *Arch Neurol* 1972;26:162–168.
4. Lothman EW, Somjen GG. Motor and electrical signs of epileptiform activity induced by penicillin in the spinal cords of decapitate cats. *Electroencephalogr Clin Neu-rophysiol* 1976;41:237–252.
5. Bussel B, Roby BA, Azouvi P, et al. Myoclonus in a pa-tient with spinal cord transection. Possible involvement of the spinal stepping generator. *Brain* 1988;111:1235–1245.
6. Fouillet N, Wiart L, Arne P, et al. Propriospinal myoclonus in tetraplegic patients: clinical, electrophysiological and therapeutic aspects. *Paraplegia* 1995;33:678–681.
7. Howell DA, Lees AJ, Toghill PJ. Spinal internuncial neurons in progressive encephalomyelitis with rigidity. *J Neurol Neurosurg Psychiatry* 1979;42:773–785.
8. Davis SM, Murray NM, Diengdoh JV, et al. Stimulus-sensitive spinal myoclonus. *J Neurol Neurosurg Psychi-atry* 1981;44:884–888.
9. Glocker FX, Deuschl G, Volk B, et al. Bilateral my-oclonus of the trapezius muscles after distal lesion of an accessory nerve. *Mov Disord* 1996;11:571–575.
10. Stayer C, Meinck HM. Stiff-man syndrome: an overview. *Neurologia* 1988;13:83–88.
11. Penry JK, Hoefnagel D, Van den Noort S, et al. Muscle spasm and abnormal postures resulting from damage to interneurones in the spinal cord. *Arch Neurol* 1960;34:500–512.
12. Rushworth G, Lishman WA, Hughes JT, et al. Intense rigidity of the arms due to isolation of motoneurones by a spinal tumour. *J Neurol Neurosurg Psychiatry* 1961;24:132–142.
13. Tarlov IM. Rigidity in man due to spinal interneuron loss. *Arch Neurol* 1967;16:536–543.
14. Whiteley AM, Swash M, Urich H. Progressive en-cephalomyelitis with rigidity. *Brain* 1976;99:27–42.
15. Shivapour E, Teasdall RD. Spinal myoclonus with vac-uolar degeneration of anterior horn cells. *Arch Neurol* 1980;37:451–453.
16. Roobol TH, Kazzaz BA, Vecht CJ. Segmental rigidity and spinal myoclonus as a paraneoplastic syndrome. *J Neurol Neurosurg Psychiatry* 1987;50:628–631.
17. Brown P. Spinal myoclonus. In: Marsden CD, Fahn S, eds. *Movement disorders 3.* London: Butterworth, 1993.
18. Halliday AM. The electrophysiological study of my-oclonus in man. *Brain* 1967;90:241–284.
19. Halliday AM. The neurophysiology of myoclonic jerk-ing: a reappraisal. In: Charlton HH, ed. *Myoclonic seizures.* Excerpta Medica International Congress Se-ries. Amsterdam: Excerpta Medica; 1975;307:1–29.
20. Fox EJ, Villanueva R, Schutta HS. Myoclonus following spinal anesthesia. *Neurology* 1979;29:379–380.
21. Levy R, Plassche W, Riggs J, et al. Spinal myoclonus re-lated to an arteriovenous malformation. Response to clonazepam therapy. *Arch Neurol* 1983;40:254–255.
22. Garcin R, Rondot P, Guiot G. Rhythmic myoclonus of the right arm as the presenting symptom of a cervical cord tumour. *Brain* 1968;91:75–84.
23. Jankovic J, Pardo R. Segmental myoclonus: clinical and pharmacologic study. *Arch Neurol* 1986;43:1025–1031.
24. Nohl M, Doose H, Gross SG, et al. Sinal myoclonus. *Eur Neurol* 1978;17:129–135.
25. Lagueny A, Tison F, Burbaud P, et al. Stimulus-sensitive spinal segmental myoclonus improved with injections of botulinum toxin type A. *Mov Disord* 1999;14:182–185.
26. Montagna P, Provini F, Plazzi G, et al. Propriospinal myoclonus upon relaxation and drowsiness: a cause of severe insomnia. *Mov Disord* 1997;12:66–72.
27. Neshige R, Kuroda Y, Oda K, et al. Reflex spinal my-oclonus. Report of a case and its physiological mecha-nism. *Rinsho Shinkeigaku* 1985;25:408–411.
28. Sagisaka H, Kakigi R, Shibasaki H, et al. A case of stimulus-sensitive segmental spinal myoclonus. *Rinsho Shinkeigaku* 1989;29:310–314.
29. Shimamura M, Livingstone RB. Longitudinal conduc-tion system serving spinal and brainstem co-ordination. *J Neurophysiol* 1963;26:258–267.
30. DiLazarro V, Restuccia D, Nardone R, et al. Changes in spinal cord excitability in a patient with rhythmic seg-mental myoclonus. *J Neurol Neurosurg Psychiatry* 1996;61:641–644.
31. Brown P, Rothwell JC, Thompson PD, et al. Pro-priospinal myoclonus: evidence for spinal "pattern" generators in humans. *Mov Disord* 1994;9:571–576.
32. Lloyd DPC. Mediation of descending long spinal reflex activity. *J Neurophysiol* 1942;5:435–458.
33. Baldissera F, Lundberg A, Udo M. Activity evoked from the mesencephalic tegmentum in descending pathways other than the rubrospinal tract. *Exp Brain Res* 1972;15:133–150.
34. Vasilenko DA. Propriospinal pathways in the ventral fu-nicles of the cat spinal cord: their effects on lum-bosacral motoneurones. *Brain Res* 1975;93:502–506.
35. Kapoor R, Brown P, Thompson PD, et al. Propriospinal myoclonus in multiple sclerosis. *J Neurol Neurosurg Psychiatry* 1992;55:1086–1088.
36. Chokroverty S. Propriospinal myoclonus. *Clin Neurosci* 1995;3:219–222.
37. Nogues M, Cammarota A, Sola C, et al. Propriospinal myoclonus in ischemic myelopathy secondary to a spinal dural arteriovenous fistula. *Mov Disord* 2000;15:355–358.
38. Vetrugno R, Provini F, Plazzi G, et al. Focal myoclonus and propriospinal propagation. *Clin Neurophysiol* 2000;111:2175–2179.
39. Schulze-Bonhage A, Knott H, Ferbert A. Pure stimulus-sensitive truncal myoclonus of propriospinal origin. *Mov Disord* 1996;11:87–90.
40. Brown P, Thompson PD, Rothwell JC, et al. Paroxysmal axial spasms of spinal origin. *Mov Disord* 1991;6:43–48.
41. Brown P, Thompson PD, Rothwell JC, et al. Axial myoclonus of propriospinal origin. *Brain* 1991;114:197–214.

Myoclonus and Paroxysmal Dyskinesias,
Advances in Neurology, Vol. 89,
edited by S. Fahn, et al.
Lippincott Williams & Wilkins, Philadelphia © 2002.

16

Restless Legs Syndrome and Periodic Limb Movements

Claudia Trenkwalder

Department of Clinical Neurophysiology, University of Goettingen, Goettingen, Germany

Restless legs syndrome (RLS) has already been described by Sir Thomas Willis, an English physician in 1672. During the centuries the term has changed several times until Karl A. Ekbom, a Swedish neurologist and surgeon, used this term for the description of nocturnal symptoms at the legs associated with sleep disorders (1). Ekbom already mentioned many aspects that have been described in past years, such as the familial component of the RLS, clinical symptomatology, and associated disorders.

The definition of the RLS comprises a clinical entity of various sensory and motor complaints that have been defined in a consensus by the International Restless Legs Syndrome Study Group (2) (IRLSSG) using four minimal criteria: (a) a desire to move the limbs, usually associated with paresthesias; (b) motor restlessness; (c) symptoms are present exclusively at rest with a partial or temporary relief by activity; (d) symptoms are worse in the evening or at night (Table 16.1). The clinical diagnosis is supported by additional criteria that may be often present but are not obligatory for the diagnosis. These additional features include sleep disturbance, with problems falling asleep and maintaining sleep; involuntary movements, the periodic limb or leg movements in sleep (PLMS) that usually affect the legs or rarely the arms; involuntary limb movements while awake and at rest; a normal neurologic examination; a

clinical course that may begin at any age, with in general a chronic condition including remissions or exacerbations; a positive family history that is suggestive for a familial disorder (2).

TABLE 16.1. *Clinical characteristics of restless legs syndrome necessary for diagnosis (minimal criteria)*

1. Desire to move the limbs usually associated with paresthesias or dysesthesias.
The paresthesias or dysesthesias are sensations that occur spontaneously during wakefulness and are often described as creeping, crawling, tingling, burning, painful, aching, cramping, knife–like, or itching. They are usually experienced as "deep seated," i.e., affecting the depth of the extremities, rather than superficially on the skin. Usually the legs alone are symptomatic or the legs are affected more than the arms. The paresthesias or dysethesias may be bilateral or unilateral, and their bodily distribution may fluctuate several times during a 24-h period.

2. Motor restlessness.
During wakefulness, patients move to relieve the paresthesias, dysesthesias, or discomfort in the limbs. The movements are involuntary in the sense that patients feel compelled to move, but the movements are voluntary in the sense that patients choose which movement to make.

3. Symptoms are worse or exclusively present at rest (i.e., lying, sitting) with at least partial and temporary relief by activity.

4. Symptoms are worse in evening or night.

Minimal criteria: 1 + 2 + 3 + 4 (all four features must be present to make the diagnosis).
Modified from Walters AS and the International Restless Legs Syndrome Study Group. Toward a better definition of the Restless Legs Syndrome. *Mov Disord* 1995;10:634–642.

CLINICAL SYMPTOMATOLOGY

The RLS is characterized by a wide range of symptoms including unpleasant sensations mostly deep in the limbs or between the ankle and knee, sometimes extending to the entire lower or even upper limb (for further details see Table 16.1). With progressive disease an involvement of the arms has been described in up to 48% of patients (3). Because pain is a frequent description in RLS, it often leads to a misdiagnosis of RLS as a chronic pain problem. Symptoms occur mostly when lying or resting and stop by moving, especially walking (4). Movements of voluntary actions such as pacing, shaking, or rubbing the limbs usually relieve symptoms temporarily, but these actions cannot replace pharmacologic treatment.

The clinical diagnosis is based on the symptomatology, the course of the disease, and findings from sleep studies, if available.

The differential diagnosis of RLS includes many other conditions that are associated with either motor restlessness, sleep disorders, or disagreeable feelings in the legs. The most important differential diagnoses are polyneuropathy, radiculopathy (5), the syndrome of painful legs and moving toes (6), myelopathies or inflammatory disorders of the spinal cord, and syndromes with increased motor restlessness. These can include panic attacks, akathisia, or myoclonic syndromes of other etiology. Other specific sleep disorders, such as sleep apnea syndrome, narcolepsy, or pure periodic limb movement disorder (PLMD) often show an increased number of periodic limb movements when investigated in the sleep laboratory (7–10).

The occurrence of PLMS associated with arousals is a frequent sign in patients with restless legs syndrome (10) but is not specific for the diagnosis. PLMS are based on the definition of the American Sleep Disorders Association (11) and are scored when there is a sequence of at least four muscle contractions recorded from the tibialis anterior muscle, each lasting 0.5 to 5 seconds and recurring at intervals of 5 to 90 seconds. These movements seem quite similar to the triple flexion movements of the hip, knee, and ankles and may also occur during relaxed wakefulness, described as dyskinesias while awake (12). During sleep, periodic leg movements may be associated with frequent arousals seen on electroencephalographic (EEG) examination and may cause the sleep disorder in RLS, which consists of light, disrupted sleep. A pathologic PLMS value is defined as more than five PLMS arousals per hour of sleep. For diagnosing RLS in the awake patient, one can also perform an immobilization test: the patients attempt to maintain a lying or sitting posture without moving the legs (suggested immobilization test [SIT]) that may provoke RLS symptoms (13). Periodic leg movements during wakefulness will then be quantified.

Actigraphy may be another method to measure the patients' motor restlessness that occurs during RLS. Actigraphic studies can be performed during the night (14), similar to polysomnographic studies of PLMS, or they can measure daytime restlessness (15).

EPIDEMIOLOGY

Recent population-based surveys showed that the prevalence of RLS in adults might range between 5% and 10% or even higher (16). In the MEMO study (17), a population-based survey of the elderly population in Germany, there was a higher prevalence of RLS in women (13%) over the age of 65 compared with elderly men (7%). A similar population-based study from the United States (18) found an age-dependent prevalence of RLS between 3% and 13% in the white Caucasian population, but no gender-specific differences. No data are currently available for prevalences of other ethnic groups such as Asian or black populations.

The prevalence of periodic limb movements ranges widely, and first reports from Lugaresi (19) revealed a prevalence of PLMS of almost 90% in RLS patients; estimations in the general population vary between 6% and almost 60% in the elderly subpopulation (15,20). These data refer to the occurrence of pure PLMS, and do not control for PLMS-associated arousals that may play an important role in RLS.

PATHOPHYSIOLOGY

The etiology and cause of the RLS is still unknown, but there are complex interactions between the integration of peripheral and central structures of the nervous system that may be important for the etiology of RLS: there is an increasing number of patients with RLS symptoms and associated peripheral nerve diseases like neuropathies and radiculopathies but also RLS patients with associated central nervous system lesions (21–25).

The occurrence of PLMS and the characterization of these movements may give further clues to the pathophysiology: polygraphically recorded periodic limb movements during the day did not elicit a cortical activity proceeding these movements, thus excluding ordinary forms of cortical myoclonus as the source of the RLS-associated involuntary movements (26). One hypothesis is that PLMS probably result from supersegmental disinhibition phenomena. The temporal and local distribution pattern of the muscles activated during PLM could also be in agreement with propriospinal phenomenons (27). In six of seven patients the onset of muscle activity was shown to occur first in the quadriceps femoris muscle, with a distribution pattern of L4/5 and S1 segments and a slow spinal propagation, described by Chokroverty as "propriospinal myoclonus" (28). In a recent study that measured 100 consecutive PLMS in RLS patients there was no stable recruitment pattern (29).

Disinhibition phenomenons of diencephalospinal pathways may also play a role in the pathophysiology of RLS. A recent study of Bara-Jimenez et al. (30) showed a pathologic flexor reflex response in RLS patients while PLMS occurred, thus pointing to an increased disinhibition level. Activated brain areas detected by functional magnetic resonance tomography (fMRT) favor brainstem generators and the involvement of the red nuclei as well as the cerebellum during the occurrence of periodic limb movement (31). The role of the basal ganglia, especially in respect to the efficacy of dopaminergic medication in RLS, remains controversial (32). In neuroimaging studies with positron emission tomography (PET) and single photon emission tomography (SPECT), subtle alterations of the dopaminergic system clearly different from the marked changes observed in Parkinson's disease could be detected (33,34). Comparing RLS patients with aged-matched controls, there was no difference between the striatal binding of Iodobenzamide (IBZM) nor the dopamine transporter binding when treated and never-treated RLS patients were compared (35). In another small study, two family members with RLS were investigated during the state of pain. The regional cerebral blood flow (RCBF-SPECT) with the tracer hexametazime (HM-PAO) before and after treatment with levodopa was measured. An increase of blood flow in the thalamus and decrease in the caudate nucleus in both patients investigated occurred only during the states of pain. With respect to the painful sensations that occur in RLS patients, the measured changes may be associated with the condition of pain and may alter basal ganglia functions as a secondary phenomenon (36). Using transcranial magnetic stimulation in a special double-stimulation technique, impaired intracortical inhibition was found in RLS patients in both a foot muscle and a hand muscle, but the latter was not involved in the clinical symptoms (37).

The role of peripheral nerve disorders may be apparent by the association of RLS with diabetes, cryoglobulinemia, amyloidosis (21,24, 38), and other neuropathies. Patients with Charcot-Marie-Tooth disease (CMT) type 1 and 2 showed RLS in 37% of the CMT2 type (39). Morphometric analysis of sural nerve biopsies revealed alterations in myelinated fiber density in patients with RLS compared with healthy controls, although RLS patients did not reveal a clinically manifest polyneuropathy. The authors suggest that an affection of small unmyelinated fibers may play a role in the development of RLS symptoms.

From treatment studies it may be obvious that the dopaminergic and opioid system is involved in the pathophysiology of the RLS (40, 41). Dopamine D2-receptor blocking agents, such as typical neuroleptic drugs, can worsen RLS or may induce symptoms (42–45). The therapeutic effect of the μ-opioid receptor agonist codeine could be blocked by the dopamine receptor antagonist pimozide in RLS patients (46), but in never-treated RLS patients an opioid antagonist, naloxone, could not provoke RLS symptoms (47). In opioid-treated patients, however, naloxone was a powerful activator of specific RLS symptoms (43,44). One may assume that a provocation of RLS symptoms by opioid antagonists in never-treated RLS patients is not possible and that the opioidergic tone in RLS may be rather low.

Endocrine investigations in RLS patients during the circadian course revealed normal levels of prolactin and growth hormone and a normal circadian rhythm of these hormones (48). The circadian rhythm of the RLS is also part of the diagnostic criteria (2) and has been investigated in recent studies. Measuring the symptoms of RLS during 3 days one could observe that there is a close relationship between the occurrence of RLS symptoms and the time of the day or night. All symptoms worsened in the evening, with a maximum increase between midnight and 3 a.m. (15,49). The measured temperature curves in these studies revealed a normal circadian core temperature that showed the minimum value at the highest PLMS numbers and vice versa. Hening et al. (15) therefore suggest that "RLS can be considered as an abnormal result linked to a normal circadian rhythm." There are many unsolved phenomenons in the clinical occurrence of RLS, for example, the role of iron (50), which may contribute to the pathophysiology of RLS as a major factor, which was assumed by Allen et al. (52). Studies of cerebrospinal fluid measurements in RLS patients showed a decrease of ferritin (51), and MRI studies revealed alterations of iron storage in several brain regions in RLS patients (51). Reports from patients with iron deficiency anemia point to iron as a pathophysiologic factor in the development of RLS. Iron supplement may lead to significant improvement in RLS patients with iron deficiency (50,53,54).

GENETICS OF RESTLESS LEGS SYNDROME

RLS often occurs in families with affected members in several generations (32). There is a wide clinical expressivity of symptoms (55), and the percentage of familial RLS varies from about 40% (56) to up to 65% (57). All these studies are based on questionnaires, sometimes by history of the patients, but direct interviews of all family members were not used, including non–affected family members (10,25,56). To analyze the mode of inheritance and to clarify the age of onset of RLS a recent study with a complex segregation analysis was performed. It showed that only patients with a younger age of onset were documented with a clear familial pattern compared with patients with a late onset of symptoms. In this study, an autosomal dominant mode of inheritance in the young-onset affected patients was the most likely model (58). A very recent study found a locus of an increased susceptibility in one French-Canadian family on chromosome 12q (59). Further studies have to elucidate if this result can also be detected in other RLS families.

SECONDARY FORMS OF RESTLESS LEGS SYNDROME

The clinical symptomatology of secondary RLS closely resembles the phenomena of the idiopathic forms. This was demonstrated when comparing patients with idiopathic and uremic RLS (60–62). Uremic RLS is the most frequent secondary form and seems to be associated with the increase of uremia and not the start of dialysis (60). No parameter that is associated with uremia and RLS could be detected to explain the occurrence of about 20% uremic patients presenting with RLS (60,62). In addition RLS is often associated with rheumatoid arthritis, disturbances of the thyroid metabolism, iron metabolism, and pregnancy (4,63).

THERAPY

The indication to treat results from subjectively reduced quality of life and quality of sleep. Treatment strategies for RLS are variable and mainly focus on dopaminergic therapy. Nonpharmacologic measures include advice on improvement of sleep hygiene and avoidance of stimulants or aggravating drugs (e.g., caffeine, alcohol, antihistamines, certain antidepressants). In physiologic conditions such as pregnancy, symptoms may resolve after delivery. In iron-deficiency anemia, iron supplementation should be given first.

Idiopathic RLS patients should be treated with dopaminergic drugs as the medication of first choice (15,64), provided the patients do not have any contraindications for dopaminergic treatment. A dosage of 50 to 100 mg of levodopa plus DDCI, such as carbidopa or benserazide, is usually effective when first administered (64,65).

Single or divided doses up to 200 to 300 mg of levodopa per night as short-acting or sustained-release preparations (66) can be titrated individually. Dopamine agonists, such as bromocriptine (67), pergolide (68,69), pramipexole (70), ropinirole (71,72), or cabergoline (73) are effective drugs in moderate to severe RLS or when rebound or augmentation occurs (74).

Opioids, especially oxycodone and tramadol, often prove to be very useful to treat sleep disorders and waking discomforts in RLS (41). Opioids generally are well tolerated and usually do not create problems with dependence. Like levodopa, they can be taken in single doses for specific situations likely to provoke RLS or as continuous long-term medication (75). Methadone can be considered for refractory cases that cannot be managed with other medications.

Benzodiazepines, especially clonazepam (76), can be used alternatively or in addition to dopaminergic agents and opioids. Other substances like carbamazepine (77), gabapentin (78), or baclofen (79) are second choice and generally have not been recognized as being as consistently efficacious as first-line agents

(80). They should be considered, however, when pharmacotherapy is indicated and patients cannot tolerate first-line agents.

A questionnaire study among sleep experts as well as a task force group of the American Sleep Disorders Association agrees that dopaminergic agents followed by opioids and benzodiazepines are the treatment of choice for RLS. In some difficult cases, combination therapies have been considered necessary as well by almost all experts, with agents generally selected from the three favored classes (80).

REFERENCES

1. Ekbom KA. Restless legs syndrome. *Acta Med Scand* 1945;158:4–122.
2. Walters A S and the International Restless Legs Syndrome Study Group. Toward a better definition of the Restless Legs Syndrome. *Mov Disord* 1995;10:634–642.
3. Michaud M, Chabli A, Lavigne G, et al. Arm restlessness in patients with restless legs syndrome. *Mov Disord* 2000;15: 289–293.
4. Collado-Seidel V, Winkelmann J, Trenkwalder C. Aetiology and treatment of restless legs syndrome. *CNS Drugs* 1999;12:9–20.
5. Walters AS, Wagner M, Hening WA. Periodic limb movements as the initial manifestation of restless legs syndrome triggered by lumbosacral radiculopathy. *Sleep* 1996;19:825–826.
6. Dressler D, Thompson PD, Gledhill RF, et al. The syndrome of painful legs and moving toes. *Mov Disord* 1994;9:13–21.
7. Boivin DB, Lorrain D, Montplaisir J. Effects of bromocriptine on periodic limb movements in human narcolepsy. *Neurology* 1993;43:2134–2136.
8. Briellmann RS, Mathis J, Bassetti C, et al. Patterns of muscle activity in legs in sleep apnea patients before and during nCPAP therapy. *Eur Neurol* 1997;38:113–118.
9. Guilleminault C, Philip P. Tiredness and somnolence despite initial treatment of obstructive sleep apnea syndrome (what to do when an OSAS patient stays hypersomnolent despite treatment). *Sleep* 1996;19: S117–S122.
10. Montplaisir J, Boucher S, Poirier G, et al. Clinical, polysomnographic, and genetic characteristics of restless legs syndrome: a study of 133 patients diagnosed with new standard criteria. *Mov Disord* 1997;12:61–65.
11. Atlas Task Force of the American Sleep Disorders Association and Guilleminault C. Recording and scoring leg movements. *Sleep* 1993;16:748–759.
12. Hening WA, Walters AS, Kavey N, et al: Dyskinesias while awake and periodic movements in sleep in restless legs syndrome: treatment with opioids. *Neurology* 1986; 36:1363–1366.
13. Montplaisir J, Boucher S, Nicolas A, et al. Immobilization tests and periodic leg movements in sleep for the diagnosis of restless leg syndrome. *Mov Disord* 1998; 13:324–329.

14. Kazenwadel J, Pollmächer T, Trenkwalder C, et al. New actigraphic assessment method for periodic leg movements (PLM). *Sleep* 1995;18:689–697.

15. Hening WA, Walters AS, Wagner M, et al. Circadian rhythm of motor restlessness and sensory symptoms in the idiopathic restless legs syndrome. *Sleep* 1999;22: 901–912.

16. Lavigne GJ, Montplaisier JY. Restless legs syndrome and sleep bruxism: prevalence and association among Canadians. *Sleep* 1994;17:739–43.

17. Rothdach A, Trenkwalder C, Haberstock J, et al. Prevalence and risk factors of RLS in an elderly population: the MEMO study. *Neurology* 2000;54:1064–1068.

18. Philips B, Young T, Finn L, et al. Epidemiology of restless legs symptoms in adults. *Arch Intern Med* 2000; 160:2137–2141.

19. Lugaresi E, Coccagna C, Tassinari CA, et al. Reliefi poligrafici sui fenomeni motori nella sindrome delle gambe senza riposo. *Riv Neurol* 1965;35:550–561.

20. Ancoli-Israel S, Kripke DM, Klauber MR, et al. Periodic limb movements in sleep in community dwelling elderly. *Sleep* 1991;14:496–500.

21. Gemignani F, Marbini A, DiGiovanni G, et al. Cryoglobulinaemic neuropathy manifesting with restless legs syndrome. *J Neurol Sci* 1997;152:218–223.

22. Hartmann M, Pfister R, Pfadenhauer K. Restless legs syndrome associated with spinal cord lesions. *J Neurol Neurosurg Psychiatry* 1999;66:688–689.

23. Hemmer B, Riemann D, Glocker FX, et al. Restless legs syndrome after a borrelia-induced myelitis. *Mov Disord* 1995;10:521–526.

24. Rutkove SB, Matheson JK, Logigian EL. Restless legs syndrome in patients with polyneuropathy. *Muscle Nerve* 1996;19:670–672.

25. Walters AS, Hickey K, Maltzman J, et al. A questionnaire study of 138 patients with restless legs syndrome: the night-walkers-survey. *Neurology* 1996;46:92–95.

26. Trenkwalder C, Bucher S, Pröckl D, et al. Bereitschaftspotential in idiopathic and symptomatic restless legs syndrome. *Electroencephalogr Clin Neurophysiol* 1993;89:95–103.

27. Trenkwalder C, Bucher SF, Oertel WH. Electrophysiological pattern of involuntary limb movements in the restless legs syndrome. *Muscle Nerve* 1993;19:155–162.

28. Chokroverty S, Walters A, Zimmerman, et al. Propriospinal myoclonus: a neurophysiologic analysis. *Neurology* 1992;42:1591–1595.

29. Provini F, Vetrugno R, Meletti S, et al. Motor pattern of periodic limb movements during sleep. *Neurology* 2001;57:300-4.

30. Bara-Jimenez W, Aksu M, Graham B, et al. Periodic limb movements in sleep: state dependent excitability of the spinal flexor reflex. *Neurology* 2000;54:1609–1616.

31. Bucher SF, Seelos KC, Oertel WH, et al. Cerebral generators involved in the pathogenesis of the restless legs syndrome. *Ann Neurol* 1997;41:639–645.

32. Trenkwalder C, Seidel VC, Gasser T, et al. Clinical symptoms and possible anticipation in a large kindred of familial restless legs syndrome. *Mov Disord* 1996; 11:389–394:

33. Routtinen HM, Partinen M, Hublin C, et al. An FDOPA PET study in patients with periodic limb movement disorder and restless legs syndrome. *Neurology* 2000;54: 502–504.

34. Turjanski N, Lees AJ, Brooks DJ. Striatal dopaminergic function in restless legs syndrome: 18F-dopa and 11C-raclopride PET studies. *Neurology* 1999;52:932–937.

35. Eisensehr I, Wetter TC, Linke R, et al. Normal IPT and IBZM SPECT in drug-naive and levodopa treated idiopathic restless legs syndrome. *Neurology* 2001;57(7): 1307–9.

36. Mountz JM, Bradley LA, Modell JG, et al. Fibromyalgia in women: abnormalities of regional blood flow in the thalamus and the caudate nucleus are associated with low pain threshold levels. *Arthritis Rheum* 1995; 138:926–938.

37. Tergau F, Wischer S, Paulus W. Motor system excitability in patients with restless legs syndrome. *Neurology* 1999;52:1060–1063.

38. Salvi F, Montagna P, Plasmati R, et al. Restless legs syndrome and nocturnal myoclonus: initial clinical manifestation of familial amyloid polyneuropathy. *J Neurol Neurosurg Psychiatry* 1999;53:522–5.

39. Gemignani F, Marbini A, Di Giovanni G, et al. Charcot-Marie-Tooth disease type 2 with restless legs syndrome. *Neurology* 1999;52:1064–1066.

40. Akpinar S. Restless legs syndrome treatment with dopaminergic drugs. *Clin Neuropharmacol* 1987;10: 69–79.

41. Walters AS, Wagner ML, Hening WA, et al. Successful treatment of the idiopathic restless legs syndrome in a randomized double-blind trial of oxycodone versus placebo. *Sleep* 1993;16:327–332.

42. Kraus T, Schuld A, Pollmächer T. Periodic leg movements in sleep and restless legs syndrome probably caused by olanzapine [Letter]. *J Clin Psychopharmacol* 1999;19:478–479.

43. Walters AS, Hening W. Review of the clinical presentation and neuropharmacology of the restless legs syndrome. *Clin Neuropharmacol* 1987;10:225–237.

44. Walters AS, Hening W, Cote L, et al. Dominantly inherited restless legs with myoclonus and periodic movements of sleep: a syndrome related to the endogenous opiates? *Adv Neurol* 1986;43:309–319.

45. Ware JC, Brown FW, Moorad PJ, et al. Nocturnal myoclonus and tricyclic antidepressants. *Sleep Res* 1984; 13:72.

46. Montplaisir J, Lorrain D, Godbout R. Restless legs syndrome and periodic movements in sleep: the primary role of dopaminergic mechanism. *Eur Neurol* 1991;31: 411–443.

47. Winkelmann J, Schadrack J, Wetter TC, et al. Opioid and dopamine antagonist drug challenges in untreated restless legs syndrome patients. *Sleep Med* 2001;2: 57–61.

48. Wetter TC, Trenkwalder C, Oertel H, et al. Endocrine rhythms in patients with restless legs syndrome. *J Neurol* 2001 (*in press*).

49. Trenkwalder C, Hening WA, Walters AS, et al. Circadian rhythm of periodic limb movements and sensory symptoms of restless legs syndrome. *Mov Disord* 1999;14:102–110.

50. Sun ER, Chen CA, Ho G, et al. Iron and the restless legs syndrome. *Sleep* 1998;21:371–377.

51. Allen RP, Barker PB, Wehrl F, et al. MRI measurement of brain iron in patients with restless legs syndrome. *Neurology* 2001;66:263–265.

52. Earley CJ, Connor JR, Beard JL, et al. Abnormalities in CSF concentrations of ferritin and transferring in restless legs syndrome. *Neurology* 2000;54:1698–1700.

53. Davis BJ, Rajput A, Rajput ML, et al. A randomized,

double-blind placebo-controlled trial of iron in restless legs syndrome. *Eur Neurol* 2000;43:70–75.

54. O'Keeffe ST, Gavin K, Lavan JN. Iron status and restless legs syndrome in the elderly. *Age Ageing* 1994;23:200–203.

55. Walters AS, Picchietti D, Hening W, et al. Variable expressivity in familial restless legs syndrome. *Arch Neurol* 1990;47:1219–1220.

56. Winkelmann J, Wetter TC, Collado-Seidel V, et al. Frequency and characteristics of the hereditary restless legs syndrome in a population of 300 patients. *Sleep* 2000;23:597–602.

57. Ondo W, Jankovic J. Restless legs syndrome: clinicoetiologic correlates. *Neurology* 1996;47:1435–1441.

58. Lazzarini A, Walters AS, Hockey K, et al. Studies of penetrance and anticipation in five autosomal-dominant restless legs syndrome pedigrees. *Mov Disord* 1999;14:111–116.

59. Desautels A, Turecki G, Montplaisir J, et al. Identification of a major susceptibility locus for restless legs syndrome on chromosome 12q. *Am J Hum Genet* 2001;69:1266–1270.

60. Collado-Seidel V, Kohnen R, Samtleben W, et al. Clinical and biochemical findings in uremic patients with and without restless legs syndrome. *Am J Kidney Dis* 1998;31:324–328.

61. Wetter TC, Stiasny K, Kohnen R, et al. Polysomnographic sleep measures in patients with uremic and idiopathic restless legs syndrome. *Mov Disord* 1998;13:820–824.

62. Winkelman JW, Chertow GM, Lazarus JM. Restless legs syndrome in end-stage renal disease. *Am J Kidney Dis* 1996;28:372–378.

63. Goodman JDS, Brodie C, Ayida GA. Restless leg syndrome in pregnancy. *Br Med J* 1988;297:1101–1102.

64. Chesson AL, Wise M, Davila D, et al. Practice parameters for the treatment of restless legs syndrome and periodic limb movement disorder: an American Academy of Sleep Medicine Report. Standards of Practice Committee of the Academy of Sleep Medicine. *Sleep* 1999;22:961–968.

65. Trenkwalder C, Stiasny K, Pollmaecher T, et al. L-dopa therapy of uremic and idiopathic restless legs syndrome: a double-blind, crossover trial. *Sleep* 1995;18:681–688.

66. Collado-Seidel V, Kazenwadel J, Wetter TC, et al. A controlled study of additional sr-L-dopa in L-dopa-responsive restless legs syndrome with late-night symptoms. *Neurology* 1999;52:285–290.

67. Walters AS, Hening W, Kavey N, et al. A double-blind randomized crossover trial of bromocriptine and placebo in restless legs syndrome. *Ann Neurol* 1988;24:455–458.

68. Earley CJ, Yaffee JB, Allen RP. Randomized, double-blind, placebo-controlled trial of pergolide in restless legs syndrome. *Neurology* 1998;51:1599–1602.

69. Wetter TC, Stiasny K, Winkelmann J, et al. A randomized controlled study of pergolide in patients with restless legs syndrome. *Neurology* 1999;52:944–950.

70. Montplaisir J, Nicolas A, Denesle R, et al. Restless legs syndrome improved by pramipexole: a double-blind randomized trial. *Neurology* 1999;52:938–943.

71. Saletu B, Gruber G, Saletu M, et al. Sleep laboratory studies in restless legs syndrome patients as compared with normals and acute effects of ropinirole. 1: findings on objective and subjective sleep and awakening quality. *Neuropsychobiology* 2000;41:181–189.

72. Saletu M, Anderer P, Saletu B, et al. Sleep laboratory studies in restless legs syndrome patients as compared with normals and acute effects of ropinirole. 2: findings on periodic leg movements arousals and respiratory variables. *Neuropsychobiology* 2000;41:190–199.

73. Stiasny K, Roebbecke J, Schüler P, et al. The treatment of idiopathic restless legs syndrome (RLS) with the D2-agonist cabergoline: an open clinical trial. *Sleep* 2000;23:349–354.

74. Allen RP, Earley CJ. Augmentation of the restless legs syndrome with carbidopa/levodopa. *Sleep* 1996;19:205–213.

75. Walters AS, Winkelmann J, Trenkwalder C, et al. Long-term opioid monotherapy in patients with restless legs syndrome. *Mov Disord* 2001 (*in press*).

76. Benes H, Kurella B, Kummer J, et al. Rapid onset of action in restless legs syndrome: a double-blind, randomized, multicenter crossover trial. *Sleep* 1999;22:1073–1081.

77. Telstad W, Sorensen O, Larsen S, et al. Treatment of the restless legs syndrome with carbamazepine: a double blind study. *Br Med J* 1984;288:444–446.

78. Adler CH. Treatment of restless legs syndrome with gabapentin. *Clin Neuropharmacol* 1997;20:148–151.

79. Guilleminault C, Flagg W. Effect of baclofen on sleep-related periodic leg movements. *Ann Neurol* 1984;15:234–239.

80. Trenkwalder C, Walters AS, Hening W. Periodic limb movements and restless legs syndrome. *Neurol Clin* 1996;14:629–650.

Myoclonus and Paroxysmal Dyskinesias,
Advances in Neurology, Vol. 89,
edited by S. Fahn, et al.
Published by Lippincott Williams & Wilkins, Philadelphia, 2002.

17

Neurophysiology of the Startle Syndrome and Hyperekplexia

Peter Brown

Sobell Department of Neurophysiology, Institute of Neurology,
London, United Kingdom

The abnormal startle consists of an exaggerated response to unexpected stimuli, particularly sounds. The classification of the startle disorders has hitherto largely relied on electrophysiologic criteria, and its clinical utility has therefore been limited. Table 17.1 gives a clinical classification of the abnormal startle. Patients are separated according to whether the clinical picture is dominated by brief body jerks that clinically seem to follow the stimulus almost immediately or by spasms that are of visibly longer latency and last a second or more. Often these spasms follow a normal or exaggerated jerk to the stimulus.

This review will focus on one cause of short latency body jerks following unexpected stimuli: hyperekplexia (pathologic exaggeration of the physiologic startle reflex). Simple clinical features distinguishing hyperekplexia from brainstem reticular reflex myoclonus are summarized in Table 17.2. Distinguishing psychogenic jerks from hyperekplexia is difficult. The former are suggested by "belle indifference," distractibility, suggestibility, and an inconsistent pattern of electromyographic (EMG) activity in the jerks (1). Hyperekplexia is distinguished from the normal startle reflex by its lower threshold, greater extent, and resistance to habituation (2–4). The normal startle response rarely involves the lower limbs in a sitting subject, whereas this is almost always the case in hyperekplexia. The

normal startle response habituates within 1 to 5 trials of auditory stimulation repeated every 20 seconds or so, leaving only an auditory blink reflex, whereas in hyperekplexia extensive jerks persist.

Hyperekplexia can be inherited, almost always as an autosomal dominant trait, or sporadic. Familial forms are due to mutations in the α_1 subunit of the glycine receptor (5). As well as startle they may have a history of stiffness as a baby, episodes of repetitive myoclonic jerks particularly during or when going off to sleep, and hyperreflexia. A hesitant wide-based gait, apneic attacks as a baby, epilepsy, and low intelligence may also occur (6–9). However, the most important aspect of the condition for the patient is the existence of attacks of generalized stiffness in response to some unexpected stimuli (6). These tend to follow the brief body jerk, last a few seconds,

TABLE 17.1. *Classification of the abnormal startle response*

Abnormal startle response	
Short latency jerks	Longer latency spasms
Exaggerated startle/ hyperekplexia	Startle epilepsy
Brainstem reticular reflex myoclonus	Stiff-man syndrome
Psychogenic	Paroxysmal dystonias Myriachit, latah, jumpers Psychogenic

TABLE 17.2. *Differential diagnosis of hyperekplexia and brainstem reticular reflex myoclonus*

	Jerks to auditory stimuli	Greatest stimulus sensitivity to taps	Presence of spontaneous and action-induced jerks	Duration of individual EMG bursts[a]
Hyperekplexia[b]	+	Mantle area[c]	−	>75 ms
Brainstem reticular reflex myoclonus	+	Distal limb	+	<75 ms

[a]Note that this refers to the duration of individual EMG bursts; bursts can be repetitive in brainstem reticular reflex myoclonus. EMG, electromyogram.
[b]Some, but not all, of these patients have infrequent tonic spasms and a family history of startle that also serve to distinguish them from brainstem reticular reflex myoclonus.
[c]The head and upper chest and back.

and are by no means elicited by every stimulus presentation (Fig. 17.1). Consciousness is preserved. Nevertheless, these spasms frequently culminate in a fall with injury. Tonic spasms, unlike the more consistent and shorter latency startle reflex, tend to improve with anticonvulsants. Opinion is divided as to whether tonic spasms are an obligate feature of genetically defined hyperekplexia. In particular, in the Dutch pedigree described by Suhren, only family members with tonic spasms were found to carry the mutation (10).

Sporadic cases of hyperekplexia do not seem to have a genetic basis (11,12); indeed many are symptomatic and a consequence of brainstem pathology such as infarct, hemorrhage, or encephalitis (2). They, too, may exhibit tonic spasms and episodes of sustained myoclonic jerks, which are therefore not unique to hereditary hyperekplexia (2,11).

Upon examination the hallmark of hyperekplexia, whether hereditary or sporadic, is a brief body jerk of short latency following unexpected stimuli. Such stimuli may be visual,

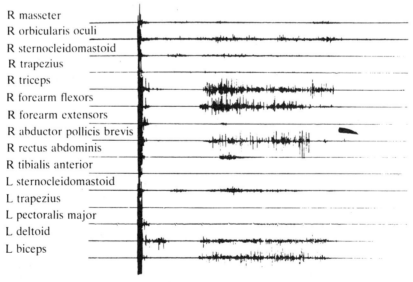

R masseter
R orbicularis oculi
R sternocleidomastoid
R trapezius
R triceps
R forearm flexors
R forearm extensors
R abductor pollicis brevis
R rectus abdominis
R tibialis anterior
L sternocleidomastoid
L trapezius
L pectoralis major
L deltoid
L biceps

FIG. 17.1. EMG record of the tonic spasm occurring after an unexpected sound in a patient with symptomatic hyperekplexia. The tonic spasm starts about 2 sec after the stimulus and is clearly separate from the very rapid and brief startle response. *L,* left; *R,* right. (From Brown P, Thompson PD, Rothwell JC, et al. The hyperekplexias and their relationship to the normal startle reflex. *Brain* 1991; 114:1903–1928, with permission.)

auditory, or somesthetic. Somesthetic stimuli are most effective when applied to the mantle area, particularly the face, when the response that results is sometimes termed a head retraction reflex.

The startle response in hyperekplexia has variously been considered to have a cortical or brainstem origin, with most current evidence favoring the latter. Two lines of evidence have been used to support a cortical origin for the startle response: the presence of giant cortical evoked potentials (13) and the presence of cortical neuronal loss on magnetic resonance spectroscopy (14). However, giant evoked potentials are only present in the minority of patients, and the study that demonstrated cortical neuronal loss did so in patients with epilepsy and without a known mutation (14). Magnetic resonance spectroscopy has been repeated in patients with a mutation in the α_1 subunit of the glycine receptor and has been found to be normal (15). The same patients were also tested with transcutaneous stimulation of the motor cortex and found to have normal stimulus response curves, cortical inhibition, and facilitation.

On the other hand, there are several lines of evidence pointing to a brainstem origin for the startle response in hyperekplexia.

- Pathology in symptomatic cases is often confined to the brainstem (2).
- Familial cases are due to mutations in the α_1 subunit of the glycine receptor, and glycine receptors are particularly concentrated in the brainstem (and spinal cord) of the mammalian central nervous system (5).
- The latency of EMG responses to taps to the head or face is often less than 20 ms (Fig. 17.2) and is in these cases only compatible with relay within the brainstem (2,4).
- The recruitment of cranial nerve innervated muscles is caudorostral in the startle, as in brainstem reticular reflex myoclonus (2).

The caudorostral recruitment of cranial nerve innervated muscles in the startle is the most contentious observation supporting a brainstem origin for the hyperekplectic startle response. There is little doubt that the shortest

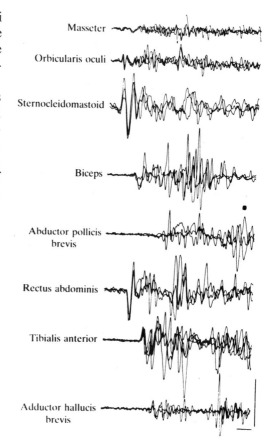

FIG. 17.2. Electromyographic (EMG) activity in the abnormal startle response elicited by taps to the head in a patient with symptomatic hyperekplexia. The unrectified EMG activity in three single trials is superimposed. Each trial was started at the point of tapping. EMG activity was recorded first in sternocleidomastoid and then later in orbicularis oculi, masseter, trunk, and limb muscles. The latencies to the intrinsic hand muscles of the hand and foot were disproportionately long. The vertical and horizontal calibration lines are 0.5 mV and 20 ms, respectively. (From Brown P, Thompson PD, Rothwell JC, et al. The hyperekplexias and their relationship to the normal startle reflex. *Brain* 1991;114:1903–1928, with permission.)

latency responses to taps to the face may follow this rule, so that the earliest muscle activity is recorded in sternocleidomastoid and later in orbicularis oculi and masseter (Fig. 17.2). However, the picture is more complicated in the startles of longer latency that follow auditory stimulation (or responses to taps in some patients). Here the earliest EMG activity is in orbicularis oculi, with sternocleidomastoid, then masseter following (Fig. 17.3). But this early response in orbicularis oculi may be due to a simultaneously induced physiologic blink

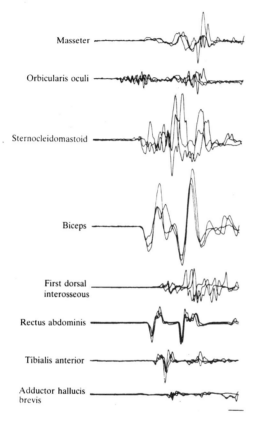

FIG. 17.3. Electromyographic (EMG) activity in the abnormal startle response elicited by auditory stimulation in a patient with symptomatic hyperekplexia. The unrectified EMG activity in three single trials is superimposed. Each trial was started at the point of presentation of a 124-dB tone. Following the normal auditory blink reflex, EMG activity was recorded first in sternocleidomastoid and then later in masseter and trunk and limb muscles.

The latencies to the intrinsic hand muscles of the hand and foot were disproportionately long. The horizontal calibration line is 20 ms. Vertical calibration is as in Figure 17.2, except for the lower five channels for which the line in Figure 17.2 represents 3 mV. (From Brown P, Thompson PD, Rothwell JC, et al. The hyperekplexias and their relationship to the normal startle reflex. *Brain* 1991;114:1903–1928, with permission.)

reflex and separate from the true generalized startle response in this muscle. Certainly two components in the EMG response in this muscle are common (Fig. 17.4), one perhaps due to the blink reflex and a later one due to the pathologic startle reflex (2–4,16).

There are other features in the recruitment order of muscles in the startle of hyperekplexia that merit comment. EMG activity in trunk and limb muscles follows that in sternocleidomastoid, usually at intervals that are a few milliseconds longer than those seen after synchronous activation of muscles through the pyramidal tract, either as in cortical myoclonus or as follows transcutaneous stimulation of the motor cortex (2). The responses recorded in the intrinsic hand and foot muscles (Figs 17.2 and 17.3) are particularly delayed relative to more proximal limb muscles (2,4). The pattern of muscle recruitment is therefore similar to that

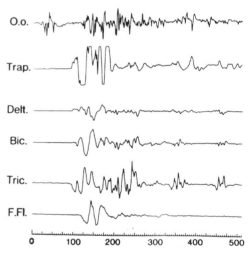

FIG. 17.4. Electromyography (EMG) during startles in a patient with idiopathic exaggerated startle following a tap to the back. Traces begin at the time of stimulus presentation. Note the two components in orbicularis oculi (*O.o*). Trapezius (*Trap*) EMG saturates at 2 mV and gain for deltoid (*delt*), biceps (*bic*), triceps, (*tric*) and forearm flexors (*F.Fl.*) is similar. Orbicularis oculi gain is doubled. The horizontal calibration lines are in milliseconds. (From Colebatch JG, Barrett G, Lees AJ. Exaggerated startle reflexes in an elderly woman. *Mov Disord* 1990;5:167– 169, with permission.)

established for the physiologic startle reflex in man, which, like that in animals, is thought to arise in the caudal reticular formation of the brainstem, particularly within the nucleus reticularis pontis caudalis (17,18).

Studies of the recruitment order of muscles in the startle response must be carefully controlled, because stimulus parameters such as intensity, repetition rate, and site may all have an influence on the absolute latency of the response (4). Even more importantly the patient's posture can have a profound effect on the pattern of the startle in

hyperekplexia. Brown et al. (19) reported two patients in whom the reflex response to sound consisted of up to three successive components (termed A, B, and C) of EMG activity. The expression of the three EMG components in the reflex response of a muscle was dependent on the postural set of that muscle (Fig. 17.5). Thus, following an auditory stimulus, the earliest latency (A) component was not recorded at rest, but was recorded when the muscle was posturally important. Conversely, the C component, which was well formed at rest, was greatly dimin-

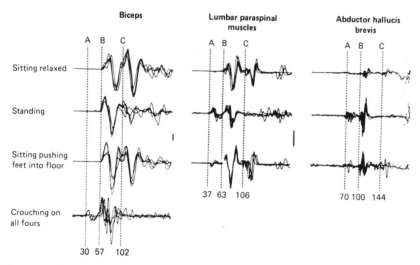

FIG. 17.5. Postural changes in the electromyographic (EMG) pattern of the reflex response to auditory stimulation in a patient with symptomatic hyperekplexia. The upper three records show the reflex EMG activity in response to auditory stimulation in each muscle when sitting relaxed. This consists of two major components, marked *B* and *C,* respectively. The middle three records show the reflex EMG activity when standing. A large short latency *A* component is seen, preceding the *B* component in the lumbar paraspinal muscles and abductor hallucis brevis. The *C* component is greatly diminished in biceps brachii and has disappeared in the lumbar paraspinal muscles and abductor hallucis brevis.

The lower three records show the reflex EMG activity in response to auditory stimulation when sitting, pushing both feet into the ground. A small short latency *A* component is visible in the lumbar paraspinal muscles and the abductor hallucis brevis. The *B* and *C* components are relatively unchanged in all three muscles, compared to sitting relaxed. The differences between the reflex EMG patterns on standing and sitting, pushing the feet into the floor, occur despite comparable levels of background EMG activity.

The bottom left record shows the reflex EMG activity in biceps brachii in response to auditory stimulation when crouching on all fours, with the center of balance shifted slightly forward. A short latency *A* component is now seen, preceding the *B* component in biceps brachii. The *C* component is absent.

Each record consists of four superimposed single trials of unrectified EMG activity. The auditory stimulus was delivered at the beginning of each trial. The total sweep duration of each trial was 200 ms. Each vertical calibration bar represents 1 mV. (From Brown P, Day BL, Rothwell JC, et al. The effect of posture on the normal and pathological auditory startle reflex. *J Neurol Neurosurg Psychiatry* 1991;54:892–897, with permission.)

ished in size or absent when standing or crouching on all fours. This change in the EMG pattern of the reflex response to sound with postural activity was striking and not simply the effect of increased background EMG activity.

The various EMG components had in common a long latency difference between biceps and tibialis anterior, about 9 ms longer than that seen after magnetic stimulation of the motor cortex, and even longer relative delays to the intrinsic hand and foot muscles. These similarities suggested that repetitive discharge within the same bulbospinal efferent system was responsible for the individual components of the reflex response to auditory stimulation. Thus postural and other influences (such as the level of facilitation from the cerebral cortex and basal ganglia) may operate independently on each component of a series of waves of bulbospinal activity, resulting in reflex responses of differing latency. Variation in absolute latency, despite preservation of the overall pattern of muscle recruitment, is a distinctive feature of both the normal and hyperekplectic startle response.

Although clinically striking, the startle response is not the only abnormality demonstrated by patents with hyperekplexia. As already mentioned, these patients may also have stimulus-induced tonic spasms and spontaneous paroxysms of jerking, often at night. The origin of either phenomenon is unknown. Cortical abnormalities such as epilepsy and giant evoked potentials may occur, but are unusual. The remaining functional abnormalities relate to brainstem and spinal function. Slowing of horizontal saccadic eye movements may be found in familial hyperekplexia and is further evidence of disturbed activity in the pontine reticular formation (20). The first period of spinal reciprocal inhibition is deficient in similar patients (Fig. 17.6), consistent with its mediation by the glycinergic Ia inhibitory interneuron (21), and spinal flexor reflexes may be exaggerated (4).

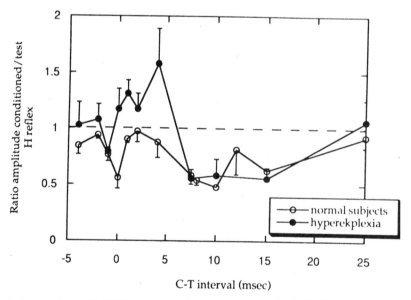

FIG. 17.6. Spinal reciprocal inhibition in hereditary hyperekplexia. Inhibition of the forearm flexor H reflex by conditioning stimulation of the radial nerve at 1.4 times motor threshold for various delays. Means and standard errors are plotted for six control subjects and three patients. Note the loss of inhibition at conditioning-test intervals of 0 to 4 ms. (From Floeter MK, Andermann F, Andermann E, et al. Physiological studies of spinal inhibitory pathways in patients with hereditary hyperekplexia. *Neurology* 1996;46:766–772, with permission.)

CONCLUSIONS

In summary, hyperekplexia is characterized by an abnormal startle response that is relayed in the brainstem and likely involves a pathologic exaggeration of the physiologic startle reflex. As such, many of the factors influencing the normal startle reflex also have a bearing on the hyperekplectic startle response, and this is most strikingly evident in the effect of posture upon the startle reflex. However, the hyperekplectic startle is but one of several abnormal features in hyperekplexia, reflecting the distributed nature of glycinergic receptors within the central nervous system.

REFERENCES

1. Thompson PD, Colebatch JG, Brown P, et al. Voluntary stimulus-sensitive jerks and jumps mimicking myoclonus or pathological startle syndromes. *Mov Disord* 1992;7:257–262.
2. Brown P, Thompson PD, Rothwell JC, et al. The hyperekplexias and their relationship to the normal startle reflex. *Brain* 1991;114:1903–1928.
3. Chokroverety S, Wakzak T, Hening W. Human startle reflex: technique and criteria for abnormal response. *Electroencephalogr Clin Neurophysiol* 1992;85:236–242.
4. Matsumoto J, Fuhr P, Nigro M, et al. Physiological abnormalities in hereditary hyperekplexia. *Ann Neurol* 1992;32:41–50.
5. Shiang R, Ryan SG, Zhu Y, et al. Mutations in the alpha1 subunit of the inhibitory glycine receptor cause the dominant neurologic disorder, hyperekplexia. *Nat Genet* 1993;5:351–357.
6. Suhren O, Bruyn GW, Tuynman JA. Hyperexplexia: a hereditary startle syndrome. *J Neurol Sci* 1966;3:577–605.
7. Andermann F, Keene DL, Andermann E, et al. Startle disease or hyperekplexia; further delineation of the syndrome. *Brain* 1980;103:985–997.
8. Kurczynski TW. Hyperekplexia. *Arch Neurol* 1983;40:246–248.
9. Saenz-Lope E, Herranz-Tanarro FJ, Masdeu JC, et al. Hyperekplexia: a syndrome of pathological startle responses. *Ann Neurol* 1984;15:36–41.
10. Tijssen MA, Shiang R, van Deutekom J, et al. Molecular genetic reevaluation of the Dutch hyperekplexia family. *Arch Neurol* 1995;52:578–582 .
11. Gastaut H, Villeneuve A. The startle disease or hyperekplexia: pathological surprise reaction. *J Neurol Sci* 1967;5:523–542.
12. Vergouwe MN, Tijssen MA, Shiang R, et al. Hyperekplexia-like syndromes without mutations in the GLRA1 gene. *Clin Neurol Neurosurg* 1997;99:172–178.
13. Markand ON, Garg BP, Weaver DD. Familial startle disease (hyperekplexia). *Arch Neurol* 1984;41:71–74.
14. Bernasconi A, Cendes F, Shoubridge EA, et al. Spectroscopic imaging of frontal neuronal dysfunction in hyperekplexia. *Brain* 1998;121:1507–1512.
15. Tijssen MAJ, Meyer BU, Davie C, et al. Motor cortex function in hereditary hyperekplexia is normal. *Mov Disord* 2000 (*in press*).
16. Colebatch JG, Barrett G, Lees AJ. Exaggerated startle reflexes in an elderly woman. *Mov Disord* 1990;5:167–169.
17. Davis M, Gendelman DS, Tischler MD, et al. Primary acoustic startle circuit: lesion and stimulation studies. *J Neurosci* 1982;2:791–805.
18. Brown P, Rothwell JC, Thompson PD, et al. New observations on the normal auditory startle reflex in man. *Brain* 1991; 114:1891–1902.
19. Brown P, Day BL, Rothwell JC, et al. The effect of posture on the normal and pathological auditory startle reflex. *J Neurol Neurosurg Psychiatry* 1991;54:892–897.
20. Tijssen MA, Bollen E, van-Exel E, et al. Saccadic eye movements in hyperekplexia. *Mov Disord* 1995;10:749–753.
21. Floeter MK, Andermann F, Andermann E, et al. Physiological studies of spinal inhibitory pathways in patients with hereditary hyperekplexia. *Neurology* 1996;46:766–772.

Myoclonus and Paroxysmal Dyskinesias,
Advances in Neurology, Vol. 89,
edited by S. Fahn, et al.
Published by Lippincott Williams & Wilkins,
Philadelphia, 2002.

18

Genetics of Idiopathic Myoclonic Epilepsies: An Overview

*Antonio V. Delgado-Escueta, †Marco T. Medina, ‡Dong Sheng Bai,
§Chung Yan Fong, ‖Miyabi Tanaka, ¶Maria Elisa Alonso

*Professor of Neurology, University of California, Los Angeles, California; †Medical Faculty of
Sciences, Honduran Association of Neurologia, Autonomous National University of Honduras,
Tegucigalpa, Honduras; ‡Chinese Academy of Sciences, Shanghai, China; §Division of Neurology,
Queen Mary Hospital, Hong Kong, China; ‖Japan; ¶Department of Genetics, National Institute of
Neurology and Neurosurgery, Mexico City, Mexico*

In the past six years, mutations in genes that encode sodium channels (1–4) and potassium ion channels (5–8), a nicotinic acetylcholine receptor subunit (9–11) and a γ subunit of GABA-A receptor (12,13) have proved to be the cause of five rare mendelian epilepsy syndromes, the mutation causing genes being unique to specific families. These include generalized epilepsy with febrile seizures plus in chromosomes 19q13 and 2q21, benign familial neonatal convulsions in chromosomes 20q13 and 8q24, autosomal dominant nocturnal frontal lobe epilepsy in chromosome 20q13, febrile seizures plus absence in chromosome 5q, and severe myoclonic epilepsy of Dravet in 2q21 (14) (Tables 18.1 to 18.4). All of these epilepsy syndromes can be mistaken for movement disorders because of their motor signs. However, only two of these syndromes have myoclonic seizures as part of their phenotype: febrile seizures plus and severe myoclonic epilepsy of Dravet. Thirty-three chromosome loci of mendelian forms of idiopathic generalized epilepsies (IGEs) of infancy, childhood, and adolescence have been reported (Tables 18.1 to 18.3). Of these, ten chromosomal loci are for idiopathic myoclonic epilepsies (Tables 18.1 and 18.2). Thus, for most of the benign/idiopathic myoclonic epilepsies, the specific gene affected by mutations has not yet been identified.

This chapter provides an overview of the new advances in molecular genetics of benign/idiopathic myoclonic epilepsies in infants, children, adolescents, and adults. It is a progress report on the nosologic classification and search for chromosomal loci of benign/idiopathic myoclonic epilepsy syndromes. After presenting an overview, this chapter focuses on the phenotypes and genotypes of these myoclonic epilepsies and the progress in our laboratories. To address their importance to the public health problem of the epilepsies, this chapter questions whether recently discovered epilepsy genes and epilepsy chromosome loci are unique to families, in rare genetic isolates, or in common outbred populations. In discussing whether epilepsy genes are evolutionarily old or new, this chapter questions whether they are "rare flora in rare soil."

Understanding the new advances in the molecular genetics of the epilepsies is important because they provide us more than a glimpse of the new practice of molecular neu-

In cooperation with the participants of the GENESS (Genetic Epilepsy Studies) International Consortium.

TABLE 18.1. *Chromosome loci of idiopathic myoclonic epilepsies of infancy, childhood, adolescence, and adults*

Reference	Phenotype	Genotype[a]	Country of origin and no. of families
40	Familial febrile seizures (FEB3) (possibly GEFS+)	2q23-24	1 family from Utah
2,37,38,39,41	Generalized epilepsies with febrile seizures plus (GEFS+ type 2)	2q23-q31	1 family from Northern Victoria, Australia
			SCN1A mutation in 2 families from France
1,4,13	Generalized epilepsies with febrile seizures plus (GEFS+ type 1)	19q13	**SCN1B mutation** in 1 Tasmanian family from Australia
	Generalized epilepsies with febrile seizures plus (GEFS+ type 3)	5q	**GABRG2 mutation** in 1 family from France
	Febrile seizures and childhood absence	5q	**GABRG2 mutation** in 1 family from Australia
44	Autosomal recessive idiopathic myoclonic epilepsy of infancy	16p13	1 family from Sardinia, Italy
15,16,28,68,69	Classic/typical juvenile myoclonic epilepsy	6p12-11 (EJM1)	42 families from Los Angeles, Belize, and Mexico
79,80	Juvenile myoclonic epilepsy with absence	6p21 between HLA-DP and HLA-B	58 families from New York
65,66	Juvenile myoclonic epilepsy with absence	6p21 between HLADW and D6S1019	29 families from Berlin, Germany, and Austria
83	IGE or JME or absences	3q26	130 families from Europe
70	JME with absence	15q14	34 families from UK and Sweden
73	Childhood absence evolving to JME	1p or 4p	10 families from Mexico and California
Delgado-Escueta et al., in progress	Photogenic childhood absence with eyelid myoclonia evolving to JME	Unknown	5 families from Mexico and California
96,97	Benign adult familial myoclonic epilepsy	8q23.3-q24.1	5 families from Japan

IGE, idiopathic generalized epilepsy; JME, juvenile myoclonic epilepsy.
[a]Unless indicated, all evidence was acquired by model-dependent linkage analyses.

rology. The epilepsies have traditionally been classified and subtyped on the basis of clinical and neurophysiologic concepts. The complexity and variability of phenotypes and overlapping clinical features limit the resolution of phenotype-based classification and confounds epilepsy nosology. Identification of tightly linked epilepsy deoxyribonucleic acid (DNA) markers and discovery of epilepsy causing mutations provide a basis for refining the classification of epilepsies. Although discovered only in rare families, so far, mutations in the $\alpha 4$ subunit of nACH receptor, SCN1A, SCN1B, KCNQ2, KCNQ3 and the $\gamma 2$ subunit of GABA-A receptor have

taught us about mechanisms of epileptogenesis. Identification of molecular lesions of common epilepsies will inevitably lead to discoveries of new treatments.

MODE OF INHERITANCE OF IDIOPATHIC MYOCLONIC EPILEPSIES

Many have long argued that the common IGEs that cause grand mal, myoclonias, and absences are genetically complex diseases. IGEs are considered to be mostly due to genetic factors with limited environmental contributions. This notion had been arrived at be-

TABLE 18.2. *Chromosome loci of other generalized epilepsies of infancy and childhood*

Reference	Phenotype	Genotype	Country of origin and no. of families
119	Infantile spasms syndrome (MIM308350)	Xp11.4-Xpter	2 families from Leuven, Belgium
5,8,20,120,121	Benign familial neonatal convulsions (EBN1)	20q	**KCNQ2 mutation** initially detected in 1 family from Sweden and then in 6 families from Newfoundland, Sweden, Quebec, USA, 6 families from France, and 1 family from Japan
8,22	Benign familial neonatal convulsions (EBN2)	8q24	**KCNQ3 mutation** in 1 family from Texas and 1 family from Japan
122	Benign familial infantile convulsions	19q13	Families from Italy
123	Familial infantile convulsions and paroxysmal choreoathetosis	16p12-q12	4 families from France and 1 family from China
42	Familial febrile seizures (FEB1)	8q13-21	1 family from Australia
43,124	Familial febrile seizures (FEB2)	19p	1 family from the Midwest (USA)
61	Familial febrile seizures (FEB4) by nonparametric GENEHUNTER and transmission linkage disequilibrium	5q14-q15	1 large and 39 nuclear families from Japan
27	Childhood absence epilepsy with or without grand mal	8q24 (ECA1)	7 families from Bombay, Argentina, Los Angeles, Spain, Saudi Arabia
82,125	Idiopathic generalized epilepsy with generalized spike waves	3p14.2-p12.1	1 family from Italy
78	Adolescent-onset idiopathic generalized epilepsies with generalized spike waves (non-JME random grand mal and juvenile absence seizures)	8p11-12	23 families (15 grand mal and 8 juvenile absence) from New York

JME, juvenile myoclonic epilepsy.

TABLE 18.3. *Chromosome loci of partial epilepsies*

Reference	Phenotype	Genotype	Country of origin and no. of families
9,10,11,24,126,127	Autosomal dominant nocturnal frontal lobe epilepsy	20q	**NACHR-α4 subunit mutation** in 2 families from Australia, 1 family from Norway, and 1 family from Japan
25,117	Autosomal dominant nocturnal frontal lobe epilepsy	15q24;	3 families from Quebec, Italy, and England
	Autosomal dominant nocturnal frontal lobe epilepsy	1cen	Calabria, Southern Italy
128,129	TLE with auditory symptoms	10q	1 family from New York; 1 family from Basque region, Spain
130	Autosomal dominant partial epilepsy with variable foci	2q (preliminary)	1 family from Australia
118	Familial partial epilepsy with variable foci	22q11-q12	2 families from Quebec; 1 family from Spain
131	Autosomal recessive rolandic epilepsy with paroxysmal exercise-induced dystonia and writer's cramp	16p12-q12	1 family from Italy
132	Centrotemporal spikes in families with rolandic epilepsy	15q14	22 families from Germany
133	Rolandic epilepsy and speech dyspraxia	?	Australia
89,90	Familial TLE	?	Australia
134	Familial TLE with hippocampal scleroses and IL-1β, IL-1α, and IL-1 receptor antagonist gene	2 (association studies)	50 patients with TLE+HS from Japan

TLE, temporal lobe epilepsy; HS, hippocampal scleroses; IL, interleukin.

TABLE 18.4. *Other epilepsies combined with other neurologic syndromes*

Reference	Phenotype	Genotype	Country of origin and no. of families
135,136	Familial spastic paraparesis and epilepsy	14q; 15q	1 family from Italy
137	Episodic ataxia type I (EA-1) and epilepsy	**Mutation in potassium channel gene KCNA1**	1 family from Glasgow
138	Frontotemporal dementia parkinsonism-17 (FTDP-17)	17q21-22 **(missense mutation at nucleotide 1137 C to T in tau gene)**	1 family from Germany

cause classical methods of human genetics such as determination of disease risks among close relatives and concordance rates of monozygotic and dizygotic twins favored a strong genetic influence on epilepsy susceptibility. Because family studies and empirical risk figures were not compatible with mendelian modes of inheritance, such epilepsies were considered complex genetic diseases. Common epilepsies, such as juvenile myoclonic epilepsy (JME), appear genetically complex when segregation analyses use small nuclear pedigrees (15,16). Results are characteristic of either an autosomal recessive (AR) (17) or autosomal dominant (AD) disorder with incomplete penetrance (18) or a two-loci model combining autosomal recessive and autosomal dominant traits (15). Thus, one could even interpret data from twin, family, and segregation studies that an oligogenic model with two or more genes interacting to produce the phenotype provided the best fit. Most recently, Durner et al. (19) performed a genome scan in 91 families ascertained through a proband with adolescent IGE. Linkage results supported an oligogenic model for IGE with strong evidence for a common susceptibility locus for IGEs in chromosome 18 that interacted with the 6p locus for JME, the 8p locus for non-JME forms of IGE, and two new loci in chromosome 5 for absence seizures. This hypothesis of an oligogenic model for IGEs was originally derived from Greenberg's segregation studies of JME (15) and could explain why grand mal only, JME only, absence only, or a combination of the three seizure types can be observed in affected members of the same family.

Accumulating evidences from linkage analyses and mutation detections that have used large families with many affected members, however, have also shown that many of these idiopathic epilepsies are, indeed, complex mendelian disorders that have locus heterogeneity (Tables 18.1 to 18.3). Even rare idiopathic epilepsy syndromes have been shown to have at least two if not more loci, such as the benign familial neonatal convulsions in chromosomes 20q (EBN1) (7,20) and 8q (EBN2) (6,8,21–23), autosomal dominant nocturnal frontal lobe epilepsy in chromosomes 20q13 (24), 15q24 (25), and 1cen (26). In other common epilepsy syndromes, such as febrile seizures and febrile seizures plus, locus heterogeneity is also present (chromosomes 8q13-21 and 19p for FEB1 and FEB2, 2q23-31 and 19q13 for GEFS+). Clear-cut autosomal dominant mendelian inheritance has been proved in multiplex and multigeneration pedigrees with childhood absence epilepsy (CAE) (27), and JME from outbred populations as well as genetic isolates (28). Autosomal recessive inheritance is present in JME from Saudi Arabia (29). Moreover, common epilepsies, such as CAE, appear even more complex when consanguinity and assortative mating is added to the mendelian inheritance (30).

There are other characteristics of the phenotypes, such as induction of seizures only with natural or electronic screen light (31), the EEG photoparoxysmal EEG spike wave traits (32), and female preponderance of the latter two traits (33), that require further strategies for disentangling environmental from genetic components of epilepsies. To the present, none of the common epilepsies have been proved to have imprinting, trinucleotide repeats, or allelic mutations as explanations for genetic complexity. Thus, aside from presenting the phenotypes and genotypes of the idiopathic myoclonic epilepsies, this chapter will illustrate families that exemplify the above factors that contribute to the complexity of epilepsy genetics.

IDIOPATHIC MYOCLONIC EPILEPSIES OF INFANCY AND EARLY CHILDHOOD

Of the 40 to 100 million persons worldwide that have epilepsy, approximately 50% are due to generalized epilepsies (34). Among the generalized epilepsies of infancy and childhood, the most common are neonatal convulsion from birth to 3 months, febrile seizures, infantile spasms of West syndrome, Lennox-Gastaut syndrome, benign myoclonic epilepsy of infancy, early childhood idiopathic myoclonic epilepsy, childhood absence epilepsy, JME, and pure grand mal tonic clonic epilepsy from 3 months to adolescence (35–36).

In the past decade, several mendelian forms of myoclonic epilepsies have been separated from these common syndromes. Hidden among the common forms of febrile convulsions is the syndrome of generalized epilepsy with febrile seizures plus (GEFS+) in chromosomes 2q23-31, 19q13 and 5q (Table 18.1). GEFS+ is a syndrome of febrile convulsions in which the affected members have various epilepsy phenotypes (37). Among the seizure phenotypes of affected family members are myoclonic seizures, myoclonic astatic, atonic, and hemiclonic seizures. GEFS+ was mapped by Wallace et al. (1) to chromosome 19q where a missense mutation in the β1 subunit gene (SCN1B) of the neuronal sodium channel was found. Three reports of GEFS+ kindreds identified a second locus, namely, chromosome 2q23-q31 (38–40). The phenotypes in two families reported by Baulac et al. (38) and by Moulard et al. (39) included myoclonic, hemiclonic hemicorporeal, and atonic seizures in addition to absences and tonic clonic. These phenotypes were similar to those of the Aus-

tralian kindred reported by Scheffer and Berkovic in 1997 (37). The phenotype in the family reported by Peiffer et al. (40) was reported as "febrile seizures" or "FS," but one member had generalized atonic seizures and the phenotype was typical of GEFS+, according to Lopes-Cendes et al. (41). Myoclonic or atonic or hemiclonic seizures were not observed in familial febrile seizures that probably remit, which was localized by Wallace et al. (42) to chromosome 8q13-21 and by Dubovsky et al. (43) to chromosome 19p. Most recently, Baulac et al. (13) reported a third locus for GEFS+ in chromosome 5q.

Autosomal recessive myoclonic epilepsy of infancy in chromosome 16p13 reported by Zara et al. (44) is distinct from infantile spasms of West syndrome, Lennox-Gastaut syndrome, severe myoclonic epilepsy of Dravet, and benign myoclonic epilepsy of Dravet. Also distinct from these syndromes is the autosomal dominant myoclonic epilepsy of early childhood that is not allelic to chromosome 16p13, 6p12-11, 8q13-21, 8q24 or 15q14 (Delgado-Escueta, 2001, *in preparation*). These myoclonic epilepsy syndromes of infancy and early childhood are rare but extremely important epilepsies. Experiments of nature, they are treasured for their illumination of the nosology of human epilepsies and the insights they may provide when we finally understand their molecular basis and pathogenesis.

Severe Myoclonic Epilepsy of Infancy

Phenotype

Severe myoclonic epilepsy of infancy (SMEI) occurs in 1 in 20,000 to 1 in 40,000 of the population. Dravet et al. (45,46) first described this syndrome of SMEI in 142 cases in 1978 and 1982. In 1982, Dalla Bernardina et al. (47) expounded on the electroencephalogram (EEG) characteristics. This syndrome represents a significant portion of the severe childhood epilepsies and is distinct from the Lennox-Gastaut syndrome and other more benign myoclonic epilepsies of infancy and early childhood. Later, Aicardi (48) suggested the term polymorphic epilepsy of infants for this syndrome because other seizure types are present. Doose et al. (49) described a similar syndrome under the term "severe idiopathic epilepsy of infancy and early childhood with generalized tonic clonic seizures and alternating hemi-grand mal." Kanazawa (50) described a similar group of infants in 1992. A family history for seizures is present in 25%.

Seizures start between 4 and 11 months, often unilateral clonic or tonic and less commonly tonic clonic. Fever triggers most attacks. Seizures are often prolonged and preceded or followed by myoclonic seizures. Later in life, afebrile seizures appear and include absences, atypical absences, and complex partial seizures in addition to myoclonic and tonic clonic seizures. Seizures are also light sensitive and may be self-induced as the child gets older. Nonconvulsive status epilepticus is frequent. Early psychomotor and speech development is normal but cognitive decline becomes evident by the second and third year and severe to moderate mental retardation follows with attention deficit and hyperactivity. Delayed speech development and ataxia is prominent as is erratic myoclonus and long tract signs. Myoclonic seizures may diminish or subside after 4 years, but 15.9% will have passed away by 11 years of age. EEG may be normal at the beginning, but eventually fast polyspike wave complexes, multifocal spikes, and photoconvulsive responses in 50% of patients with slow background rhythms suggest the diagnosis of SMEI in infants with myoclonias. In general, SMEI is very resistant to all forms of antiepileptic drug treatment (51).

Genotype

Recently, Claes et al. (14) identified *de novo* mutations in seven unrelated patients from Belgium with sporadic SMEI. After confirming paternity using microsatellites, all parents were tested for the patient's mutations. The mutations were absent in all parents as well as in 92 control individuals. The severity of the SMEI phenotype could be reflected by the nature of the SCN1A mutations identified in the patients. In five of seven patient's

frameshifts, deletions or an insertion or a nonsense mutation was identified. More specifically, four patients had frameshift mutations, one had a nonsense mutation, one had a splice donor mutation, and one had a missense mutation. All occurred in SCN1A or the α subunit of a neuronal voltage gated sodium channel, specifically exons 5, 16, 22, and 26. Thus, in the majority of patients with SMEI, mutations would theoretically result in early termination of translation. This would then produce a C-truncated protein. Rapid degradation of these truncated proteins could then lead to a loss of function similar to haploinsufficiency. Claes et al. (14) also suggests the alternative explanation that some of the transcripts could lead to abnormal proteins with a toxic increase in function. Interestingly, similar heterozygous SCN1A mutations had originally been found in a milder form of epilepsy, namely, autosomal dominant GEFS+. However, all GEFS+ mutations were missense mutations that have reduced penetrance.

Benign Myoclonic Epilepsy of Infancy

In benign myoclonic epilepsy of infancy (BMEI), myoclonic seizures that are distinct from tonic seizures or atonic seizures, characteristically saccadic and associated with EEG diffuse polyspikes, often axial and massive with head drops or segmental and mild, usually on awakening, occurring many times in a day with normal EEG background, is distinguished from severe syndromes by the normal psychomotor development of the child and the almost exclusive presence of myoclonias. Starting from 4 months to 3 years, boys are more commonly affected. Absences may be present but tonic clonic seizures are rare. First described by Dravet et al. (51,52), it is rare to infrequent and has a genetic component in 31% of cases. Twenty-eight percent are preceded by febrile seizures. EEG polyspikes with myoclonias may be photosensitive. Myoclonias are controlled by valproate and prognosis is good. Lombroso and Fejerman (53) may have described similar cases in 1977 under the term "benign nonepileptic myoclonus in early infancy" where ictal EEGs were normal. Single cases were also described by Colomaria et al. in 1987 (54) and by Salas Puig et al. in 1990 (55). A cohort of families, ascertained through a proband with "early childhood myoclonic epilepsy" collected for genetic studies, was described by Delgado-Escueta et al. in 1990 (56). The chromosome locus or site of mutations for BMEI has not been identified.

Idiopathic Epilepsy with Myoclonic Astatic Seizures

Doose et al. (57) proposed to divide myoclonic astatic epilepsy into centrencephalic or cryptogenic and symptomatic types. Because of family histories of seizures in 37% of cases, genetic factors are postulated to play an important role in the centrencephalic type. Seizures, photosensitivity, biparietal θ rhythms and spike wave complexes are increased in siblings and parents (58,59). Myoclonic astatic seizures (jerks of arms and legs with head nodding) start during the second to fifth years of life and are associated with absences and nonconvulsive status epilepticus. Astatic seizures with abrupt loss of tone occur as part of and after myoclonias of arms and face. Myoclonic static/absence status is not uncommon. Febrile or afebrile seizures can precede the appearance of myoclonic astatic seizures. Aside from the spike wave complexes, monomorphic biparietal θ rhythms are described by Doose and Baier (58,59) as characteristic of the genetic or centrencephalic type of myoclonic astatic epilepsy. Because both normal and abnormal psychomotor development is described in the reports of Doose et al. (57), mixtures of other subsyndromes are suspected to be present in this group.

It is likely that cases of benign myoclonic epilepsy as described by Dravet et al. (46,51,52) are included in the group of centrencephalic myoclonic astatic epilepsy described by Doose et al. (60). The syndrome of early childhood myoclonic epilepsy, which we reported in 1990, is probably also a subgroup of the syndrome of Doose because almost all of our cases had myoclonic astatic drop seizures at onset together

with frequent myoclonic seizures and absences beginning at 1 to 4 years of age. Tonic clonic seizures were rare or absent. EEGs showed diffuse 4- to 6-Hz polyspike wave complexes. Magnetic resonance imaging and positron emission tomography studies were normal except in one proband who had difficult birth process in addition to a family with tonic clonic seizures. We studied 13 families, all of whom had a positive family history for seizures (56, Delgado-Escueta et al., *in preparation*).

The symptomatic form of myoclonic astatic epilepsy is similar to the Lennox-Gastaut syndrome since mental retardation is always present and lesions are demonstrated on brain imaging in 90% of cases (57).

Generalized Epilepsy with Febrile Seizures Plus

Phenotypes

The first report of GEFS+ by Scheffer and Berkovic (37) involved two large Australian families with an autosomal dominant epilepsy trait that started in infancy and early childhood and that remitted by midchildhood. This syndrome in the majority of patients is therefore benign. Scheffer and Berkovic ascertained families through probands with infantile febrile convulsions. Affected family members had myoclonic astatic seizures or febrile seizures plus myoclonic astatic seizures, atonic seizures, and absences in infancy and early childhood. Hence, depending on who is considered the index case, these families could as readily been classified as idiopathic myoclonic astatic epilepsy of Doose or idiopathic or primary myoclonic epilepsy of infancy and early childhood or absence epilepsy in early childhood. Myoclonic or astatic seizures are easily mistaken for movement disorders. Affected family members who were older than 6 years gave a history of multiple febrile seizures during infancy and early childhood, afebrile seizures, and grand mal tonic clonic seizures. Since then, more families with febrile convulsions with similar phenotypes have been reported from northern Victoria, Australia; Utah, United States; Geneva, Switzerland; Strasbourg, France; and Israel (Table 18.1). In all these families, mutations in the β subunit (SCN1B) or α subunit (SCN1A) of neuronal voltage gated sodium channels have been observed (1–3). Interestingly, three levels of consanguinity are present in the large family from Victoria (1). In five of nine families reported from Australia, bilineal inheritance is also present, adding more complexity to the modes of inheritance. Lately, the phenotype of febrile seizures plus has been expanded to include absence seizures only or tonic clonic seizures only as the sole phenotypes in affected family members. In the latest reports, a mutation in the γ subunit of GABA-A receptor was observed instead of SCN1A or SCN1B (13).

Genotypes

The first locus for the GEFS+ syndrome (GEFS+ type 1) was reported by Wallace et al. in 1998 (1) who mapped one large Tasmanian family from Australia to 19q13.1, assuming a monogenic model with 64% penetrance and a phenocopy rate of 3%. Positional cloning strategies were successful in proving that the β subunit of the voltage gated sodium channel gene (SCN1B) was responsible for the 19q13 locus and the "febrile convulsions plus syndrome" in the Tasmanian family. The nucleotide variation consisted of a cysteine to tryptophan amino acid change. Because the β1 subunit of the voltage gated sodium channel also mapped to the same 19q13 region, mutation analyses was performed in the β1 subunit and a point mutation segregated with affected members. Six of the 12 members affected with febrile seizures did not have the mutation in the SCN1B gene. The β1 subunit modulates channel gating properties and sodium inactivation. Mutant β subunits are hypothesized to alter the disulfide bond that maintain the extracellular fold motif of the β1 subunit, produce slower inactivation, slower recovery from inactivation, persistent inward sodium currents, and recurrent depolarizations.

A sobering result was observed when the mutation in SCN1B was not found in 25 other GEFS+ families or in 25 other febrile convulsion families, indicating that the SCN1B mutations are rare contributors to GEFS+ or febrile convulsions (61).

Lopes-Cendes et al. in 1996 and 2000 (41) linked one Australian family to chromosome 2q23-24 and hence identified GEFS+ type 2. Most recently, four separate groups from Australia, Utah, Switzerland, and France have reported four unrelated families with the GEFS+ 2 phenotype that show linkage to the same interval of 2q23-31 (Table 18.1). Two missense mutations (Thr875Met and Arg1648His) in the α1 subunit of the sodium channel (SCN1A) was recently reported by Escayg et al. (2) in the two French families. Similar mutations in SCN1A were not detected in 100 controls. The mutant residues Thr875 and Arg1648 are located in the S4 transmembrane domain of the α subunit of the sodium channel. The S4 segments have a role in channel gating and introduction of Arg1648His mutation into SCN2A causes a decrease in the rate of channel inactivation. This suggests that a similar mutation in SCN1A may reduce the rate of inactivation of SCN1A producing increased sodium influx and increased neuronal excitability. A loss of function mutation in the β subunit of the sodium channel in GEFS+ type 1 also indirectly decreases the rate of inactivation of sodium channel α subunits (1).

In yet another major advance in the identification of genes for idiopathic epilepsy, Baulac et al. (13) studied a large French family with a phenotype compatible with GEFS+ comprising 17 affected members and provided strong evidence for linkage to chromosome 5q34, thus identifying GEFS+ type 3. Baulac et al. (13) initially tested two affected individuals of this large French family for mutations in GABRG2 by direct sequencing of the nine exons. They found an A to T transversion in exon 8, resulting in the substitution of a positively charged lysine residue for a neutral methionine (K289M) and creating a NcoI restriction that cosegregated with the disease in the family. The authors then analyzed one proband each from ten GEFS+ families for the GABRG2 mutation and found no other disease causing mutations. They then analyzed GABA mediated currents in *Xenopus laevis* oocytes expressing mutant GABA-A receptors. Oocytes receiving the ribonucleic acids (RNAs) encoding the mutant $\alpha1\beta2\gamma2$ –K289M receptor expressed 10% of the maximal current amplitude compared to wild type subunit combinations. GABA-evoked currents in oocytes with the mutation were decreased compared to wild type responses at all concentrations tested. Baulac et al. (13) thus provided the first evidence that GABA-A receptor is directly involved in human idiopathic epilepsy.

Autosomal Recessive Idiopathic Myoclonic Epilepsy of Infancy in Chromosome 16p13

Phenotype

Autosomal recessive idiopathic myoclonic epilepsy of infancy in chromosome 16p13 was described in one 4-generation Italian family by Zara et al. (44). The family had two related branches that originated from the same area of Naples. Eight members from the third generation were affected with myoclonic seizures that started between 5 and 36 months of age. The myoclonic seizures persisted to adulthood. Febrile convulsions were present between 5 months and 3 years of age in five members, four of which also had afebrile generalized tonic clonic seizures at 4 to 8 months of age. Ictal EEGs showed bisynchronous spike waves. All seizures were well controlled by valproate.

Genotype

After screening the genome with 304 STRPs, a maximum lod score of 4.48 was obtained for D16S3027 at $\theta=0$ (44). Recombinations defined a candidate region spanning 3.4 cM between D16S3024 and D16S423. Candidate genes include a voltage dependent chloride channel 7 gene (CLCN7), sodium/hydrogen exchanger isoform 3 (SLC9AR2), and synaptogyrin III gene.

IDIOPATHIC MYOCLONIC EPILEPSIES OF ADOLESCENCE

Juvenile myoclonic epilepsy is probably the most common form of IGEs, accounting for 10% to 30% of all epilepsies (62–64). Four chromosomal loci have been identified in JME, namely, (a) chromosome 6 within or approximately 10 cM below the HLADQ region observed in families from New York, Austria, and Germany (15–16,65–67); (b) chromosome 6p12-11 some 30 cM below HLA in families from Los Angeles, Mexico, Belize (28,68–69), and Japan (*unpublished personal communication*); (c) chromosome 15q14 observed in families from the United Kingdom and Sweden (70); and (d) chromosome 6q toward the telomeric end for two consanguineous families from Saudi Arabia (29).

Of the five chromosomal loci that underlie the syndrome of CAE, two phenotypes evolve into JME during adolescence. The five syndromes and their chromosome loci are (a) remitting pyknoleptic childhood absence in 15q12 (71,72); (b) CAE that evolves to and persists as JME in 1por 4q or both as observed in one large family from the cities of Guadalajara and Mexico City (73); (c) 8q24 for CAE that persists with grand mal seizures as observed in one large family from Bombay, India, and medium-sized families from Argentina, Spain, Saudi Arabia, and California (27); (d) the syndrome of photogenic CAE with eyelid myoclonia that evolves and persists as JME and is not allelic to the 6p11, 1p, 3p14.2-12.1, 8p11-12, 8q13-21, 8q23-24.1or 8q24 loci and hence is another separate epilepsy locus (Delgado-Escueta, *unpublished observation*); and (e) a separate locus in chromosome 21q22.3 that had been suggested for juvenile absence by Sander at al. (74) by association studies with GluR5 kainate receptor gene (GR1K1).

Phenotypes of Juvenile Myoclonic Epilepsy

Two major phenotypic subsyndromes form the majority of JME, namely, JME without absence seizures and JME with absence seizures. The first subsyndrome—JME with no absences—accounts for 55% of all cases of JME. This subsyndrome usually starts with awakening myoclonias during adolescence, most commonly at 13 to 15 years of age. Two years later, grand mal convulsions appear. As emphasized above, in this first subsyndrome there are no absence seizures in probands or family members. The second phenotype is JME mixed with absences. In 36% of JMEs, pyknoleptic absences, myoclonias, and grand mal convulsions all start during adolescence. In another 5% of all JMEs, the disorder starts during mid or late childhood as pyknoleptic absences with 3 Hz spike and wave complexes as well as 4 to 6 Hz spike or polyspike waves complexes. During adolescence, myoclonias and grand mal convulsions follow. In a still-smaller group (4%), absences start after 18 years of age and follow myoclonic and grand mal seizures that start at adolescence (75).

Autosomal Dominant Juvenile Myoclonic Epilepsy or "Classic/Typical" Juvenile Myoclonic Epilepsy in Chromosome 6p12-11

Phenotypes

In our initial studies, we genotyped families ascertained through a proband with classic JME or only adolescent -onset myoclonias and grand mal seizures with or without rare spanioleptic absences. Affected members who were not probands had JME, or grand mal seizures only, or myoclonias only and rarely absences only. It is important to note that linkage to chromosome 6p was initially observed studying classic/typical JME (16). We subsequently studied families ascertained through a proband with JME mixed with late childhood or adolescent pyknoleptic absences. Affected nonproband members in these families also have JME, myoclonias only, grand mal seizures only and rarely absences only. Clinically asymptomatic members who had the EEG trait of 3- to 6-Hz multispike wave complexes were also considered affected for purposes of linkage analyses (75).

Genotypes

The chromosome 6p12-11 locus or EJM1 is found in classic/typical JME families from Los Angeles, Belize, and Mexico.

At the Human Gene Mapping 9 Workshop in 1987, we reported for the first time the existence of an epilepsy gene by showing that families with JME from Los Angeles may be linked to the Bf-HLA loci in 6p (15,16). Using clinical and EEG characteristics of affected family members, we reported a pooled maximum lod score of 3.04 at recombination fractions of $\theta_m=0.01$ and $\theta_f=0.10$ under a recessive model of inheritance assuming full penetrance using HLA and Bf (properdin factor) as markers. Because we subsequently found no significant association with any specific alleles of HLA and because of one recombinant family, we suggested that the JME locus might lie outside the HLA region.

Following the initial studies with BF-HLA, pairwise, multipoint, and recombination analyses in a large family from Belize (28) and 22 small/medium sized families from Los Angeles proved that a JME gene is located in 6p12-11, centromeric to HLA (68,76). Autosomal dominant inheritance with 70% penetrance was assumed in this analysis. When lod scores for small and medium sized multiplex families are added to lod scores of the LA-Belize pedigree, Zmax values for D6S294 and D6S257 are greater than 7 ($\theta_{m=f}=000$). The admixture test (H_2 vs. H_1) was significant ($p=0.0234$ for D6S294 and 0.0128 for D6S272), supporting the hypotheses of linkage with heterogeneity. Estimated proportion of linked families was 0.50 (95% confidence interval 0.05 to 0.99) for D6S294 and D6S272 (76). Low posterior probability of linkage was observed in families who had JME mixed with absences and EEG 3 Hz spike waves. Thus, for subsequent studies designed to narrow the 6p12-11 region we excluded any families that has members affected with absence seizures as the sole phenotype and ascertained only thru probands with classic/typical JME.

Between 1987 and 1995, we identified and narrowed the locus for classic/typical juvenile myoclonic epilepsy to a 7 cM area in chromosome 6p12-11 using the 28 families from Belize and Los Angeles (28,68,76). Between 1998 to 2000, analyses of 16 newly recruited medium-sized multiplex and multigenerational families (155 members and 35 affected) from Mexico again confirmed the 6p12-11 locus and reduced the area to 3 cM through new informative recombinations (69). A YAC/BAC physical map of the 6p12-11 area was constructed and six new dinucleotide repeats were used to narrow the candidate region of EJM1 further to 500KB. We are now isolating gene exons from BACs using direct cDNA selection, characterizing candidate genes and analyzing for mutations using heteroduplex analyses and direct sequencing. Mutation analyses have eliminated six candidate genes that map to the critical 500-kb area. (77).

Juvenile Myoclinic Epilepsy Mixed with Absences

Phenotype

There are clear differences between the JME phenotypes of chromosomes 15q14, 6p21.3, and 6p12-11. Differences consist of how often absences as the only phenotype and how often clinically asymptomatics with EEG multispike wave traits only occur in probands and family members and whether the JME trait is transmitted more often by mothers. Absences with JME or absences as the sole phenotype or absences with grand mal seizures are relatively more frequent in phenotypes of probands of the 15q14 and 6p21.3 loci compared to the 6p12-11 locus. For example, 21 out of 85 JME probands from New York City whose locus is in 6p21.3 had absences (78,79) while 11 of 59 affected members had either childhood or juvenile-onset absences in families from Sweden and United Kingdom whose locus is in 15q14 (70). Seven CAE and 12 juvenile-onset absence epilepsy or a total of 19 absence epilepsies is present in 76 affected members of 35 JME families from Germany and Austria whose locus is in 6p21.3 (65). Thus, these JME reports from New York City, Germany/Austria, and United Kingdom/Sweden are linkage analyses of families with JME mixed with absences (CAE and JAE). In our studies on classic/typical JME, families who have a member affected with CAE with or without grand mal

or juvenile absence with or without grand mal are excluded (28,68,76).

Genotypes

Is There a Separate Juvenile Myoclinic Epilepsy/Absence Locus in the 6p21.3/HLADQ Area in Families from New York and Berlin?

In 1991, Weissbecker et al. (66), in a replication study of the chromosome 6p JME gene, analyzed 23 families from Berlin and confirmed the linkage to 6p. However, they excluded *tight* linkage to HLA, in agreement with our original suggestions in 1988 that the JME gene is outside the HLA region. Sander et al. (74) enlarged the family number to 29 with 277 members from Germany and Austria. Individuals with IGEs were considered affected, but asymptomatic members with the EEG trait of spike wave complexes were considered unknown. Sander et al. (74) reported peak lod scores of 3.08 at the HLADQ, assuming dominant inheritance with 70% penetrance. Multipoint lod scores peaked at a map position 3.3 cM centromeric to HLADQ (Zmax=3.27). These authors also observed five recombinations that define a JME candidate region spanning 10.1 cM flanked by HLADQ telomeric and D6S1019 centromeric.

In 1996, Greenberg et al. (80), using families from New York, suggested that the JME locus resides within the HLA region, between HLA-DP and HLA-B loci. The phenotype of these families from New York are different from the Los Angeles, Belize, and Mexico families in that affected members had absences as the sole seizure type in addition to JME and grand mal tonic clonic seizures. Persons who were clinically asymptomatic but who had the EEG trait of paroxysmal parietal θ rhythm were also considered affected. These investigators also claim that the chromosome 6p locus expresses both grand mal seizures on awakening and JME. The New York group studied HLA-DR and DQ frequencies in 24 JME patients and in 24 non-JME forms of adolescent-onset IGEs and found the frequency of DR13 and DQB1 alleles to be significantly higher in JME. In 1994, Obeid et al. (81) also noted that DR13 was associated with JME in families from Saudi Arabia with an odds ratio of 4.5. The HLA association studies by Greenberg et al. (80) and Obeid et al. (81) suggest that a second epilepsy gene may be present in chromosome 6p, lying within the HLA complex. JME families from Los Angeles, Belize, Mexico, and Germany do not have significant association with HLA alleles.

It is likely that still other chromosomal loci exist for JME since some JME families from Spain do not link to either chromosomes 6p, 8q24 or 15q14. In 1999, Durner et al. (78) reported a separate chromosome 8p11-12 locus for a non-JME form of IGEs with random grand mal, absences, and asymptomatics with generalized spike waves. Earlier, Pandolfo et al. (82) from the Italian League Against Epilepsy observed in one large family from Italy a susceptibility locus for IGEs with generalized spike waves in 3p14.2-12.1. In a recent collaborative study from Europe involving 130 multiplex families ascertained through a proband with JME or idiopathic absence epilepsy, nonparametric multipoint linkage analyses using the GeneHunter program provided significant evidence for linkage on chromosome 3q26 (Znpl=4.19 at D3S3725) and suggestive evidence on chromosomes 14q23 (Znpl=3.28 at D14S63) and 2q36 (Znpl=2.98 at D2S1371; p =0.000535) (83). This collaborative study from Europe suggests that at least three genetic factors confer susceptibility to generalized seizures in a broad spectrum of idiopathic generalized epilepsy syndromes.

Is Juvenile Myoclonic Epilepsy Mixed with Absence Oligogenic?

Two recent linkage studies tested the hypotheses that shared genetic factors contribute to the epileptogenesis of common IGEs such as JME mixed with absences. The first study involved five European research groups from Germany, United Kingdom, France, Italy, and the Netherlands that combined efforts to collect 130 IGEs multiplex families. Sander et al. (83) scanned the genome of these 130 IGEs-multiplex families ascertained through a proband with either absence epilepsy (CAE or JAE) or JME and one or more siblings affected with one of a variety of IGE traits. A total of 617 family members were genotyped. Of these, 351 were clinically affected, 116 with CAE, 59 with JAE, 95 with JME, 6 with idiopathic absences, 50 with grand mal tonic clonic epilepsy, 7 with awakening grand mal tonic clonic epilepsy, 7 with one tonic clonic seizure, 1 with photosensitive epilepsy, 1 with Lennox-Gastaut syndrome, 1 with West syndrome, 3 with symptomatic epilepsies, and 5 with febrile convulsions. There were also 20 asymptomatic persons with the EEG spike wave trait. Results suggested a novel IGE susceptibility locus on chromosome 3q26 and suggestive evidence for two IGE loci on chromosomes 14q23 and 2q36.1. Nonparametric multipoint linkage analyses using GeneHunter program provided significant scores of Z_{NPL}= 4.19 at D3S3725; p=0.000017 and suggestive evidence for linkage for two loci on 14q23 (Z_{NPL}=3.28 at D14S63; p=0.000566) and chromosome 2q36 (Z_{NPL}=2.98 at D2S1371; p=0.000535). Parametric two point linkage analyses provided significant evidence for linkage at two adjacent markers D3S1574 (Zmax=4.43 at θmax=0.14) and D3S3725 (Zmax=3.31 at θmax=0.18) assuming a broad affectedness model, an autosomal dominant mode of inheritance, and genetic homogeneity.

The second genome scan study involved 91 families collected by Mount Sinai, Montefiore, Columbia Presbyterian, Beth Israel, New York Hospital medical centers, Elmhurst Hospital, and Hospital for Joint Diseases, all from New York and the Sinai Hospital of Baltimore (19). Thirty-eight families (42%) were multiplex or multigenerational. Fifty-three families were presumably simplex. Fifty-three probands had JME, 10 had JAE, and 21 had epilepsy with tonic clonic seizures. Seven probands had IGEs that could not be assigned to any of the above three IGE groups. Fifty-two members among 388 family members in addition to probands were affected with IGE. Nineteen had myoclonic seizures, 20 had absences, and

37 had tonic clonic seizures. Linkage results supported a locus common to IGEs on chromosome 18 (lod score 4.4/5.2 multipoint/two point at θm/f=0.1/0.01) when only family members with IGEs were considered affected under an autosomal recessive mode of inheritance. By stratifying the families by dominant seizure type and investigating for linkage for subforms of IGEs, a locus on chromosome 8 for non JME forms (multipoint homogeneity lod score 3.8 and two point lod score of 1.9 assuming a recessive mode of inheritance with 70% penetrance), on chromosome 6 for JME (two point lod score of 4.2 at a low female but high male recombination fraction θm/f= 0.5/0.01 and multipoint heterogeneity lod score of 2.3 at α=0.50) and 2 possible loci on chromosome 5 for absence. Multipoint lod score of 3.8 was observed between D5S406 and D5S416 assuming autosomal recessive inheritance with 50% penetrance. The highest two point lod score was 2.8 at D5S406 with θm/f=0.01/0.1. Another marker D5S2027 gave a multipoint lod score of 3.4 assuming dominant inheritance with 50% penetrance. Two point lod score at D5S2027 was lower at 1.9 with θm/f=0.01/0.1. Durner et al. (19) conclude that their results favor an oligogenic model for IGEs with a common susceptibility gene in chromosome 18 and interactions of different loci producing JME (chromosome 6) or non-JME forms of IGEs (chromosome 8) and absences (chromosome 5).

Autosomal Recessive Juvenile Myoclonic Epilepsy in Chromosome 15q14

Phenotypes

The phenotype of JME in 15q14 is different from the phenotype of JME in 6p11. In the study (70) of 34 JME families with 165 members ascertained from United Kingdom and Sweden and enrolled in a European collaborative effort, individuals with pyknoleptic absences only as well as individuals with JME or tonic clonic seizures only were considered affected. Pyknoleptic absences as the sole seizure type are not part of the phenotype of JME in 6p12-11. Unlike families that map to 6p12-11, there were no clinically asymptomatic members in families from Sweden and United Kingdom that had the EEG trait of spike wave complexes. Persons with clinical seizures did show generalized spike and waves or polyspike and wave discharges on their EEGs. Like the linkage study from Los Angeles, persons with febrile seizures or single seizures were considered unaffected (70).

Genotype

Using the GeneHunter program, significant evidence in favor of heterogeneity was obtained. Multipoint parametric linkage analyses gave a maximum lod score of 4.42 at a region 1.7 cM telomeric to D15S144 at α=0.65, assuming autosomal recessive inheritance. Nonparametric analyses gave a maximum total score of Zall=2.94; p=0.00048 at marker A CTC (70). Candidate genes include the α7 neuronal acetylcholine receptor (CHRNA7).

Autosomal Recessive Juvenile Myoclonic Epilepsy in Chromosome 6q24

Bate et al. (29) studied previously ascertained consanguineous Saudi Arabian families in which JME segregated as an autosomal recessive trait (84). In two large consanguineous pedigrees, linkage analyses using GeneHunter program gave a multipoint lod score of 4.6 assuming an autosomal recessive inheritance with 0.9 penetrance. A region of haplotype sharing is being investigated and the region has been reduced to a 3.2 to 10.8 cM on chromosome 6q24.

Pyknoleptic Childhood Absence Epilepsy Evolving to Juvenile Myoclonic Epilepsy–Is This a Two-Locus Model?

Because non-6p linked families had phenotypes of JME mixed with pyknoleptic absences, our laboratories proceeded to recruit families with such phenotypes for genome wide screens. When we analyze the phenotypes of all of our probands ascertained as JME, pyknoleptic absences appear in late childhood in 27%, in adolescence in 23%, and after 18 years in 5% (75). When we analyze all our probands ascertained as pyknoleptic childhood absence epilepsy, about 10% to 12% evolve into JME. Put in another way, one subsyndrome of childhood absences starts between 5 to 10 years of age as frequent daily flurries of absences just like classic childhood pyknoleptic absences, but myoclonic seizures and grand mal convulsions appear during adolescence, making it difficult to distinguish from JME. Their EEGs also show irregular spike and polyspike wave complexes in addition to classic or typical 3-Hz spike and slow wave complexes during absences. Mai et al. (85) estimates 5.3% and Janz (64) mentions 4.6 % of JMEs evolve out of childhood pyknoleptic absences.

We studied one large family (M17) from Mexico City and Guadalajara whose members had mixtures of pyknoleptic absence, JME, and grand mal seizures. The family was ascertained through a proband with pyknoleptic childhood absence and typical 3-Hz spike waves and also irregular polyspike waves. During adolescence she developed grand mal convulsions and myoclonias. In other words, her illness of CAE had evolved into JME. After performing EEGs in 109 family members, we initially genotyped 43 members belonging to three generations of which 6 members were considered affected in all analyses. Affected members had either juvenile absences only (female cousin) or grand mal only (brother) or absence with grand mal (grandmother, mother, female cousin) or JME (female cousin). One female cousin (member no. 50) was asymptomatic but had typical 3-Hz spike and multispike waves that was spontaneous as well as photic induced. In addition, two first-degree male cousins had partial seizures of temporal lobe origin and one has cysticercosis (73). Westling et al. (73) performed sib pair analyses of 286 polymorphic DNA markers located throughout the genome using the S.A.G.E. program SIBPAL and then model based linkage analyses of the 22 markers of interest (73). Five markers (D1S448, D1S550, D1S500, D1S465, D1S207) showed indications of linkage

($p<0.01$) and were within approximately 7 cM on chromosome 1p. D1S305 showed positive scores when members affected with partial epilepsies were considered affected. D1S305 is 34 cM centromeric to the cluster of markers that showed significant scores. Other markers, which showed significance ($p<0.01$), were D2S427, D9S303, D12S61 and D21S156. Evidence for linkage for marker D1S207 disappeared when members with "partial epilepsies" or member no. 50 were considered affected. The strongest evidence for linkage was obtained for D2S427 ($p<0.00005$ under all definitions).

We (86) subsequently analyzed 22 markers of interest using an autosomal dominant inheritance model with 70% penetrance and a narrow diagnostic model that considered members with partial epilepsy and member no. 50 as unaffected. They obtained the best lod score of 3.8 for D1S207. Multipoint analyses showed 3.803 lod score when the epilepsy locus was directly at D1S207. One recombination between the epilepsy and D1S550, D1S465, and D1S448 suggest the epilepsy gene is centromeric to these markers at or below D1S207 and D1S488. Using the Bonferroni correction for multiple testing (87,88) where lod score after it is increased by log 10(k) is 3.78, the score of 3.799 obtained for D1S207 remained significant.

Gee performed a second and independent analysis in our laboratories in 1998. Segregation ratio across sibships best fit autosomal dominant inheritance with 45% penetrance. Using this autosomal dominant inheritance model for linkage analyses, three diagnostic models were tested. In the first model, members who have IGEs, such as childhood absence that evolves to JME, or JME with pyknoleptic absences, juvenile absence only, childhood absence plus grand mal convulsions, JME only, and grand mal only were considered affected. In the second model, all members who have generalized epilepsies as listed in the first model plus one asymptomatic child with EEG typical 3-Hz spike wave complexes (member M17-50) were considered affected. In the third model, members who have partial epilepsies of temporal lobe origin were also considered affected. This model was used because a familial form of temporal lobe epilepsy had recently been described to be genetic in origin (89,90).

Exclusionary evidence was first obtained for chromosome 6p microsatellites including TNF and D6S291 (20 cM region); D6S426 (5 cM region); D6S271, D6S269, D6S294 (10 cM region); and D6S282, D6S295 (1 cM region). An exclusion map of approximately 50% of the genome was then generated in family M-17 by testing 220 microsatellite STRPs. This was true under all three models.

Significant linkage was then obtained with STRPs in chromosome 1p (D1S207) Zmax $\theta_{m=f}=0.001$) being greater than 3.60 using the first diagnostic model. Haplotypes of family members were also analyzed and three recombinations in three affected members supported the results of pairwise analyses. Although partial seizures from the temporal lobe were considered unlikely to be part of the family M17 phenotype, one computational linkage analysis considered members suffering from partial epilepsies to be affected, and Zmax dropped to 3.0. A first cousin (M17-50) of the proband is asymptomatic and has the EEG 3-Hz spike wave complexes typical for remitting childhood absence. The child is now 10 years of age and is still asymptomatic. When she is included among those who are affected, Zmax dropped to −2.66 and significant linkage scores disappeared (73).

Thus, two separate analyses of these data both pointed to a chromosomal locus in 1p. We have now extended this family to 28 more members including 14 members of the fourth generation. We have completed their EEGs and identified 4 EEG affected members (3- to 5-Hz spike waves) in the third generation and 3 members with epilepsies (1 with childhood absences evolve to JME; 2 with grand mal seizures only) in the fourth generation. We hope to reduce the size of the critical epilepsy region as we genotype new members with more chromosome 1p markers.

Photogenic Childhood Absences with Eyelid Myoclonias Evolving to Juvenile Myoclonic Epilepsies–Female Preponderance

Another dilemma in the diagnosis of JME are patients whose photogenic pyknoleptic absences have eyelid myoclonia and who develop grand mal and myoclonic seizures during late childhood or adolescence consistent with the diagnosis of JME. Affected members are mostly females. Absence seizures may be self-induced. First reported by Radovici et al. in 1932 (91) and Andermann et al. in 1962 (92), this syndrome is also called eyelid myoclonia with absences by Jeavons et al. (33). Panayiotopoulos (93,94) describes its key features as (a) eye closure induced eyelid myoclonia with absences starting during childhood with grand mal tonic clonic seizures developing in adult life; half also have myoclonic seizures; (b) photosensitivity; and (c) 3- to 6-Hz polyspike waves are triggered by eye closure and eliminated in darkness.

We agree with Panayiotopoulos et al. (93,94) that this syndrome is a distinct entity. Important evidence supporting this concept is the chromosome locus we have found for this syndrome. These patients are often grouped as a subsyndrome within JME or within childhood absence epilepsy. Because their epilepsies start as childhood absence, we had originally recruited these probands within the childhood absence syndromes where they form 3% of all our childhood absence probands. However, it is a syndrome that persists into adult life where their main problems then become grand mal and myoclonic seizures. Moreover, as shown in the large family we describe below, the majority of affected family members have JME (adolescent-onset myoclonias only or with grand mal seizures) or absences with eyelid myoclonia and myoclonic and grand mal seizures. For these reasons, we favor considering them as a clinical subsyndrome of JME.

Our laboratories identified a 133-member multiplex-multigenerational family (LA40) ascertained through a photosensitive CAE proband whose childhood pyknoleptic absences started at three years of age and are associated with eyelid myoclonia. CCTV-EEG telemetry caught her inducing absences by looking at the sunlight and waving the outstretched fingers of her hands in front of the sunlight. This was also described earlier by Andermann et al. in 1962 (92). Between 8 and 10 years of age, she started to have tonic clonic convulsions. At 12 years of age, myoclonic seizures were more often. Four members of this family are affected; EEG shows spike wave discharges and myoclonias during photic stimulation but are otherwise clinically asymptomatic. Thirteen other family members are affected clinically with seizures. Her sister and mother both have spontaneous or photic-induced myoclonias and grand mal seizures that started at 11 years of age. Two other members have childhood absences that persisted with grand mal and myoclonic seizures during adolescence. Two have childhood absence plus grand mal; two have childhood absence only; three have grand mal only; and two have myoclonic seizures only. We demonstrated pyknoleptic absences with 2.5- to 3.5-Hz spike waves with eyelid myoclonia and myoclonic seizures with 5- to 15-Hz rapid spikes during photic stimulation in 9 of these 13 patients. All affected members were females except for two males (one with absence and one with myoclonias.)

Segregation pattern best fit an autosomal dominant trait with incomplete penetrance, SLINK, version 2.60 (95) assuming an autosomal dominant model with a penetrance of 0.9, and a linked codominant four-allele marker with equal allele frequencies ($p=0.25$), showed maximum lod scores ranged from 11.2 at $\theta=0.001$ to 6.2 at $\theta0.3$. The estimated probability of obtaining a maximum total lod score greater than +3 was 85.2% (interpolating all recombination fractions). Results of computer simulation indicate that family LA40 will demonstrate linkage, if a closely linked marker is found.

Our laboratories screened 65 family members with the sixth version of the Weber lab screening set, which consists of 169 microsatellites with average heterozygosity of 0.78 and an average spacing of 24.2 cM. Lod scores of more than 1.5 at $\theta=0$ identified four chromosomal regions, namely, 1p, 2p, 12p. and 19q. Other areas that showed positive lod scores were D2S406 with lod of 1.5 at $\theta=0.15$ and D1S318 with lod score of 2.33 at $\theta=0.001$. As far as markers in chromosome 6p, none of the seven markers studied gave evidence of tight linkage to the clinical epilepsies, CAE, or the clinical epilepsies plus the paroxysmal EEG patterns under any of the models studied (autosomal dominant or autosomal recessive with penetrances of 90%, 70%, or 50%) when the total lod scores were considered.

IDIOPATHIC MYOCLONIC EPILEPSIES OF ADULTS

Autosomal Dominant Benign Adult Familial Myoclonic Epilepsy in 8q23-24.1

Phenotype

One large family from Japan was first reported by Mikami et al. in 1999 (96) to map to 18q23-24.1. This single family had 27 members, 17 of whom were affected with tremulous finger movements and myoclonus of the upper and/or lower extremities by 30.5 years of age. Generalized tonic clonic seizures occurred infrequently. Follow-up studies over nearly 15 years suggest that myoclonus may increase late in the disease. None of the patients developed cerebellar ataxia or dementia. Generalized polyspikes and waves were present in EEGs. Photomyoclonus were induced by photic stimulation in some patients. The amplitudes of components P25 and N33 of the sensory evoked potentials were increased in all patients. Valproate and clonazepam were effective in stopping myoclonus and epilepsy.

Four other previously reported Japanese kindreds with similar phenotypes were studied by Plaster et al. in 1999 (97). In most of the reported families SSEP, VEP, and long loop C reflexes indicated "cortical reflex myoclonus." Skeletal muscle biopsy, rectal biopsy, and chromosome analyses were normal.

Genotype

A separate chromosomal site for the syndrome of familial adult myoclonus epilepsy (FAME) was localized in 8q23-24.1 by Mikami et al. and Plaster et al. in 1999 (96,97). Interestingly, this locus for FAME in 8q24 is presumed to be separate from the 8q24 locus for benign family neonatal convulsions (EBN2) responsible for the KCNQ3 mutation, the 8q24 locus for childhood absence epilepsy, the 8q24 locus of idiopathic generalized epilepsy, and the 8q13-21 locus for familial febrile seizures (Table 18.1).

Mikami et al. (96) first genotyped microsatellites in regions corresponding to previously mapped epilepsies and obtained preliminary evidence for linkage with D8S284. After 17 other STRPs were typed, maximum lod scores were obtained, namely, 4.314 at θ=0 with D8S1779 in two-point analyses. Maximum multipoint lod score of 5.42 was obtained for the interval between D8S555 and D8S1779, using the program LINKMAP. Plaster et al. (97) performed a genome wide linkage screen using 98 markers from the Utah marker development group. The LOD score for one large family was greater than 3.0 at θ=0. The summed lod scores for the other three families was 1.78 at θ=0. Obligate recombinants defined D8S514 as centromeric boundary and D8S1804 as telomeric boundary. Candidate genes include the glutamate binding subunit ionotropic receptor, NMDA receptor (GRINA), the β3 subunit of the neuronal nicotinic acetylcholine receptor, Tax interaction protein 43 and phosphodiesterase I/nucleotide pyrophosphatase 2 (PDNP2).

DISCUSSION

Are Recently Discovered Epilepsy Genes Unique to a Family, in Rare Genetic Isolates, or Common on Outbred Populations?

As the experience in Alzheimer disease has taught us, genes may be unique to a family or a few families or to a restricted genetic isolate or they may be susceptibility genes for the common variety of diseases. Much excitement was initially stirred by the localization of the β-amyloid precursor gene in chromosome 21 and the subsequent identification of mutations in the gene encoding β-amyloid precursor protein in one family (98). This mutation in the β-amyloid precursor gene turned out to be unique to this single family. Rare families with early-onset familial autosomal dominant Alzheimer disease (EOFAD) from France and Italy map to chromosome 14q24.3 and demonstrate more than 50 missense mutations and a splice site mutation in the presenilin 1 gene that cosegregate with EOFAD (99–101). In yet another rare variety of the EOFAD among Germans in the Volga river region, another gene with mutations segregating with affected members of early-onset Alzheimer's disease families resides in chromosome 1 and resembles presenilin 1 and is hence called presenilin 2. Perhaps most important from the public health point of view is the discovery that carriers of the apolipoprotein E4 (APO E4) allele have a significantly increased risk for the common variety of late-onset sporadic Alzheimer disease (LOAD) that is found in most populations of the world. The risk for developing Alzheimer disease is at least three to four times increased and much higher still in E4 homozygotes (102). In Finland, the combination of myeloperoxidase A and ApoE4 alleles increase the risk for men at 11.4 as compared to 3.0 for APO E4 alone (103). Because 50% of LOAD cases carry no APOE4 alleles, three separate and independent groups searched for additional risk factors using parametric and nonparametric linkage analyses and recently identified an Alzheimer disease locus in chromosome 10 (104–106). A similar understanding needs to be attained among the 5 epilepsy genes, so far defined and the more than 24 epilepsy chromosomal sites localized for various epilepsy syndromes. Tables 18.1 18.3 list the number of families that have been studied in localizing these chromosomal loci and the number of families that have been proved to have mutations in epilepsy genes.

Epilepsy Genes: Evolutionarily Old and Ancient Versus New and Younger

Whether an epilepsy gene is unique to a family, in rare genetic isolates with a founder or in common outbred populations may be gleaned from their geographic location, their presence in specific racial/ethnic groups, their evolution and their young or ancient age. Over the past decade, the nonrecombining part of the Y chromosome, inherited patrilineally (107), and the matrilineal mitochondrial DNA (mtDNA) (108–109) have become critical tools in the study of human migration and evolution (110–111). In addition to genealogic resolution, nonrecombining euchromatic part of the Y chromosome and mtDNA both show geographic structure, demographic history, and genealogic depth for assessment of the date of origin of humans. For instance, sequence polymorphisms estimate expansion of modern humans to have occurred between 50,000 and 200,000 years before the present, from an effective estimated population of about 10,000 individuals. Most current neutral polymorphisms are less than 800,000 years old. The initial dispersal of modern humans from Africa (112–114) on a coastal route through North and East Africa into Saudi Arabia through Iraq and Iran to Pakistan along Indian coastlines and then into Western India is based on the African mitochondrial haplogroup M. The first Americans started migration to the continent about 43,000 years before the present. The presence of epilepsy genes in these various racial/ethnic groups provide a clue as to the age of the epilepsy gene and time of occurrence of mutation(s). For instance, in Unverricht-Lundborg myoclonic epilepsy, a putative founding 3-2-4-4 haplotype was seen in 75/87 Finnish chromosomes with expansions of the promoter region of cystatin B gene suggesting a single origin of the expansion mutation in the Finnish population. Among Mediterraneans, Unverricht-Lundbord disease (EPM1) patients, 14 of 22 chromosomes had either the Finnish haplotype or a haplotype that could have arisen from it by a single recombination. In four Saudi Arabian chromosomes, more recombinations may have

occurred. The history of the Finnish population dates the mutation to at least some 2000 years back, and one interpretation of these results is that the mutation arose only once in an individual whose descendants spread over the Mediterranean region and Northern Europe (115).

Epilepsy Allele Enrichment in Affected Populations: Are They "Rare Flora in Rare Soil"?

The genetic complexity that underlies the epilepsies is still largely unknown. One group of common epilepsies could be represented by a relatively small pool of common polymorphic epilepsy alleles with a frequency of more than 0.01 that represents a number of highly restricted alleles from a limited number of epilepsy loci. Such common epilepsy alleles could have undergone expansion after passing thru a bottleneck in population migration and elimination. This may be the case in autosomal dominant JME in 6p12-11, and autosomal dominant febrile seizures in 8q, 19p, 5q14-15 that have a high expression rate. Another group is probably represented by a pool of epilepsy alleles at a large number of loci, at a low population frequency of less than 0.01 with varying intermediate and small effects on risk requiring interactions between epilepsy genes for actual phenotypic expression. It is likely that such conditions apply to the common IGEs susceptibility loci in chromosomes 3q26, 14q23, and 2q36 as reported by Sander et al. (83) and in chromosomes 18, 6, 8, and 5 as reported by Durner et al. (19). In addition, there are common forms of genetic epilepsies whose EEG traits are clearly mendelian (the 3 Hz spike waves, the EEG photoparoxysmal spike wave trait, and the centrotemporal spikes) but whose clinical seizures have relatively lower expression, such as absences and rolandic seizures. What is clear is that a growing body of information is showing that the number of epilepsy genes (nonallelic heterogeneity) is high. Whether these alleles represent "rare flora in rare soil" or "rare flora in common soil" or "common flora in common soil" will have to be determined for each epilepsy gene.

There are some regularly recurring regions where epilepsy genes have been harvested, namely, Australia, Quebec, France, Italy, Sardinia, Japan, Finland, and Sweden, as in the rare syndromes of autosomal dominant nocturnal frontal lobe epilepsy (ADNFLE) and autosomal dominant partial epilepsy with variable foci (ADPEVF), the common syndrome of rolandic epilepsy with centrotemporal spikes, febrile seizures, generalized epilepsy with febrile seizures plus and febrile seizures plus absence epilepsy (Tables 18.1 to 18.3). California, Mexico, and Central America are countries where the common JME 6p12-11 allele seems to be concentrated although they have been reported in Germany, Austria, and Japan. The KCNQ2 mutation of the rare benign familial neonatal convulsions was initially detected in a family from Newfoundland and then also observed in a family from Norway. Success in defining epilepsy alleles in these countries could partly be a reflection of where epilepsy alleles have been enriched by stratification of populations, consanguinity, assortative mating, and prolonged inbreeding. Australia, Quebec, Newfoundland, Mexico, and Central America represent relatively very young and new founder populations (less than 20 generations). Relatively speaking, Sardinia and Japan represent less recent founder populations (less than 200 generations). Sardinia and Japan are calculated to have expanded from founders of perhaps 1,000 individuals about 100 generations ago. The founder pool size must be very low (less than 100) if epilepsy allele frequencies are high (116). It will be important to determine if the common epilepsy alleles are common or rare in these countries with founder populations and if the epilepsy alleles so far reported are rare epilepsy alleles in a rare population. So far the majority of ADNFLE families do not map to the site of the CHRNA4 20q gene (25,26,117). Also, ADNFLE and ADPEVF (118) represent relatively rare diseases in the inbred populations of Europe and Canada. Likewise, the SCN1B mutation is not found in most GEFS+ families and in febrile convulsion families. The GABRG2 mutation was not found in a larger number of GEFS+ families from France (13). Epilepsy alleles of common epilepsies like JME and CAE should be studied in the founder populations of Australia and Quebec. Alleles of common epilepsies are not expected to be found in large numbers in the founder populations of Australia and Quebec.

Not All Alleles That Lead to Epilepsies Are as Yet Known and Many Are to Come

It is difficult to form an expectation for the distribution of epilepsy alleles that could be used for designing a mapping strategy for epilepsy alleles, given the presence of a high degree of heterogeneity. In addition, we do not know if the epilepsy alleles recently identified are evolutionarily ancient or genetically young and new. If the epilepsy alleles recently discovered represents epilepsy alleles in outbred populations that predated the divergence of the human population more than 100,000 years ago, such epilepsy alleles would have been destined to be lost through generations or fixated at a low frequency in outbred populations. However, such ancient genes could reach high frequencies in inbred groups or founder populations. An epilepsy gene that has reached a relatively high frequency in inbred groups could be exemplified by Lafora disease in Bangalore, India, Saudi Arabia, and in pockets of Palestinian immigrants. In some situations, population expansion in local areas would have frozen any change in frequency by minimizing genetic drift and we would be detecting epilepsy alleles mainly in special populations. The rare genotypes of autosomal dominant nocturnal frontal lobe epilepsy in chromosome 20q and the generalized epilepsy with febrile seizures plus in chromosome 19q could be examples. On the other hand, if the newly discovered epilepsy mutations are new risk alleles, they could stabilize and lead to high frequencies within a short time if the population is inbred and there is reduced allelic diversity and fixation of otherwise segregating epilepsy risk alleles. This could be exemplified by the absence and grand mal seizures found in Guaymi Indians in the Boca del Toros region of Panama. Such epilepsy allelic enrichment is affected by shared environment and by the interaction of such shared environment with the epilepsy alleles.

The considerations of these above discussions and the list of epilepsy loci in Tables 18.1 to 18.3 plus the accelerating progress in completing the sequence of the human genome all show why there should be even more epilepsy alleles to be discovered. Recent discoveries in Australia, France, Spain, Japan, and Quebec, not to mention California and Mexico, demonstrate that this is not merely a theoretical speculation. Founder effects in special population groups can lead to unusually high frequencies of otherwise rare epilepsy alleles. To discover more common epilepsy alleles with a high degree of nonallelic heterogeneity in outbred populations and to detect more epilepsy alleles with major, intermediate, and small effects, we will need to perform model-based linkage analyses as well as sib pair analyses and perhaps an SNP based consortium for association and transmission linkage disequilibrium studies. To acquire large populations for such large-scale genetic studies, an international collaboration is needed. Such epilepsy genetics studies must include very young founder populations like Costa Rica, Quebec, and Newfoundland as well as admixed populations of Mexico.

ACKNOWLEDGMENTS

We acknowledge the contributions and participation of my many colleagues who have participated as part of the GENESS (Genetic Epilepsy Studies) international consortium. Specifically, we wish to mention Drs. Astrid Rasmussen, Francisco Rubio Donnadieu; and Sergio Cordova (National Institute of Neurology and Neurosurgery, Mexico City, Mexico); Dr. Pravina Shah and her team (K.E.M. Hospital, Bombay, India); Dr. Ignacio Pascual-Castroviejo (Hospital La Paz, Madrid, Spain); Dr. Sonia Khan (Al Kharj Military Hospital, Riyadh, Saudi Arabia); and Drs. Gregorio Pineda and Gregory Walsh (California). Others have played an important role as physician scientists (Drs. Jose Serratosa and Berge Minassian), neuroscientists (Lucy Treiman, PhD and Jesus Sainz, PhD), geneticists (Robert Sparkes, PhD), coordinators (Joan Spellman, Adriana Lopez, and Bernadette Sakamoto), laboratory technicians (Aurelio Jara Prado, Susan Shih, Reza Iranmanesh) and EEG technicians (Nancy Kjeldgaard and Charlotte McTerrell). Most importantly, our international collaboration would not be possible without the participation and commitment of individuals and families who volunteer to participate as study subjects.

REFERENCES

1. Wallace RH, Wang DW, Singh R, et al. Febrile seizures and generalized epilepsy associated with a mutation in the Na+ channel β1 subunit gene SCN1B. Nat Genet 1998;19:366–370.
2. Escayg A, MacDonald BT, Meisler MH, et al. Mutations of SCN1A, encoding a neuronal sodium channel in two families with GEFS+2. Nat Genet 2000;24:343–345.
3. Escayg A, Heils A, MacDonald BT, et al. A novel SCN1A mutation associated with generalized epilepsy with febrile seizures plus–and prevalence of variants in patients with epilepsy. Am J Hum Genet 2001;68:866–873.
4. Wallace RH, Scheffer IE, Barnett S, et al. Neuronal sodium-channel α1-subunit mutations in generalized epilepsy with febrile seizures plus. Am J Hum Genet 2001;68:859–865.
5. Biervert C, Steinlein OK. Structural and mutational analysis of KCNQ2, the major gene locus for benign familial neonatal convulsions. Hum Genet 1999;104:234–240.
6. Charlier C, Singh NA, Ryan SG, et al. A pore mutation in a novel KQT-like potassium channel gene in an idiopathic epilepsy family. Nat Genet 1998;18:53–55.
7. Singh NA, Charlier C, Stauffer D, et al. A novel potassium channel gene, KCNQ2, is mutated in an inherited epilepsy of newborns. Nat Genet 1998;18:25–29.
8. Hirose S, Zenri F, Akiyoshi H, et al. A novel mutation of KCNQ3 (c.925T→C) in a Japanese family with benign familial neonatal convulsions. Ann Neurol 2000;47:822–826.
9. Steinlein O, Mulley JC, Propping P, et al. A missense mutation in the neuronal nicotinic acetylcholine receptor α 4 subunit is associated with autosomal dominant nocturnal frontal lobe epilepsy. Nat Genet 1995;11:201–203.
10. Steinlein OK, Mgnusson A, Stoodt J, et al. An insertion mutation of the CHRNA4 gene in a family with autosomal dominant nocturnal frontal lobe epilepsy. Hum Mol Genet 1997;6:943–947.
11. Hirose S, Iwata H, Akiyoshi H, et al. A novel mutation of CHRNA4 responsible for autosomal dominant nocturnal frontal lobe epilepsy. Neurology 1999;53:1749–1753.

12. Wallace RH, Marini C, Petrou S, et al. Mutant GABAA receptor γ2-subunit in childhood absence epilepsy and febrile seizures. *Nat Genet* May 2001; 28(1):49-52.

13. Baulac S, Huberfeld G, Gourfinkel-An I, et al. First genetic evidence of GABAA receptor dysfunction in epilepsy: A mutation in the γ2-subunit gene. *Nat Genet* 2001;28:46-48.

14. Claes L, Del-Favero J, Ceulemans B, et al. De Novo mutations in the sodium-channel gene SCN1A cause severe myoclonic epilepsy of infancy. *Am J Hum Genet* 2001; 68:1327-1332.

15. Greenberg DA, Delgado-Escueta AV, Maldonado HM, et al. Segregation analysis of juvenile myoclonic epilepsy. *Genet Epidemiol* 1988;5:81-94.

16. Greenberg DA, Delgado-Escueta AV, Widelitz H, et al. Juvenile myoclonic epilepsy (JME) may be linked to the BF and HLA loci on human chromosome 6. *Am J Med Genet* 1988;31:185-192.

17. Obeid T, Panayiotopoulos CP. Juvenile myoclonic epilepsy: a study in Saudi Arabia, *Epilepsia* 1988;29: 280-282.

18. Greenberg DA. Inferring mode of inheritance by comparison of lod scores. *Am J Hum Genet* 1989;59: 653-663.

19. Durner M, Keddache MA, Tomasini L, et al. Genome scan of idiopathic generalized epilepsy: evidence for major susceptibility gene and modifying genes influencing the seizure type. *Ann Neurol* 2001;49: 328-335.

20. Leppert M, Anderson VE, Quattlebaum T, et al. Benign familial neonatal convulsions linked to genetic markers on chromosome 20. *Nature* 1989;337;647-648.

21. Steinlein O, Schuster V, Fischer C, et al. Benign familial neonatal convulsions: Confirmation of genetic heterogeneity and further evidence for a second locus on chromosome 8q. *Hum Genet* 1995;95:411-415.

22. Lewis TB, Leach RJ, Ward K, et al. Genetic heterogeneity in benign familial neonatal convulsions: Identification of a new locus on chromosome 8q. *Am J Hum Genet* 1993;53:670-675.

23. Ryan SG, Wiznitzer M, Hollman C, et al. Benign familial neonatal convulsions: Evidence for clinical and genetic heterogeneity. *Ann Neurol* 1991;29:469-473.

24. Phillips HA, Scheffer IE, Berkovic SF, et al. Localization of a gene for autosomal dominant nocturnal frontal lobe epilepsy to chromosome 20q13.2. *Nat Genet* 1995;10:117-118.

25. Phillips HA, Scheffer IE, Crossland KM, et al. Autosomal dominant nocturnal frontal lobe epilepsy: Genetic heterogeneity and evidence for a second locus at 15q24. *Am J Hum Genet* 1998;63:1108-1116.

26. De Fusco M, Becchetti A, Patrignani A, et al. The nicotinic receptor β2 subunit is mutant in nocturnal frontal lobe epilepsy. *Nat Genet* 2000;26:275-276.

27. Fong GCY, Shah PU, Gee MN, et al. Childhood absence epilepsy with tonic-clonic seizures and electroencephalogram 3-4-Hz spike and slow wave complexes: linkage to chromosome 8q24. *Am J Hum Genet* 1998;63:1117-1129.

28. Serratosa JM, Delgado-Escueta AV, Medina MT, et al. Juvenile myoclonic epilepsy: D6S313 and D6S258 flank a 40 cM JME region. *Ann Neurol* 1996;39:58-66.

29. Bate L, Mitchell W, Williamson M, et al. Molecular genetic analysis of juvenile myoclonic epilepsy in the Saudi Arabian population. *Epilepsia* 2000;41(7):72 (abst).

30. Sugimoto Y, Morita R, Amano K, et al. Childhood absence epilepsy in 8q24: Refinement of candidate region and construction of physical map. *Genomics* 2000;68:264-272.

31. Kasteleijn-Nolst Trenite DGA, Binnie CD, Meinardi H. Photosensitive patients: symptoms and signs during intermittent photic stimulation and their relation to seizures in daily life. *J Neurol Neurosurg Psychiatry* 1987;50:1546-1549.

32. Wolf P, Goosses R. Relation of photosensitivity to epileptic seizures. *J Neurol Neurosurg Psychiatry* 1986;49:1386-1391.

33. Jeavons PM, Harding GFA. *Photosensitive epilepsy.* London: Heinemann, 1975.

34. Hauser WA, Hesdorfer DC. *Epilepsy: frequency, causes and consequences.* Landover, MD: Demos Publications, 1990.

35. Commission on Classification and Terminology of the International League Against Epilepsy. Proposal for revised classification of epilepsies and epileptic syndromes. *Epilepsia* 1989;30:389-399.

36. Commission on Classification and Terminology of the International League Against Epilepsy. Proposed revisions clinical and electroencephalographic classification of epileptic seizures. *Epilepsia* 1981;22:480-501.

37. Scheffer IE, Berkovic SF. Generalized epilepsy with febrile seizures plus: a genetic disorder with heterogeneous clinical phenotypes. *Brain* 1987;120:479-490.

38. Baulac S, Gourfinkel-An I, Picard F, et al. A second locus for familial generalized epilepsy with febrile seizures plus maps to chromosome 2q21-q33. *Am J Hum Genet* 1999;65:1078-1085.

39. Moulard B, Guipponi M, Chaigne D, et al. Identification of a new locus for generalized epilepsy with febrile seizures plus (GEFS+) on chromosome 2q24-q33. *Am J Hum Genet* 1999;65:1396-1400.

40. Peiffer A, Thompson J, Charlier C, et al. A locus for febrile seizures (FEB3) maps to chromosome 2q23-24. *Ann Neurol* 1999;46:671-678.

41. Lopes-Cendes I, Scheffer IE, Berkovic SF, et al. A new locus for generalized epilepsy with febrile seizures plus maps to chromosome 2. *Am J Hum Genet* 2000; 66:698-701.

42. Wallace RH, Berkovic SF, Howell RA, et al. Suggestion of a major gene for familial febrile convulsions mapping to 8q13-21. *J Med Genet* 1996;33:308-312.

43. Dubovsky J, Weber JL, Orr HT, et al. A second gene for familial febrile convulsions maps on chromosome 19p. *Am J Hum Genet* 1996;59(Suppl 4):A223.

44. Zara F, Gennaro E, Stabile M, et al. Mapping of a locus for familial autosomal recessive idiopathic myoclonic epilepsy of infancy to chromosome 16p13. *Am J Hum Genet* 2000;66:1552-1557.

45. Dravet C. Les epilepsies graves de l'enfant. *Vie Med* 1978;8:543-548.

46. Dravet C, Roger J, Bureau M, et al. Myoclonic epilepsies in childhood. In: Akimoto H, Kazamatsuri H, Seino M, et al., eds. *Advances in epileptology: XIIIth Epilepsy International Symposium.* New York: Raven Press, 1982:135-140.

47. Dalla Bernardina B, Capovilla G, Gattoni MB, et al. Epilepsie myoclonique grave de la premiere annee. *Rev EEG Neurophysiol* 1982;12:21-25.

48. Aicardi J. *Epilepsy in children.* New York: Raven Press, 1994.
49. Doose H, Gerken H, Hien-Volpel, et al. Genetics of photosensitive epilepsy. *Neuropadiatrie*1969:1:56–73.
50. Kanazawa O. Medically intractable generalized tonic-clonic or clonic seizures in infancy. *J Epilepsy* 1992;5: 143–148.
51. Dravet C, Bureau M, Genton P. Benign myoclonic epilepsy of infancy: electroclinical symptomatology and differential diagnosis from the other types of generalized epilepsies of infancy. *Epilepsy Res Suppl* 1992;6:131–135.
52. Dravet C, Giraud N, Bureau M, et al. Benign myoclonus of early infancy or benign non-epileptic spasms. *Neuropediatrics* 1986;17:33–38.
53. Lombroso CT, Fejerman N. Benign myoclonus in early infancy. *Ann Neurol* 1977;1:138–143.
54. Colamaria V, Plouin P, Dulac O, et al. Kojewnikow's epilepsia partialis continua: Two cases associated with striatal necrosis. *Neurophysiol Clin* 1988;18:535–539.
55. Salas Puig, Ramos E, Macarron J, et al., Benign myoclonic epilepsy of infancy. *Acta Paediatr (Scand)* 1990;79(11):1128–30.
56. Delgado-Escueta AV, Greenberg D, Weissbecker K, et al. Gene mapping in the idiopathic generalized epilepsies: Juvenile myoclonic epilepsy, childhood absence epilepsy, epilepsy with grand mal seizures and early childhood myoclonic epilepsy. *Epilepsia* 1990;31(S3): 19–29.
57. Doose H. Myoclonic astatic epilepsy of early childhood. In: Roger J, Bureau M, Dravet C, et al., eds. *Epileptic syndromes in infancy, childhood and adolescence*, 2nd ed. London: John Libbey, 1992:103–114.
58. Doose H, Baier WK. Genetic factors in epilepsies with primary generalized minor seizures. *Neuropediatrics* 1987;18(Suppl 1):1–64.
59. Doose H, Baier WK. Theta rhythms in the EEG: a genetic trait in childhood epilepsy. *Brain Dev* 1988;10: 347–354.
60. Doose H, Gerken H, Leonhardt R, et al. Centrencephalic myoclonic-astatic petit mal, *Neuropadiatrie* 1970;2:59–78.
61. Nakayama J, Hamano K, Iwasaki N, et al. Significant evidence for linkage of febrile seizures to chromosome 15q14-q15. *Hum Mol Genet* 2000;9(1):87–91.
62. Gooses R. *Die Beziehung der Fotosensibilitat zu den verschiedenen epileptischen syndromen* [Thesis]. Freie Berlin University, West Berlin, 1984.
63. Janz D. *Die epilepsien.* Stuttgart: Thieme Medical Publishers, 1969.
64. Janz D. Epilepsy with impulsive petit mal (juvenile myoclonic epilepsy). *Acta Neurol Scand* 1985;72:449–459.
65. Durner M. Sander T, Greenberg DA, et al. Localization of idiopathic generalized epilepsy on chromosome 6p in families of juvenile myoclonic epilepsy patients. *Neurology* 1991;41:1651–1655.
66. Sander T, Bockenkamp B, Hildmann T, et al. Refined mapping of the epilepsy susceptibility locus EJM1 on chromosome 6. *Neurology* 1997;49:842–847.
67. Weissbecker KA, Durner M, Janz D, et al. Confirmation of linkage between juvenile myoclonic epilepsy and the HLA-region on chromosome 6. *Am J Med Genet* 1991;39:32–39.
68. Liu AW, Delgado-Escueta AV, Serratosa JM, et al. Juvenile myoclonic epilepsy locus in chromosome 6p21.2-p11:linkage to convulsions and EEG trait. *Am J Hum Genet* 1995; 57:368–381.
69. Bai D, Alonso M-E, Morita R, et al. Juvenile myoclonic epilepsy in Mexico linked to chromosome 6p21-11. 54th Annual Meeting of the American Epilepsy Society, December 2000.
70. Elmslie FV, Rees M, Williamson MP, et al. Genetic mapping of a major susceptibility locus for juvenile myoclonic epilepsy on chromosome 15q. *Hum Mol Genet* 1997;6:1329–1334.
71. Tanaka M, Pascual Castroviejo I, Medina MT, et al. Linkage analysis between subsyndromes of childhood absence epilepsy (CAE) and the GABAA recepter β3 subunit (GABRB3) on chromosome 15q11.2-12. 54th Annual Meeting of the American Epilepsy Society. *Epilepsia* 1999;41(Suppl 7):250.
72. Feutch M, Fuchs K, Fichlbauer E, et al. Possible association between childhood absence epilepsy and the gene encoding GABRB3. *Biol Psychiatry* 1999; 46:997–1002.
73. Westling B, Weissbecker K, Serratosa JM, et al. Evidence for linkage of Juvenile myoclonic epilepsy with absence to chromosome 1p. *Am J Hum Genet* 1996;59 (Suppl 4):A1392.
74. Sander T, Hildmann T, Kretz R, et al. Allelic association of juvenile absence epilepsy with GluR5 kainate receptor gene (GRIK1) polymorphism. *Am J Med Genet* 1997;74:416–421.
75. Delgado-Escueta AV, Medina MT, Serratosa JM, et al. Mapping and positional cloning of common idiopathic generalized epilepsies: juvenile myoclonus epilepsy and childhood absence epilepsy. *Adv Neurol* 1999;79: 351–374.
76. Liu AW, Delgado-Escueta AV, Gee MN, et al. Juvenile myoclonic epilepsy in chromosome 6p12-p11:locus heterogeneity and recombinations. *Am J Med Genet* 1996;63:438–446.
77. Morita R, Miyazaki E, Shah PU, et al. Exclusion of the JRK/3H8 gene as a candidate for human childhood absence epilepsy mapped on 8q24. *Epilepsy Res* 1999; 37:151–158.
78. Durner M, Zhou G, Dingyi F, et al. Evidence for linkage of adolescent-onset idiopathic generalized epilepsies to chromosome 8 – and genetic heterogeneity *Am J Hum Genet* 1999;64:1411–1419.
79. Greenberg DA, Durner M, Keddache M, et al. Reproducibility and complications in gene searches: linkage on chromosome 6, heterogeneity, association, and maternal inheritance in juvenile myoclonic epilepsy. *Am J Hum Genet* 2000;66:2 508–516.
80. Greenberg DA, Durner M, Shinnar S, et al. Association of HLA class II alleles in patients with juvenile myoclonic epilepsy compared to patients with other forms of adolescent onset generalized epilepsy. *Neurology* 1996;47:750–755.
81. Obeid T, el Rab MO, Daif AK, et al. Is HLA-DRW13 (W6) associated with juvenile myoclonic epilepsy in Arab patients? *Epilepsia* 1994;35:319–321.
82. Zara F, Labuda M, Pandolfo M, et al. Unusual EEG pattern linkage to chromosome 3p in a family with idiopathic generalized epilepsy. *Neurology* 1998;51: 493–498. [Published erratum appears in *Neurology* 1998;51:1520.]
83. Sander T, Berlin W, Ostapowicz A, et al. Variation of the genes encoding the human glutamate EAAT2,

serotonin and dopamine transporters and susceptibility to idiopathic generalized epilepsy. *Epilepsy Res* 2000; 41:1 75–81.

84. Panayiotopoulos CT, Obeid T. Juvenile myoclonic epilepsy: an autosomal recessive disease. *Ann Neurol* 1989;25:440–443.

85. Mai R, Canevini MP, Pontrelli V, et al. L'epilepssia mioclonica giovanile di Janz: analisi prospettica di un campione di 57 pazienti. *Boll Lega It Epil* 1990;70/71: 307–309.

86. Delgado-Escueta AV, Medina MT, Serratosa JM, et al. Mapping and positional cloning of common idiopathic generalized epilepsies: juvenile myoclonus epilepsy and childhood absence epilepsy. *Adv Neurol* 1999; 79:351–374.

87. Risch N, Merikangas K. The future of genetic studies of complex human diseases. *Science* 1996;273: 1516–1517.

88. Lander ES, Schork NJ. Genetic dissection of complex traits. *Science* 1994;265:2037–2048.

89. Berkovic SF, Howell RC, Hopper JL. Familial temporal lobe epilepsy: a new syndrome with adolescent/adult onset and a benign course. In: Wolf P, ed. *A new syndrome with adolescent/adult onset and a benign course: epileptic seizures and syndromes.* London: John Libbey, 1994:257–263.

90. Berkovic SF, McIntosh AM, Howell RA, et al. Familial temporal lobe epilepsy: a common disorder identified in twins. *Ann Neurol* 1996;40:227–235.

91. Radovici A, Misirliou V, Gluckman M. Epilepsie reflexe provoquee par excitation des rayons solaires. *Rev Neurol* 1932;57:1305–1308.

92. Andermann K, Oaks G, Berman S, et al. Self-induced epilepsy. *Arch Neurol* 1962;6:49–79.

93. Panayiotopoulos C. Fixation-off-sensitive epilepsy in eyelid myoclonia with absence seizures. *Ann Neurol* 1987;22:87–89.

94. Duncan JS, Panayiotopoulos CP. *Eyelid myoclonia with absences.* London: John Libbey, 1996.

95. Ott J. *Analysis of human genetic linkage.* Baltimore: The Johns Hopkins University Press, 1991.

96. Mikami M, Yasuda T, Terao A, et al. Localization of a gene for benign myoclonic epilepsy to chromosome 8q23.2-q24.1. *Am J Hum Genet* 1999;65:745–751.

97. Plaster NM, Uyama E, Uchino M, et al. Genetic localization of the familial adult myoclonic epilepsy (FAME) gene to chromosome 8q24. *Neurology* 1999; 53:1180–1183.

98. Lendon CL, Ashall F, Goate AM. Exploring the etiology of Alzheimer disease using molecular genetics. *JAMA* 1997;277:825–831.

99. Campion D, Flaman JM, Brice A, et al. Mutations of the presenilin I gene in families with early-onset Alzheimer's disease. *Hum Mol Genet* 1995;4:2373–2377.

100. Champion D, Dumanchin C, Hannequin D, et al. Early-onset autosomal dominant Alzheimer disease: Prevalence, genetic heterogeneity and mutation spectrum. *Am J Hum Genet* 1999;65:664-670.

101. Sorbi S, Nacmias B, Forleo P, et al. Missense mutation of S182 gene in Italian families with early-onset Alzheimer's disease. *Lancet* 1995;346:439–440.

102. Corder EH, Saunders AM, Strittmatter WJ, et al. Gene dose of apolipoprotein E type 4 allele and the risk of Alzheimer's disease in late onset families. *Science* 1993;261:921–923.

103. Reynolds WF, Hiltunen M, Pirskamen M, et al. MPO and APOE epilepsy 4 polymorphisms interact to increase risk for AD in Finnish males. *Neurology* 2000; 55:1284–1290.

104. Myers A, Holmans P, Marshall H, et al. Susceptibility locus for Alzheimer's disease on chromosome 10. *Science* 2000;290(5500):2304–2305.

105. Ertekin-Taner N, Graff-Radford N, Younkin LH, et al. Linkage of plasma Ab42 to a quantitative locus on chromosome 10 in late-onset Alzheimer's disease pedigrees. *Science* 2000;290(5500):2303–2304.

106. Bertram L, Blacker D, Mullin K, et al. Evidence for genetic linkage of Alzheimer's Disease to chromosome 10q. *Science* 2000;290(5500):2302–2303.

107. Casalotti R, Simoni L, Belledi M, et al. Y-chromosome polymorphism and the origins of the European gene pool. *Proc R Soc Lond B Biol Sci* 1999;266:1959–1965.

108. Torroni A, Lott MT, Cabell MF, et al. MtDNA and the origin of Caucasians: Identification of ancient Caucasian-specific haplogroups, one of which is prone to a recurrent somatic duplication in the D-loop region. *Am J Hum Genet* 1994;55: 760–776.

109. Simoni L, Calafell F, Pettener D, et al. Geographic patterns of mtDNA diversity in Europe. *Am J Hum Genet* 2000;66:262–278.

110. Stumpf MPH, Goldstein DB. Genealogical and evolutionary interference with the human Y chromosome. *Science* 2001;291:1738–1742.

111. Cann RL. Genetic clues to dispersal in human populations: retracing the past from the present. *Science* 2001;291:1742–1748.

112. Quintana-Murci L, Semino O, Bandelt HJ, et al. Genetic evidence of an early exit of Homo Sapiens from Africa through Eastern Africa. *Nat Genet* 1999;23: 437–441.

113. Ingman M, Kaessmann H, Paabo S, et al. Mitochondrial genome variation and the origin of modern humans. *Nature* 2000;408(6813):708-13.

114. Underhill PA, Shen P, Lin AA, et al. Y chromosome sequence variation and the history of human populations. *Nat Genet* 2000;26(3):358-61.

115. Virtaneva K, D'Amato E, Miao J, et al. Unstable minisatellite expansion causing recessively inherited myoclonus epilepsy, EPM1. *Nat Genet* 1997;15:393–396.

116. Kruglyak L. Prospects of whole-genome linkage disequilibrium mapping of common disease genes. *Nat Genet* 1999;22:139–144.

117. Gambardella A, Annesi G, De Fusco M, et al. A new locus for autosomal dominant nocturnal frontal lobe epilepsy maps to chromosome 1. *Neurology* 2000;28: 1467–1471.

118. Xiong L, Labuda M, Li D, et al. Mapping of a gene determining familial partial epilepsy with variable foci to chromosome 22q11-q12. *Am J Hum Genet* 2000;65: 1698–1710.

119. Claes S, Devriendt K, Lagae L, et al. The X–linked infantile spasms syndrome (MIM 308350) maps to Xp11.4-Xpter in two pedigrees. *Ann Neurol* 1997;42: 360–364.

120. Malafosse A, Leboyer M, Dulac O, et al. Confirmation of linkage of benign familial neonatal convulsions to D20S19 and D20S20. *Hum Genet* 1992;89:54–58.

121. Bievert C, Schroeder BC, Kubisch C, et al. A potassium channel mutation in neonatal human epilepsy. *Science* 1998;279:403–406.

122. Guipponi M, Rivier F, Vigevano F, et al. Linkage mapping of benign familial infantile convulsions (BFIC) to chromosome 19q. *Hum Mol Genet* 1997;6: 473–477.

123. Szepetowski P, Rochette J, Berquin P, et al. Benign infantile convulsions and paroxysmal chorioathetosis: a new neurological syndrome linked to the pericentromeric region of human chromosome 16. *Am J Hum Genet* 1997;61:889–898.

124. Kugler SL, Stenroos ES, Mandelbaum DE, et al. Hereditary febrile seizures: phenotype and evidence for a chromosome 19p locus. *Am J Med Genet* 1998; 79:354–361.

125. Zara F, Bianchi A, Avanzini G, et al. Mapping of genes predisposing to idiopathic generalized epilepsy. *Hum Mol Genet* 1995;4:1201–1207.

126. Ito M, Kobayashi K, Fujii T, et al. Electroclinical picture of autosomal dominant nocturnal frontal lobe epilepsy in a Japanese family. *Epilepsia* 2000;41:52–58.

127. Scheffer IE, Bhatia KP, Lopes-Cendes I, et al. Autosomal dominant nocturnal frontal lobe epilepsy. A distinctive clinical disorder. *Brain* 1995;118:61–73.

128. Ottman R, Risch N, Hauser WA, et al. Localization of a gene for partial epilepsy to chromosome 10q. *Nat Genet* 1995;10:56–60.

129. Poza JJ, Saenz A, Martinez-Gil A, et al. Autosomal dominant lateral temporal epilepsy: clinical and genetic study of a large Basque pedigree linked to chromosome 10q. *Ann Neurol* 1999;42:182–188.

130. Scheffer IE, Phillips HA, O'Brien CE, et al. Familial partial epilepsy with variable foci: a new partial epilepsy syndrome with suggestion of linkage to chromosome 2. *Ann Neurol* 1998;44:890–899.

131. Guerrini R, Bonanni P, Nardocci N, et al. Autosomal recessive rolandic epilepsy with paroxysmal exercise-induced dystonia and writer's cramp: delineation of the syndrome and gene mapping to chromosome 16p12-11.2. *Ann Neurol* 1999;45:344–352.

132. Neubauer BA, Fiedler B, Himmelein B, et al. Centrotemporal spikes in families with rolandic epilepsy: linkage to chromosome 15q14. *Neurology* 1998;51: 1608–1612.

133. Scheffer IE, Jones L, Pozzebon M, et al. Autosomal dominant rolandic epilepsy and speech dyspraxia: a new syndrome with anticipation. *Ann Neurol* 1995;38: 633–642.

134. Kanemoto K, Kawasaki J, Miyamoto T, et al. Interleukin (IL)-1β, IL-1α, and IL-1 receptor antagonist gene polymorphisms in patients with temporal lobe epilepsy. *Ann Neurol* 2000;47:571–574.

135. Gigli et al., 1998.

136. Fink JK, Wu C-TB, Jones SM, et al. Autosomal dominant family spastic paraplegia: Tight linkage to chromosome 15q. *Am J Hum Genet* 1995;56:188–192.

137. Zuberi SM, Eunson LH, Spauschus A, et al. A novel mutation in the human voltage-gated potassium channel gene (Kv1.1) associates with episodic ataxia type 1 and sometimes with partial epilepsy. *Brain* 122:817–825.

138. Sperfeld AD, Collatz MB, Baier H, et al. FTDP-17: An early-onset phenotype with Parkinsonism and epileptic seizures caused by a novel mutation. *Ann Neurol* 1999; 46:708–715.

Myoclonus and Paroxysmal Dyskinesias,
Advances in Neurology, Vol. 89,
edited by S. Fahn, et al.
Lippincott Williams & Wilkins, Philadelphia © 2002.

19

Inherited Myoclonus-Dystonia

*Rachel Saunders-Pullman, †Laurie Ozelius, and *Susan B. Bressman

*Department of Neurology, Beth Israel Medical Center, New York, New York; and †Department of
Molecular Neurogenetics, Massachusetts General Hospital, Charlestown, Massachusetts*

The nomenclature of benign hereditary myoclonic syndromes in the literature has been confusing because families with similar phenotypes have been variably described as hereditary myoclonus-dystonia, hereditary essential myoclonus, and alcohol-responsive myoclonic-dystonia (1,2). From genetic studies, we know that at least one family labeled with each of these entities has been linked to a locus on 7q21 (3–5); therefore, the regrouping of families from each of these entities under the term "inherited myoclonus dystonia syndrome" appears valid.

Dystonia is characterized by sustained twisting or posturing movements, usually directional in nature (6). Myoclonus describes fast, lightning-like jerks (7). Myoclonus and dystonia may occur together in several genetic diseases with subtle clinical differences. Some patients with dystonia may have fast dystonic movements that are as quick as 100 ms (8). This may occur in DYT1 and other forms of primary dystonia (9). Conversely, occasional myoclonic jerks may occur superimposed on dystonic movements, particularly in the upper arms with writer's cramp. When dystonia is the prominent feature, and there are mild myoclonic-like associated jerks, this has been defined as myoclonus-dystonia (M-D) (10) (Table 19.1). However, in some individuals myoclonus may also be the prominent feature that is inherited (1). It is in these individuals with myoclonus as the primary prevalent movement that we consider M-D.

Myoclonus may be primary or essential if the only neurologic feature is myoclonus and there is no known etiology. Most essential myoclonus is not hereditary (11), and there is clinical variability, suggesting a heterogeneity between hereditary and apparently nongenetic forms. While not the first to report hereditary myoclonus (for a descriptive history, see Gasser [2]), Mahloudjhi and Pikielny (8) were instrumental in defining the clinical entity of M-D, which they termed hereditary essential myoclonus. In an attempt to systematically distinguish this benign hereditary myoclonus from other forms of myoclonus, particularly progressive myoclonias, such as those with ataxia or epilepsy, they set criteria for benign hereditary myoclonus with their description of a family with six affected family members.

TABLE 19.1. *Characteristics of myoclonus-dystonia*

1. Myoclonus as primary feature; dystonia may also be seen but is rarely sole feature.
2. Autosomal dominant with incomplete penetrance and variable expressivity.
3. Onset usually in the first or second decade.
4. No associated neurologic features, such as gross ataxia, dementia, epilepsy, and a normal electroencephalogram and somatosensory evoked potentials.
5. Usually a benign clinical course, compatible with long life span.

Adapted from Mahloudji M, Pikielny RT. Hereditary essential myoclonus. *Brain* 1967;90:669–674; and Gasser T. Inherited myoclonus-dystonia syndrome. *Adv Neurol* 1998;78:325–334.

Mahloudjhi and Pikielny defined the syndrome as onset of myoclonus in the first or second decade, a benign course, autosomal dominant inheritance, the absence of seizures, dementia, gross ataxia or other neurologic deficits, and a normal electroencephalogram (EEG). While dystonia *per se* is not mentioned, one of their patients is described as having "tendency to turn his head to the right especially when concentrating," suggestive of cervical dystonia (8). Thus, already in these early descriptions, comorbid myoclonus and dystonia are described.

Families are now characterized as having M-D when an individual has prominent early-onset myoclonus, which may or may not be associated with dystonia, and there are no other neurologic features. Infrequently, one family member may demonstrate only mild dystonia (2). Unlike DYT1 families where dystonia is the predominant feature and dystonic jerks may be myoclonic in nature, myoclonus is a prominent feature in this syndrome (2,12). Gasser revised the original criteria in a manner that describes all chromosome 7q21 linked families to date. These revisions include (a) in addition to myoclonus, mild dystonic features may be present in some individuals, either in the presence of predominant dystonia, or rarely, as the sole movement; (b) symptoms usually, but not always, start in the first and second decade; and (c) in addition to normal EEG, somatosensory evoked potentials should be normal, thereby distinguishing this syndrome from familial cortical myoclonic tremor (FCMT). While the myoclonus of M-D may be very oscillatory (13), FCMT has very rhythmic myoclonus, which meets the definition of tremor (14).

MOLECULAR GENETICS

An M-D locus on chromosome 7q21 (HUGO designation DYT11) was mapped in a North American family with ten affected individuals with clinical features typical for this disorder (3). Obligate recombinations restricted the disease to an interval of about 28 cM. This locus has been confirmed in eight other M-D families, and the region containing DYT11 has been narrowed to 14 cM (4). Three candidate genes were screened (metabotropic glutamate receptor type 3 and two γ subunits of guanine nucleotide-binding proteins, GNG11 and GNGT1) (3,4) and did not reveal any mutations. Four French families with M-D also demonstrated linkage to this region (15), but did not narrow the region. Four German families were reported who further confirmed the locus and narrowed the region to a 7.2 cM area, flanked by the markers D7S652 and D7S2480. When recombination events from all papers are combined, this narrows the region containing the M-D gene to a 4.26cM region between markers D7S652 and D7S821. There has been no shared (partial) haplotype reported within the linked region among these families, rendering a recent common founder mutation unlikely (4,5). The pedigree structure in these families supports an autosomal dominant mode of inheritance with reduced penetrance and variable expressivity. Although exclusion to this region cannot be tested in smaller families, the absence of excluded families supports a major etiologic role for the 7q locus in M-D.

Concurrent with the report of linkage to chromosome 7q21, a missense change (Val54Ile) in a conserved region of the dopamine D2 receptor (DRD2) on 11q23 was found to cosegregate with M-D in one family (16). However, this change has not been identified in other families or singleton cases, and there is no evidence of linkage to 11q23, or of the missense change in other M-D families (4,16–19). Further, receptor binding and signal transduction assays of the D2 dopamine mutant and wild type receptors reveal identical agonist and antagonist affinities and functional responses (17). Thus, the role of this missense change including the molecular mechanisms through which the Val→Ile mutation may contribute to M-D remains to be determined.

Recently, mutations in the epsilon-sarcoglycan (SCGE) gene, located within the candidate interval on chromosome 7q21, were re-ported to cause M-D in six families from Germany (20). The mutations included two non-sense changes in exon three (289C→T; R97X and 304C→T;R102X), the latter of which was found in two families, a one base pair deletion (565delA), a 10 base pair deletion (488-97del), and a splice site mutation at the exon-intron junction of exon 6 (907+1G→A) (20). Our group has confirmed these findings as we have screened ten M-D families for mu-tations in the SGCE gene and identified a mutation in each family (unpublished data). The SGCE gene clearly represents the major M-D locus, mutations which probably ac-count for most cases of clinically typical M-D. The orthologous SGCE mouse gene shows maternal imprinting, i.e. it is predominantly expressed from its paternal allele (21). Zim-prich et al. (20) examined M-D pedigrees dis-playing linkage to chromosome 7q markers and noted a marked difference in penetrance dependent on the parent of origin of the dis-ease allele. If the disease gene is inherited from the father the disease is expressed, but if inherited from the mother the disease is not expressed (non-penetrant). However, some of the family members did not follow the im-printing pattern and further study is required as to the role of parental gender on expres-sion of M-D.

SGCE is the fifth member of the sarcogly-can family. It contains twelve exons and en-codes a protein of 405 amino acids that is highly homologous to alpha-sarcoglycan (22, 23). It is widely expressed in both embryonic and adult tissues (22), including the brain (20, 23). The other members of the sarcogly-can family encode transmembrane compo-nents of the dystrophin-glycoprotein com-plex that link the cytoskeleton to the extracellular matrix. Mutations in the genes encoding the other sarcoglycans, which are mainly expressed in muscle, cause autosomal recessive limb-girdle muscular dystrophies (24). SGCE appears to be functionally simi-lar to alpha-sarcoglycan in skeletal muscle (25); however, nothing is known about its function in the brain as yet.

CLINICAL COURSE

Symptom onset of M-D is usually in the first or second decade and may be as early as 6 months (1,2). Although cases as late as onset at ages 37 and 38 (4,15) have been reported, indi-viduals may be asymptomatic at the time of ex-amination, and subjects may recall even later ages of onset. The neck and arms are involved most commonly with myoclonus, followed by the trunk and bulbar muscles, with less com-mon involvement of the legs. When mild dys-tonia is observed in some family members, it may occur in the same or a different distribu-tion as the myoclonus. Rarely, dystonia is the only manifestation, and then it is usually writer's cramp, or less frequently, torticollis.

Postural tremor has also been variably re-ported in some families and can be estimated at approximately 10%. Hand or head tremor were present in 7 of 15 individuals thought to be af-fected in one large family (three individuals had isolated tremor) (26). Other families with tremor have also been reported (13,27,28).

Most affected adults often report that the muscle jerks respond dramatically to alcohol (1,8,12), although there is heterogeneity among and between families. In one study with eight reported families, seven had at least one family member with dramatic re-sponse to alcohol (4), and in another with four families, only two had a family member with clear response to alcohol, but these were smaller families (15). M-D is compatible with a normal lifespan and often compatible with normal lifestyle. Sequelae of alcohol used to self-medicate symptoms may be socially much more disabling than the myoclonus and dystonia. The disorder tends to plateau in adulthood. Spontaneous remissions have been reported, and individuals have been noted to have transient leg dystonia in early childhood, which has resolved (8,12).

In the first reported chromosome 7q-linked M-D family, which is characteristic of these families, there were ten affected individuals (3). Of seven male and three female subjects, four had myoclonus and definite dystonia, four had myoclonus and probable dystonia, one had only myoclonus, and one had only writer's cramp. The mean age of onset was 6.5 years with a range of 4–15 years; one individual had unknown age of onset. He self-reported age of onset at 62, although it is unclear whether symptoms predated his sixties. The myoclonus occurred at rest, but was worsened with action, especially in muscles not directly involved in the task, such as overflow to the neck when writing or pouring. The jerks were variable, in some individuals they were focal, others multifocal, or isolated trunk jerks, and at times were small amplitude and oscillatory. The movements worsened with stress, sudden noise, caffeine, and tactile stimuli. There was marked improvement with alcohol, moderate improvement with clonazepam and valproate, and no response to carbidopa/levodopa. The observed dystonia in this family included writer's cramp, torticollis, and mild leg involvement. There was a question of postural stability in several affected family members, raising the possibility of parkinsonian features or mild cerebellar disturbance. However, no response to carbidopa/levodopa was reported, and mild cerebellar features may be part of the M-D syndrome (8).

Clinical features in the second group of 7-q linked families were similar (4). Among the eight families, there were 42 affected, 27 males and 15 females. There was myoclonus and dystonia in 23, myoclonus in 15, and dystonia in 4. Myoclonus affected primarily the trunk, neck, proximal limbs (arms more than legs), and face. Dystonia involved the arms and neck, with mild infrequent leg. The mean age of onset was 8.1 years, with a range of 1 to 37 years.

In the family associated with the DRD2 change, clinical features were indistinguishable from the 7q-linked families. There were eight affected, five male and three female. M-D was present in four, myoclonus alone in three, and dystonia alone in one. Myoclonus was prominent in the trunk, neck, and arms and responded to ingestion of alcohol (16).

NONMOTOR CLINICAL FEATURES

In addition to myoclonus and dystonia, nonmotor features have been reported in some families. Kyllerman et al. (29) reported cognitive slowing in some of their family members (29). However, the prominent nonmotor features have been psychiatric disease reported in some (3,16,29) but not all (5) families. Nygaard et al. (3) reported that nine of ten affected individuals reported psychiatric problems, including diagnoses and treatment for depression, anxiety, and obsessive-compulsive disorder (OCD) (3). Depression, personality disorders, and addiction were reported in other families (16), and treatment of the panic attacks in one individual with familial M-D with Nefazadone led to the improvement of both the panic attacks and the myoclonus (30). However, systematic study for psychiatric illness has not been performed in these M-D families, and it is unknown whether these features segregate with the M-D locus.

In order to determine whether the same genetic etiology underlies both neurologic and psychiatric signs, we studied psychiatric symptoms in nonmanifesting carriers (NMCs), non-carriers (NCs), and manifesting carriers (MCs) in three families demonstrating linkage of M-D to the 7q21 locus (3,4). Carrier status was assigned by comparing the haplotypes of each family member to the disease bearing haplotype showing linkage in that family. Whether an individual manifested neurologic symptoms was determined by review of a standardized videotaped exam; an individual was defined as manifesting M-D only if there were definite signs of myoclonus, dystonia, or both (31). Trained clinical interviewers, who were blind to the individual's position in the pedigree and carrier status, administered the computerized version of the Composite International Diagnostic Interview (CIDI)–WHO version (*http://wwwlive.who.ch /msa/cidi/computerizedcidi.htm*) via the telephone. The CIDI is a comprehensive, fully standardized diagnostic interview used to assess psychiatric symptomatology and has been used in large epidemiologic studies of psychiatric disorders (32). The instrument has excellent reliability (33), and diagnostic algorithms have been developed for *Diagnostic and Statistical Manual of Mental Disorders* (DSM-IV) diagnoses.

Algorithms for the DSM-IV diagnosis of OCD (300.3), generalized anxiety disorder (GAD, 300.02), major affective disorder (MAD, recurrent depression 296.31-.33 or bipolar mania 296.41-.43), alcohol abuse without alcohol dependence (305.00), alcohol dependence (303.90), drug abuse without drug dependence (305.2-7, .90I, 90O, 90P), and drug dependence (304.00,304.1-6,9, .9O), were used (33).

To determine whether DSM-IV diagnoses segregate with the linked 7q21 haplotype within families, we assigned diagnoses to all interviewed family members using the CIDI algorithms. We compared rates of disorders between the MCs, NMCs, and NCs by testing two hypotheses: (a) whether the psychiatric condition is associated with the M-D mutation and (b) whether the psychiatric condition is associated with the neurologic symptomatology. For the first hypothesis, we compared rates in all carriers (MCs and NMCs) versus noncarriers. For the second hypothesis, we compared rates in neurologically symptomatic carriers (MCs) with asymptomatic individuals (NMCs and NCs).

Of 55 participating individuals, 16 were MCs, 11 were NMCs, and 28 were NCs. The carrier and noncarrier groups did not differ significantly in gender, age or education, nor did the manifesting and nonmanifesting carrier groups. The rate of OCD was significantly higher in carriers compared to noncarriers (p=0.023). It was also higher in the symptomatic gene carriers (MC) (25.0%) compared to the asymptomatic group (NMC and NC combined) (2.6%, p=0.022). Alcohol dependence was increased in the symptomatic

carriers (43.8% versus 12.8%, p=0.027), but not in the carrier group overall (MC and NMC versus NC). Alcohol abuse was not increased in either the symptomatic carriers or the carriers overall. The rate of GAD was elevated in symptomatic carriers compared to asymptomatic individuals (37.5% versus 12.8%) (p=0.061), but was not increased in the gene carriers overall. There was also more drug use in the symptomatic carriers (31.3%) versus the asymptomatic group (12.8%), but this difference was not statistically significant. MAD was increased in the symptomatic carriers (31.3%) versus the asymptomatic group (17.9%), but this was also not significant (Table 19.2).

Thus, OCD is associated with the DYT11 M-D gene. OCD was increased both in the carrier group overall (MC and NMC) and the symptomatic carrier group (MC). Eighty percent of individuals with OCD were symptomatic for M-D. With this small sample size we cannot conclusively determine whether the association with OCD is a gene effect or is associated with having neurologic symptoms of myoclonus and dystonia. If it is the latter, OCD may be reactive to having the neurologic disorder or may be indicative of diminished penetrance for both psychiatric and neurologic signs. We postulate that OCD may be an expression of the DYT11 gene and is not a reactive phenomenon. In support of this idea, OCD was not observed among the probands, who were the most severely affected family members. OCD or obsessive-compulsive symptoms are also not usually reported as reactive to medical disability. OCD is also increased in TS, another movement

TABLE 19.2. *Obsessive-compulsive disorder and alcohol abuse and dependence among DYT11 family members*

	Alcohol abuse disorder (abuse or dependence) (%)	Alcohol dependence (%)	OCD (%)
Carriers (n = 27)	40.0	25.9	18.5
MC (n = 16)	33.3	43.8	25.0
NMC (n = 11)	45.5	0.0	9.1
Noncarriers (n = 28)	17.4	17.9	0.0

MC, manifesting carriers; NMC, nonmanifesting carriers; OCD, obsessive-compulsive disorder.

disorder of unclear etiology. Dystonia and TS may share basal ganglia pathophysiology, including a relative state of dopamine excess (34,35), and the significance of the relationship between OCD and M-D is unclear. It is of interest that both TS and M-D show moderate male predominance, although OCD may be a feature associated with TS, which is more frequent in girls.

In contrast to the effect seen with OCD, we believe the association with alcohol use is due to the palliative effect of alcohol on the motor symptoms, rather than a direct effect of the gene. We found a significant difference only in the most severe form of alcohol use, alcohol dependence, which is more frequent in symptomatic individuals. Thus, we believe it is likely that the pattern of alcohol dependence may begin when alcohol is used to self-treat motor symptoms.

Because our results are based on only three M-D families with a limited number of individuals, the analysis needs to be replicated in other M-D families. Until the DYT11 gene is elucidated, these studies will be limited to multiplex families demonstrating linkage to this locus. Once the gene is cloned, a much larger M-D population, including simplex families, may be suitable for study. Further studies of other linked families are necessary to lend greater insight into the relationship of myoclonus dystonia and psychiatric disorders.

TREATMENT

Although the symptoms of M-D usually resolve with ingestion of alcohol, the risk of long-term effects of alcohol dependence far exceeds the benefits, rendering it an unacceptable treatment option. γ-Hydroxybutyric acid (GHB) has been reported to markedly improve symptoms of myoclonus, in a manner similar to alcohol (36). Larger placebo-controlled studies are warranted, because GHB is the most promising treatment for M-D. Multiple other medications have been tried, including clonazepam and valproate, with moderate efficacy (3). Anticholinergics have been reported useful by one group (37), but

others have not found similar efficacy (1). We treated a single patient with levetiracetam, but this was less effective than valproate. In parallel to essential tremor, which may also respond to alcohol, primidone, and propanolol have also been tried, but with limited benefits. Improvement with 5-hydroxytryptophan has been reported in some cases (30).

Stereotactic thalamotomy has diminished myoclonus, but was accompanied by dysarthria in one patient and mild hemiparesis in another (38). In two others, myoclonus was improved, but without significant gain in function (39). Deep brain stimulation (DBS) of the medial globus pallidus improved dystonia and myoclonus; however, only 8-week follow-up was reported (40). Cloning of the DYT11 gene as well as further trials with GHB and DBS represent windows of treatment for this disorder.

REFERENCES

1. Quinn NP. Essential myoclonus and myoclonic dystonia. *Mov Disord* 1996;11:119–124.
2. Gasser T. Inherited myoclonus-dystonia syndrome. *Adv Neurol* 1998;78:325–334.
3. Nygaard TG, Raymond D, Chen C, et al. Localization of a gene for myoclonus-dystonia to chromosome 7q21-q31. *Ann Neurol* 1999;46:794–798.
4. Klein C, Schilling K, Saunders-Pullman R, et al. A major locus for myoclonus-dystonia maps to chromosome 7q in eight families. *Am J Hum Genet* 2000;67:1314–1319.
5. Asmus F, Zimprich A, Naumann M, et al. Inherited myoclonus-dystonia syndrome: narrowing the 7q21-q31 locus in German families. *Ann Neurol* 2001;49:121–124.
6. Fahn S. Concept and classification of dystonia. *Adv Neurol* 1988;50:1–8.
7. Marsden CD, Hallet M, Fahn S. The nosology and pathophysiology of myoclonus. In: Marsden CD, Fahn S, eds. *Movement disorders.* London: Butterworths, 1982:196–248.
8. Mahloudji M, Pikielny RT. Hereditary essential myoclonus. *Brain* 1967;90:669–674.
9. Obeso JA, Rothwell JC, Lang AE, et al. Myoclonic dystonia. *Neurology* 1983;33: 825–830.
10. Quinn NP, Rothwell JC, Thompson PD, et al. Hereditary myoclonic dystonia, hereditary torsion dystonia and hereditary essential myoclonus: an area of confusion. *Adv Neurol* 1988;50:391–401.
11. Bressman S, Fahn S. Essential myoclonus. *Adv Neurol* 1986;43: 287–294.
12. Kyllerman M, Forsgren L, Sanner G, et al. Alcohol-responsive myoclonic dystonia in a large family: dominant inheritance and phenotypic variation. *Mov Disord* 1990;5:270–279.
13. Fahn S, Sjaastad O. Hereditary essential myoclonus in a large Norwegian family. *Mov Disord* 1991;6:237–247.

14. Terada K, Ikeda A, Mima T, et al. Familial cortical myoclonic tremor as a unique form of cortical reflex myoclonus. *Mov Disord* 1997;12:370–377.
15. Vidailhet M, Tassin J, Durif F, et al. A major locus for several phenotypes of myoclonus-dystonia on chromosome 7q. *Neurology* 2001;56:1213–1216.
16. Klein C, Brin MF, Kramer P, et al. Association of a missense change in the D2 dopamine receptor with myoclonus dystonia. *Proc Natl Acad Sci USA* 1999;96 (9):5173–5176.
17. Klein C, Gurvich N, Sena-Esteves M, et al. Evaluation of the role of the D2 dopamine receptor in myoclonus dystonia. *Ann Neurol* 2000;47:369–373.
18. Durr A, Tassin J, Vidaihlet M, et al. D2 receptor gene in myoclonic dystonia and essential myoclonus. *Ann Neurol* 2000;48:127–128.
19. Grimes DA, Bulman D, George-Hyslop PS, et al. Inherited myoclonus-dystonia: evidence supporting genetic heterogeneity. *Mov Disord* 2001:16:106–110.
20. Zimprich A, Grabowski M, Asmus F, et al. Mutations in the gene encoding epsilon-sarcoglycan cause myoclonus-dystonia syndrome. *Nat Genet* 2001;29: 66-69.
21. Piras G, El Kharroubi A, Kozlov S, et al. Zac1 (Lot1), a potential tumor suppressor gene, and the gene for epsilon-sarcoglycan are maternally imprinted genes: identification by a subtractive screen of novel uniparental fibroblast lines. *Mol Cell Biol* 2000;20:3308-3315.
22. Ettinger AJ, Feng G, Sanes JR. Epsilon-Sarcoglycan, a broadly expressed homologue of the gene mutated in limb-girdle muscular dystrophy 2D. *J Biol Chem* 1997;272:32534-32538.
23. McNally EM, Ly CT, Kunkel LM. Human epsilon-sarcoglycan is highly related to alpha-sarcoglycan (adhalin), the limb girdle muscular dystrophy 2D gene. *FEBS Lett* 1998;422:27-32.
24. Angelini C, Fanin M, Freda MP, et al. The clinical spectrum of sarcoglycanopathies. *Neurology* 1999;52:176-179.
25. Liu LA, Engvall E. Sarcoglycan isoforms in skeletal muscle. *J Biol Chem*1999;274:38171-38176.
26. Korten JJ, Notermans SL, Frenken CW, et al. Familial essential myoclonus. *Brain* 1974;97:131–138.
27. Kurlan R, Behr J, Medved L, et al. Myoclonus and dystonia: a family study. *Adv Neurol* 1988;50:385–389.
28. Schaefer KP, Wieser S. Neurophysiologische Untersuchungen zur essentiellen Myoklonie. *Arch Psychiat Nerv Krankh* 1964;205:572–590.
29. Kyllerman M, Sanner G, Forsgren L, et al. Early onset dystonia decreasing with development: case report of two children with familial myoclonic dystonia. *Brain Dev* 1993;15:295–298.
30. Scheidtmann K, Muller F, Hartmann E, et al. Familial myoclonus-dystonia syndrome associated with panic attacks. *Nervenarzt* 2000;71:839–842.
31. Bressman SB, deLeon D, Kramer PL, et al. Dystonia in Ashkenazi Jews: clinical characterization of a founder mutation. *Ann Neurol* 1994;36:771–777.
32. Kessler RC, McGonagle KA, Zhao S, et al. Lifetime and 12-month prevalence of DSM-III-R psychiatric disorders in the United States. Results from the National Comorbidity Survey. *Arch Gen Psychiatry* 1994;51:8–19.
33. Wittchen HU. Reliability and validity studies of the WHO Composite International Diagnostic Interview (CIDI): a critical review. *J Psychiat Res* 1994;28:57–84.
34. Jankovic J, Rohaidy H. Motor, behavioral and pharmacologic findings in Tourette's syndrome. *Can J Neurol Sci* 1987;14:541–546.
35. Jankovic J, Orman J. Tetrabenazine therapy of dystonia, chorea, tics and other dyskinesias. *Neurology* 1988; 38: 391–394.
36. Priori A, Bertolasi L, Pesenti A, et al. Gamma-hydroxybutyric acid for alcohol-sensitive myoclonus with dystonia. *Neurology* 2000;54:1706.
37. Duvoisin RC. Essential myoclonus: response to anticholingeric therapy. *Clin Neuropharmacol* 1984;7: 141–147.
38. Gasser T, Bereznai, Mueller B, et al. Linkage studies in alcohol-responsive myoclonic dystonia. *Mov Disord* 1996;11:363–370.
39. Suchowerksy O, Davis J, Furtado S, et al. Thalamic surgery for essential myoclonus results in clinical but not functional improvement. *Mov Disord* 2000;15(Suppl 3): 44.
40. Liu X, Griffin I, Miall C, et al. *Mov Disord* 2000;15 (Suppl 3): 81.

Myoclonus and Paroxysmal Dyskinesias,
Advances in Neurology, Vol. 89,
edited by S. Fahn, et al.
Lippincott Williams & Wilkins, Philadelphia © 2002.

20

Clinical Features and Genetics of Unverricht-Lundborg Disease

Anna-Elina Lehesjoki

Department of Medical Genetics, University of Helsinki, Helsinki, Finland

Progressive myoclonic epilepsies (PMEs) are a heterogeneous group of rare, mostly autosomal recessive inherited disorders that are characterized by the association of epilepsy, myoclonus, and progressive neurologic deterioration, in particular ataxia and dementia (1,2). Despite a common name, PMEs differ in clinical features, etiology, and pathogenesis as well as prognosis. Many PMEs display accumulation of abnormal storage material. The most common forms of PME are Unverricht-Lundborg disease, Lafora disease, the neuronal ceroid lipofuscinoses, myoclonus epilepsy with ragged-red fibers, and the sialidoses. In addition, a number of rarer disorders manifest as PME. The molecular genetics of several forms of PME have been understood in the past decade, which has resulted in advances in diagnostics and classification.

EPIDEMIOLOGY AND CLINICAL CHARACTERISTICS

Unverricht-Lundborg disease (EPM1) is inherited autosomal recessively. It occurs worldwide and is the most common single disease entity among the PMEs. EPM1 is enriched in Finland, where the incidence is 1:20,000 births (3). The prevalence of EPM1 appears to be increasing due to the more benign course of the disease during the past few decades. EPM1 is relatively frequent also in the Western Mediterranean region.

The age of onset of the symptoms is 6 to 15 years (3–5). The symptoms progress insidiously and in general become prominent in the teenage years. Stimulus-sensitive myoclonic jerks are an essential feature for the diagnosis of EPM1 and are the first symptoms in at least half of the patients. The course is initially progressive. Previously, myoclonus tended to be progressive throughout life. However, as a result of the advances in the medical treatment of EPM1 patients, the development of myoclonus may stabilize or even improve over time (5,6).

Generalized tonic-clonic seizures are the presenting feature in nearly half of the patients (3–5). In rare cases tonic-clonic seizures do not appear at all. Some patients experience absence seizures, psychomotor seizures, or focal motor signs. Epileptic seizures are most frequent 3 to 7 years after the onset and may later cease entirely.

Neurologic findings are initially normal, but patients later develop ataxia and incoordination as well as intention tremor and dysarthria (3–5). EPM1 patients are mentally alert, but show a slow decline in intelligence over time (5,7). Their mood is often labile and depression is common. Due to better medication as well as improvements in the whole therapy regimen, the prognosis of EPM1 patients has improved significantly and patients now live to their 60s.

The electroencephalogram (EEG) is always abnormal in EPM1 patients even before the symptoms appear (5,8). It is most characteristic before antiepilepsy drug medication. Background activity is slower than normal and symmetric, generalized and high-voltaged spike and wave and polyspike and wave paroxysms are characteristic. Marked photosensitivity is the most prominent feature.

On histopathologic examination, widespread nonspecific degenerative changes, but no intracellular inclusions, have been seen in the central nervous system (4,9). Loss of Purkinje cells has been observed, but this may have resulted from treatment with phenytoin (10).

THERAPY

Valproic acid (VPA) has been considered the drug of choice for EPM1 (3,4,11,12). If started immediately after the onset of symptoms, VPA delays or even stops the progression of the disease process and it also seems to suppress the photoconvulsive response. Clonazepam has been reported effective (11,13) as add-on therapy to VPA and occasional exacerbations of seizure activity are best treated by a brief course of diazepam. Piracetam has been used for years to treat patients with PME, and the response has been favorable in many cases (14–16). In addition to the medication, attention should be paid to the proper psychosocial rehabilitation of EPM1 patients.

MOLECULAR GENETICS

The mutated gene on chromosome 21q22.3 responsible for EPM1 was identified using a positional cloning strategy. A genome-wide search for linkage was undertaken in 12 Finnish EPM1 families to localize the EPM1 gene to chromosome 21q22.3 (17). Using linkage disequilibrium and by exploiting historical recombinations in haplotype analysis, the EPM1 gene localization was narrowed to an approximately 175-kb region (18). A systematic search for genes in this region resulted in the identification of previously described but unmapped protein, cystatin B (CSTB), a cysteine protease inhibitor (19).

Northern blot analysis of lymphoblastoid cell mRNA revealed dramatically reduced levels of CSTB mRNA in EPM1 patients. The role of CSTB in EPM1 was confirmed by demonstrating mutations in patients.

An unstable expansion of a dodecamer (12 bp) repeat unit of 5′-ccccgccccgcg-3′ located 175 bp upstream from the translation initiation codon in the promoter region of the CSTB gene is the most common EPM1-associated mutation (20–22). It accounts for approximately 90% of disease alleles worldwide. This repeat is normally polymorphic, with 2 to 3 copies, but expanded alleles associated with the EPM1 phenotype contain at least 30 repeat copies (23). All except one patient so far reported carry the expansion mutation on at least one disease chromosome, and the majority are homozygous for it. No correlation between the repeat size and the age of onset or the severity of the clinical phenotype has been reported (20–23). Expanded alleles of the EPM1 minisatellite show a high mutation rate with contractions or expansions of the minisatellite typically by a single repeat unit (24). The expansion of the dodecamer repeat in EPM1 represents the first case of instability of a repeat unit other than trinucleotides in association with human diseases.

Five other mutations that affect 1 to 2 nucleotides in the CSTB gene have been reported (19,25). Two of the mutations affect splice sites: a G to C transversion at the last nucleotide of intron 1 alters the 3′ splice site AG dinucleotide and an A to G change affects the invariant AG dinucleotide of the acceptor splice site of intron 2. Two mutations predict a truncated protein: a C to T transition at codon 68 generates an early stop codon and a deletion of two nucleotides (TC) in exon 3 causes a frameshift and results in the introduction of a stop codon at position 75. An G to C change in exon 1 that results in the substitution of a highly conserved glycine to an arginine at amino acid position 4 is the only missense mutation so far reported in EPM1. Analysis of the CSTB gene mutations, notably the minisatellite expansion mutation can be used to confirm the clinical diagnosis of EPM1.

CYSTATIN B IN UNVERRICHT-LUNDBORG DISEASE

In vitro analysis of the CSTB promoter activity has shown that the minisatellite repeat expansion mutation results in reduced transcriptional activity (26,27) compatible with the reduced CSTB messenger ribonucleic acid (mRNA) levels observed in patients (19–22,26). However, the subsequent molecular pathogenetic mechanisms remain unknown. CSTB is a ubiquitously expressed 98 amino acid nonglycosylated protein of approximately 12 kD that belongs to a large superfamily of protease inhibitors, the cystatins (28–31). The cystatins inhibit *in vitro* several papain-family cysteine proteases, cathepsins, by tight and reversible binding (32–35). The cysteine cathepsins are lysosomal proteases that have acidic pH-optima with the exception of cathepsin S, which retains its proteolytic activity also in physiological pH (36). CSTB is ubiquitously expressed, and it has been suggested to counteract inappropriate proteolysis of the cell due to cathepsins that leak out of the lysosomes, but CSTB may also interact with other cellular proteins.

In lymphoblastoid cells of EPM1 patients the papain inhibitory activity, corresponding to CSTB activity in these cells, has been found to be significantly reduced or absent (Lehesjoki et al., *unpublished findings*). Decreased CSTB activity correlates with significantly increased cathepsin activity, especially of cathepsins B, L, and S. These data suggest that increased protease activity may play a role in the pathogenesis of EPM1.

CYSTATIN B–DEFICIENT MOUSE–A MODEL FOR UNVERRICHT-LUNDBORG DISEASE

Mice deficient for CSTB have been produced by targeted disruption of the mouse Cstb gene (37). These mice develop a phenotype that resembles the human phenotype (Table 20.1). The mice show progressive ataxia and myoclonic seizures. However, in contrast to the human phenotype in which the myoclonic seizures are stimulus sensitive, they only occur during sleep in mice. No tonic-clonic seizures, photosensitivity or spike wave complexes in EEG, typical in human patients, have been observed in the mice. The clinical features in mice are associated with apoptotic death of cerebellar granule cells, suggesting that CSTB has a role in preventing apoptosis in specific mammalian cells. The mechanism by which CSTB blocks apoptosis is unknown and may occur either directly, by inhibition of caspases, a family of evolutionarily related cysteine proteases that are involved in the initiation of apoptosis or indirectly, by inhibition of cathepsins, which may activate caspases (37). The finding of increased cathepsin activity in EPM1 patients would favor the latter hypothesis. In addition to the neurologic symptoms, approximately 40% of the mice develop ocular opacity as a result of corneal lesions that have not been reported in human EPM1 patients. The findings in Cstb-deficient mice suggest that CSTB has a neuroprotective mechanism of action and that EPM1 should be classified as a primary neurodegenerative disorder that selectively targets specific mammalian cells.

TABLE 20.1. *Comparison of human and mouse EPM1 phenotypes*

Feature	Human	Mouse
Myoclonic seizures	Present; stimulus sensitive	Present; during sleep
Ataxia	Present	Present
Electroencephalogram	Spike wave and polyspike wave	4–5 Hz spike
Tonic-clonic seizures	Present	Absent
Photosensitivity	Marked	Absent
Cerebellar apoptosis	Not reported	Present
Corneal lesions	Not reported	Present in approximately 40%

Further evidence supporting the hypothesis of an endogenous neuroprotective role of CSTB arises from studies in a rat kindling model of epilepsy (38), in which seizure activity has been shown to induce marked and widespread up-regulation of CSTB mRNA and protein in forebrain neurons.

CONCLUSION

The recent advances in the molecular understanding of EPM1 have important implications. An etiologic diagnosis of EPM1 is now possible, and the clinical suspicion of EPM1 can be easily confirmed by demonstrating mutations in the CSTB gene. The identification of CSTB as the defective gene in EPM1 and the development of the Cstb-deficient mouse model provide the basis for further studies on the biochemical and pathologic pathways underlying this disease, which should eventually help patients more directly by revealing molecular targets for treatment.

REFERENCES

1. Berkovic SF, Andermann F, Carpenter S, et al. Progressive myoclonus epilepsies: specific causes and diagnosis. *N Engl J Med* 1986;315:296–304.
2. Marseille Consensus Group. Classification of progressive myoclonus epilepsies and related disorders. *Ann Neurol* 1990;28:113–116.
3. Norio R, Koskiniemi M. Progressive myoclonus epilepsy; genetic and nosological aspects with special reference to 107 Finnish patients. *Clin Genet* 1979;15: 382–398.
4. Koskiniemi M, Donner M, Majuri H, et al. Progressive myoclonus epilepsy: a clinical and histopathologic study. *Acta Neurol Scand* 1974;50:307–332.
5. Lehesjoki AE, Koskiniemi M. Clinical features and genetics of progressive myoclonus epilepsy of the Unverricht-Lundborg type. *Ann Med* 1998;30:474–480.
6. Kyllerman M, Sommerfelt TK, Hedström A, et al. Clinical and neurophysiological development of Unverricht-Lundborg disease in four Swedish siblings. *Epilepsia* 1991;32:900–909.
7. Koskiniemi M. Psychological findings in progressive myoclonus epilepsy without Lafora bodies. *Epilepsia* 1974;15:537–545.
8. Koskiniemi M, Toivakka E, Donner M. Progressive myoclonus epilepsy: electroencephalographical findings. *Acta Neurol Scand* 1974;30:333–359.
9. Haltia M, Kristensson K, Sourander P. Neuropathological studies in three Scandinavian cases of progressive myoclonus epilepsy. *Acta Neurol Scand* 1969;45:63–77.
10. Eldridge R, Iivanainen M, Stern R, et al. 'Baltic' myoclonus epilepsy: hereditary disorder of childhood made worse by phenytoin. *Lancet* 1983;2:838–842.
11. Iivanainen M, Himberg JJ. Valproate and clonazepam in the treatment of severe progressive myoclonus epilepsy. *Arch Neurol* 1982;39:236–238.
12. Somerville ER, Olanow W. Valproic acid: treatment of myoclonus in dyssynergia cerebellaris myoclonica. *Arch Neurol* 1982;39:527–528.
13. Goldberg MA, Dorman JD. Intention myoclonus: successful treatment with clonazepam. *Neurology* 1976;26: 24–26.
14. Remy C, Genton P. Effect of high dose of oral piracetam on myoclonus in progressive myoclonus epilepsy (Mediterranean myoclonus). *Epilepsia* 1991;32:6.
15. Gouliaev AH, Senning A. Piracetam and other structurally related nootropics. *Brain Res* Rev 1994;19: 180–222.
16. Koskiniemi M, Van Vleymen B, Hakamies L, et al. Piracetam relieves symptoms in progressive myoclonus epilepsy: a multicentre, randomised, double blind, crossover study comparing the efficacy and safety of three dosages of oral piracetam with placebo. *J Neurol Neurosurg Psychiatry* 1998;64:344–348.
17. Lehesjoki A-E, Koskiniemi M, Sistonen P, et al. Localization of a gene for progressive myoclonus epilepsy to chromosome 21q22. *Proc Natl Acad Sci USA* 1991;88: 3696–3699.
18. Virtaneva K, Miao J, Träskelin, et al. Progressive myoclonus epilepsy EPM1 locus maps to a 175 kb interval in distal 21q. *Am J Hum Genet* 1996;58:1247–1253.
19. Pennacchio LA, Lehesjoki A-E, Stone NE, et al. Mutations in the gene encoding cystatin B in progressive myoclonus epilepsy (EPM1). *Science* 1996;271:1731–1734.
20. Lafreniere RG, Rochefort DL, Chretien N, et al. Unstable insertion in the 5′-flanking region of the cystatin-B gene is the most common mutation in progressive myoclonus epilepsy type-1, EPM1. *Nat Genet* 1997;15:298–302.
21. Virtaneva K, D'Amato E, Miao J, et al. Unstable minisatellite expansion causing recessively inherited myoclonus epilepsy, EPM1. *Nat Genet* 1997;15:393–396.
22. Lalioti MD, Scott HS, Buresi C, et al. Dodecamer repeat expansion in cystatin B gene in progressive myoclonus epilepsy. *Nature* 1997;386:847–851.
23. Lalioti MD, Scott HS, Genton P, et al. A PCR amplification method reveals instability of the dodecamer repeat in progressive myoclonus epilepsy (EPM1) and no correlation between the size of the repeat and age at onset. *Am J Hum Genet* 1997;62:842–847.
24. Larson GP, Ding S, Lafrenière RG, et al. Instability of the EPM1 minisatellite. *Hum Mol Genet* 1999;8: 1985–1988.
25. Lalioti MD, Mirotsou M, Buresi C, et al. Identification of mutations in cystatin B, the gene responsible for the Unverricht-Lundborg type of progressive myoclonus epilepsy (EPM1). *Am J Hum Genet* 1997;60:342–351.
26. Alakurtti K, Virtaneva K, Joensuu T, et al. Characterization of the cystatin B gene promoter harboring the dodecamer repeat expanded in progressive myoclonus epilepsy, EPM1. *Gene* 2000;242:65–73.
27. Lalioti MD, Scott HS, Antonarakis SE. Altered spacing of promoter elements due to the dodecamer repeat expansion contributes to reduced expression of the cystatin B gene in EPM1. *Hum Mol Genet* 1999;8:1791–1798.
28. Järvinen M, Rinne A. Human spleen cysteine protease

inhibitor: purification, fractionation into isoelectric variants and some properties of the variants. *Biochim Biophys Acta* 1982;708:210–217.

29. Ritonja A, Machleidt W, Barrett AJ. Amino acid sequence of the intracellular cysteine proteinase inhibitor cystatin B from human liver. *Biochem Biophys Res Commun* 1985;131:1187–1192.

30. Barrett AJ. The cystatins, a diverse superfamily of cysteine peptidase inhibitors. *Biomed Biochim Acta* 1986;45:1363–1373.

31. Jerala R, Trstenjak M, Lenarcic, et al. Cloning a synthetic gene for human stefin B and its expression in E. coli. *FEBS Lett* 1988;239:41–44.

32. Abrahamson M, Barrett AJ, Salvesen G, et al. Isolation of six cysteine proteinase inhibitors from human urine: their physicochemical and enzyme kinetic properties and concentrations in biological fluids. *J Biol Chem* 1986;261:11282–11289.

33. Machleidt W, Thiele U, Assfalg-Machleidt I, et al. Molecular mechanism of inhibition of cysteine proteinases by their protein inhibitors: kinetic studies with natural and recombinant variants of cystatins and stefins. *Biomed Biochim Acta* 1991;50:613–620.

34. Brömme D, Rinne R, Kirschke H. Tight-binding inhibition of cathepsin S by cystatins. *Biomed Biochim Acta* 1991;50:631–635.

35. Lenarcic B, Krizaj I, Zunec P, et al. Differences in specificity for the interactions of stefins A, B, and D with cysteine proteinases. *FEBS Lett* 1996;395:113–118.

36. Kirschke H, Wiederanders B. Cathepsin S and related lysosomal endopeptidases. *Method Enzymol* 1994;244:500–511.

37. Pennacchio LA, Bouley DM, Higgins KM, et al. Progressive ataxia, myoclonic epilepsy and cerebellar apoptosis in cystatin B-deficient mice. *Nat Genet* 1998;20:251–258.

38. D'Amato E, Kokaia Z, Nanobashvili A, et al. Seizures induce widespread upregulation of cystatin B, the gene mutated in progressive myoclonus epilepsy, in rat forebrain neurons. *Eur J Neurosci* 2000;12:1687–1695.

Myoclonus and Paroxysmal Dyskinesias,
Advances in Neurology, Vol. 89,
edited by S. Fahn, et al.
Lippincott Williams & Wilkins, Philadelphia © 2002.

21

Progressive Myoclonus Epilepsy with Polyglucosan Bodies: Lafora Disease

Berge A. Minassian

*Department of Pediatrics (Neurology), Hospital for Sick Children
and University of Toronto, Toronto, Ontario, Canada*

The progressive myoclonus epilepsies (PMEs) are devastating inherited neurodegenerative disorders associated with progressively worsening myoclonus, myoclonic epilepsy, early dementia, and death. Studies in PME patients have contributed substantially to our understanding of myoclonus, especially cortical myoclonus (see chapter 12). The defective genes for most of the PME are known and are allowing the generation of knockout mouse models. These animals will be an invaluable resource in future explorations of myoclonus.

There are five main forms of PME: the neuronal ceroid lipofuscinoses (NCLs) (chapter 22), type I sialidosis, Unverricht-Lundborg disease (ULD) (chapter 20), myoclonic epilepsy with ragged red fibers (MERRF) (chapter 23), and Lafora disease (LD) (Table 21.1). NCL and sialidosis are lysosomal lipid storage diseases; ULD is due to deficiency of cystatin B, an inhibitor of lysosomal cathepsins; MERRF is a mitochondrial disorder; and LD is a glycogen storage disease. NCLs are primarily diseases of childhood (less than 10 years of age). The other PMEs have onsets or major disease burden in adolescence or young adulthood.

This chapter focuses on LD, the story of which begins with Gonzalo Lafora in 1911. Lafora was studying autopsy brains of patients with teenage-onset PME and dementia when he observed striking bilayered spherical structures, sometimes as large as the neurons containing them (1). This had not been seen in the PME cases studied previously by Unverricht (2) and Lundborg (3). During the following decades, Lafora's PME served as a prototypical condition from which the other nonearly childhood PME (ULD, sialidosis [4], adult forms of NCL [5] and MERRF [6]) were distinguished by virtue of not containing Lafora inclusions.

In the following sections, we review the clinical, neurophysiologic, pathologic, and genetic features of LD. We also attempt to place together all the known pieces of the jigsaw puzzle of the pathogenesis of this condition, starting with the first, largest and oldest piece, the Lafora body.

THE CLINICAL SYNDROME (7–25)

The typical patient with LD is a normal teenager who presents with one or more of the following symptoms. He or she may exhibit myoclonic jerks usually precipitated by action or excitement, may experience (ictal) visual hallucinations, may be noticed to be depressed and performing poorly at school, or may experience a generalized convulsion.

In most patients, the obviously progressive disease sets in between 12 and 17 years of age. Many would have had isolated febrile or nonfebrile convulsions earlier in infancy or childhood (13,22–24). Rarely, the progres-

TABLE 21.1. *Inherited progressive myoclonus epilepsies*

Syndrome	Genes	Age at onset (year)	Suggestive clinical signs	Characteristic pathologic features
Neuronal ceroid lipofuscinoses (see chapter 22)	7 genes: CLN1-6 and CLN8	0–9, except CLN4 (adult form)	Visual loss due to macular degeneration	Lipopigment deposits: granular osmiophilic, curvilinear, or fingerprint profile forms
Unverricht-Lundborg disease (see chapter 20)	EPM1	6–15	Prominent cerebellar signs; slow progression	None
Lafora disease	EPM2A[a]	6–19	Visual hallucinations due to occipital seizures	Lafora polyglucosan inclusion bodies
Sialidosis, type 1 (4)	NEU1	8–15	Cherry-red spot	Urinary oligosaccharides, fibroblast neuraminidase deficit
Myoclonic epilepsy with ragged red fibers (see chapter 23)	MTTK[b]	3–65	Short stature, lactic acidosis	Ragged red fibers; mitochondrial respiratory chain abnormalities

[a]Mutations in at least one other unknown gene also cause Lafora disease (see text).
[b]MTTK mutations are responsible for 80% to 90% of cases. Other cases are due to mutations in the MTTL1 gene.

sively worsening epilepsy begins as early as six years of age (23,24).

Following onset, there is a variable rate of clinical worsening partly depending on the severity of the epilepsy. Seizures and myoclonus respond temporarily to valproic acid and piracetam, but gradually become intractable. Frequency of generalized convulsions is variable, but all patients will develop almost continuous myoclonus during wakeful hours and frequent occipital lobe seizures. Mental decline continues unabated with appearance of agitation, psychosis, and dementia. Dysarthria and ataxia occur early in the course of the disease, but spasticity sets in only in the later stages. By their mid-20s most patients are in a tube-fed vegetative state with continuous myoclonus. Some will maintain minimal reactions with the family such as a reflex-like smiling upon cajoling. Non-tube-fed patients have frequent aspirations due to seizures, and death from aspiration pneumonia is common.

Myoclonus and occipital seizures are cardinal features of LD. Myoclonus can be fragmentary, symmetric, or generalized. It occurs at rest and is exaggerated with excitement, by action, or by photic stimulation. Myoclonus usually disappears with sleep. Trains of massive myoclonias with relative preservation of consciousness occur, mimicking generalized convulsions (13,24,25). Myoclonus is the primary reason for early wheelchair dependency prior to any motor deficits.

Occipital seizures are very common presenting as transient blindness, simple or complex visual hallucinations, photomyoclonic or photoconvulsive seizures, or classic migraine with scintillating scotomata (13,18,24). Prominence of occipital seizures is not a feature of other PMEs such as the NCLs. On the other hand, clinically significant retinal pathology is not a feature of LD, but is an early severe characteristic of the NCLs and sialidosis.

NEUROPHYSIOLOGIC STUDIES

Abnormalities on electroencephalography (EEG) precede clinical symptoms as seen in affected younger siblings of confirmed cases (13,23). The EEG background slows, α-rhythm and sleep features are lost with progression, and photosensitivity is common. Increasingly, the record becomes replete with paroxysms of generalized irregular spike wave discharges with occipital predominance and focal, especially occipital, abnormalities (18,24). Unlike juvenile myoclonic epilepsy (JME), epileptiform discharges decrease during sleep (24).

Myoclonus is primarily cortical, although subcortical myoclonus cannot be ruled out. Both positive and negative myoclonus have been documented (chapter 12). Photomyoclonus has been shown to proceed by a rapid spread of electrical transients from the occiput (Fig. 21.1) to the ipsilateral rolandic

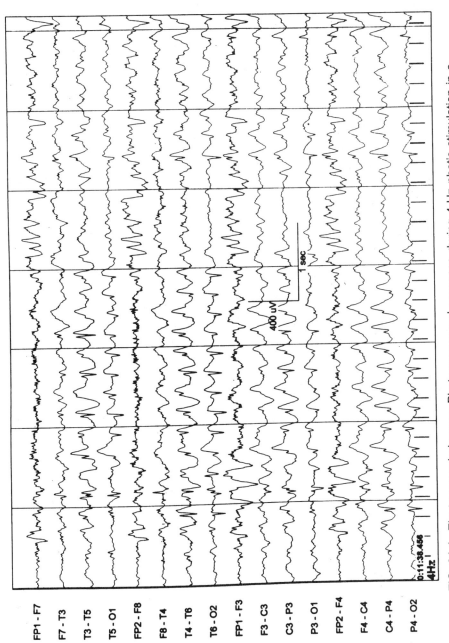

FP1 - F7
F7 - T3
T3 - T5
T5 - O1
FP2 - F8
F8 - T4
T4 - T6
T6 - O2
FP1 - F3
F3 - C3
C3 - P3
P3 - O1
FP2 - F4
F4 - C4
C4 - P4
P4 - O2

400 uV

1 sec

0:11:38.456
4Hz

FIG. 21.1. Electroencephalogram: Photoparoxysmal response during 4-Hz photic stimulation in a 14-year-old girl with new onset LD (several-months history of early morning myoclonia, dysarthria, and mild cognitive). The patient's sister, with biopsy-proven LD, died of seizure-induced aspiration pneumonia at the age of 22 years at the time of the writing of this article. Both sisters have a homozygous single nucleotide insertion at nucleotide 800 of the EPM2A gene that disturbs laforin's catalytic PTP domain and truncates the protein.

area, and from there to the contralateral sensorimotor cortex (26,27).

High voltage somatosensory and visual evoked potentials are recorded especially in the early years of the disease. Progressive prolongation of central latencies in the above as well as in auditory brainstem responses occur as time goes on (16,24).

DIAGNOSIS: DIFFERENTIAL AND CONFIRMATION

Myoclonic seizures in a teenager invoke the very common diagnosis of JME. This comes rapidly into doubt with the persistently slow background and the irregular occipital spike waves on the EEG. Visual hallucinations and "negative" symptoms (withdrawal, cognitive decline) conjure concerns of schizophrenia, which is ruled out with the onset of convulsions and an EEG with epileptiform activities. Normal funduscopic and electroretinographic evaluations go against sialidosis and NCLs. Absence of cerebrospinal fluid (CSF) measles antibody and normal CSF lactate exclude subacute sclerosing panencephalitis and MERRF, respectively.

Diagnostic confirmation in most PME relies on pathologic analysis, although this is gradually shifting to genetic testing. This is especially the case in ULD in which pathologic analysis is not revealing, and most patients have a common gene mutation (chapter 20). In LD, biopsy of brain (1,7–25, 28,29), liver (15), muscle (30), or skin (31, 32) will reveal the pathognomonic Lafora bodies.

Although in skin Lafora bodies can sometimes be found in myoepithelial cells of both eccrine (salty sweat) and apocrine (odorous sweat) glands (32), their predominant location is in the duct cells of the former but not the latter (31). The axilla (replete with apocrine glands) has therefore no advantage over biopsy at any other skin site. In fact, apocrine cells normally have periodic acid-Schiff (PAS)–positive inclusions, which the uninitiated sometimes misinterpret as Lafora bodies (S. Carpenter, *personal communication*). There-

fore, avoiding the axilla as a site of biopsy is preferred.

Biopsy in LD can be negative due to sampling error (20,33). Genetic testing at present detects mutations in approximately 70% of cases (see below).

PATHOLOGY

At a time when brain biopsies were thought the only way for definitive diagnosis of LD, several papers reported little neuronal loss in patients with already intractable myoclonus (12,14). This indicates that factors in addition to cortical neuronal loss are likely involved in the epilepsy of LD. With disease progression, at autopsy, substantial neuronal loss is seen. All regions of the central nervous system (CNS) are involved, including cerebral and cerebellar cortex, basal ganglia, cerebellar nuclei, thalamus, hippocampus, and retina as well as anterior and posterior horn cells of the spinal cord (1,8–14,28).

The Lafora Bodies

In the CNS, Lafora bodies are present predominantly in neurons (13,29). They range in size from 3 to 40 μ and often occupy the entire cytoplasm. They have a dense core and a less dense periphery (Fig. 21.2; see Color Plate 1 following page 288), and they stain strongly positive with PAS. PAS staining also reveals numerous small dustlike granules that are composed of the same material as the larger Lafora bodies. The subcellular distribution of these two accumulations is as follows. The larger Lafora bodies are in the perikaryal region near the nucleus (Fig. 21.2C; see Color Plate 1 following page 288), and the dustlike granules are within dendrites (Fig. 21.2D; see Color Plate 1 following page 288) (1,8–14,25,28,29,34,35). The cumulative size of the dendritic dustlike granules has been estimated to exceed that of the large spherical perikaryal Lafora bodies. Axons rarely contain Lafora bodies or any PAS-positive accumulations (29).

Lafora bodies outside the CNS have been found in most other organs, including skin (see

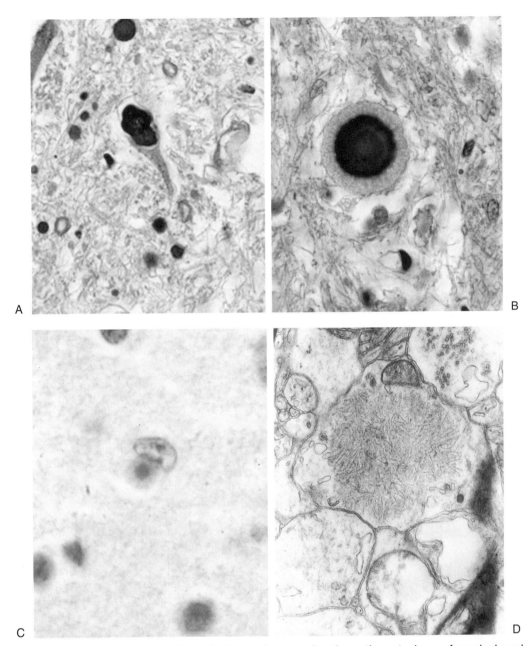

FIG. 21.2. Lafora bodies: **A:** A large Lafora body occupying the entire cytoplasm of a spinal cord neuron (center of figure); several other Lafora bodies are also seen. Periodic acid-Shiff (PAS), ×1000. **B:** A Lafora body that has outgrown its neuron and is free in the neuropil, hemalum-phloxine-saffrin, ×1000. **C:** A Lafora body (center of figure) with typical appearance (dense core and looser periphery) and typical juxtanuclear (perikaryal) localization, PAS, ×2000. **D:** Electron micrograph of a Lafora body in a dendrite, ×30,000 (see Color Plate 1 following page 288).

above), but are most prominent in liver and muscle (especially cardiac muscle) (15,30–32). Despite the massive accumulations in liver and to a lesser degree in muscle, to my knowledge there have been no reports of hepatic or skeletal or cardiac muscle disease.

In muscle, Lafora bodies are enclosed within a surrounding membrane (12). In liver, the presence of a membrane remains controversial (15,36). In brain, most authors (8–14) reported that Lafora bodies are free in the cytoplasm. Cajal et al. (37) contended that during early phases of their maturation, Lafora bodies are encapsulated within a membranous structure.

Composition of the Lafora Bodies

Positivity on PAS staining indicates an important content of carbohydrate. With electron microscopy, Lafora bodies are seen to be made up of short fibrils of 50 to 100 Å diameter. Many fibrils appear to be in physical association with the endoplasmic reticulum (ER) (38) or ribosomes (39). Acid hydrolysis dissolves the fibrils and reveals that they consist of glucose molecules. The PAS-positive accumulations in LD are therefore glucose polymers (polyglucosans). Polyglucosans differ from glycogen (the physiologic mammalian glucose polymer) in that they lack the regular branching pattern that allows glycogen to go into suspension in the cytoplasm (8–21,25,34,35). Glycogen branching requires the coordinated action of a number of enzymes, defects of which may be relevant to LD (discussed below).

THE LAFORA DISEASE GENE: EPM2A

EPM2A was identified in 1998 using a standard positional cloning approach (40,41). It is composed of four exons and codes for a 331 amino acid protein called laforin. More than 20 mutations have been reported, all in the coding region of the gene (23,40,41). Only three mutations have been found to occur in more than two families (23).

Genotype-phenotype correlation studies have been hampered by the rarity of the disease because most centers follow a small number of patients. It appears that the mutation type does not correlate with any specific seizure type at onset or age of onset (23).

The mouse (42) and dog (*unpublished*) homologues of EPM2A have been identified and show greater than 90% sequence identity with the human gene at the amino acid sequence level.

Finally, it has also been shown that at least one other, yet unknown, gene also causes LD (43). Mutations in this second gene are predicted to be present in the cluster of French Canadian patients and other LD patients whose disease gene locus does not link to the EPM2A locus on chromosome 6q24.

THE LAFORA DISEASE PROTEIN: LAFORIN

Laforin has experimentally been shown to be a dual-specificity protein tyrosine phosphatase (PTP) (40,44,45). PTPs are a greater than 500 member strong family of regulatory proteins that adjust the functions of their substrates by regulating the phosphorylation status of key tyrosine residues (46–49). All PTPs contain the amino acid sequence motif HCxAGxxRS/T, usually in their carboxy terminus half (46) (x represents any amino acid). This motif and surrounding sequences form the catalytic domain utilized in the phosphatase reaction (47). Although all PTPs utilize the same catalytic mechanism, they each have only one or a few target substrates. This specificity is usually conferred by the amino terminus half of the protein, the sequence of which is unique to the particular PTP (48). Dual-specificity PTPs can exert their regulatory function by dephosphorylating not only tyrosine but also serine and threonine residues (49). Laforin's target phosphoprotein(s) are not known.

Based on sequence analysis, laforin's N terminus half contains a carbohydrate binding module (CBM) (23). CBMs are evolutionarily conserved sequences found in a variety of proteins from prokaryotes to humans that digest or otherwise interact with a variety of carbohydrates, including starch and glycogen. A printed review of CBMs is not available, but extensive annotations can be found at *http://afmb.cnrs-mrs.fr/pedro/CAZY/cbm.html.*

Laforin's expression profile was determined at the messenger ribonucleic acid (mRNA) level and found to be ubiquitous (40). Laforin's subcellular localization was established in nonneural tissue cultures. The protein was found to localize at the ER (44, 45) and the plasma membrane (45). Laforin is likely not an integral membrane protein, because it lacks any predicted transmembrane domains (23). It is also likely not an intra-ER resident protein, because it lacks an ER signal peptide (23). Ganesh et al. (44) showed that at the ER laforin is actually localized on ribosomes in a protein-protein interaction with unidentified ribosomal components.

PATHOGENESIS OF LAFORA DISEASE: AN EMERGING PICTURE

The available pieces of the jigsaw puzzle of the pathogenesis of LD were identified above. How these pieces might fit together will be explored in this section, starting with further probing of the known data.

Do polyglucosan bodies (PGBs) occur in conditions other than LD? PGB bodies occur in the following conditions. In Andersen disease (glycogen storage disease type IV), all tissues, including brain, are replete with polyglucosan accumulations. Patients usually die in early childhood from cirrhosis (50). The disease is caused by mutations in the gene coding for glycogen branching enzyme (BE) that either completely or almost completely abolish the enzyme's activity (51,52).

Polyglucosans accumulate in muscle in patients with Tarui disease (glycogen storage disease type VII) caused by deficiency of muscle phosphofructokinase activity (52–54).

Large PGBs form in axons (Fig. 21.3) or axon hillocks of neurons in patients with adult PGB disease (APBD), a neurologic disorder characterized by upper and lower motor neuron signs and dementia, but no seizures or myoclonias (55). APBD is caused by milder mutations of the Andersen disease gene that result in decreased BE activity (56,57).

Comparatively small amounts of polyglucosans normally form with aging in many tis-

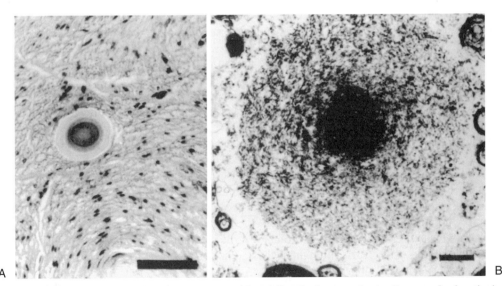

FIG. 21.3. Polyglucosan bodies from a case with adult polyglucosan body disease. **A:** A polyglucosan body in a lateral popliteal nerve fascicle, bar=50μm. **B:** An electron micrograph of a polyglucosan body with a bilayered structure indistinguishable from Lafora bodies, bar=1μm.

sues, including neurons and glia. These aggregate with advanced aging into PGBs called corpora amylacea (CA). CA are most prominent in astrocytes, in the glial feltwork under the ependymal lining of the ventricles, and in subpial regions on the surface of the brain. Neuronal CA, like APBD PGBs, are found exclusively in axons and never in soma or dendrites (29). In both CA and APBD it appears that the polyglucosans form in the neuronal body and are then taken into axons by axoplasmic flow in what seems to be part of a physiologic clearing mechanism. Some evidence exists suggesting that CA are further cleared out of axons into glia by cell-to-cell transfer mechanisms (29).

Finally, PGBs are seen in the globus pallidus in long-standing basal ganglia disease with status marmoratus (Bielchowsky body disease) (29,58) and in rare cases of a disorder akin to amyotrophic lateral sclerosis (29, 59). Again, disruption of neuron to glia polyglucosan transfer has been suggested in the formation of Bielchowsky bodies (29).

What are the differences in the PGBs between the different conditions? Polyglucosans in all the above including LD are glucose polymers. They most probably originate from a defect in glycogen metabolism, because there is no other source of glucose polymers in animal tissues. They differ from glycogen in lacking an organized branching pattern (13–15,18,23,25,29,34,35,38,39,45,54,55,58, 59). This appears to render them insoluble and resistant to digestion (34,35). Small differences in extents of phosphorylation and sulfation between Lafora bodies and CA have been reported but are of unknown significance and reproducibility (34).

Whereas the composition of the PGB does not appear to differ among the different conditions, the intracellular location of the PGB does. The comparison is most relevant between LD and APBD because both are neurologic disorders with neuronal PGBs throughout the CNS, but with different clinical presentations. In LD, the PGBs are in the perikaryal region or in the dendrites and rarely in axons (12,29, 34,35). In APBD, they are in axons or axon

hillocks and never in the soma or dendrites (55). The composition, size, morphology (Fig. 21.3) and numbers of APBD PGBs and Lafora bodies being similar, it is likely that their differing subcellular locations are responsible for their different neurologic symptoms. The neuronal hyperexcitability in the myoclonus and epilepsy of LD may therefore be due to the dendritic accumulations. The motor and sensory deficits and dementia in APBD may be due to disruption of axonal function (55).

Why do LD polyglucosans not migrate into axons like CA or APBD polyglucosans? As mentioned, electron microscopic studies showed that LD polyglucosans appear to be associated with ER and their ribosomes (13, 38,39). In neurons, rough ER (RER), i.e., ER with ribosomes, is present only in the perikaryal region and in dendrites but not in axons. It is possible that RER-associated polyglucosan formation and deposition in LD restricts their accumulation in perikarya and dendrites and prevents their translocation into axons.

What are the defects in glycogen metabolism that result in polyglucosan formation in the non-LD PGB diseases, and what clues into the pathogenesis of LD can be gleaned from them? There are four cytoplasmic enzymes that act directly on the glycogen particle (Fig. 21.4). Glycogen synthase (GS) adds units of glucose-6-phosphate (G6P) to elongate a glycogen strand. BE detects lengthening, and transfers six or more residues from the end of the long chain to other segments of the particle, thus maintaining its globularity and preventing asymmetrically elongated arms (Fig. 21.4A). On the catabolic side, when glucose is needed, glycogen phosphorylase digests off one unit at a time then stops and comes off when the branch it is acting on is down to four glucose units. Debranching enzyme removes this remaining tetrasaccharide stump and places it on a longer chain for renewed digestion by glycogen phosphorylase (Fig. 4B) (52).

By virtue of the order in which the catabolic enzymes proceed (Fig. 21.4B), deficiencies or hyperactivities of their functions would not be

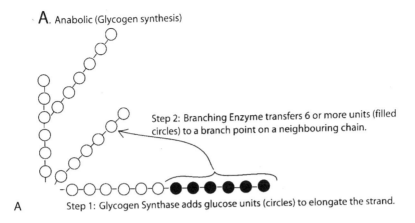

Step 2: Branching Enzyme transfers 6 or more units (filled circles) to a branch point on a neighbouring chain.

A   Step 1: Glycogen Synthase adds glucose units (circles) to elongate the strand.

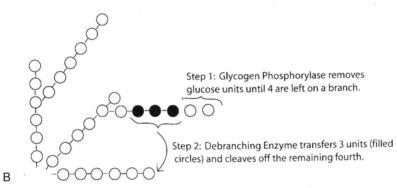

Step 1: Glycogen Phosphorylase removes glucose units until 4 are left on a branch.

Step 2: Debranching Enzyme transfers 3 units (filled circles) and cleaves off the remaining fourth.

B

FIG. 21.4. Glycogen metabolism. **A:** Glycogen synthesis. **B:** Glycogen breakdown.

expected to, and do not, result in asymmetrically long glycogen strands (polyglucosans). In contrast, the anabolic enzymes need to act in a balanced concerted fashion; strand elongation not balanced by adequate branching would result in polyglucosans, as proposed by DiMauro et al. (Fig. 21.4A) (54). For this reason, in Andersen disease and APBD, deficient branching due to defective BE causes polyglucosan formation and accumulation. In Tarui disease, polyglucosan accumulation is likely due to GS hyperactivity (54). In this condition, phosphofructokinase deficiency results in accumulation of its upstream substrate G6P, and G6P is the most potent allosteric activator of GS (60). Finally, Raben et al. (61) added further support to the DiMauro theory by genetically overexpressing GS in muscle and showing that this results in PGB formation in muscle (61).

There is one lysosomal enzyme, acid maltase, that can also act directly on the glycogen particle (52). Although this maltase can digest normal glycogen, it appears unable to rid the cell from polyglucosan accumulations in all the above PGB diseases. This is likely due to the insolubility of the polyglucosans and consistent with their relative high resistance to digestion with amylases *in vitro* (34,35).

If the pathogenesis of LD polyglucosans also comprises an imbalance between BE and GS, it is more likely that the mechanism involves GS hyperactivity rather than BE deficiency, because BE deficiency does not result in LD, but in APBD and Andersen disease.

How could GS become hyperactive in LD, and where does laforin fit in? In addition to the allosteric regulation by G6P, GS activity is tightly regulated through phosphorylation at a number of specific serine residues. This phosphorylation state can be affected by a number of kinases and phosphatases including casein kinase I, casein kinase II, cAMP-dependent kinase, glycogen synthase kinase, and protein phosphatase-1 (PP1) (62). These enzymes are themselves regulated by phosphorylation (62,63) and are likely downstream elements of signal transduction pathways initiated by insulin, glucagon, adrenergic hormones, and other factors. Laforin, by virtue of being a PTP, could well be involved in the phosphoregulation of the above or other GS-controlling enzymes. Laforin would not be expected to act directly on GS, because dephosphorylation inhibits GS (62).

The kinases and phosphatases that control GS activity are multipurpose enzymes employed by many cellular signaling cascades. One means by which they acquire specificity to particular functions, e.g., control of glycogen synthase activity, is through specific binding proteins that target them to the site in which they are required. Confirmed examples of this include several PP-1 binding proteins that contain carbohydrate binding modules that target PP-1 to GS on the glycogen particle (64) (see also *http://afmb.cnrs–mrs.fr/pedro/CAZY/cbm_21.html*). It is of note that laforin also contains a carbohydrate-binding module similar to that of these PP-1 interactors (see above).

The glycogen particle (64,65), its tightly bound GS (64), glycogen synthase kinase (66), PP-1 (67), and laforin (see above) have all been shown to associate with the ER. The physical possibilities are therefore in place for the interactions that might result in ER-associated GS hyperfunction and the ER-associated polyglucosan depositions seen in LD.

What is the role of laforin at the plasma membrane? For long, as exposed above, because of the delayed onset and subsequent progressive nature of the disease, the storage material has been considered pathogenic in the epilepsy of LD. Could defective membrane-associated laforin have a more direct role on neuronal excitability? Of note in this respect is that many LD patients have isolated febrile or non-febrile convulsions in infancy and early childhood years prior to the onset of the progressive syndrome (13,22–24). Forays into theories of epileptogenesis by defective laforin would be highly speculative at this time. However, one intriguing possibility is involvement in the insulin-mediated regulation of neuronal excitability (68–70) (see below). One preliminary piece of data in support of this came at the conference from which the present volume originated; Bara-Jimenez et al. reported hyperinsulinism in a patient with LD. In brain, separate from and more important than its role in carbohydrate metabolism, insulin is involved in the regulation of synaptic transmission. The insulin receptor is localized at dendrites and other postsynaptic terminal sites on the neuron body. It is a tyrosine kinase that when activated by insulin regulates AMPA and GABA-A receptor numbers at the synapse (68–70). At what level insulin signaling diverges into its various paths is not known. It is possible that laforin acts at a common point, thus influencing both glycogen metabolism and resulting in Lafora bodies and insulin-mediated synaptic transmission, resulting in epilepsy.

FUTURE PROSPECTS

A cure for LD will come via one or both of two avenues. A more complete understanding of the pathogenesis of the disease will expose openings for medical interventions. Advances in gene, protein, or stem cell therapies will allow replacement of the defective protein. Important missing pieces from the pathogenesis puzzle include the second LD gene, laforin-interacting proteins, measures of the activities of enzymes regulating glycogen metabolism, and measures of neuronal membrane excitabilities in neurons deficient of laforin and not replete with polyglucosans.

Knockout mouse and natural dog models of the disease are presently being evaluated. These animals will be important not only for new insights into pathogenesis, but also for testing new therapeutic approaches. Meanwhile, based on the knowledge that Lafora bodies are carbohydrate compounds, an international collaborative clinical trial based at the National Institutes of Health in the United States (Bara-Jimenez et al.) has been initiated to test whether carbohydrate restriction will diminish Lafora body formation and disease progression.

ACKNOWLEDGMENTS

I would like to acknowledge Elayne Chan, BSc., for stimulating discussions, Dr. Stephen W. Scherer for his support, and Drs. Yves Robitaille, Patrick Shannon and Stirling Carpenter for the Lafora and APBD photomicrographs.

REFERENCES

1. Lafora GR. Uber das vorkommen amyloider korperchen im innern der ganglienzellen;zugleich ein zum studium der amyloiden substanz im nervensystem. *Virchows Arch [Pathol Anat]* 1911;205:295–303.
2. Unverricht H. *Die myoclonie.* Leipzig: Franz Deuticke, 1891:1–128.
3. Lundborg H. Die progressive myoklonus epilepsie (Unverricht's Myoklonie). Uppsala: Almquist and Wiksell, 1903:1–207.
4. Federico A, Cecio A, Apponi Battini G, et al. Macular cherry-red spot and myoclonus syndrome: juvenile form of sialidosis. *J Neurol Sci* 1980;48:157–169.
5. Kufs H. Uber eine Spatform der amaurotischen Idiotie und ihre heredofamiliaren Grundlagen. *Z Ges Neurol Psychiat* 1925;95:169–188.
6. Fukuhara N, Tokiguchi S, Shirakawa K, et al. Myoclonus epilepsy associated with ragged-red fibers (mitochondrial abnormalities): disease entity or a syndrome? Light- and electron-microscopic studies of two cases and a review of the literature. *J Neurol Sci* 1980;47:117–133.
7. Minassian BA, Sainz J, Delgado-Escueta AV. Genetics of myoclonic and myoclonus epilepsies. *Clin Neurosci* 1996;223–235.
8. Schwarz G, Yanoff M. Lafora's disease. *Arch Neurol* 1965;12:173–188.
9. Janeway R, Ravens J, Rupert P, et al. Progressive myoclonus epilepsy with Lafora inclusion bodies. *Arch Neurol* 1967;16:565–582.
10. Gambetti P, Di Mauro S, Hirt L, et al. Myoclonic epilepsy with Lafora bodies. *Arch Neurol* 1971;25:483–493.
11. Neville HE, Brooke MH, Austin JH. Studies in myoclonus epilepsy (Lafora body form). *Arch Neurol* 1974;30:466–474.
12. Carpenter S, Karpati G, Andermann F, et al. Lafora's disease: Peroxisomal storage in skeletal muscle. *Neurology* 1974;24:531–538.
13. Van Heycop ten Ham MW. Lafora disease, a form of progressive myoclonus epilepsy. Magnus O, Lorentz de Haas, eds. Handbook of Clinical Neurology. Amsterdam: North Holland Publishing Company, 1974;15: 382–422.

14. Busard HL, Renier WO, Gabreels FJ, et al. Lafora disease: a quantitative morphological and biochemical study of the cerebral cortex. *Clin Neuropathol* 1987;6:1–6.
15. Nishimura RN, Ishak KG, Reddick R, et al. Lafora disease: diagnosis by liver biopsy. *Ann Neurol* 1980;8: 409–415.
16. Kobayashi K, Iyoda K, Ohtsuka Y, et al. Longitudinal clinicoelectrophysiologic study of a case of Lafora disease proven by skin biopsy. *Epilepsia* 1990;31: 194–201.
17. Baumann RJ, Kocoshis SA, Wilson S. Lafora disease: liver histopathology in presymptomatic children. *Ann Neurol* 1983;4:86–89.
18. Roger J, Pellissier JF, Bureau M, et al. Le diagnostic precoce de la maladie de Lafora. Importance des manifestations paroxystiques visuelles et interet de la biopsie cutanee. *Rev Neurol (Paris)* 1983;139:115–124.
19. Busard BLSM, Renier WO, Gabreels FJM, et al. Lafora's disease. *Arch Neurol* 1986;43:296–299.
20. Drury I, Blaivas M, Abou-Khalil B, et al. Biopsy results in a kindred with Lafora disease. *Arch Neurol* 1993; 50;102–105.
21. Berkovic SF, Cochius J, Andermann E, et al. Progressive myoclonus epilepsies: clinical and genetic aspects. *Epilepsia* 1993;34(Suppl 3):S19–S30.
22. Acharya JN, Satishchandra P, Shankar SK. Familial progressive myoclonus epilepsy: clinical and electrophysiologic observations. *Epilepsia* 1995;36:429–434.
23. Minassian BA, Ianzano L, Meloche M, et al. Mutation spectrum and predicted function of laforin in Lafora's progressive myoclonus epilepsy. *Neurology* 2000;55: 341–346.
24. Roger J, Genton P, Bureau M, et al. Progressive myoclonus epilepsies in childhood and adolescence. In: Roger J, Bureau M, Dravet C, et al., eds. *Epileptic syndromes in infancy, childhood and adolescence,* 2nd ed. London: Libbey, 1992:381–400.
25. Roger J, Gastaut H, Boudouresques J, et al. Epilepsie–myoclonie progressive avec corps de Lafora. Etude clinique et polygraphique. Controle anatomique ultra–structural. *Rev Neurol (Paris)* 1967;116:197–212.
26. Shibasaki H, Neshige R. Photic cortical reflex myoclonus. *Ann Neurol* 1987;22:252–257.
27. Rubboli G, Meletti S, Gardella E, et al. Photic reflex myoclonus: a neurophysiologic study in progressive myoclonus epilepsy. *Epilepsia* 1999;40(Suppl 4):50–58.
28. Lafora GR, Gluck B. Beitrag zur histopathologie der myoklonischen epilepsie. *Z Ges Neurol Psychiat* 1911; 6:1–14.
29. Cavanagh JB. Corpora-amylacea and the family of polyglucosan diseases. *Brain Res Rev* 1999;29:265–295.
30. Harriman DGF, Millar JHD. Progressive familial myoclonic epilepsy in three families: its clinical features and pathological basis. *Brain* 1955;78:325–349.
31. Carpenter S, Karpati G. Sweat gland duct cells in Lafora disease: diagnosis by skin biopsy. *Neurology* 1981;31:1564–1568.
32. Busard HLSM, Gobreels-Festen AAWM, Renih WU, et al. Axilla skin biopsy; a reliable test for the diagnosis of Lafora's disease. *Ann Neurol* 1987;21:599–601.
33. Minassian BA, Ianzano L, Delgado-Escueta AV, et al. New deletion mutations in *EPM2A* and the genetic diagnosis of Lafora's disease. *Neurology* 2000;54:488–490.
34. Sakai M, Austin J, Witmer F, et al. Studies in myoclonus epilepsy (Lafora body form); II. Polyglucosans in the

systemic deposits of myoclonus epilepsy and in corpora amylacea. *Neurology* 1970;20:160–176.

35. Nikaido T, Austin J, Stukenbrok H. Studies in myoclonus epilepsy. III: the effects of amylolytic enzymes on the ultrastructure of Lafora bodies. *J Histochem Cytochem* 1971;19:382–385.

36. Carpenter S, Karpati G. Ultrastructural findings in Lafora disease. *Ann Neurol* 1981;10:63–64.

37. Cajal RYS, Blanes A, Martinez A, et al. Lafora's disease: an ultrastructural and histochemical study. *Acta Neuropathol (Berl)* 1975;30:189–196.

38. Collins GH, Cowden RR, Nevis AH. Myoclonus epilepsy with Lafora bodies: an ultrastructural and cytochemical study. *Arch Neurol* 1968;86:239–254.

39. Toga M, Dubois D, Hassoun J. Ultra-structure des corps de Lafora. *Acta Neuropathol* 1968;10:132–142.

40. Minassian BA, Lee JR, Herbrick JA, et al. Mutations in a gene encoding a novel protein tyrosine phosphatase cause progressive myoclonus epilepsy. *Nat Genet* 1998; 20:171–174.

41. Serratosa JM, Gomez-Garre P, Gallardo ME, et al. A novel protein tyrosine phosphatase gene is mutated in progressive myoclonus epilepsy of the Lafora type (EPM2). *Hum Mol Genet* 1999;8:345–352.

42. Ganesh S, Amano K, Delgado-Escueta AV, et al. Isolation and characterization of mouse homologue for the human epilepsy gene, EPM2A. *Biochem Biophys Res Commun* 1999;257:24–28.

43. Minassian BA, Sainz J, Serratosa JM, et al: Genetic locus heterogeneity in Lafora's progressive myoclonus epilepsy. *Ann Neurol* 1999;45:262–265.

44. Ganesh S, Agarwala KL, Ueda K, et al. Laforin, defective in the progressive myoclonus epilepsy of lafora type, is a dual-specificity phosphatase associated with polyribosomes. *Hum Mol Genet* 2000;9:2251–2261.

45. Minassian BA, Andrade D, Ianzano L, et al. Laforin is a cell membrane and endoplasmic reticulum associated protein tyrosine phosphatase. *Ann Neurol* 2001; 49:271–275.

46. Denu JM, Stuckey JA, Saper MA, et al. Form and function in protein dephosphorylation. *Cell* 1996;87: 361–364.

47. Tonks NK, Neel BG. From form to function: signaling by protein tyrosine phosphatases. *Cell* 1996;87:365–368.

48. Hafen E. Kinases and phosphatases: a marriage is consummated. *Science* 1998;280:1212–1213.

49. Martell KJ, Angelotti T, Ullrich A. The "VH1-like" dual-specificity protein tyrosine phosphatases. *Mol Cell* 1998;8:2–11.

50. Schochet SS, McCormick WF, Zellweger H. Type IV glycogenosis (amylopectinosis): light and electron microscopic observations. *Arch Pathol* 1970;90:354–363.

51. Thon VJ, Khalil M, Cannon JF. Isolation of human glycogen branching enzyme cDNAs by screening complementation in yeast. *J Biol Chem* 1993;268:7509–7513.

52. Chen YT, Burchell A. Glycogen storage diseases. In: Scriver CR, Beaudet AL, Sly WS, et al., eds. *The metabolic and molecular bases of inherited disease,* 7th ed. New York: McGraw-Hill, 1995:935–965.

53. Tarui S, Okuno G, Ikura Y. Phosphofructokinase deficiency in skeletal muscle: a new type of glycogenosis. *Biochem Biophys Res Commun* 1965;19:517–523.

54. Hays AP, Hallett M, DiMauro S, et al. Muscle phosphofructokinase deficiency: Abnormal polysaccharide in a case of late-onset myopathy. *Neurology* 1981;31: 1077–1086.

55. Robitaille Y, Carpenter S, Karpati G, et al. A distinct form of adult polyglucosan body disease with massive involvement of central and peripheral neuronal processes and astrocytes: a report of four cases and a review of the occurrence of polyglucosan bodies in other conditions such as Lafora's disease and normal ageing. *Brain* 1980;103:315–336.

56. Lossos A, Meiner Z, Barash V, et al. Adult polyglucosan body disease in Ashkenazi Jewish patients carrying the Tyr329Ser mutation in the glycogen-branching enzyme gene. *Ann Neurol* 1998;44:867–872.

57. Ziemssen F, Sindern E, Schroder JM, et al. Novel missense mutations in the glycogen-branching enzyme gene in adult polyglucosan body disease. *Ann Neurol* 2000;47:536–540.

58. DeLeon GA. Bielchowsky bodies: Lafora–like inclusions associated with atrophy of the lateral pallidum. *Acta Neuropathol* 1974;30:183–188.

59. Orthner H, Becher PE, Muller D. Recessive erbliche amyotrophische Lateralsklerose mit Lafora-Korpern. *Arch Psychiatr Nerv* 1973;217:387–412.

60. Villar-Palasi C, Guinovart JJ. The role of glucose 6-phosphate in the control of glycogen synthase. *FASEB J* 1997;11:544–558.

61. Raben N, Danon M, Lu N, et al. Surprises of genetic engineering: a possible model of polyglucosan body (Lafora) disease. *Neurology* 2000;54(Suppl 3):A359–A360.

62. Roach PJ, Cao Y, Corbett A, et al. Glycogen metabolism and signal transduction in mammals and yeast. *Adv Enzyme Regul* 1991;31:101–120.

63. Woodgett JR. Regulation and functions of the glycogen synthase kinase-3 subfamily. *Semin Cancer Biol* 1994; 5:269–275.

64. DiMauro S, Trojaborg W, Gambetti P, et al. Binding of enzymes of glycogen metabolism to glycogen in skeletal muscle. *Arch Biochem Biophys* 1971;144:413–422.

65. Chamlian A, Benkoel L, Minko D, et al. Ultrastructural heterogeneity of glycogen in human liver. *Liver* 1989; 9:346–350.

66. Angenstein F, Greenough WT, Weiler IJ. Metabotropic glutamate receptor-initiated translocation of protein kinase p90rsk to polyribosomes: a possible factor regulating synaptic protein synthesis. *Proc Natl Acad Sci USA* 1998;95:15078–15083.

67. Liu J, Brautigan DL. Insulin-stimulated phosphorylation of the protein phosphatase-1 striated muscle glycogen-targeting subunit and activation of glycogen synthase. *J Biol Chem* 2000;275:15940–15947.

68. Abbott MA, Wells DG, Fallon JR. The insulin receptor tyrosine kinase substrate p58/53 and the insulin receptor are components of CNS synapses. *J Neurosci* 1999; 19:7300–7308.

69. Zhao W, Chen H, Xu H, et al. Brain insulin receptors and spatial memory: correlated changes in gene expression, tyrosine phosphorylation, and signaling molecules in the hippocampus of water maze trained rats. *J Biol Chem* 1999;274:34893–34902.

70. Man YH, Lin JW, Ju WH, et al. Regulation of AMPA receptor-mediated synaptic transmission by clathrin-dependent receptor internalization. *Neuron* 2000;25:649–662.

Myoclonus and Paroxysmal Dyskinesias,
Advances in Neurology, Vol. 89,
edited by S. Fahn, et al.
Lippincott Williams & Wilkins, Philadelphia © 2002.

22

Clinical Features and Molecular Genetic Basis of the Neuronal Ceroid Lipofuscinoses

R. Mark Gardiner

Department of Pediatrics, University College London, The Rayne Institute,
London, United Kingdom

The neuronal ceroid lipofuscinoses (NCLs) are a group of neurodegenerative disorders characterized by psychomotor deterioration, visual failure, and the accumulation of autofluorescent lipopigment in neurons and other cell types. Several recent reviews are available (1,2), and the proceedings of the Eighth International Congress on NCLs will be published soon (3). There are five types that may include progressive myoclonus epilepsy: classical late infantile or *CLN2* (Jansky-Bielschowsky disease), juvenile or *CLN3* (Spielmeyer-Vogt-Sjögren or Batten disease), adult or *CLN4* (Kufs or Parry disease), late infantile Finnish variant or *CLN5*, and late infantile variant or *CLN6*. Inheritance is autosomal recessive except for the adult form, which may display autosomal dominant inheritance. The main clinical features include failure of psychomotor development, impaired vision, and epilepsy. The biochemical basis of this group of diseases has until recently remained obscure. Studies of storage bodies have demonstrated that the major component in both late-infantile and juvenile (but not infantile) NCL is the protein subunit c of the mitochondrial adenosine triphosphate synthase complex (4,5).

Advances in human molecular genetic techniques have allowed positional cloning strategies to be applied to identification of the defective genes and their protein products. So far, six disease gene loci have been mapped, and five of these genes have been isolated.

INFANTILE NEURONAL CEROID LIPOFUSCINOSES, HALTIA-SANTAVUORI DISEASE (CLN1)

The infantile subtype of NCL (INCL) is characterized by early blindness and rapid neurologic deterioration, leading to death at 8 to 11 years. In most children with INCL, normal development begins to slow down during the second year of life. Examination reveals hypotonia, clumsiness in fine motor control, and retarded head growth. Additional signs, including dystonia, choreoathetosis, myoclonic jerks, or epileptic seizures, may have their onset in the second or third years. Magnetic resonance imaging (MRI) shows hypointense thalami on T2-weighted images, and electroencephalography (EEG) indicates thalamic dysfunction. The characteristic storage bodies—granular osmiophilic deposits—are found in brain and other tissues, and the major storage materials are saposins (6). The disease locus was assigned to human chromosome 1p32 (7) by a random linkage approach. Linkage disequilibrium mapping suggested that *CLN1* was close to a marker HY-TM1 (8), and haplotype analysis suggested one founder mutation in the Finnish population. The *CLN1* gene was shown to encode palmitoyl protein thioesterase (PPT1) by a positional candidate approach (9).

More than 30 mutations have been described, including Arg 122 Trp, which accounts for 98% of Finnish INCL disease chromosomes. PPT is an approximately 37 kD glycoprotein that is postulated to play a role in the catabolism of lipid modified proteins (10), and there is evidence that PPT is a lysosomal enzyme (11).

It is now known that a small number of patients with late-infantile, juvenile, or even adult-onset but granular osmiophilic deposits on histology have mutations in the gene encoding PPT1. It has been possible to correlate the site of missense mutations with these phenotypic effects in the context of the recently solved crystal structure of PPT. Missense mutations near the active site that disrupt PPT folding lead to an inactive enzyme and a severe, early-onset phenotype. Mutations associated with late-onset, such as T75P, D79G, Q177E, and G250V, are remote from the active site and affect V_{max} or K_m.

The PPT enzyme activity can be assayed in leukocytes or fibroblasts as a diagnostic procedure.

LATE-INFANTILE NEURONAL CEROID LIPOFUSCINOSES: *CLN2, CLN5, CLN6*

There is considerable phenotypic variation within the category of NCL with onset in late infancy. At least three subtypes exist, including classical late-infantile NCL (Jansky-Bielschowsky disease, *CLN2*), variant late-infantile NCL (sometimes called "early juvenile," *CLN6*), and a specific Finnish form of variant late-infantile NCL (*CLN5*).

CLN2

Children with classical late-infantile NCL (LINCL) usually present with epilepsy at the age of 2 to 3 years. This is quickly followed by ataxia, myoclonic jerks, and progressive mental deterioration. Visual failure usually becomes apparent after the age of 2 to 3 years.

Seizures may be partial, generalized tonic-clonic, secondary generalized, or absences. A specific EEG feature is posterior spikes to low-frequency photic stimulation and the giant visual evoked potential (VEP) elicited only with flash stimulation. Brain atrophy, especially infratentorial, is found on imaging.

The gene for classical LINCL was mapped by linkage analysis to chromosome 11p15 (12) using homozygosity mapping in five consanguineous families. The *CLN2* gene product—which is defective or missing in LINCL—was recently identified using an integrated biochemical genomic strategy (13).

Mutations in the gene encoding tripeptidyl peptidase 1 (TPP1) on chromosome 11p15 cause classical LINCL. This is a pepstatin-insensitive lysosomal enzyme with homology to bacterial carboxypeptidases. More than 30 mutations have been found so far, including missense, nonsense, deletion, insertion, and splicing mutations (14). TPP1 processively removes tripeptides from the N terminal of proteins undergoing degradation in the lysosome. The specificity and substrate range of TPP1 is under investigation. Available evidence indicates cleavage of peptides, with an Mr above 5,000 and involvement in the initial degradation of subunit c in lysosomes.

Analysis of TPP1 enzyme activity is available as a diagnostic test. This works best in fibroblasts but is applicable to leukocytes.

CLN5

A variant of late NCL is found almost exclusively in Finland and is caused by mutations in the gene *CLN5*. In Finnish variant LINCL, the first symptom is usually clumsiness and hypotonia at around 5 years of age. This is followed by visual impairment between 5 and 7 years, ataxia at 7 to 10 years, myoclonia at 8 to 9 years, and epilepsy between 5 and 11 years. In the second decade, dystonia and extrapyramidal signs become apparent.

Both MRI and computed tomography demonstrate generalized brain atrophy, more severe in the cerebellum. The *CLN5* gene was assigned to chromosome 13q21-q32 by linkage analysis in 16 Finnish families with common ancestors (15). The gene was subsequently identified by positional cloning (16).

CLN5 encodes a putative transmembrane protein of 407 amino acids. Predicted features include two transmembrane helices, suggesting that the protein is a transmembrane protein with an intraluminal loop.

Three mutations have been identified. The Finnish major mutation (*CLN5* Fin major) occurs on 94% of Finnish disease chromosomes and is a 2bp deletion in exon 4 predicted to result in a truncated polypeptide of 391 amino acids. The Fin minor mutation, identified in a single family is a G> A transversion in exon 1 predicted to result in a truncated protein of only 74 amino acids. One non-Finnish mutation has been detected in a Dutch patient, a missense mutation in exon 4. The function of *CLN5* is unknown.

JUVENILE ONSET NEURONAL CEROID LIPOFUSCINOSES, BATTEN DISEASE *(CLN3)*

Batten disease or juvenile-onset NCL (JNCL) is the most common neurodegenerative disorder of childhood and has an incidence of up to 1 in 25,000 births and an increased prevalence in the Northern European populations. Onset usually begins with visual failure at age 5 to 10 years, followed by epilepsy and deterioration to a vegetative state.

Most patients become blind during the second decade of life. Cognitive decline begins early. Epilepsy has its onset around 10 to 11 years in most patients. The most common seizure type is primary or secondary generalized tonic-clonic seizures. Myoclonus is usually subtle. A parkinsonian type of extrapyramidal dysfunction develops with ataxia, dysarthria, and rigidity. Behavioral and psychiatric problems, including psychosis with hallucination, are common. A number of patients who are compound heterozygotes for missense mutations have a milder phenotype dominated by visual failure with preserved cognition and motor function.

In JNCL, the EEG develops a progressive background abnormality with paroxysms. The electroretinogram (ERG) is usually very low or unrecordable at diagnosis, and the VEP attenuates slowly over 5 to 15 years. Brain imaging is usually normal in patients under the age of 10 years and thereafter shows progressive cerebral and cerebellar atrophy. Vacuolated lymphocytes are a hallmark of classical JNCL.

Following initial assignment of *CLN3* to chromosome 16 (17), additional genetic analysis refined the location of the gene to within a 2 cM interval (18–20). The gene was identified by positional cloning (21). Subsequent work has defined the genomic organization of *CLN3*, identified a range of mutations and established genotype-phenotype correlation, and explored the structure and function of the protein product that *CLN3*encodes.

At the time of writing, a total of 25 different disease-causing mutations have been detected. About 80% carry the 1.02 kb deletion, which is the common founder mutation. This mutation is predicted to produce a truncated protein consisting of the first 153 residues of the protein followed by 28 novel amino acids before the stop codon. An additional three deletions have been identified, and the remaining include 1 to 2 bp insertions or deletions and single-base changes causing missense, nonsense, or splice-site mutations. Thirteen of these are predicted to result in severe truncation of the native protein. All six missense mutations in *CLN3* affect residues that are completely conserved between the human protein and its homologues in yeast, dog, and mouse. It is noteworthy that all eight patients with a milder phenotype comprising visual failure but relatively preserved cognitive and motor function were found to have missense mutations in *CLN3* on at least one disease chromosome.

The *CLN3* gene encodes a 438 amino acid protein of as yet unknown function (22). Hydrophobicity plots are consistent with the existence of 5 to 7 transmembrane domains of a length (22 to 23 amino acids) sufficient to span a lipid bilayer. A homology search has identified a yeast protein in *Saccharomyces cerevisiae* that has 36% identity and 56% similarity with the *CLN3* protein. All of the known single-point mutation sites in Batten disease patients are found at sites that have identical residues in the yeast protein.

It has recently been demonstrated that a subtype of JNCL with granular osmiophilic deposits is caused by mutations in the PPT gene (23).

NORTHERN EPILEPSY: *CLN8*

Northern epilepsy, also known as progressive epilepsy with mental retardation (EPMR), was recently delineated as a new autosomal recessive childhood-onset epilepsy syndrome. Subsequent neuropathologic studies have established this as a novel, unusually protracted form of NCL, and the designation *CLN8* has been assigned to the disease gene locus.

In most patients, development up to school age is normal. Onset occurs with epilepsy at age 5 to 10 years. All patients have generalized tonic-clonic seizures, and one-third have complex partial seizures. Myoclonic epilepsy does not occur. Progressive mental deterioration follows and continues slowly into adulthood. After age 30 years, patients have difficulties with equilibrium and walking. Although decreased visual activity has been detected in some patients, retinal degeneration has not been reported.

The EEG shows progressive slowing of background activity and scanty interictal epileptiform activity. Brain imaging shows progressive cerebellar and brainstem atrophy in young adulthood with subsequent cerebral atrophy.

The 23 patients of the original series were identified within a small geographic area in Northeastern Finland. The gene locus *CLN8* was assigned to the telomeric region of chromosome 8, 8p23 by linkage studies (24,25).

Transcript identification and mutation scanning of candidate genes has led to the identification of the *CLN8* gene (26). The gene encodes a putative transmembrane protein of 286 amino acids, and the mutation is a missense mutation (R24G). A naturally occurring mouse model of NCL, the motor neuron degeneration

(mnd) mouse, was shown to map to the corresponding chromosomal region in the mouse. The murine orthologue of *CLN8* was therefore screened for mutations and a homozygous change (267-268 ins C) identified in *mnd/mnd* mice. This represents the first example of a human and animal model of NCL being caused by mutations in orthologous genes.

The *CLN8* protein contains an ER-retrieval signal in its C terminus, and available evidence indicates that it is an ER resident protein that recycles between the ER and ER-Golgi intermediate compartment (ERGIC) (27). Its function is unknown.

CONCLUSIONS

The NCLs comprise a heterogenous group of inherited disorders, several of which are PMEs. Five underlying human genes have been isolated, two of which encode lysosomal enzymes. Biochemical and deoxyribonucleic acid–based diagnostic tests are now available. A mutation database is available at: *http://www.ucl.ac.uk/NCL*. A unifying theory of pathogenesis remains elusive.

REFERENCES

1. Goebel HH, Mole SE, Lake BD, eds. *The neuronal ceroid lipofuscinoses (Batten disease)*. Amsterdam: IOS Press, 1999;211.
2. Goebel HH, Nardocci N, eds. The neuronal ceroid lipofuscinoses: current knowledge and perspectives. Neurological Sciences Vol 21. Supplement to No. 3: 2000.
3. Proceedings of the 8th International Congress on Neuronal Ceroid Lipofuscinoses. *Eur J Paediatr Neurol* 2001;5(supp. A)
4. Fearnley IM, Walker JE, Martinus RD, et al. The sequence of the major protein stored in ovine ceroid lipofuscinosis is identical with that of the dicyclohexylcarbodiimide-reactive proteolipid of mitochondrial ATP synthase. *Biochem J* 1990;268:751–758.
5. Palmer DN, Fearnley IM, Walker JE, et al. Mitochondrial ATP synthase subunit c storage in the ceroid-lipofuscinoses (Batten disease). *Am J Med Genet* 1992;42: 561–567.
6. Tyynela J, Palmer DN, Baumann M, et al. Storage of saposins A and D in infantile neuronal ceroid-lipofuscinosis. *FEBS Lett* 1993;330:8–12.
7. Jarvela I, Schleutker J, Haataja L, et al. Infantile form of neuronal ceroid lipofuscinosis (CLN1) maps to the short arm of chromosome 1. *Genomics* 1991;9:170–173.
8. Hellsten E, Vesa J, Speer M, et al. Refined assignment of the infantile neuronal ceroid lipofuscinosis (CLN1)

locus at 1p32: incorporation of linkage disequilibrium in multipoint analysis. *Genomics* 1993;16:720–725.

9. Vesa J, Hellsten E, Verkruyse LA, et al. Mutations in the palmitoyl protein thioesterase gene causing infantile neuronal ceroid lipofuscinosis. *Nature* 1995;376: 584–587.

10. Camp LA, Verkruyse LA, Afendis SJ, et al. Molecular cloning and expression of palmitoyl-protein thioesterase. *J Biol Chem* 1994;269:23212–23219.

11. Verkruyse LA, Hofmann SL. Lysosomal targeting of palmitoyl-protein thioesterase. *J Biol Chem* 1996;271: 15831–15836.

12. Sharp JD, Wheeler RB, Lake BD, et al. Loci for classical and a variant late infantile neuronal ceroid lipofuscinosis map to chromosomes 11p15 and 15q21-23. *Hum Mol Genet* 1997;6:591–595.

13. Sleat DE, Donnelly RJ, Lackland H, et al. Association of mutations in a lysosomal protein with classical late-infantile neuronal ceroid lipofuscinosis. *Science* 1997; 277:1802–1805.

14. Sleat DE, Gin RM, Sohar I, et al. Mutational analysis of the defective protease in classic late-infantile neuronal ceroid lipofuscinosis, a neurodegenerative lysosomal storage disorder. *Am J Hum Genet* 1999;64:1511–1523.

15. Savukoski M, Kestilä M, Williams R, et al. Defined chromosomal assignment of CLN5 demonstrates that at least four genetic loci are involved in the pathogenesis of human ceroid lipofuscinoses. *Am J Hum Genet* 1994; 55:695–701.

16. Savukoski M, Klockars T, Holmberg V, et al. *CLN5*, a novel gene encoding putative transmembrane protein mutated in Finnish variant late infantile neuronal ceroid lipofuscinosis. *Nat Genet* 1998;19:286–288.

17. Eiberg H, Gardiner RM, Mohr J. Batten disease (Spielmeyer-Sjogren disease) and haptoglobins (HP): indication of linkage and assignment to chromosome 16. *Clin Genet* 1989;36:217–218.

18. Gardiner RM, Sandford A, Deadman M, et al. Batten disease (Spielmeyer-Vogt; juvenile-onset neuronal ceroid lipofuscinosis) maps to human chromosome 16. *Genomics* 1990;8:387–390.

19. Callen DF, Baker E, Lane S, et al. Regional mapping of the Batten Disease locus (CLN3) to human chromosome 16p12. *Am J Hum Genet* 1991;49:1372–1377.

20. Mitchison HM, Thompson AD, Mulley JC, et al. Fine genetic mapping of the Batten disease locus (CLN3) by haplotype analysis and demonstration of allelic association with chromosome 16p microsatellite loci. *Genomics* 1993;16:455–460.

21. The International Batten Disease Consortium. Isolation of a novel gene underlying Batten Disease, CLN3. *Cell* 1995;82:949–957.

22. Janes RW, Munroe PB, Mitchison HM, et al. A model for Batten disease protein CLN3: functional implications from homology and mutations. *FEBS Lett* 1996; 399:75–77.

23. Mitchison HM, Hofmann SL, Becerra CHR, et al. Mutations in the palmitoyl-protein thioesterase gene (*PPT; CLN1*) causing juvenile neuronal ceroid lipofuscinosis with granular osmiophilic deposits. *Hum Mol Genet* 1998;7:291–297.

24. Tahvanainen E, Ranta S, Hirvasniemi A, et al. The gene for a recessively inherited human childhood progressive epilepsy with mental retardation maps to the distal short arm of chromosome 8. *Proc Natl Acad Sci USA* 1994; 91:7267–7270.

25. Ranta S, Lehesjoki A-E, Bonaldo M de F, et al. High-resolution mapping and transcript identification at the progressive epilepsy with mental retardation locus on chromosome 8p. *Genome Res* 1997;7:887–896.

26. Ranta S, Zhang Y, Ross B, et al. The neuronal ceroid lipofuscinoses in human EPMR and *mnd* mutant mice are associated with mutations in *CLN8*. *Nat Genet* 1999;23:1–4.

27. Lonka L, Kyttala A, Ranta S, et al. The neuronal ceroid lipofuscinosis *CLN8* membrane protein is a resident of the endoplasmic reticulum. *Hum Mol Genet* 2000;9: 1691–1697.

Myoclonus and Paroxysmal Dyskinesias,
Advances in Neurology, Vol. 89,
edited by S. Fahn, et al.
Lippincott Williams & Wilkins, Philadelphia © 2002.

23

Clinical Features and Genetics of Myoclonic Epilepsy with Ragged Red Fibers

*Salvatore DiMauro, *Michio Hirano, ††Petra Kaufmann, †Kurenai Tanji,
*Mary Sano, *§Dikoma C. Shungu, ††Eduardo Bonilla, and *Darryl C. DeVivo

*Departments of *Neurology, †Pathology, and §Radiology,
Columbia University College of Physicians and Surgeons, New York, New York
††Department of Neurology, Columbia University, New York, New York*

In 1921, Ramsey Hunt described six patients with a disorder characterized by ataxia, myoclonus, and epilepsy, which he called "dyssynergia cerebellaris myoclonica" (1). More than 50 years passed before Tsairis et al. (2) associated familial myoclonic epilepsy with mitochondrial abnormalities in the muscle biopsy (ragged red fibers), although this family was not described in detail until 1989 (3). The clinical syndrome was clearly identified and labeled myoclonic epilepsy with ragged red fibers (MERRF) by Fukuhara et al. in 1980 (4). MERRF was one of the three major discrete multisystem disorders first classified as "mitochondrial encephalomyopathy"; the other two were Kearns-Sayre syndrome (KSS) and mitochondrial encephalopathy, lactic acidosis, and strokelike episodes (MELAS) (5).

MERRF has two other historical distinctions: (a) it was the first well-defined human disease in which maternal inheritance was clearly demonstrated, thus suggesting a defect of the mitochondrial DNA (mtDNA) (6); and (2) it was the first disorder in which a molecular defect was associated with epilepsy (7).

Thirteen years after the birth of mitochondrial genetics (8,9) and after the initially spirited controversy between "lumpers" and "splitters" has largely subsided (10), MERRF remains a distinct clinical syndrome and one of the most common mitochondrial encephalomyopathies. In this chapter, we review the clinical, morphologic, and biochemical features of MERRF, discuss molecular genetics and pathophysiology (to the limited extent that we understand it), and consider therapeutic options (to the even more limited extent that these are possible).

CLINICAL FEATURES

MERRF is a multisystem disorder characterized by (a) myoclonus, (b) generalized epilepsy, (c) ataxia, and (d) ragged red fibers (RRFs) in the muscle biopsy (4). In a recent review, we found 62 patients who fulfilled these diagnostic criteria, and their symptoms and signs are listed in Table 23.1 in order of frequency (11). Although onset is usually in childhood, early development is normal and adult onset is not uncommon. Besides the defining criteria, common clinical manifestations include hearing loss, peripheral neuropathy, dementia, short stature, exercise intolerance, and optic atrophy. Less common clinical signs (seen in less than half of the patients) include cardiomyopathy, pigmentary retinopathy, pyramidal signs, ophthalmoparesis, and multiple lipomas. As usual in mi-

TABLE 23.1. *Clinical features of 62 MERRF patients*

Symptom/sign	Present	Recorded	Percent
Myoclonus	62	62	100
Epilepsy	62	62	100
Normal early development	17	17	100
Ragged-red fibers	47	51	92
Hearing loss	41	45	91
Lactic acidosis	24	29	83
Family history	34	42	81
Exercise intolerance	8	10	80
Dementia	39	52	75
Neuropathy	17	27	63
Short stature	4	7	57
Impaired sensation	9	18	50
Optic nerve atrophy	14	36	39
Cardiomyopathy	2	6	33
Wolff-Parkinson-White syndrome	2	9	22
Pigmentary retinopathy	4	26	15
Pyramidal signs	8	60	13
Ophthalomoparesis	3	28	11
Pes cavus	5	60	8
Multiple lipomas	2	60	3

The following symptoms and signs were reported once each in 60 patients: migraine headaches, hypothyroidism, irregular menses, elevated creatine kinase, extrapyramidal signs, and hepatomegaly. Diabetes mellitus, hypoparathyroidism, strokes, cerebrospinal fluid protein >100 mg/dL, and heart block were not noted in these patients. (From Hirano M, DiMauro S. Clinical features of mitochondrial myopathies and encephalomyopathies. In: Lane RJM, ed. *Handbook of Muscle Disease.* New York: Marcel Dekker, 1996:479–504, with permission.)

tochondrial encephalomyopathies, maternal family members may be oligosymptomatic or asymptomatic. The family initially reported by Tsairis et al. (2) and later by Lombes et al. (3) is a good example of intrafamiliar clinical heterogeneity. The mother, at age 33, presented with a myopathy that was diagnosed as limb-girdle muscular dystrophy despite the presence of RRFs, and died of a lymphoma 13 years later without ever developing brain symptoms. Of her four children, a son had RRFs at age 22 but was still asymptomatic at age 40. Two daughters died at 12 and 16 years of age after rapidly progressive encephalopathy compatible with MERRF. The fourth child, a son in whom we documented the typical mutation, also had typical MERRF with onset in childhood, but the course was relatively slow and he died at age 36.

After molecular defects in the tRNA[Lys] gene of mtDNA, and especially the A8344G mutation, were defined, a few unusual clinical presentations were noted, either in isolation or, more often, in pedigrees in which typical MERRF was also manifested. Several papers have described the wide spectrum of clinical presentations associated with the A8334G mutation (12–15), but a few entities deserve special attention.

Spinocerebellar degeneration and neuropathologically proven Leigh syndrome (LS) were diagnosed in several members of two families, in both of which autosomal dominant transmission had been initially suspected (15,16). It is noteworthy that in one of these families the molecular diagnosis was established using paraffin-embedded samples 23 years after the initial clinical report (17), a good example of "archeopathology."

Considering the variety of etiologies of LS—albeit all related to oxidative metabolism (18)—it is not surprising that mtDNA mutations causing typical MERRF can also cause LS. Besides the two families mentioned above, LS has been reported in many other patients carrying the A8344G mutation (12–14,19). We have studied two half-sisters of different fathers who harbored a different mutation (G8363A) in the tRNA[Lys] gene and died in infancy of LS: their mother developed typical MERRF in her late 20s (20).

Peripheral neuropathy is not uncommon (Table 23.1) and is usually sensorimotor, with impairment of position and vibration sense as well as weakness and areflexia, but at least in one case motor symptoms predominated, simulating Charcot-Marie-Tooth disease (15).

In 1975, long before the molecular defects of MERRF became known, Karl Ekbom (21) described multiple lipomas in association with hereditary ataxia, photomyoclonus, and skeletal deformities in a family in which the A8344G mutation was later documented (22). These tumors, varying in size from small subcutaneous nodules to disfiguring masses and usually located in the nape of the neck and in the shoulder area, have been reported in multiple patients with the A8344G mutation (12,14,15,23–27). Interestingly, multiple lipomas were also seen in a family with cerebellar ataxia and a different mutation (G8363A) in the tRNA^Lys gene (28), but were described only in two other patients with mtDNA alterations, a 60-year-old woman with a single deletion (29) and a 53-year-old man with multiple deletions (30).

We are conducting a longitudinal study of patients with MERRF-8344 and MELAS-3243, the two major syndromes due to mtDNA point mutations. Although this study is still in progress, preliminary comparative data of clinical, neurobehavioral, and neuroradiologic features from 5 patients with MERRF and 19 with MELAS are showing interesting differences. For patients with MERRF, mean age at onset is 21 years (range, 7 to 30), and it is also 21 years (range, 3 to 46) for patients with MELAS. At entry into the study, all patients with MERRF had only mild cognitive impairment, including attention and memory deficits. In contrast, 63% of the MELAS patients had had severe cognitive deficits that included reasoning, memory, language, attention, and visuospatial orientation. The only psychiatric diagnosis in our MERRF population is depression, occurring in two-thirds of the probands. In the MELAS population, depression is somewhat less prevalent, affecting one-third of the probands. However, more than half of the MELAS probands have other psychiatric difficulties, including behavioral abnormalities, disinhibition, substance abuse, delusions, and psychotic features. Only 2 patients with MERRF require assistance with activities of daily living (ADL), whereas 12 patients with MELAS are totally dependent for ADL. Five MELAS patients died within one decade of symptom onset. The average disease duration for MELAS patients in our study is 6 years (range, less than 1 to 22). In contrast, the disease duration in MERRF patients is 19 years (range, 7 to 42), and the mortality is low (0 of 5 patients). In conclusion, it appears that MERRF has a relatively long course and only mild behavioral and cognitive deficits, whereas MELAS is associated with progressive cognitive impairment, significant psychiatric and behavioral disturbances, and a more truncated course.

Laboratory Tests

Patients with typical MERRF have elevated blood lactate and pyruvate at rest, which increase excessively with moderate exercise. Lumbar puncture shows elevated cerebrospinal fluid (CSF) protein levels, but these rarely surpass 100 mg per dL. Electromyography and nerve conduction studies are usually compatible with a myopathic process, except when peripheral neuropathy is also part of the clinical picture. Electroencephalography shows generalized spike and wave discharges with background slowing, but focal epileptiform discharges may also be seen.

Brain computed tomography or magnetic resonance imaging scans may show brain atrophy and basal ganglia calcifications. Phosphorus magnetic resonance spectroscopy of the gastrocnemius muscle in eight patients (only three of whom had signs of myopathy) documented mitochondrial dysfunction in all, as evidenced by increased relative intracellular inorganic phosphate (Pi) concentration and decreased phosphocreatine to Pi ratio (31). However, no mitochondrial dysfunction was seen in the brain by the same technique.

We compared the severity of cerebral lactic acidosis in our patients with MERRF and MELAS by magnetic resonance spectroscopic imaging in a voxel mainly containing lateral ventricular fluid. The institutional unit (IU) of measurement was determined by dividing the lactate peak area by the root mean square deviation of the background noise in each voxel. MERRF probands showed increased lactate in both the CSF and the cerebral cortex, whereas in oligosymptomatic carriers of the A8344G mutation increased lactate was only detectable in the CSF (Fig. 23.1). Brain lactate was significantly lower in MERRF than in MELAS patients ($p < 0.005$). The correlation (0.33) between neuropsychologic scores and brain lactate levels approached significance in both MERRF and MELAS patients.

Muscle biopsy shows RRFs with the modified Gomori trichrome stain in over 90% of typical patients (11). These fibers react intensely with the succinate dehydrogenase (SDH) stain, a more sensitive indicator of excessive mitochondrial proliferation. Both RRFs and some non-RRFs fail to stain with the histochemical reaction for cytochrome *c* oxidase (COX). Muscle biopsies from five MERRF patients also showed strongly SDH-reactive blood vessels (SSVs), which are characteristically seen in muscle biopsies from patients with typical MELAS (32). However, in contrast to SSVs of MELAS patients, which stain positively for COX, the SSVs in the MERRF patients were uniformly COX-negative (33).

Biochemical studies of respiratory chain enzymes in muscle extracts usually show decreased activities of respiratory chain complexes containing mtDNA-encoded subunits, and especially COX deficiency (3,14,34–36).

GENETICS

Maternal inheritance was evident in a large family (6), in which, 5 years later, Shoffner et al. (7) documented the "typical" molecular defect, an A-to-G transition at nt 8344 in the tRNA[Lys] gene of mtDNA. As mentioned above, this was the first molecular defect associated with a specific form of epilepsy. The A8344G mutation is present in about 90% of patients with MERRF.

Two more mutations have been associated with MERRF. Interestingly, and certainly not by chance, both are in the tRNA[Lys] gene. The first mutation, T8356C, was discovered almost simultaneously in an American family with typical MERRF (37), and in an Italian family in which typical MERRF symptoms coexisted with strokelike episodes and migrainous headache, thus justifying the label "MERRF/MELAS overlap syndrome" (38). A common clinical feature of both families was hyperthyroidism, which is rather unusual in mitochondrial diseases and may, therefore, be related to this specific mutation. A third family with this mutation was reported from Japan: the proband had typical MERRF, but a maternal aunt had strokelike episodes, another example of MERRF/MELAS overlap (39).

The second mutation, G8363A, was first identified in two unrelated American families with maternally inherited cardiomyopathy, which was severe enough to cause early death in several members of one family (40). Although cardiomyopathy dominated the clinical picture, encephalomyopathy was also present, with neurosensory hearing loss, progressive external ophthalmoparesis, mental retardation, limb weakness, and peripheral neuropathy variably affecting members of both families. Interestingly, cerebellar symptoms were frequent, including ataxia, dysmetria, slurred speech, and gait instability. It is also noteworthy (and, again, probably not an accidental finding) that one proband had "horse collar" lipomas. The following year, Ozawa et al. (41) found the same mutation in two unrelated Japanese patients with typical MERRF, one of whom also had cardiomyopathy. We studied a family with the G8363A mutation in which two girls (from different fathers) died in infancy of LS whereas their mother developed typical MERRF around age 30 (20).

There is consensus that the A8344G mutation is heteroplasmic and has to be present in very high abundance (about 90% of total mtDNA) to cause symptoms; in other words,

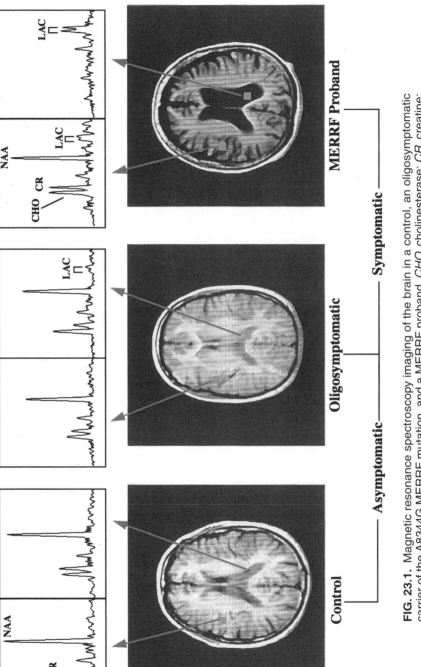

FIG. 23.1. Magnetic resonance spectroscopy imaging of the brain in a control, an oligosymptomatic carrier of the A8344G MERRF mutation, and a MERRF proband. *CHO*, cholinesterase; *CR*, creatine; *NAA*, N-acetyl-L-aspartate; *LAC*, lactate.

it is a relatively benign mutation (7). In four MERRF patients studied postmortem, we found that the mutation was present in similar amounts in different tissues (14), an observation shared by others (19,42–44). Longitudinal studies are rare, but in two patients muscle biopsies were repeated after intervals of 3 and 10 years: the percentage of mutated genomes did not change in either patient (14,45). We also found that the proportion of mutated mtDNA was similar in muscle and blood from four patients. This led us to conclude that analysis of mtDNA in blood is a more reliable diagnostic test in MERRF than in MELAS, where the percentages of mutant genomes is considerably lower in blood than in muscle (14). However, Larsson et al. (23) and Hammans et al. (13) found slightly but consistently lower proportions of mutant genomes in blood than in muscle in MERRF patients. In patients with typical symptoms, the mutation is almost invariably detectable in blood; in oligosymptomatic individuals, a negative blood test does not exclude the diagnosis.

Predictably, oligosymptomatic patients have lower mutation loads. In one such patient with an overall mutation load in muscle of 18%, single fiber analysis revealed a wide variation of heteroplasmy, ranging from 0% to 80% (46). In this same study, the high threshold of the A8344G mutation was confirmed by the finding that histochemically COX-negative single fibers had levels of heteroplasmy greater than 95%.

All three mutations associated with MERRF affect highly conserved base pairs in the tRNA^{Lys} gene: the A8344G and the T8356C mutations are in the TψC stem (7,37), and the G8363A mutation is in the aminoacyl acceptor stem of the gene (40) (Fig. 23.2).

A single patient with myoclonus, seizures, ataxia, and RRFs, but also peripheral neuropathy, dementia, and neuroradiologic evidence of cerebral and especially cerebellar atrophy, did not have any mutation in the tRNA^{Lys} gene, but did have multiple mtDNA deletions in muscle (47). Family history was not available because he was adopted.

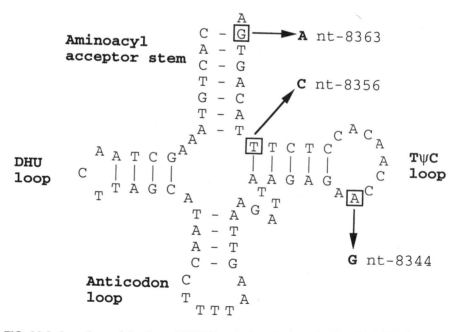

FIG. 23.2. Locations of the three MERRF mutations in the mitochondrial tRNA^{Lys} gene.

Genetic Counseling

Prenatal diagnosis poses special problems for mtDNA-related diseases because of two main concerns: (a) the mutational load in amniocytes or chorionic villi will not correspond to that of other fetal tissues and (b) the mutational load in prenatal samples may shift *in utero* or after birth due to mitotic segregation. These concerns still impede prenatal diagnosis for disorders due to tRNA mutations, including MERRF.

NEUROPATHOLOGY

The histopathologic lesions in mitochondrial encephalomyopathies are nonspecific and include spongiform degeneration, neuronal loss, focal necrosis, astrocytosis, demyelination, and mineral deposition. All of these changes are present to some extent in the three major syndromes: MERRF, MELAS, and KSS. What characterizes each syndrome is the topographic pattern of the lesions (48). As shown in Figure 23.3, neuronal loss and gliosis predominate in MERRF, involving preferentially cerebellum, brainstem, and spinal cord. In the cerebellum, neuronal loss is

especially severe in the dentate nucleus—an observation originally made by Ramsey Hunt, who, in 1921, described "primary atrophy of the dentate system" in patients with "dyssynergia cerebellaris myoclonica" (1). The inferior olivary nucleus is the most severely affected structure in the brainstem, followed by the red nucleus and the substantia nigra. In the spinal cord, cell loss is considerable in the Clarke nucleus and less severe in the anterior and posterior horns. Demyelination affects preferentially the superior cerebellar peduncles and posterior columns. In the spinal cord, degeneration of the posterior spinocerebellar tracts is common, whereas pyramidal involvement is usually mild.

To gain a better insight on the involvement of the respiratory chain in MERRF, we studied by immunohistochemistry the expression of different subunits in the frontal cortex, cerebellum, and medulla from a patient with typical MERRF (49). We used antibodies against the mtDNA-encoded subunit 1 (ND1) of complex I; the nDNA-encoded iron-sulfur (FeS) protein of complex III; the mtDNA-encoded subunit II of COX (COX II); the nDNA-encoded subunit IV of COX (COX

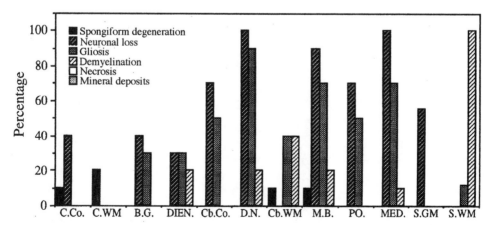

FIG. 23.3. Topographic distribution of brain lesions in MERRF. *C.Co,* cerebral cortex; *C.WM,* cerebral white matter; *B.G.,* basal ganglia; *DIEN.,* diencephalon; *Cb.Co.,* cerebellar cortex; *D.N.,* dentate nucleus; *Cb.WM,* cerebellar white matter; *M.B.,* midbrain; *PO,* pons; *MED.,* medulla; *S.GM,* spinal cord gray matter; *S.WM,* spinal cord white matter. (Adapted from Sparaco M, Bonilla E, DiMauro S, et al. Neuropathology of mitochondrial encephalomyopathies due to mitochondrial DNA defects. *J Neuropathol Exp Neurol* 1993;52:1–10.)

IV); and the mtDNA-encoded subunit 8 (AT-Pase 8) of complex V. We found a selective decrease of COX II expression in all areas studied, but especially in regions more affected by degenerative changes, such as the dentate nucleus and the inferior olivary nucleus. These results were rather surprising be-cause studies of the MERRF mutation *in vitro* had suggested a generalized defect of mitochondrial protein synthesis (see below). On the other hand, the selective involvement of COX II was in agreement with biochemical and immunologic data obtained by Lombes et al. (3) in the brain of the same patient. We ob-

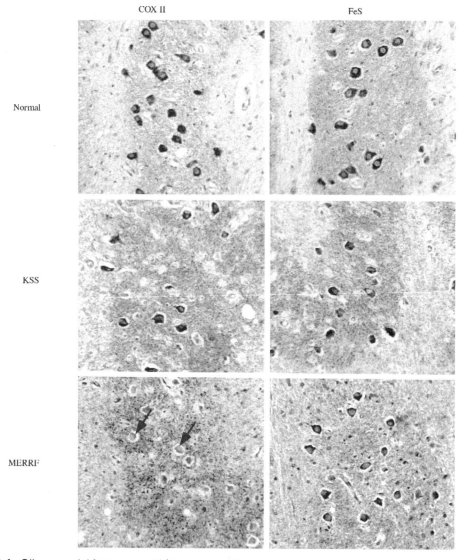

FIG. 23.4. Olivary nuclei from a control **(upper panel)**, a patient with Kearns-Sayre syndrome (KSS) **(middle panel)**, and a patient with MERRF **(lower panel)**. The samples were immunostained for the detection of mtDNA-encoded COX II and nDNA-encoded non-heme iron-sulfur protein (FeS) of complex III. The immunostain for COX II is markedly reduced only in olivary neurons *(black arrows)* of the MERRF patient while the immunoreactivity for FeS is normal in the same patient. ×120 (see Color Plate 2 following page 288).

tained similar data in a second patient with typical MERRF, in whom a selective decrease of COX II expression was seen in the olivary nucleus, contrasting with a normal expression of the same subunit in the olivary nucleus of a patient with KSS (Fig. 23.4; see Color Plate 2 following page 288).

The study of Sparaco et al. (49) also revealed that the immunohistochemical abnormalities were more widespread than the lesions seen by traditional histopathology. For example, COX II expression was decreased in the cerebral cortex, which could explain the mild cognitive impairment observed in many of our patients.

PATHOGENESIS

Although our knowledge of the molecular etiologies of mitochondrial encephalomyopathies has progressed at a breakneck pace since 1988, when mutations in mtDNA were first associated with human disease (8,9), our understanding of pathogenesis has lagged behind and remains incomplete, at best. Clinical expression of any mtDNA point mutation, including A8344G, depends on three factors: degree of heteroplasmy (mutation load); tissue distribution of the mutation; and tissue threshold, that is, the vulnerability of different tissues to a specific mutation.

As discussed above, the A8344G mutation is present in very high abundance in all tissues of typical patients, and there is no clear correlation between mutation load in muscle and clinical severity (14). However, it is still possible that even small differences in mutation load among tissues may have large functional consequences. An example of this situation is offered by the A3243G MELAS mutation. In patients with typical MELAS, fibers containing very high levels (90% to 95%) of the mutation are histochemically COX-positive, whereas in patients with maternally inherited progressive external ophthalmoplegia (PEO) fibers containing yet higher levels (95% to 98%) of the same mutation are COX-negative (50). By the same token, small differences in mutation load between muscle and brain might explain why of

two members of the same family, one may present with typical MERRF and the other with a "limb-girdle" myopathy (2,3).

Detailed studies of pathogenesis have been hindered by the lack of animal models for mtDNA-related disorders. This situation is now changing, as both large-scale deletions and point mutations have been introduced in heteroplasmic amounts into mice (51,52). It is likely that one strain of "mitomice" will soon harbor the A8344G mutation, thus allowing us to compare mutation load, clinical involvement, and biochemical features in different tissues. Until now, however, the best alternative to animal models has been cybrid cell cultures. These are established human cell lines that are first emptied of their mtDNA through exposure to ethidium bromide, then repopulated with various percentages of mutated mtDNA through fusion with enucleated cells from patients (cytoplasts) (53). Chomyn et al. (54) found that cybrids harboring high proportions of the A8344G mutation had decreased protein synthesis, decreased oxygen consumption, and COX deficiency. The polypeptides containing higher numbers of lysine residues were more severely affected, suggesting that the mutation inhibits protein synthesis directly. Similarly, cultured myotubes containing more than 85% mutant mtDNA showed decreased translation, affecting more severely proteins that contained larger numbers of lysine residues (36). Here, however, we may see the danger of extrapolating cybrid data to the *in vivo* situation (and the promise of mitomice). Contrary to expectations, the immunohistochemical study of a patient's brain showed that although the ATPase 8 subunit is large and contains a high proportion of lysine residues, its expression was not as severely impaired as that of COX II (49).

Additional studies in cybrid cell lines harboring the A8344G mutation showed decreased levels of tRNA[Lys] and of aminoacylated tRNA[Lys] (55). Masucci et al. (56) found decreased protein synthesis and oxygen consumption not only in cybrids harboring the A8344G mutation but also in cybrids harboring the G8356A mutation. In addition, they identified aberrant mitochondrial translation products in both cybrid cell lines, which they attributed to ribosomal frameshifting. Shifting of the ribosome forward or backward is seen in certain viruses, bacteria, and yeast when an amino acid is limiting.

An even more perplexing problem is the preferential association of mutations in tRNA^{Lys} with certain clinical manifestations, such as myoclonus and multiple lipomas. Myoclonus may be due, in part at least, to the selective involvement of the inferior olivary nuclei and of the cerebellar dentate nucleus, which have both been implicated in the genesis of reticular reflex myoclonus and segmental myoclonus (57–59). However, even if the immunohistochemical data suggest that the A8344G mutation may be more abundant in the inferior olives and in the dentate nucleus, the question still remains why should this particular mutation (or mutations in this particular gene) "prefer" these anatomic structures.

In 1991, Berkovic et al. (60) described four patients with multiple symmetrical lipomatosis, of whom three had RRFs in their muscle biopsies and two had clinical histories compatible with MERRF. Although the authors only performed Southern blot analysis of mtDNA (which was normal), they postulated that the lipomas may consist of brown fat and that mitochondrial dysfunction may impair lipolysis in this tissue and result in excessive lipid accumulation and tumor formation. Very high mutation loads for the A8344G or the G8363A mutation (≥90%) were documented in the adipose tissue from lipomas in several studies (22,24,28,61). In fact, the degree of heteroplasmy was higher in the lipomas than in blood and even muscle in some patients (22,24), and, in one patient, it was 96% in the lipoma and 86% in normal subcutaneous fat (61). The expression of uncoupling protein-1, a marker of brown fat, was documented in the lipoma from one patient with the A8344G mutation but not in the lipoma from another patient with the G8363A mutation (61). Though these findings partially vindicate the original hypothesis of Berkovic et al. (60), a simple defect of mitochondrial energy production cannot explain excessive lipid accu-

mulation in brown fat because high mitochondrial activity in this tissue is not associated with high ATP requirement. In fact, mitochondria in brown adipose tissue are involved in thermogenesis and their respiratory activity is uncoupled from ATP production (61).

Of course, other aspects of mitochondrial dysfunction may be operative in causing lipomas, but the fact that these tumors have been associated only with point mutations in the tRNA^{Lys} suggests that this gene may play some kind of specific role. We know that there may be more to tRNA genes than their role in mtDNA translation because tRNA$^{Leu(UUR)}$, for example, contains a transcription termination site for rRNA synthesis (62). An additional interesting observation is that certain mutation sites in the generic "cloverleaf" structure of tRNA molecules (Fig. 23.2) seem to be preferentially associated with certain clinical phenotypes, such as cardiomyopathy, progressive external ophthalmoplegia, or encephalopathy (63). In this respect, it is noteworthy that the G8363A mutation is often associated with cardiomyopathy (see above) and the C3303T mutation in a very similar position on the aminoacyl acceptor stem of the tRNA$^{Leu(UUR)}$ gene is also typically associated with cardiomyopathy (64,65).

In conclusion, the tissue-specific manifestations of some mtDNA mutations remain a puzzle. Possible explanations include interaction of the mutant gene with nuclear-encoded tissue-specific mitochondrial proteins, an unknown tissue-specific function of the gene product, or a local environmental factor increasing the vulnerability of a given tissue to the gene defect, such as a relatively poor defense system against oxidative stress. Clearly, more work is needed to understand the relationship between tRNA^{Lys} mutations and some characteristic manifestations of MERRF, including myoclonus, multiple lipomas, hyperthyroidism (37,38), and hypertension (22,27).

THERAPY

As with other mitochondrial encephalomyopathies, there is no specific therapy for

MERRF, and most patients are empirically treated with "cocktails" of vitamins and cofactors, including coenzyme Q10 (CoQ10) (50 to 100 mg three times a day) and L-carnitine (1,000 mg three times a day) (66).

Palliative management includes conventional anticonvulsant therapy, although there are no controlled studies comparing the efficacy of different antiepilepsy regimens. Myoclonus can be controlled with clonazepam (0.5 to 1 mg three times a day) or with zonisamide. As with all mitochondrial diseases, valproate has to be used with caution and always in association with L-carnitine because of its well-documented inhibition of carnitine uptake (67).

Lactic acidosis can be controlled with bicarbonate, which, however, has only a transient buffering effect and may exacerbate the cerebral symptoms (68). Despite the evidence of mild lactate accumulation in the brain of MERRF patients (Fig. 23.1), lactic acidosis is only rarely a clinical concern in MERRF. For this reason, dichloroacetate (DCA), which can be beneficial to MELAS patients, is not indicated in MERRF patients (66). In addition, there are drawbacks to DCA treatment: (a) the drug is not yet commercially available in the United States; (b) there are no controlled studies of its efficacy in mitochondrial encephalomyopathies, although one is underway in our Center in a homogeneous population of patients with MELAS; and (c) DCA may cause peripheral neuropathy even when administered together with thiamine (8.6 mg per kg).

Gene therapy for mtDNA-related diseases is in its infancy and is fraught with problems because of polyplasmy and heteroplasmy (69). In this regard the newly available "mitomice" will be invaluable tools. One promising approach is based on our understanding of heteroplasmy and the threshold effect. If we could cause even a small shift in the relative proportion of mutant and wild-type mtDNAs, we might improve the clinical phenotype dramatically. To achieve this goal, various approaches have been taken, including the use of peptide nucleic acids (PNAs) to inhibit selectively the replication of complementary mtDNAs harboring the A8344G mutation (70). Successful delivery of PNAs into mitochondria *in vitro* bodes well for the future applicability of this approach *in vivo* (71).

Satellite cells and myoblasts contain lesser amounts of pathogenic mtDNA mutations than do mature muscle fibers (72–74). This observation has suggested two different therapeutic approaches. The first is to cause limited muscle necrosis by injection of myotoxic agents, such as bupivacaine (75); the second is to induce muscle damage through isometric exercise (76,77): both conditions would be followed by regeneration of muscle fibers harboring lower mutation loads. Both therapeutic modalities are still in the experimental stage and would seem to be more applicable to patients with isolated mitochondrial myopathy than to those with a multisystem disorder such as MERRF.

ACKNOWLEDGMENTS

Part of the work described here was funded by NIH grants PO1HD32062 and NS11766 and by a grant from the Muscular Dystrophy Association.

REFERENCES

1. Hunt JR. Dyssynergia cerebellaris myoclonica–primary atrophy of the dentate system: a contribution to the pathology and symptomatology of the cerebellum. *Brain* 1921;44:490–538.
2. Tsairis P, Engel WK, Kark P. Familial myoclonic epilepsy syndrome associated with skeletal muscle mitochondrial abnormalities. *Neurology* 1973;23:408.
3. Lombes A, Mendell JR, Nakase H, et al. Myoclonic epilepsy and ragged-red fibers with cytochrome oxidase deficiency: neuropathology, biochemistry, and molecular genetics. *Ann Neurol* 1989;26:20–33.
4. Fukuhara N, Tokiguchi S, Shirakawa K, et al. Myoclonus epilepsy associated with ragged-red fibers (mitochondrial abnormalities): disease entity or a syndrome? *J Neurol Sci* 1980;47:117–133.
5. DiMauro S, Bonilla E, Zeviani M, et al. Mitochondrial myopathies. *Ann Neurol* 1985;17:521–538.
6. Rosing HS, Hopkins LC, Wallace DC, et al. Maternally inherited mitochondrial myopathy and myoclonic epilepsy. *Ann Neurol* 1985;17:228–237.
7. Shoffner JM, Lott MT, Lezza A, et al. Myoclonic epilepsy and ragged-red fiber disease (MERRF) is associated with a mitochondrial DNA tRNALys mutation. *Cell* 1990;61:931–937.
8. Holt IJ, Harding AE, Morgan Hughes JA. Deletions of

muscle mitochondrial DNA in patients with mitochondrial myopathies. *Nat* 1988;331:717–719.

9. Wallace DC, Singh G, Lott MT, et al. Mitochondrial DNA mutation associated with Leber's hereditary optic neuropathy. *Science* 1988;242:1427–1430.

10. Rowland LP. Mitochondrial encephalomyopathies: lumping, splitting, and melding. In: Schapira AHV, DiMauro S, eds. *Mitochondrial disorders in neurology.* Oxford: Butterworth-Heinemann, 1994:116–129.

11. Hirano M, DiMauro S. Clinical features of mitochondrial myopathies and encephalomyopathies. In: Lane RJM, ed. *Handbook of muscle disease.* New York: Marcel Dekker Inc., 1996:479–504.

12. Berkovic S, Shoubridge E, Andermann F, et al. Clinical spectrum of mitochondrial DNA mutations at base pair 8344. *Lancet* 1991;338:457.

13. Hammans SR, Sweeney MG, Brockington M, et al. The mitochondrial DNA transfer RNALys A->G(8344) mutation and the syndrome of myoclonic epilepsy with ragged red fibers (MERRF). *Brain* 1993;116:617–632.

14. Silvestri G, Ciafaloni E, Santorelli F, et al. Clinical features associated with the AφG transition at nucleotide 8344 of mtDNA ("MERRF mutation"). *Neurology* 1993;43:1200–1206.

15. Howell N, Kubacka I, Smith R, et al. Association of the mitochondrial 8344 MERRF mutation with maternally inherited spinocerebellar degeneration and Leigh disease. *Neurology* 1996;46:219–222.

16. Santorelli FM, Tanji K, Shanske S, et al. The mitochondrial DNA A8344G mutation in Leigh syndrome revealed by analysis in paraffin-embedded sections: revisiting the past.*Ann Neurol* 1998;44:962–964.

17. Greenwood RS, De Vivo DC, Nelson JS, et al. An autosomal dominant form of necrotizing encephalomyelopathy resembling a spinocerebellar degeneration. *Trans Am Neurol Assoc* 1975;100:47–51.

18. DiMauro S, De Vivo DC. Genetic heterogeneity in Leigh syndrome. *Ann Neurol* 1996;40:5–7.

19. Sweeney MG, Hammans SR, Duchen LW, et al. Mitochondrial DNA mutation underlying Leigh's syndrome: clinical, pathological, biochemical, and genetic studies of a patient presenting with progressive myoclonic epilepsy. *J Neurol Sci* 1994;121:57–65.

20. Shtilbahns A, Shanske S, Goodman S, et al. G8363A mutation in the mitochondrial DNA transfer ribonucleic acid Lys gene: another cause of Leigh syndrome. *J Child Neurol* 2000;15:759–761.

21. Ekbom K. Hereditary ataxia, photomyoclonus, skeletal deformities and lipoma. *Acta Neurol Scand* 1975;51:393–404.

22. Traff J, Holme E, Nilsson BY. Ekbom's syndrome of photomyoclonus, cerebellar ataxia and cervical lipoma is associated with tRNALys A8344G mutation in mitochondrial DNA. *Acta Neurol Scand* 1995;92:394–397.

23. Larsson NG, Tulinius MH, Holme E, et al. Segregation and manifestations of the mtDNA tRNALys A->G(8344) mutation of myoclonus epilepsy and ragged-red fibers (MERRF) syndrome. *Am J Hum Genet* 1992;51:1201–1212.

24. Holme E, Larsson NG, Oldfors A, et al. Multiple symmetric lipomas with high levels of mtDNA with the tRNALys A>G(8344) mutation as the only manifestation of disease in a carrier of myoclonus epilepsy and ragged-red fibers (MERRF) syndrome. *Am J Hum Genet* 1993;52:551–556.

25. Calabresi PA, Silvestri G, DiMauro S, et al. Ekbom's syndrome: lipomas, ataxia, and neuropathy with MERRF. *Muscle Nerve* 1994;17:943–945.

26. Naumann M, Reiners K, Gold R, et al. Mitochondrial dysfunction in adult-onset myopathies with structural abnormalities. *Acta Neuropathol* 1995;89:152–157.

27. Austin SA, Vriesendorp FJ, Thandroyen FT, et al. Expanding phenotype of the 8334 transfer tRNAlysine mitochondrial DNA mutation. *Neurology*1998;51:1447–1450.

28. Casali C, Fabrizi GM, Santorelli FM, et al. Mitochondrial G8363A mutation presenting as cerebellar ataxia and lipomas in an Italian family.*Neurology* 1999;52:1103–1104.

29. Campos Y, Martin MA, Navarro C, et al. Single large-scale mitochondrial DNA deletion in a patient with mitochondrial myopathy associated with multiple symmetric lipomatosis. *Neurology* 1996;47:1012–1014.

30. Klopstock T, Naumann M, Schalke B, et al. Multiple symmetric lipomatosis: abnormalities in complex IV and multiple deletions in mitochondrial DNA. *Neurology* 1994;44:862–866.

31. Matthews PM, Berkovic SF, Shoubridge EA, et al. In vivo magnetic resonance spectroscopy of brain and muscle in a type of mitochondrial encephalomyopathy (MERRF). *Ann Neurol* 1991;29:435–438.

32. Hasegawa H, Matsuoka T, Goto I, et al. Strongly succinate dehydrogenase-reactive blood vessels in muscles from patients with mitochondrial myopathy, encephalopathy, lactic acidosis, and stroke-like episodes. *Ann Neurol* 1991;29:601–605.

33. Hasegawa H, Matsuoka T, Goto Y, et al. Cytochrome c oxidase activity is deficient in blood vessels of patients with myoclonus epilepsy with ragged-red fibers. *Acta Neuropathol* 1993;85:280–284.

34. Wallace DC, Zheng X, Lott MT, et al. Familial mitochondrial encephalomyopathy (MERRF): genetic, pathophysiological and biochemical characterization of a mitochondrial DNA disease. *Cell* 1988;55:601–610.

35. Yoneda M, Tanno Y, Horai S, et al. A common mitochondrial DNA mutation in the tRNALys of patients with myoclonus epilepsy associated with ragged-red fibers. *Biochem Int* 1990;21:789–796.

36. Boulet L, Karpati G, Shoubridge EA. Distribution and threshold expression of the tRNALys mutation in skeletal muscle of patients with myoclonic epilepsy and ragged-red fibers (MERRF). *Am J Hum Genet* 1992;51:1187–1200.

37. Silvestri G, Moraes CT, Shanske S, et al. A new mtDNA mutation in the tRNALys gene associated with myoclonic epilepsy and ragged-red fibers (MERRF). *Am J Hum Genet* 1992;51:1213–1217.

38. Zeviani M, Muntoni F, Savarese N, et al. A MERRF/MELAS overlap syndrome associated with a new point mutation in the mitochondrial DNA tRNALys gene. *Eur J Hum Genet* 1993;1:80–87.

39. Sano M, Ozawa M, Shiota S, et al. The T-C (8356) mitochondrial DNA mutation in a Japanese family. *J Neurol* 1996;243:441–444.

40. Santorelli FM, Mak S-C, El-Schahawi M, et al. Maternally inherited cardiomyopathy and hearing loss associated with a novel mutation in the mitochondrial DNA tRNALys gene (G8363A). *Am J Hum Genet* 1996;58:933–939.

41. Ozawa M, Nishino I, Horai S, et al. Myoclonus epilepsy associated with ragged-red fibers: a G-to-A mutation at nucleotide pair 8363 in mitochondrial tRNALys in two families. *Muscle Nerve* 1997;20:271–278.

42. Lombes A, Diaz C, Romero NB, et al. Analysis of the tissue distribution and inheritance of heteroplasmic mitochondrial DNA point mutation by denaturing gradient gel electrophoresis in MERRF syndrome. *Neuromuscul Disord* 1992;2:323–330.

43. Tanno Y, Yoneda M, Tanaka K, et al. Uniform tissue distribution of tRNA(Lys) mutation in mitochondrial DNA in MERRF patients. *Neurology* 1993;43:1198–1200.

44. Chen R-S, Huang C-C, Chu N-S, et al. Tissue distribution of mutant mitochondrial DNA in a patient with MERRF syndrome. *Muscle Nerve* 1996;19:519–521.

45. Mita S, Tokunaga M, Uyama E, et al. Single muscle fiber analysis of myoclonus epilepsy with ragged-red fibers. *Muscle Nerve* 1998;21:490–497.

46. Moslemi A-R, Tulinius M, Holme E, et al. Threshold expression of the tRNALys A8344G mutation in single muscle fibres. *Neuromuscul Disord* 1998;8:345–349.

47. Blumenthal DT, Shanske S, Schochet SS, et al. Myoclonus epilepsy with ragged red fibers and multiple mtDNA deletions. *Neurology* 1998;50:524–525.

48. Sparaco M, Bonilla E, DiMauro S, et al. Neuropathology of mitochondrial encephalomyopathies due to mitochondrial DNA defects. *J Neuropathol Exp Neurol* 1993;52:1–10.

49. Sparaco M, Schon EA, DiMauro S, et al. Myoclonic epilepsy with ragged-red fibers (MERRF): an immunohistochemical study of the brain. *Brain Pathol* 1995;5: 125–133.

50. Petruzzella V, Moraes CT, Sano MC, et al. Extremely high levels of mutant mtDNAs co-localize with cytochrome c oxidase-negative ragged-red fibers in patients harboring a point mutation at nt 3243. *Hum Mol Genet* 1994;3:449–454.

51. Inoue K, Nakada K, Ogura A, et al. Generation of mice with mitochondrial dysfunction by introducing mouse mtDNA carrying a deletion into zygotes. *Nat Genet* 2000;26:176–181.

52. Sligh JE, Levy SE, Waymire KG, et al. Maternal germline transmission of mutant mtDNAs from embryonic stem cell-derived chimeric mice. *Proc Natl Acad Sci USA* 2000;97:14461–14466.

53. King MP, Attardi G. Human cells lacking mtDNA: repopulation with exogenous mitochondria by complementation. *Science* 1989;246:500–503.

54. Chomyn A, Meola G, Bresolin N, et al. In vitro genetic transfer of protein synthesis and respiration defects to mitochondrial DNA-less cells with myopathy-patient mitochondria. *Mol Cell Biol* 1991;11:2236–2244.

55. Enriquez JA, Chomyn A, Attardi G. MtDNA mutation in MERRF syndrome causes defective aminoacylation of tRNA(Lys) and premature translation termination. *Nat Genet* 1995;10:47–55.

56. Masucci JP, Davidson M, Koga Y, et al. In vitro analysis of mutations causing myoclonus epilepsy with ragged-red fibers in the mitochondrial tRNALys gene: two genotypes produce similar phenotypes. *Mol Cell Biol* 1995;15:2872–2881.

57. Geller BD, Hallett M. A physiologic and pharmacologic approach to the diagnosis and treatment of myoclonus. In: Chokroverty S, ed. *Movement disorders*. New York: PMA Publishing, 1990:201–235.

58. Chung E, Van Woert MH. Myoclonus: sites and mechanism of action. *Exp Neurol* 1984;85:273–282.

59. Pranzatelli MR, Snodgrass SR. The pharmacology of myoclonus. *Clin Neuropharmacol* 1985;8:99–130.

60. Berkovic SF, Andermann F, Shoubridge EA, et al. Mitochondrial dysfunction in multiple symmetrical lipomatosis. *Ann Neurol* 1991;29:566–569.

61. Vila MR, Gamez J, Solano A, et al. Uncoupling protein-1 mRNA expression in lipomas from patients bearing pathogenic mitochondrial DNA mutations. *Biochem Biophys Res Comm* 2000;278:800–802.

62. Kruse B, Narasimhan N, Attardi G. Termination of transcription in human mitochondria: identification and purification of a DNA binding protein factor that promotes termination. *Cell* 1989;58:391–397.

63. Schon EA, Bonilla E, DiMauro S. Mitochondrial DNA mutations and pathogenesis. *J Bioenerg Biomembr* 1997;29:131–149.

64. Silvestri G, Santorelli FM, Shanske S, et al. A new mtDNA mutation in the tRNA(LeuUUR) gene associated with maternally inherited cardiomyopathy. *Hum Mutat* 1994;3:37–43.

65. Bruno C, Kirby DM, Koga Y, et al. The mitochondrial DNA C3303T mutation can cause cardiomyopathy and/or skeletal myopathy. *J Pediatr* 1999;135:197–202.

66. DiMauro S, Hirano M, Schon EA. Mitochondrial encephalomyopathies: therapeutic approaches. *Neurol Sci* 2000;21:S901–S908.

67. Tein I, DiMauro S, Xie Z-W, et al. Valproic acid impairs carnitine uptake in cultured human skin fibroblasts: an in vitro model for pathogenesis of valproic acid-associated carnitine deficiency. *Pediatr Res* 1993;34:281–287.

68. De Vivo DC, DiMauro S. Mitochondrial diseases. In: Swaiman KF, Ashwal S, ed. *Pediatrc neurology: principles and practice*. St Louis: Mosby, 1999: 494–509.

69. Murphy MP, Smith RAJ. Drug delivery to mitochondria: the key to mitochondrial medicine. *Adv Drug Deliv Rev* 2000;41:235–250.

70. Taylor RW, Chinnery PF, Turnbull DM, et al. Selective inhibition of mutant human mitochondrial DNA replication in vitro by peptide nucleic acids. *Nat Genet* 1997;15:212–215.

71. Chinnery PF, Taylor RW, Diekert K, et al. Peptic nucleic acid delivery to human mitochondria. *Gene Ther* 1999; 6:1919–1928.

72. Clark KM, Bindoff LA, Lightowlers RN, et al. Reversal of a mitochondrial DNA defect in human skeletal muscle. *Nat Genet* 1997;16:222–224.

73. Fu K, Hartlen R, Johns T, et al. A novel heteroplasmic tRNAleu(CUN) mtDNA point mutation in a sporadic patient with mitochondrial encephalomyopathy segregates rapidly in skeletal muscle and suggests an approach to therapy. *Hum Mol Genet* 1996;5:1835–1840.

74. Shoubridge EA, Johns T, Karpati G. Complete restoration of a wild-type mtDNA genotype in regenerating muscle fibers in a patient with a tRNA point mutation and mitochondrial encephalomyopathy. *Hum Mol Genet* 1997;6:2239–2242.

75. Andrews RM, Griffiths PG, Chinnery PF, et al. Evaluation of bupivacaine-induced muscle regeneration in the treatment of ptosis in patients with chronic progressive external ophthalmoplegia and Kearns-Sayre syndrome. *Eye* 1999;13:769–772.

76. Taivassalo T, Fu K, Johns T, et al. Gene shifting: a novel therapy for mitochondrial myopathy. *Hum Mol Genet* 1999;8:1047–1052.

77. Taivassalo T, Reddy H, Matthews PM. Muscle response to exercise in health and disease. *Neurol Clin* 2000;18: 15–34.

Myoclonus and Paroxysmal Dyskinesias,
Advances in Neurology, Vol. 89,
edited by S. Fahn, et al.
Lippincott Williams & Wilkins, Philadelphia © 2002.

24

Dentatorubral-Pallidoluysian Atrophy: Clinical Aspects and Molecular Genetics

Shoji Tsuji

Department of Neurology, Brain Research Institute, Niigata University, Niigata, Japan

Dentatorubral-pallidoluysian atrophy (DRPLA) is a rare autosomal dominant neurodegenerative disorder clinically characterized by various combinations of cerebellar ataxia, choreoathetosis, myoclonus, epilepsy, dementia, and psychiatric symptoms (MIM#125370) (1). The term DRPLA was originally used by Smith et al. to describe a neuropathologic condition associated with severe neuronal loss, particularly in the dentatorubral and pallidoluysian systems of the central nervous system, in a sporadic case without a family history (2,3). The hereditary form of DRPLA was first described in 1972 by Naito et al. (4). Since then, a number of reports on Japanese pedigrees with similar clinical presentations have been published (5–14), and DRPLA has been established as a distinct disease entity.

The gene for DRPLA was discovered in 1994, and an unstable CAG trinucleotide repeat expansion in the protein-coding region of this gene was found to be the causative mutation for DRPLA (15,16). To date, at least eight diseases have been found as being caused by expansion of CAG repeats coding for polyglutamine stretches, which include spinal and bulbar muscular atrophy (SBMA) (17), Huntington's disease (HD) (18), spinocerebellar ataxia type 1 (SCA1) (19), DRPLA (15,16), Machado-Joseph disease (20), spinocerebellar ataxia type 2 (SCA2) (21–23), spinocerebellar ataxia type 6 (SCA6) (24) and spinocerebellar ataxia type 7 (SCA7) (25).

In this chapter, the clinical and molecular genetic aspects of DRPLA are described. Recent progress in the study of the molecular mechanisms of neurodegeneration caused by expanded polyglutamine stretches is also discussed.

CLINICAL FEATURES OF DENTATORUBRAL-PALLIDOLUYSIAN ATROPHY

The most striking clinical characteristic features of DRPLA are the considerable heterogeneity in clinical presentation depending on the age of onset and the prominent genetic anticipation. Naito and Oyanagi (26) reported that juvenile-onset patients (onset before the age of 20) frequently exhibit a phenotype of progressive myoclonic epilepsy (PME), characterized by ataxia, seizures, myoclonus, and progressive intellectual deterioration. Epileptic seizures are a feature in all patients with onset before the age of 20, and the frequency of seizures decreases with age after 20. Occurrence of seizures in patients with onset after the age of 40 is rare. Various forms of generalized seizures including tonic, clonic, or tonic-clonic seizures are observed in DRPLA. Myoclonic epilepsy and absence or atonic seizures are occasionally observed in patients with onset before the age of 20.

In contrast, patients with onset after the age of 20 tend to develop cerebellar ataxia, choreoathetosis, and dementia, thereby making this disease occasionally difficult to differentiate from HD and other spinocerebellar ataxias (26). Some patients were occasionally diagnosed as having HD, since the main clinical presentations were involuntary movements and dementia, which masked the presence of ataxia. The evaluation of preceding ataxia and atrophy of the cerebellum and brainstem, in particular the pontine tegmentum, as detected by sagittal MRI scan, is crucial for the differential diagnosis.

The mode of inheritance of DRPLA is autosomal dominant with a high penetrance. The prevalence rate of DRPLA in the Japanese population has been estimated to be 0.2 to 0.7 per 100,000, which is comparable with that of HD in the Japanese population (27). Although DRPLA has been reported to occur predominantly in Japanese individuals, several cases with similar clinical features have been described in other ethnic groups (28–30). Since the discovery of the gene for DRPLA (15,16), CAG repeat expansion of the DRPLA gene has been demonstrated by molecular analysis in several European and North American families (31–36).

The discovery of the gene for DRPLA has made it possible to analyze the diverse clinical presentations based on the size of expanded CAG repeats. There is an inverse correlation between the age at onset and the size of expanded CAG repeats. To clarify the clinical presentations of DRPLA, we analyzed the relationship between the common clinical features of DRPLA (ataxia, dementia or mental retardation, myoclonus, epilepsy, choreoathetosis, and psychiatric changes including character changes, delusions, or hallucinations) and the age at onset (37–39). We found that ataxia and dementia are cardinal features irrespective of the age at onset. Patients with onset before the age of 20 frequently exhibit myoclonus and epilepsy in addition to ataxia and dementia. The combination of these clinical features corresponds to the PME phenotype. On the other hand, patients with onset after the age of 20 frequently exhibit choreoathetosis and psychiatric disturbances in addition to ataxia and dementia. Since the age at onset is inversely correlated with the size of expanded CAG repeats, the above observations imply that the clinical presentation is strongly correlated with the expanded CAG repeat size. A similar correlation between the clinical features and the expanded CAG repeat size has been demonstrated in other diseases caused by CAG repeat expansions.

A clear genotype-phenotype correlation was also observed in magnetic resonance imaging (MRI) findings of DRPLA patients (40). To clarify the relationship between the size of expanded CAG repeat of DRPLA gene and the atrophic changes of the brainstem and cerebellum, we quantitatively analyzed the MRI findings of 26 patients with DRPLA with the diagnosis confirmed by molecular analysis of the DRPLA gene. When the DRPLA patients were classified into two groups based on the size of the expanded CAG repeat of the DRPLA gene (group 1, number of CAG repeat units ≥66; group 2, number of CAG repeat units ≤65), we found strong inverse correlations between the age at MRI and the areas of midsagittal structures of the cerebellum and brainstem in group 1 but not in group 2, suggesting that a clear genotype-phenotype correlation was observed in patients with largely expanded CAG repeats. Furthermore, multiple regression analysis of the overall groups revealed that both the patient's age at MRI and the size of the expanded CAG repeat correlated with the areas of the midsagittal structures. Taken together, these results suggest that both the age and the size of expanded CAG repeats independently affect the atrophic changes in the midsagittal structures of the cerebellum and brainstem. Involvement of the cerebral white matter detected as areas with high intensity signals on T2-weighted images was occasionally observed in DRPLA patients. We found that the involvement of cerebral white matter is more frequently observed in patients belonging to group 2 than in group 1 patients, suggesting that the disease duration is a major determinant for the white matter involvement.

MOLECULAR GENETICS OF DENTATORUBRAL-PALLIDOLUYSIAN ATROPHY

DRPLA is characterized by prominent anticipation (15,16,37,41,42). Paternal transmission results in more prominent anticipation (26 to 29 years per generation) than does maternal transmission (14 to 15 years per generation). Given the strong parental bias on the degree of anticipation observed in HD (18) and spinocerebellar ataxia type 1 (SCA1) (19), we speculated that DRPLA must be a disease caused by unstable CAG repeat expansion of an as yet unidentified gene. Using cDNA clones known to carry CAG repeats as candidate genes, we and another study group independently discovered that the CAG repeat of a gene on chromosome 12, which had been reported as CTG-B37, was expanded in patients with DRPLA (15,16). The CAG repeats in patients with DRPLA were expanded to 54 to 79 repeat units, as compared to 6 to 35 repeat units in normal individuals (15,37–39).

The detailed structure of the full-length cDNA of the human DRPLA gene has been determined (43,44). The DRPLA cDNA is predicted to code for 1,185 amino acids. The CAG repeat expansion in the DRPLA gene is located 1,462 bp downstream from the putative methionine initiation codon and is predicted to code for a polyglutamine stretch. Interestingly, polyserine and polyproline stretches exist near the CAG repeat. In contrast to the length of the polyglutamine stretch, the lengths of these polyserine and polyproline stretches are not highly polymorphic (43). Putative nuclear localizing signals have been identified near the amino-terminus of DRPLA protein (45), which is compatible with recent observations that DRPLA protein is translocated into nucleus, preferentially in neuronal cells (46). The physiologic functions of DRPLA protein, however, remain to be elucidated.

The gene for RPLA was mapped to 12p13.31 by *in situ* hybridization (47). The human DRPLA gene spans approximately 20 kbp and consists of 10 exons, with the CAG repeats located in exon 5 (44).

Northern blot analysis revealed that a 4.7-kb transcript is widely expressed in various tissues, including the heart, lung, kidney, placenta, skeletal muscle, and brain, without predilection for regions exhibiting neurodegeneration (43,44). Reverse transcription polymerase chain reaction (RT-PCR) analysis of mRNA extracted from various regions of autopsied brains of patients with DRPLA demonstrated that DRPLA mRNA from a mutant DRPLA gene with expanded CAG repeats is expressed at levels comparable to the wild-type DRPLA gene, suggesting that CAG repeat expansion does not alter the transcriptional efficiency of the DRPLA gene (43). The expression levels of the mutant DRPLA proteins were also analyzed by Western blot analysis, which indicated that mutant DRPLA proteins are expressed at levels similar to those of wild-type DRPLA proteins (48). These studies strongly indicate that CAG repeat expansion does not alter the transcription or translation efficiency of the mutant DRPLA gene. Therefore, it seems likely that mutant DRPLA proteins with expanded polyglutamine stretches are toxic to neuronal cells, suggesting "gain of toxic functions."

MOLECULAR BASIS OF GENETIC ANTICIPATION AND MOLECULAR MECHANISMS OF INSTABILITY OF CAG REPEATS

As described above, DRPLA is characterized by a prominent genetic anticipation with a mean acceleration of age at onset of 25.6 ± 2.4 years in paternal transmission and 14.0 ± 4.0 years in maternal transmission (15,16, 37–39). In accordance with the strong parental bias for genetic anticipation, a much larger intergenerational increase was observed for paternal transmission ($5.8 + 0.9$ repeat units per generation, n = 16) compared to maternal transmission ($1.3 + 1.6$ repeat units per generation, n = 4) (15,37–39). This phenomenon has also been described for HD (18, 49–51), SCA1 (19,52), and SCA7 (25). These results strongly indicate that similar mechanisms must underlie the intergenerational instability of the expanded CAG repeats during male gametogenesis. In fact, it has been demonstrated that DNA from the sperm of patients with HD shows considerable variations in the size of expanded CAG repeats compared to DNA from somatic cells (53).

To investigate the molecular mechanisms of instability of CAG repeats, we generated transgenic mice harboring a single copy of a mutant DRPLA gene (54). The transgenic mice in fact exhibited an age-dependent increase (+0.31 per year) in male transmission and an age-dependent contraction in female transmission (−1.21 per year). Such age-dependent increase in the intergenerational changes in the sizes of expanded CAG repeats in paternal transmission and age-dependent contraction in maternal transmission were also observed in 83 parent-offspring pairs of DRPLA patients (56 paternal and 27 maternal transmissions).

Based on a linear regression model and the continuous cell divisions required for spermatogenesis throughout adult life, the mean increase in the size of CAG repeats in male transmission in mice was calculated to be +0.31 per year and +0.0073 per spermatogenesis cycle. These values were comparable to those observed in DRPLA patients, which were calculated to be +0.27 and +0.012, respectively. These results strongly indicate that the difference in the actual intergenerational changes between humans and mice is due to the reproductive lifespan variations and that a common mechanism underlies the age-dependent increase in the sizes of CAG repeats both in humans and in mice.

In contrast to spermatogenesis, oogenesis occurs only during fetal life and ceases at the diplotene stage of the first meiotic prophase by 5 days after birth, suggesting that age-dependent contraction of CAG repeats occurs after the cessation of meiotic DNA replication. Similar observations have been made in transgenic mice for SCA1 and SBMA (55,56). These results strongly suggest that contraction of the CAG repeats occurs during the prolonged resting stage, and mechanisms such as repair of damaged DNA or selective degeneration of the primary oocyte with

larger CAG repeats might be involved in the contraction process.

The transgenic mice also exhibited somatic instabilities of CAG repeats, similar to those observed in DRPLA patients (54). The size range of the CAG repeats was smallest in the cerebellum compared to that in the cerebrum and various somatic tissues. This observation has been well documented in HD, SCA1, MJD, and DRPLA (42,53,57–59). Since the cerebellum contains a dense population of granule cells, which are neuronal cells, it is assumed that neuronal cells exhibit the least instability because they do not undergo cell divisions and that cell divisions are required for the development of somatic instabilities of CAG repeats (58). Similar phenomena were observed in the granular layers of the cerebellar cortex and hippocampal formation in autopsied DRPLA brains (59). Another interesting finding of this study is the age-dependent increase in the degree of somatic mosaicism. The size ranges of CAG repeats were much larger at 64 weeks compared to those at 3 weeks. These data strongly support the fact that the degree of somatic mosaicism increases with age. However, it remains to be elucidated how the age-dependent increase in the degree of the somatic mosaicism is involved in the pathogenesis of DRPLA.

Manley et al. (60) recently examined instability of the HD CAG repeat by crossing transgenic mice carrying exon 1 of human HD with Msh2−/− mice and demonstrated that the mismatch repair enzyme MSH2 is required for somatic instability of the CAG repeat.

MECHANISMS OF NEURODEGENERATION CAUSED BY CAG REPEAT EXPANSION

There is increasing evidence suggesting "gain of toxic functions" of mutant proteins with expanded polyglutamine stretches, in particular, truncated mutant proteins containing expanded polyglutamine stretches. Such toxicities have been demonstrated not only in transient expression systems (61–65), but also in transgenic mice (61,66–68).

Initial studies in transient expression systems demonstrated that expression of expanded polyglutamine stretches led to aggregate formation and concomitant apoptotic cell death (61–65). Presence of aggregate bodies was subsequently confirmed as neuronal intranuclear inclusions (NIIs) in HD and SCA1 transgenic mice (67,69,70). Subsequent studies revealed NIIs in postmortem human brains, including cases of HD (69,71), SCA1 (70), MJD/SCA3 (62), DRPLA (63,72), SCA7 (73), SBMA (74), and SCA2 (75). These results have led to the paradigm that expression of expanded polyglutamine stretches result in aggregate formation and apoptotic cell death.

Recent studies, however, suggest that this is not the case. Interestingly, neuronal death was not observed in transgenic mice for HD (66,76) and SBMA (68). Recent studies on a transgenic mouse model for HD using inducible promoters clearly demonstrated reversibility of neuropathology and phenotypic expressions (77). These data strongly support that neuronal dysfunction but not apoptotic cell death is the primary event in polyglutamine diseases.

Detailed immunohistochemical analysis of autopsied brains of DRPLA patients using 1C2 monoclonal antibody that recognizes preferentially expanded polyglutamine stretches has demonstrated that diffuse accumulation of mutant DRPLA protein/atrophin-1 in the neuronal nuclei, rather than the formation of NIIs, was the predominant pathologic condition and involved a wide range of central nervous system regions far beyond the systems previously reported to be affected (78).

Although the physiologic functions remain unclear, full-length wild-type DRPLA protein has recently been demonstrated to be localized predominantly in the nuclei of cultured cells (45,46). Such nuclear localization is presumably mediated by putative nuclear localization signals (NLSs) in these. In fact, we found that mutant DRPLA protein is expressed predominantly in the nucleus of neuronally differentiated PC12 cells using an adenovirus expression system. We furthermore demonstrated that intranuclear aggregate bodies are preferentially formed in neuronally differentiated PC12 cells and that these cells are more vulnerable than fibroblasts to the toxic effects of expanded polyglutamine stretches of the DRPLA protein (46). These observations emphasize the importance of nuclear translocation of full-length or truncated DRPLA proteins with expanded polyglutamine stretches. The observations that transgenic mice expressing mutant ataxin-1 with a mutated NLS did not develop ataxia (79), and that addition of a nuclear export signal to mutant Huntingtin suppressed the formation of NIIs and apoptosis (80), further emphasize the role of nuclear translocation of mutant proteins with expanded polyglutamine stretches. These findings suggest that interaction of polyglutamine stretches and some nuclear proteins may be involved in the cytotoxicity caused by expanded polyglutamine stretches.

To date, a number of proteins have been found to associate with the gene products for polyglutamine diseases (70,81–99). As described above, recent studies have emphasized the role of nuclear transport and nuclear accumulation of mutant proteins with expanded polyglutamine stretches prior to intranuclear inclusion formation in the pathogenesis of polyglutamine disease (78). These findings raise a new paradigm that interaction of mutant proteins containing expanded polyglutamine stretches with nuclear proteins may lead to neuronal dysfunction, in particular, transcriptional dysfunction. Recent discovery of sequestration of nuclear proteins by expanded polyglutamine stretches (70,94–99) strongly support this hypothesis. To further support this hypothesis, down-regulation of selective genes has been demonstrated in the transgenic mice for HD (100) and SCA1 (101). These results suggest that intranuclear accumulation of mutant proteins and transcriptional dysregulation are the primary pathogenic mechanisms of polyglutamine diseases (Fig. 24.1). Given the reversibility of disease process in polyglutamine disease (77),

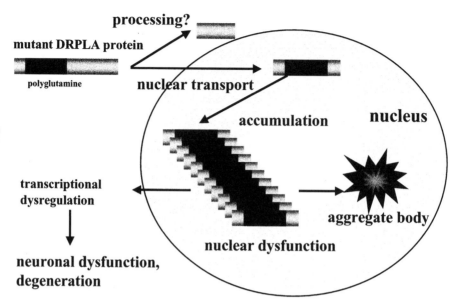

FIG. 24.1. A hypothetical model of neuronal dysfunction caused by mutant dentatorubral-pallidoluysian atrophy protein with expanded polyglutamine stretches.

there seems to be a wide time window for therapeutic approaches, and therapeutic strategies aimed against transcriptional dysregulation will be a challenging approach.

ACKNOWLEDGMENTS

This study was supported in part by the Research for the Future Program from the Japan Society for the Promotion of Science (JSPS-RFTF96L00103); a Grant-in-Aid for Scientific Research on Priority Areas (Human Genome Program) from the Ministry of Education, Science, Sports and Culture, Japan; a grant from the Research Committee for Ataxic Diseases, the Ministry of Health and Welfare, Japan; a grant for Surveys and Research on Specific Diseases, the Ministry of Health and Welfare, Japan; and special coordination funds from the Japanese Science and Technology Agency.

REFERENCES

1. Naito N, Oyanagi S. Familial myoclonus epilepsy and choreoathetosis: hereditary dentatorubral-pallidoluysian atrophy. *Neurology* 1982;32:789–817.

2. Smith JK, Gonda VE, Malamud N. Unusual form of cerebellar ataxia: combined dentato-rubral and pallido-Luysian degeneration. *Neurology* 1958;8:205–209.

3. Smith JK. Dentatorubropallidoluysian atrophy. In Vinken PJ, Bruyn GW, eds. *Handbook of clinical neurology.* Amsterdam: North-Holland 1975;21:519–534.

4. Naito H, Izawa K, Kurosaki T, et al. Two families of progressive myoclonus epilepsy with Mendelian dominant heredity [Japanese]. *Psychiatr Neurol Jpn* 1972;74:871–897.

5. Naito H, Ohama E, Nagai H. A family of dentatorubropallidoluysian atrophy (DRPLA) including two cases with schizophrenic symptoms [Japanese]. *Psychiatr Neurol Jpn* 1987;89:144–158.

6. Oyanagi S, Naito H. A clinico-neuropathological study on four autopsy cases of degenerative type of myoclonus epilepsy with Mendelian dominant heredity [Japanese]. *Psychiatr Neurol Jpn* 1977;79:113–129.

7. Tanaka Y, Murobushi K, Ando S, et al. Combined degeneration of the globus pallidus and the cerebellar nuclei and their efferent systems in two siblings of one family: primary system degeneration of the globus pallidus and the cerebellar nuclei. [Japanese]. *Brain Nerve* 1977;29:95–104.

8. Hirayama K, Iizuka R, Maehara K, et al. Clinico-pathological study of dentatorubropallidoluysian atrophy. Part I: its clinical form and analysis of symptomatology [Japanese]. *Adv Neurol* 1981;25:725–736.

9. Iizuka R, Hirayama K, Maehara KA. Dentato-rubro-pallido-luysian atrophy: a clinico-pathological study. *J Neurol Neurosurg Psychiatry* 1984;47:1288–1298.

10. Suzuki S, Kamoshita S, Ninomura S. Ramsay Hunt syndrome in dentatorubral-pallidoluysian atrophy. *Pediatr Neurol* 1985;1:298–301.

11. Iizuka R, Hirayama K. Dentato-rubro-pallido-luysian atrophy. In Vinken PJ, Bruyn GW, Klawans HL, eds. *Handbook of clinical neurology.* Amsterdam: North-Holland 1986;5:437–443.

12. Iwabuchi K. Clinico-pathological studies on dentato-rubro-pallido-luysian atrophy (DRPLA). *Yokohama Med J* 1987;38:291–301.

13. Iwabuchi K, Amano N, Yagishita S, et al. A clinico-pathological study on familial cases of dentatorubro-pallidoluysian atrophy (DRPLA). *Clin Neurol* 1987; 27:1002–1012.

14. Akashi T, Ando S, Inose T, et al. Dentato-rubro-pallido-luysian atrophy: a clinicopathological study [Japanese]. *Rinsho Seishin Igaku* 1987;29:523–531.

15. Koide R, Ikeuchi T, Onodera O, et al. Unstable expansion of CAG repeat in hereditary dentatorubral-pallidoluysian atrophy (DRPLA). *Nat Genet* 1994;6:9–13.

16. Nagafuchi S, Yanagisawa H, Sato K, et al. Expansion of an unstable CAG trinucleotide on chromosome 12p in dentatorubral and pallidoluysian atrophy. *Nat Genet* 1994;6:14–18.

17. La Spada AR, Wilson EM, Lubahn DB, et al. Androgen receptor gene mutations in X-linked spinal and bulbar muscular atrophy. *Nature* 1991;352:77–79.

18. The Huntington's Disease Collaborative Research Group. A novel gene containing a trinucleotide repeat that is expanded and unstable on Huntington's disease chromosomes. *Cell* 1993;72:971–983.

19. Orr HT, Chung MY, Banfi S, et al. Expansion of an unstable trinucleotide CAG repeat in spinocerebellar ataxia type 1. *Nat Genet* 1993;4:221–226.

20. Kawakami H, Maruyama H, Nakamura S, et al. Unique features of the CAG repeats in Machado-Joseph disease. *Nat Genet* 1995;9:344–345.

21. Sanpei K, Takano H, Igarashi S, et al. Identification of the spinocerebellar ataxia type 2 gene using a direct identification of repeat expansion and cloning technique, DIRECT. *Nat Genet* 1996;14:277–284.

22. Pulst SM, Nechiporuk A, Nechiporuk T, et al. Moderate expansion of a normally biallelic trinucleotide repeat in spinocerebellar ataxia type 2. *Nat Genet* 1996; 14:269–276.

23. Imbert G, Saudou F, Yvert G, et al. Cloning of the gene for spinocerebellar ataxia 2 reveals a locus with high sensitivity to expanded CAG/glutamine repeats. *Nat Genet* 1996;14:285–291.

24. Zhuchenko O, Bailey J, Bonnen P, et al. Autosomal dominant cerebellar ataxia (SCA6) associated with small polyglutamine expansions in the alpha 1a-voltage-dependent calcium channel. *Nat Genet* 1997;15:62–69.

25. David G, Abbas N, Stevanin G, et al. Cloning of the SCA7 gene reveals a highly unstable CAG repeat expansion. *Nat Genet* 1997;17:65–70.

26. Naito H, Oyanagi S. Familial myoclonus epilepsy and choreoathetosis: hereditary dentatorubral-pallidoluysian atrophy. *Neurology* 1982;32:798–807.

27. Inazuki G, Kumagai K, Naito H. Dentatorubral-pallidoluysian atrophy (DRPLA): its distribution in Japan and prevalence rate in Niigata. *Seishin Igaku* 1990;32:1135–1138.

28. Titica J, van Bogaert L. Heredo-degenerative hemiballismus: a contribution to the question of primary atrophy of the corpus Luysii. *Brain* 1946;69:251–263.

29. De Barsy TH, Myle G, Troch C, et al. La Dyssynergie cerebelleuse myoclonique (R. Hunt): affection au-tonome ou rariante du type degeneratif de l'epilepsie-myoclonie progressive (Unvericht-Lundborg) appoche anatomo-alinique. *J Neurol Sci* 1968;8:111–127.

30. Farmer TW, Wingfield MS, Lynch SA, et al. Ataxia, chorea, seizures, and dementia: pathologic features of a newly defined familial disorder. *Arch Neurol* 1989; 46:774–779.

31. Warner TT, Williams L, Harding AE. DRPLA in Europe. *Nat Genet* 1994;6:225.

32. Warner TT, Lennox GG, Janota I, et al. Autosomal-dominant dentatorubropallidoluysian atrophy in the united kingdom. *Mov Disord* 1994;9:289–296.

33. Norremolle A, Nielsen JE, Sorensen SA, et al. Elongated CAG repeats of the B37 gene in a Danish family with dentato-rubro-pallido-luysian atrophy. *Hum Genet* 1995;95:313–318.

34. Connarty M, Dennis NR, Patch C, et al. Molecular re-investigation of patients with Huntington's disease in Wessex reveals a family with dentatorubral and pallidoluysian atrophy. *Hum Genet* 1996;97:76–78.

35. Burke JR, Wingfield MS, Lewis KE, et al. The Haw River syndrome: dentatorubropallidoluysian atrophy (DRPLA) in an African-American family. *Nat Genet* 1994;7:521–524.

36. Potter NT. The relationship between (CAG)n repeat number and age of onset in a family with dentatorubral-pallidoluysian atrophy (DRPLA): diagnostic implications of confirmatory and predictive testing. *J Med Genet* 1996;33:168–170.

37. Ikeuchi T, Koide R, Tanaka H, et al. Dentatorubral-pallidoluysian atrophy (DRPLA): clinical features are closely related to unstable expansions of trinucleotide (CAG) repeat. *Ann Neurol* 1995;37:769–775.

38. Ikeuchi T, Onodera O, Oyake M, et al. Dentatorubral-pallidoluysian atrophy (DRPLA): close correlation of CAG repeat expansions with the wide spectrum of clinical presentations and prominent anticipation. *Semin Cell Biol* 1995;6:37–44.

39. Ikeuchi T, Koide R, Onodera O, et al. Dentatorubral-pallidoluysian atrophy (DRPLA): molecular basis for wide clinical features of DRPLA. *Clin Neurosci* 1995; 3:23–27.

40. Koide R, Onodera O, Ikeuchi T, et al. Atrophy of the cerebellum and brainstem in dentatorubral pallidoluysian atrophy: influence of CAG repeat size on MRI findings. *Neurology* 1997;49:1605–1612.

41. Naito H. [Clinical picture of DRPLA] [Review] [Japanese]. *No To Shinkei* 1995;47:931–938.

42. Ueno S, Kondoh K, Kotani Y, et al. Somatic mosaicism of CAG repeat in dentatorubral-pallidoluysian atrophy (DRPLA). *Hum Mol Genet* 1995;4:663–666.

43. Onodera O, Oyake M, Takano H, et al. Molecular cloning of a full-length cDNA for dentatorubral-pallidoluysian atrophy and regional expressions of the expanded alleles in the CNS. *Am J Hum Genet* 1995;57:1050–1060.

44. Nagafuchi S, Yanagisawa H, Ohsaki E, et al. Structure and expression of the gene responsible for the triplet repeat disorder, dentatorubral and pallidoluysian atrophy (DRPLA). *Nat Genet* 1994;8:177–182.

45. Miyashita T, Nagao K, Ohmi K, et al. Intracellular aggregate formation of dentatorubral-pallidoluysian atrophy (DRPLA) protein with the extended polyglutamine. *Biochem Biophys Res Commun* 1998;249:96–102.

46. Sato A, Shimohata T, Koide R, et al. Adenovirus-mediated expression of mutant DRPLA proteins with expanded polyglutamine stretches in neuronally differentiated PC12 cells: preferential intranuclear aggregate formation and apoptosis. *Hum Mol Genet* 1999;8: 997–1006.

47. Takano T, Yamanouchi Y, Nagafuchi S, et al. Assignment of the dentatorubral and pallidoluysian atrophy (DRPLA) gene to 12p 13.31 by fluorescence in situ hybridization. *Genomics* 1996;32:171–172.

48. Yazawa I, Nukina N, Hashida H, et al. Abnormal gene product identified in hereditary dentatorubral-pallidoluysian atrophy (DRPLA) brain. *Nat Genet* 1995; 10:99–103.

49. Duyao M, Ambrose C, Myers R, et al. Trinucleotide repeat length instability and age of onset in Huntington's disease. *Nat Genet* 1993;4:387–392.

50. Snell RG, MacMillan JC, Cheadle JP, et al. Relationship between trinucleotide repeat expansion and phenotypic variation in Huntington's disease. *Nat Genet* 1993;4:393–397.

51. Andrew SE, Goldberg YP, Kremer B, et al. The relationship between trinucleotide (CAG) repeat length and clinical features of Huntington's disease. *Nat Genet* 1993;4:398–403.

52. Chung MY, Ranum LP, Duvick LA, et al. Evidence for a mechanism predisposing to intergenerational CAG repeat instability in spinocerebellar ataxia type I. *Nat Genet* 1993;5:254–258.

53. Telenius H, Kremer B, Goldberg YP, et al. Somatic and gonadal mosaicism of the Huntington disease gene CAG repeat in brain and sperm. *Nat Genet* 1994; 6:409–414.

54. Sato T, Oyake M, Nakamura K, et al. Transgenic mice harboring a full length human mutant DRPLA gene reveal CAG repeat instability. *Hum Mol Genet* 1999;8: 99–106.

55. La Spada AR, Peterson KR, Meadows SA, et al. Androgen receptor YAC transgenic mice carrying CAG 45 alleles show trinucleotide repeat instability. *Hum Mol Genet* 1998;7:959–967.

56. Kaytor MD, Burright EN, Duvick LA, et al. Increased trinucleotide repeat instability with advanced maternal age. *Hum Mol Genet* 1997;6:2135–2139.

57. Chong SS, McCall AE, Cota J, et al. Gametic and somatic tissue-specific heterogeneity of the expanded SCA1 CAG repeat in spinocerebellar ataxia type 1. *Nat Genet* 1995;10:344–350.

58. Takano H, Onodera O, Takahashi H, et al. Somatic mosaicism of expanded CAG repeats in brains of patients with dentatorubral-pallidoluysian atrophy: cellular population-dependent dynamics of mitotic instability. *Am J Hum Genet* 1996;58:1212–1222.

59. Hashida H, Goto J, Kurisaki H, et al. Brain regional differences in the expansion of a CAG repeat in the spinocerebellar ataxias: dentatorubral-pallidoluysian atrophy, Machado-Joseph disease, and spinocerebellar ataxia type 1. *Ann Neurol* 1997;41:505–511.

60. Manley K, Shirley TL, Flaherty L, et al. Msh2 deficiency prevents in vivo somatic instability of the CAG repeat in Huntington disease transgenic mice. *Nat Genet* 1999;23:471–473.

61. Ikeda H, Yamaguchi M, Sugai S, et al. Expanded polyglutamine in the Machado-Joseph disease protein induces cell death in vitro and in vivo. *Nat Genet* 1996;13:196–202.

62. Paulson HL, Perez MK, Trottier Y, et al. Intranuclear inclusions of expanded polyglutamine protein in spinocerebellar ataxia type 3. *Neuron* 1997;19:333–344.

63. Igarashi S, Koide R, Shimohata T, et al. Suppression of aggregate formation and apoptosis by transglutaminase inhibitors in cells expressing truncated DRPLA protein with an expanded polyglutamine stretch. *Nat Genet* 1998;18:111–117.

64. Martindale D, Hackam A, Wieczorek A, et al. Length of huntingtin and its polyglutamine tract influences localization and frequency of intracellular aggregates. *Nat Genet* 1998;18:150–154.

65. Cooper JK, Schilling G, Peters MF, et al. Truncated N-terminal fragments of huntingtin with expanded glutamine repeats form nuclear and cytoplasmic aggregates in cell culture. *Hum Mol Genet* 1998;7:783–790.

66. Mangiarini L, Sathasivam K, Seller M, et al. Exon 1 of the HD gene with an expanded CAG repeat is sufficient to cause a progressive neurological phenotype in transgenic mice. *Cell* 1996;87:493–506.

67. Hodgson JG, Agopyan N, Gutekunst CA, et al. A YAC mouse model for Huntington's disease with full-length mutant huntingtin, cytoplasmic toxicity, and selective striatal neurodegeneration. *Neuron* 1999;23:181–192.

68. Adachi H, Kume A, Li M, et al. Transgenic mice with an expanded CAG repeat controlled by the human AR promoter show polyglutamine nuclear inclusions and neuronal dysfunction without neuronal cell death. *Hum Mol Genet* 2001;10:1039–1048.

69. Davies SW, Turmaine M, Cozens BA, et al. Formation of neuronal intranuclear inclusions underlies the neurological dysfunction in mice transgenic for the HD mutation. *Cell* 1997;90:537–548.

70. Skinner PJ, Koshy BT, Cummings CJ, et al. Ataxin-1 with an expanded glutamine tract alters nuclear matrix-associated structures. *Nature* 1997;389:971–974.

71. Difiglia M, Sapp E, Chase KO, et al. Aggregation of huntingtin in neuronal intranuclear inclusions and dystrophic neurites in brain. *Science* 1997;277: 1990–1993.

72. Hayashi Y, Kakita A, Yamada M, et al. Hereditary dentatorubral-pallidoluysian atrophy: ubiquitinated filamentous inclusions in the cerebellar dentate nucleus neurons. *Acta Neuropathol (Berl)* 1998;95:479–482.

73. Holmberg M, Duyckaerts C, Durr A, et al. Spinocerebellar ataxia type 7 (SCA7): a neurodegenerative disorder with neuronal intranuclear inclusions. *Hum Mol Genet* 1998;7:913–918.

74. Li M, Miwa S, Kobayashi Y, et al. Nuclear inclusions of the androgen receptor protein in spinal and bulbar muscular atrophy. *Ann Neurol* 1998;44:249–254.

75. Koyano S, Uchihara T, Fujigasaki H, et al. Neuronal intranuclear inclusions in spinocerebellar ataxia type 2: triple-labeling immunofluorescent study. *Neurosci Lett* 1999;273:117–120.

76. Turmaine M, Raza A, Mahal A, et al. Nonapoptotic neurodegeneration in a transgenic mouse model of Huntington's disease. *Proc Natl Acad Sci USA* 2000; 97:8093–8097.

77. Yamamoto A, Lucas JJ, Hen R. Reversal of neuropathology and motor dysfunction in a conditional model of Huntington's disease. *Cell* 2000;101:57–66.

78. Yamada M, Wood JD, Shimohata T, et al. Widespread occurrence of intranuclear atrophin-1 accumulation in the central nervous system neurons of patients with dentatorubral-pallidoluysian atrophy. *Ann Neurol* 2001;49:14–23.

79. Klement IA, Skinner PJ, Kaytor MD, et al. Ataxin-1 nuclear localization and aggregation: role in polyglutamine-induced disease in SCA1 transgenic mice. *Cell* 1998;95:41–53.

80. Saudou F, Finkbeiner S, Devys D, et al. Huntingtin acts in the nucleus to induce apoptosis but death does not correlate with the formation of intranuclear inclusions. *Cell* 1998;95:55–66.

81. Li XJ, Li SH, Sharp AH, et al. A huntingtin-associated protein enriched in brain with implications for pathology. *Nature* 1995;378:398–402.

82. Burke JR, Enghild JJ, Martin ME, et al. Huntingtin and DRPLA proteins selectively interact with the enzyme GAPDH. *Nat Med* 1996;2:347–350.

83. Kalchman MA, Graham RK, Xia G, et al. Huntingtin is ubiquitinated and interacts with a specific ubiquitin-conjugating enzyme. *J Biol Chem* 1996;271:19385–19394.

84. Koshy B, Matilla T, Burright EN, et al. Spinocerebellar ataxia type-1 and spinobulbar muscular atrophy gene products interact with glyceraldehyde-3-phosphate dehydrogenase. *Hum Mol Genet* 1996;5:1311–1318.

85. Bao J, Sharp AH, Wagster MV, et al. Expansion of polyglutamine repeat in huntingtin leads to abnormal protein interactions involving calmodulin. *Proc Natl Acad Sci USA* 1996;93:5037–5042.

86. Matilla A, Koshy BT, Cummings CJ, et al. The cerebellar leucine-rich acidic nuclear protein interacts with ataxin-1. *Nature* 1997;389:974–978.

87. Onodera O, Burke JR, Miller SE, et al. Oligomerization of expanded-polyglutamine domain fluorescent fusion proteins in cultured mammalian cells. *Biochem Biophys Res Commun* 1997;238:599–605.

88. Wanker EE, Rovira C, Scherzinger E, et al. HIP-I: a huntingtin interacting protein isolated by the yeast two-hybrid system. *Hum Mol Genet* 1997;6:487–495.

89. Sittler A, Walter S, Wedemeyer N, et al. SH3GL3 associates with the Huntingtin exon 1 protein and promotes the formation of polygln-containing protein aggregates. *Mol Cell* 1998;2:427–436.

90. Faber PW, Barnes GT, Srinidhi J, et al. Huntingtin interacts with a family of WW domain proteins. *Hum Mol Genet* 1998;7:1463–1474.

91. Boutell JM, Wood JD, Harper PS, et al. Huntingtin interacts with cystathionine beta-synthase. *Hum Mol Genet* 1998;7:371–378.

92. Wood JD, Yuan J, Margolis RL, et al. Atrophin-1, the DRPLA gene product, interacts with two families of WW domain-containing proteins. *Mol Cell Neurosci* 1998;11:149–160.

93. Nagai Y, Onodera O, Strittmatter WJ, et al. Polyglutamine domain proteins with expanded repeats bind neurofilament, altering the neurofilament network. *Ann N Y Acad Sci* 1999;893:192–202.

94. Wood JD, Nucifora Jr FC, Duan K, et al. Atrophin-1, the dentato-rubral and pallido-luysian atrophy gene product, interacts with ETO/MTG8 in the nuclear matrix and represses transcription. *J Cell Biol* 2000;150:939–948.

95. McCampbell A, Taylor JP, Taye AA, et al. CREB-binding protein sequestration by expanded polyglutamine. *Hum Mol Genet* 2000;9:2197–2202.

96. Waragai M, Junn E, Kajikawa M, et al. PQBP-1/Npw38, a nuclear protein binding to the polyglutamine tract, interacts with U5-15kD/dim1p via the carboxyl-terminal domain. *Biochem Biophys Res Commun* 2000;273:592–595.

97. Steffan JS, Kazantsev A, Spasic-Boskovic O, et al. The Huntington's disease protein interacts with p53 and CREB-binding protein and represses transcription. *Proc Natl Acad Sci U S A* 2000;97:6763–6768.

98. Shimohata T, Nakajima T, Yamada M, et al. Expanded polyglutamine stretches interact with TAFII130, interfering with CREB-dependent transcription. *Nat Genet* 2000;26:29–36.

99. Nucifora Jr FC, Sasaki M, Peters MF, et al. Interference by huntingtin and atrophin-1 with cbp-mediated transcription leading to cellular toxicity. *Science* 2001;291:2423–2428.

100. Luthi-Carter R, Strand A, Peters NL, et al. Decreased expression of striatal signaling genes in a mouse model of Huntington's disease. *Hum Mol Genet* 2000;9:1259–1271.

101. Lin X, Antalffy B, Kang D, et al. Polyglutamine expansion down-regulates specific neuronal genes before pathologic changes in SCA1. *Nat Neurosci* 2000;3:157–163.

Myoclonus and Paroxysmal Dyskinesias,
Advances in Neurology, Vol. 89,
edited by S. Fahn, et al.
Lippincott Williams & Wilkins, Philadelphia © 2002.

25

The Role of the Serotonin System in Animal Models of Myoclonus

*Christopher G. Goetz, *Paul M. Carvey,
§Eric J. Pappert, ‡Toan Q. Vu, and *†Sue E. Leurgans

*Department of Neurological Sciences, †Department of Preventive Medicine, Rush University,
Rush-Presbyterian-St. Luke's Medical Center, Chicago, Illinois; §Neurology Associates, Austin, Texas;
and ‡Department of Neurology, University of Missouri Health Care, Columbia, Missouri

In 1971, Lhermitte et al. empirically and successfully treated patients with 5-hydroxytryptophan (5-HTP) and improved their posthypoxic myoclonus (1). This observation opened an era of interest in the serotonin system and its relationship to myoclonus as a movement disorder. The discovery that posthypoxic patients with myoclonus (Lance-Adams syndrome) had low levels of 5-hydroxy-indole acetic acid (5-HIAA), the cerebrospinal fluid metabolite of serotonin, further supported a hypothesis that this disorder related to low central nervous system serotonin activity (2). However, other reports linked high serotonergic function to myoclonus, especially drug-induced forms (3). To amplify these early clinical reports and examine the mechanism of serotonergic influences in myoclonus, a number of animal models have been developed. These models predominantly involve small laboratory mammals and have served to define anatomic and neuropharmacologic mechanisms related to myoclonus. They also suggest therapeutic options and areas of future research in humans with this movement disorder.

NEUROCHEMISTRY OF THE SEROTONERGIC SYSTEM

Serotonin is synthesized from the dietary amino acid tryptophan and the intermediate metabolite 5-HTP. Tryptophan hydroxylase is the rate-limiting enzyme for serotonin synthesis that transforms tryptophan to 5-HTP, and the second reaction to form serotonin from 5-HTP involves the nonspecific enzyme aromatic amino acid decarboxylase. This latter enzyme is the same enzyme that converts levodopa to dopamine (4). The primary cell bodies of most serotonergic neurons are located in the raphe nuclei, and projection sites include the forebrain, basal ganglia, brainstem, and spinal cord (5). Subclasses of serotonin receptors are unequally distributed in these various regions (6). Serotonin is metabolized by presynaptic reuptake and then degradation by monoamine oxidase to 5-HIAA.

ANIMAL MODELS

Whereas there are many behaviors associated with high or low nervous system serotonin, four primary serotonergic models have been developed for myoclonus. P, p-DDT (P, p-dicholorophenyltrichloroethane) is a toxin that induces stimulus-sensitive myoclonus in the rat (7). The movement disorder is improved by augmentation of serotonergic activity through various pharmacologic agents and exacerbated by serotonergic antagonists (8). Because of the highly toxic nature of p, p-DDT and the self-limited nature of the myoclonus, this is a complicated model to use and has not been adopted extensively in behavioral and biochemical research efforts. A second, technically complex model of myoclonus involves the intracisternal or intraventricular injection of dihydroxylated indole compounds that destroy serotonergic terminals (9). In this lesion model, subsequent systemic administration of serotonergic agonists or intracerebral infusions of serotonin induce myoclonus, whereas the abnormal behavior can be prevented by prior inhibition of serotonin synthesis. The multiple steps involved in the generation of this model and its unclear direct extrapolation to human disease have limited its application (10).

In our laboratory, we have worked with two other models, one involving systemic injections of 5-HTP in the guinea pig and the other involving cardiac arrest in the rat with subsequent spontaneous development of audiosensitive myoclonus. In each of these, we and other investigators have studied the serotonergic system pharmacologically.

5-HYDROXYTRYPTOPHAN-INDUCED MYOCLONUS IN YOUNG GUINEA PIGS

In the intact young guinea pig, subcutaneous injections of 5-HTP lead to symmetric, generalized, rhythmic myoclonic jerks (11). At low intensity, these movements involve the head and trunk, but in a dose-dependent manner, they progress over 60 to 90 minutes to involve the entire body and provoke myoclonic jerks that cause the animal to jump from the laboratory floor (12). Myoclonus frequency can be rated over 1 minute every 10 minutes and expressed over time to give a total score or an area under the curve (Fig. 25.1). Both intensity and duration of the myoclonus correlate with brain serotonin levels (11). The myoclonus can be augmented by serotonin agonists, by serotonin reuptake inhibitors, or with tryptophan in conjunction with monoamine oxidase inhibition (13). Conversely, myoclonus is blocked by serotonergic receptor antagonists

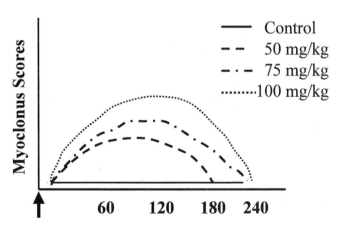

FIG. 25.1. Dose-response curves for 5-hydroxytryptophan-induced myoclonus in young guinea pigs. The *arrow* indicates injection time and the horizontal axis represents the number of minutes. To test for enhancement and reduction of the behavior by a pharmacologic agent, drugs are usually tested in the context of the middle dose (75 mg per kg). (From, Carvey P, Paulseth JE, Goetz CG, et al. 5-HTP-induced myoclonic jumping behavior in guinea pigs. *Adv Neurol* 1986;43:509–516.)

and specifically antagonized in dose-dependent fashion by agents that block the 5-hydroxytryptamine$_{1/2}$ (5-HT$_{1/2}$) subsystems (14). Of an array of serotonergic receptor antagonists, only mesulergine and methiothepin antagonized myoclonus (Fig. 25.2).

Whereas the behavior is directly related to serotonergic activation, modifying effects occur with manipulation of nonserotonergic systems. Dopamine receptor agonists diminish myoclonus when given acutely, although chronic treatment can augment the behavior (15). Low-dose neuroleptics enhance the intensity of myoclonus (15) (Fig. 25.3).

Future work with this model will focus on precise identification of the anatomic locus responsible for this serotonergic behavior. Because a large variety of drugs used in clinical practice can provoke myoclonus, this animal model may be most applicable to studying the pathophysiology and pharmacology of drug-induced myoclonus. Pharmacologic agents

that can induce myoclonus in humans include antidepressants that block presynaptic reuptake of serotonin and medications that have serotonin receptor agonist properties, such as lisuride (16). Because dopaminergic pharmacology influences serotonergic function, dopamine agents that induce myoclonus, such as levodopa, bromocriptine, and amantadine, may do so by indirectly involving serotonergic systems (3,17). Levodopa-induced myoclonus in Parkinson disease has been hypothesized to relate to serotonin displacement from terminals by large doses of levodopa (3).

5-HTP-induced myoclonus has also been posited to serve as a model for myoclonic syndromes seen particularly in young patients. Because the animal behavior is most marked in young guinea pigs, the original report on the model suggested that the behavior might serve best as a model for infantile spasms, a pediatric condition associated with myoclonus (11). In a series of Down syn-

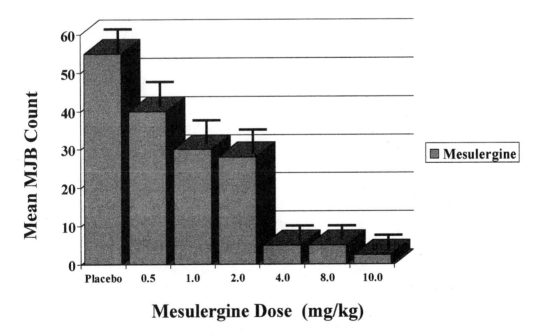

FIG. 25.2. Effects of the serotonin receptor-specific antagonist mesulergine on 5-hydroxytryptophan-induced myoclonus. Mesulergine and methiothepin were effective antagonists of the behavior in contrast to the others tested. (From, Pappert EJ, Goetz CG, Stebbins GT, et al. 5-HTP-induced myoclonus in guinea pigs: mediation through 5HT$_{1/2}$ receptor subtypes. *Eur J Pharmacol* 1998;347: 51–56.)

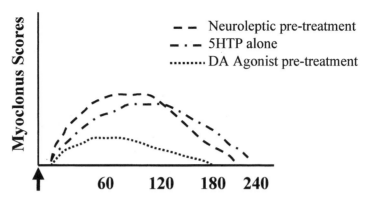

FIG. 25.3. Effects of dopaminergic manipulation on 5-hydroxytryptophan-induced myoclonus. Neuroleptic pretreatment augments the peak intensity of myoclonus and acute pretreatment with a dopamine agonist inhibits the behavior. The *arrow* represents time of 5HTP injection and the horizontal axis represents minutes. (From, Weiner WJ, Carvey PM, Nausieda PA, et al. Dopaminergic antagonism of 5-HTP-induced myoclonic jumping behavior. *Neurology* 1979;29:1622–1627.)

drome patients treated with 5-HTP, 9 of 60 developed infantile spasms with myoclonus syndrome that abated or improved when 5-HTP was stopped (18). Furthermore, in cases of infantile spasms without Down syndrome, high serum serotonin levels can be detected in some patients (19). Altered tryptophan metabolism with increased excretion of xanthurenic acids has frequently been reported in infantile spasms (20,21). The model may also be applied to study the mechanism of myoclonus in neuroblastomas, tumors that produce catecholamines, and, on occasion, indolaminergic products (11).

POSTHYPOXIC AUDIOGENIC MYOCLONUS IN THE RAT

The second model that has been a focus of our laboratory research involves rats that undergo cardiac arrest and develop posthypoxic audiosensitive myoclonus. This behavior is posited to be a model for posthypoxic myoclonus in humans, a sequel of cardiac or pulmonary arrest and also known as Lance-Adams syndrome. Normal rats demonstrate low levels of myoclonic jerks when exposed to sudden sound. Cardiac arrest induced by surgical kinking of the great vessels in the rat provokes a marked enhancement of this be-

havior that is quantifiable by a standardized rating scale (22). The protocol developed by Truong et al. (22) exposes animals to a 95-dB, 40-ms, 1-Hz click that is generated by a metronome. The resultant myoclonic behavior is rated from 0 (no reaction) to 5 (whole body jerk of such severity that the animal jumps). A set of 45 auditory stimuli provides a total myoclonus score that can range from 0 to 225. A series of five to ten sets, each separated by a 10-minute rest period, generates a mean myoclonus score for that day. When the cardiac arrests last 8 minutes, myoclonus is markedly enhanced over presurgical scores and lasts in a relatively stable condition above the baseline levels for 1 week (23) (Fig. 25.4). These features provide the opportunity for both acute and more chronic pharmacologic testing of the serotonergic system.

In this model, myoclonus improves with 5-HTP treatment, and the severity scores inversely correlate with striatal serotonin and cortical 5-HIAA levels (24). Conversely, myoclonus is blocked by two serotonergic receptor antagonists, mesulergine and methiothepin, in a dose-dependent manner (25). These antagonists, the same ones that selectively inhibited myoclonus in the guinea pig model (see above), primarily affect the 5-$HT_{1/2}$ subsystems, suggesting that brain areas

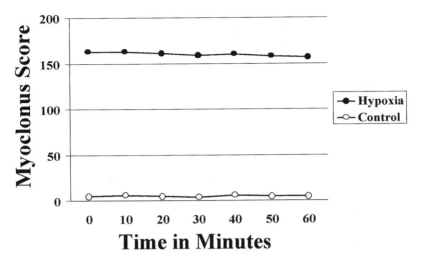

FIG. 25.4. Postanoxic myoclonus in the rat. *Upper line* shows high myoclonus scores after hypoxia, compared to normal controls. (From, Goetz CG, Vu TQ, Carvey PM, et al. Post-hypoxic myoclonus in the rat: natural history, stability and serotonergic influences. *Mov Disord* 2000;15(Suppl 1):39–46.)

rich in these populations may be primarily affected by hypoxia (Fig. 25.5). Mesulergine blocks primarily 5-HT$_2$ receptors, and the three highest doses tests (9 to 15 mg per kg) reduced the myoclonic responses compared with placebo. Methiothepin affects both 5-HT$_1$ and 5-HT$_2$ receptors, and all doses studied (0.5 to 5 mg per kg) significantly antagonized myoclonus. The more substantial effect of methiothepin compared with mesulergine may relate to the former drug's ability to block both receptor subtypes. GR 127935, a relatively specific antagonist of the 5-HT$_{1D}$ receptors without marked activity at 5-HT$_2$ receptors induced a trend toward reduction in myoclonus. Serotonergic antagonists that primarily block other subtypes of receptors do not inhibit the myoclonus in these posthypoxic animals.

The model has also been used in pharmacologic studies of serotonergic agonists. Acute treatment with 5-HT$_{1C}$ agonists and chronic treatment with 5-HT$_{1A}$ agonists decrease posthypoxic myoclonus (26). Furthermore, a significant reduction in KCl-stimulated and N–methyl–D–asparate (NMDA)-stimulated release of serotonin occurs as a consequence of cardiac arrest and myoclonus

in this model (27). Together, the serotonin agonist and antagonist studies suggest that a focus on the brain regions dense in 5-HT$_{1/2}$ receptors may be key to understanding the anatomic substrate of posthypoxic myoclonus. The fact that the same influence on myoclonus can be affected by agonists and antagonists depending on duration of treatment suggests a high level of plasticity or feedback control within the involved receptor populations. Current work using this model and 2-deoxyglucose autoradiography is aimed at defining regions of interest with high densities of 5-HT$_{1/2}$ receptors most affected by hypoxia.

The primary advantage of this animal model is its close behavioral correlation with a human condition. Unlike the guinea pig and toxin-induced models, this behavior occurs as a direct consequence of cardiac arrest, the same precipitant that provokes Lance-Adams syndrome in humans. No other pharmacologic manipulation is necessary to provoke the myoclonus. Furthermore, like Lance-Adams syndrome, the myoclonus is stimulus sensitive, in this case, particularly by sound stimuli. In addition to these clinical parallels, the stability of the behavior over 1 week allows for acute pharmacologic studies as well

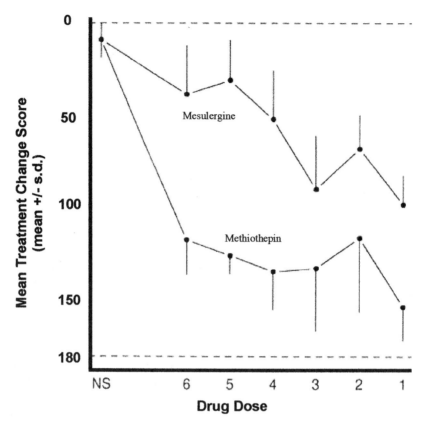

FIG. 25.5. Dose-response curves for mesulergine (dose range, 1.5 to 15 mg per kg) and methio-thepin (dose range, 0.5 to 5.0 mg per kg) and reduction of postanoxic myoclonus in the rat. (From, Pappert EJ, Goetz CG, Vu TQ, et al. Animal model of post-hypoxic myoclonus: effects of serotonergic antagonists. *Neurology* 1999;52:16–21.)

as longer treatments that would mimic chronic therapies in humans.

Final explanations generated by this rat model in regard to the pathophysiology of posthypoxic myoclonus, however, must integrate the simultaneous observations that the myoclonus is aborted by agents that augment (5-HTP) as well as antagonize (selective receptor blockers) serotonergic activity. Pathologic studies in humans demonstrate that serotonergic cell populations are not destroyed in patients with Lance-Adams syndrome, suggesting that neurochemical rather than structural changes underlie the behavioral alterations (20). Several different neuropharmacologic hypotheses can be offered for this apparent paradox. First, the amount of 5-HTP delivered to the brain and the consequent degree of serotonergic stimulation are sufficient to cause a depolarization blockade that inhibits receptors effectively in a comparable fashion with selected receptor blockade. In this way, the two pharmacologic interventions produce a similar final inhibition on the movement disorder. Second 5-HTP could be transformed into serotonin and could activate selectively yet-to-be-identified hypersensitive serotonergic receptor populations that are in antagonistic equilibrium with 5-HT$_1$ and 5-HT$_2$ receptors. The same therapeutic benefit thus could result from either 5-HTP treatment or blockade of the antagonistic 5-HT$_1$ and 5-HT$_2$ receptor subtypes. Additionally, 5-HT$_{1B/1D}$ receptors are primarily autoreceptors, and their activation decreases serotonin release (21).

Hence, antagonism would increase serotonin release possibly similar to the effects of 5-HTP. Finally, serotonin receptors are coupled to other neurotransmitters, for example, dopamine in the striatum, so that some effects of serotonin antagonism can relate to activation or inhibition of these chemicals.

FUTURE PERSPECTIVES

Serotonergic neurochemistry has been implicated in the pathophysiology of several human neurobehavioral disorders besides myoclonus, specifically migraine headaches, hallucinations, and depression. Though myoclonus is relatively rare, the prevalence of these more common disorders has stimulated the study and development of therapeutic agents that augment or diminish serotonergic activity in the central nervous system. Some such agents are currently available for human use and several others are in development. A systematic evaluation of these agents in the animal models of myoclonus will help delineate their specific mechanisms of action *in vivo* and help to define efficacy and screening data on drug safety in the context of myoclonus. Data derived from animal models can then be applied to human myoclonus to rank the chemical agents most likely to be applicable and safe for clinical use. Ultimately, well-designed, randomized, and placebo-controlled clinical trials of such agents will define their safety and efficacy in humans. In this way, the basic science laboratory and clinical neurologic centers work in concert, the former to define chemical systems and mechanisms of action of various agents, the latter to define safety and efficacy in patients with myoclonic disorders. Animal models of human neurologic disorders form the interface between these two scientific disciplines.

ACKNOWLEDGMENTS

The authors acknowledge the support of the Myoclonus Research Foundation and the United Parkinson Foundation (Parkinson Disease Foundation).

REFERENCES

1. Lhermitte F, Peterfalvi M, Marteau R, et al. Analyse pharmacologique d'un cas de myoclonie d'attention. *Rev Neurol* 1971;124:21–31.
2. Growdon JH, Young RR, Shahani BT. 5-HTP in treatment of several different syndromes in which myoclonus is prominent. *Neurology* 1976;26:1135–1140.
3. Klawans HL, Goetz C, Bergen D. Levodopa-induced myoclonus. *Arch Neurol* 1975;32:330–334.
4. Cooper JR, Bloom FE, Roth RH. *The biochemical basis of neuropharmacology.* New York: Oxford University Press, 1996.
5. Descarries L, Audet MA, Coucet G. Morphology of central serotonin receptors. In: Whitaker-Azmitia P, Peroutka BL, eds. *Neuropharmacology of serotonin.* New York: New York Academy of Sciences Press, 1990:81–92.
6. Glennon RA, Dukat M. Serotonin receptor subtypes. In: Bloom FE, Kupfer DJ, eds. *Psychopharmacology, The Fourth Generation of Progress.* New York: Raven Press, 1995.
7. Chung HE, Van Woert MH. P, p-DDT-induced neurotoxic syndrome: experimental myoclonus. *Neurology* 1978;28:1020–1023.
8. Chung HE, Van Woert MH. P, p-DDT-induced alterations in brain serotonin metabolism. *Neurotoxicology* 1981;2:649–655.
9. Stewart RM, Growdon JH, Cancian D, et al. Myoclonus after 5-HTP in rats with lesions of indoleamine neurons in the CNS. *Neurology* 1976;26:690–694.
10. Gerson SC, Baldessarini RJ. Motor effects of serotonin in the central nervous system. *Life Sci* 1980;27:1435–1439.
11. Klawans HL, Goetz C, Weiner WJ. 5-HTP-induced myoclonus in guinea pigs and the possible role of serotonin in infantile spasms. *Neurology* 1973;23:1234–1240.
12. Carvey P, Paulseth JE, Goetz CG, et al. 5-HTP-induced myoclonic jumping behavior in guinea pigs. *Adv Neurol* 1986;43:509–516.
13. Chadwick D, Hallett M, Jenner P, et al. 5-HTP induced myoclonus in guinea pigs: physiological and pharmacological investigation. *J Neurol Sci* 1978;35:157–163.
14. Pappert EJ, Goetz CG, Stebbins GT, et al. 5-HTP-induced myoclonus in guinea pigs: mediation through $5HT_{1/2}$ receptor subtypes. *Eur J Pharmacol* 1998;347:51–56.
15. Weiner WJ, Carvey PM, Nausieda PA, et al. Dopaminergic antagonism of 5-HTP-induced myoclonic jumping behavior. *Neurology* 1979;29:1622–1627.
16. Pappert EJ, Goetz CG. Treatment of myoclonus In: Kurlan R, ed. *Treatment of movement disorders.* Philadelphia: JB Lippincott, 1995:247–336.
17. Buchman AS, Bennett DA, Goetz CG. Bromocriptine-induced myoclonus. *Neurology* 1987;37:885–886.
18. Coleman M. Infantile spasms associated with 5-HTP administration in patients with Down's syndrome. *Neurology* 1971;21:911–919.
19. Coleman M, Boullin D, Davis M. Serotonin abnormalities in the infantile spasm syndrome. *Neurology* 1971;21:421.
20. Jeune M, Cotte J, Nermier M. L'épreuve de charge au tryptophane comme moyen de détection des apyridoxinoses chez l'enfant. *Pédiatrie* 1959;14:853–857.
21. Bower BD. Tryptophan load test in the syndrome of infantile spasms. *Proc R Soc Med* 1961;54:540–542.
22. Truong DD, Matsumoto RR, Schwartz PH, et al. Novel

rat cardiac arrest model of post-hypoxic myoclonus. *Mov Disord* 1994;9:201–206.

23. Goetz CG, Vu TQ, Carvey PM, et al. Post-hypoxic myoclonus in the rat: natural history, stability and serotonergic influences. *Mov Disord* 2000;15(Suppl 1):39–46.

24. Matsumoto RR, Aziz N, Truong DD. Association between brain indole levels and severity of posthypoxic myoclonus in rats. *Pharmacol Biochem Behav* 1995;50:553–558.

25. Pappert EJ, Goetz CG, Vu TQ, et al. Animal model of post-hypoxic myoclonus: effects of serotonergic antagonists. *Neurology* 1999;52:16–21.

26. Fleshler M. Adequate acoustic stimulus for startle reaction in the rat. *J Comp Physiol Psychol* 1965;69:200–207.

27. Kanthasamy AG, Vu TQ, Truong DD, et al. Neurochemical and behavioral correlates of posthypoxic myoclonus: a microdialysis study. *Soc Neurosci Abstr* 1995;21:2058.

Myoclonus and Paroxysmal Dyskinesias,
Advances in Neurology, Vol. 89,
edited by S. Fahn, et al.
Lippincott Williams & Wilkins, Philadelphia © 2002.

26

Involvement of γ-Aminobutyric Acid in Myoclonus

Rae R. Matsumoto

Department of Pharmaceutical Sciences, University of Oklahoma Health Sciences Center,
Oklahoma City, Oklahoma

γ-Aminobutyric acid (GABA) is a major inhibitory neurotransmitter. GABA is present in virtually every region of the brain (1), and it can act through one of three subtypes of receptors: $GABA_A$, $GABA_B$, and $GABA_C$ (2). The GABA receptor subtype that appears important in the context of myoclonus is the $GABA_A$ receptor.

This chapter is divided into four sections. First, background on $GABA_A$ receptor structure and pharmacology is provided. Second, evidence of an involvement of $GABA_A$ receptors in myoclonus, based on studies in experimental animals, is summarized. Third, clinical evidence for a role of GABA in myoclonus in humans and antimyoclonic pharmacotherapies that target GABA receptors are presented. Fourth, the interaction of GABA with other neurochemical systems involved in myoclonus is briefly reviewed.

GABA_A RECEPTORS: BACKGROUND

The three subtypes of GABA receptors ($GABA_A$, $GABA_B$, and $GABA_C$) can be distinguished from one another based on their amino acid sequences, signal transduction mechanisms, sensitivity to drugs, distribution in the body, and functional effects (Table 26.1). Several excellent reviews are available for reference (3–7). Therefore, only the

$GABA_A$ receptor will be summarized here because of its relevance to myoclonus.

GABA_A Receptor Structure

Recent advances in molecular biology have demonstrated that the $GABA_A$ receptor is a heteropentameric protein assembled from a combination of subunits. These subunits may include α, β, δ, γ, ε, θ, and π, some of which can be expressed as multiple isoforms and/or splice variants (3,5,6,8). Each of the five subunits that assemble together to form a $GABA_A$ receptor contains four transmembrane spanning domains, with the second transmembrane spanning region of each subunit forming the walls of the Cl^- ionophore (Fig. 26.1) (6,7). The specific subunit combinations that come together to form the $GABA_A$ receptor can vary, with individual subunits exhibiting different regional distributions in the brain (7,9–11). Differences in the subunit stoichiometry of $GABA_A$ receptors affect not only the responsiveness of the receptor to different drug classes, but also the potency of GABA itself (7). Furthermore, changing the order in which the subunits are assembled in the pentameric receptor sequence may also have functional consequences for the response of the receptor to drugs. Although the consequences of this

TABLE 26.1. *Differences between GABA receptor subtypes*

Type of receptor	GABA$_A$ ionotropic	GABA$_B$ metabotropic	GABA$_C$ ionotropic
Channels			
Cl$^-$	inc I$_{Cl}$	N/E	inc I$_{Cl}$
Ca^{2+}	N/E	dec I$_{Ca}$	N/E
K$^+$	N/E	inc I$_K$	N/E
Subunits	$\alpha,\beta,\gamma,\delta$	GABA$_B$1	ρ
	ϵ,π,θ	GABA$_B$2	
Ligands			
Bicuculline	Antagonist	N/E	N/E
Benzodiazepines	Enhance	N/E	N/E
Barbiturates	Enhance	N/E	N/E
Neurosteroids	Enhance	N/E	N/E
Picrotoxinin	Antagonist	N/E	Antagonist
Baclofen	N/E	Agonist	N/E
Phaclofen	N/E	Antagonist	N/E
CACA	N/E	N/E	Agonist
TPMPA	N/E	N/E	Antagonist
Distribution	CNS	CNS	Retina

CACA, cis-4-aminocrotonic acid; CNS, central nervous system; GABA, γ-aminobutyric acid; I, conductance; N/E, no effect; TPMPA, (1,2,5,6-tetrahydropyridine-4-yl)methylphosphinic acid.

molecular heterogeneity has yet to be studied in the context of myoclonus, it is likely that certain subtypes or subfamilies of GABA$_A$ receptors have important ramifications for the development and treatment of myoclonus, whereas others do not.

GABA$_A$ Receptor Pharmacology

In terms of the pharmacology related to this receptor, it has long been known that the GABA$_A$ receptor is a complex protein with multiple recognition sites. It contains, minimally, a GABA binding site coupled to a Cl$^-$ channel. In addition, the receptor complex may also contain binding sites for benzodiazepines, barbiturates, convulsants, neurosteroids, and/or ethanol (Fig. 26.1).

Convulsants, such as picrotoxin, are thought to bind within the Cl$^-$ ionophore, where they inhibit the activity of the channel (6,7). GABA, on the other hand, appears capable of interacting with several subunits that comprise GABA$_A$ receptors. Recombinant expression studies demonstrate that homooligomeric α, β, γ, or δ subunits form functional channels, but that channel assemblies comprised of combinations of two different subunits are often more responsive to

GABA (4,7). Furthermore, some subunits, such as ϵ, θ, and π, do not appear to form functional receptors when expressed alone, although they do so when coexpressed with α and β subunits (12–15). Therefore, some subunits have an integral role in the GABA$_A$ receptor complex, while other subunits may contribute to functional heterogeneity, including the differential responsiveness of the receptor complex to different drug classes.

Benzodiazepines, which enhance the effects of GABA by increasing the frequency of Cl$^-$ channel openings (16,17), appear to bind at the interface of α ($\alpha_{1,2,5}$) and γ ($\gamma_{2,3}$) subunits (5) and require a minimum of $\alpha\beta\gamma$ subunits in their pentameric structure to achieve a GABA-enhancing effect (18). Similarly to benzodiazepines, barbiturates have a GABA-enhancing effect when they interact with the GABA$_A$ receptor complex (6). However, unlike benzodiazepines that increase the frequency of Cl$^-$ channel openings, barbiturates act by prolonging the open duration of the channels and can do so even in the absence of GABA (7,16,17). Barbiturates can interact with multiple subunits that assemble together to form a functional GABA$_A$ receptor (7,19–21). Of the many subunits with which these drugs may interact, the specific binding

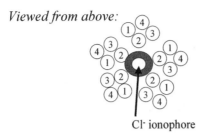

Viewed from above:

Cl⁻ ionophore

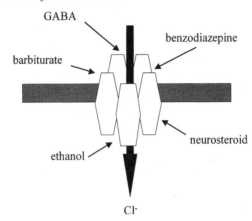

Viewed from the side:

GABA

benzodiazepine

barbiturate

neurosteroid

ethanol

Cl⁻

FIG. 26.1. Structure of GABA$_A$ receptor. GABA$_A$ receptors are heteropentameric proteins with the five subunits assembled around a Cl⁻ ionophore. The second transmembrane spanning region of each subunit is thought to form the walls of the ionophore. There are multiple isoforms of GABA$_A$ receptors, composed of different combinations of subunits, which convey variations in sensitivity and responsivity to GABA and different drug classes that interact with the receptor. The example shown here possesses the full spectrum of responses exhibited by GABA$_A$ receptors, including interactions with GABA, benzodiazepines, barbiturates, convulsants, neurosteroids, and ethanol. Convulsants bind within the Cl⁻ ionophore. Benzodiazepines bind at the interface of α and γ subunits. GABA, barbiturates, and neurosteroids can all activate any number of oligomeric subunits, and when presented in combinations are thought to bind to different sites from one another and benzodiazepines. Therefore, each of the drug classes that act at GABA$_A$ receptors is shown interacting with a different subunit in this figure.

site for barbiturates is thought to be one that is distinct from both the GABA and benzodiazepine sites, when the receptors are in their native states (6). In addition to benzodiazepines and barbiturates, modulation of GABA$_A$ receptors can be achieved by ethanol and neurosteroids (6,7,22).

GABA AND MYOCLONUS: ANIMAL MODELS

A role for GABA in myoclonus is supported by data from studies involving experimental animals. This section summarizes studies demonstrating that disruption of GABA$_A$ function can elicit myoclonus. The specific regions of the central nervous system that can mediate these effects are also reviewed.

Effects of GABA$_A$ Antagonists Compared to Other Drugs

The importance of GABA in myoclonus is best illustrated by examining the consequences of disrupting GABA-ergic activity in the brains of rats, relative to comparable manipulations of other neurotransmitter systems. This section thus summarizes the consequences of microinjecting drugs that target specific neurotransmitter systems, including those that alter GABA function, into the lateral ventricles where they would get widely distributed throughout the brain along with the flow of cerebrospinal fluid. If disruptions in GABA-ergic function are responsible for myoclonus, then it should be possible to induce the jerking movements in animals that are otherwise normal by mimicking the appropriate neurochemical pathology.

Infusion of $GABA_A$ antagonists, such as SR-95531 and bicuculline, into the lateral ventricles of rats elicits myoclonus in a dose-dependent manner. There appears to be some neurochemical specificity to this effect because similar injections of a vehicle control or the following 13 compounds are unable to elicit myoclonus under comparable conditions: picrotoxin or t–butylbicyclophosphorothionate (TBPS) ($GABA_A$ channel blockers), muscimol ($GABA_A$ agonist), baclofen ($GABA_B$ agonist), apomorphine (dopamine agonist), methysergide (5-HT $_2$ [5-hydroxytryptamine] antagonist), clonidine (α_1-adrenergic agonist), phentolamine (α_1-adrenergic antagonist), propranolol (β-adrenergic antagonist), histamine, l-glutamic acid, and N-methyl-D-aspartate (NMDA receptor agonist) (23).

In contrast to the $GABA_A$ antagonists, the $GABA_A$ channel blockers, picrotoxin and TBPS, only produce clonic-tonic generalized convulsions in this animal model (23). Even after administering low doses of the $GABA_A$ receptor channel blockers, myoclonic movements are not elicited; all that is observed at lower doses are full blown convulsions in fewer animals. Therefore, although myoclonus often exists on a continuum with seizures, these data provide further evidence that they can occur independently of one another.

The myoclonus generated by $GABA_A$ antagonists following microinjection into the lateral ventricles cannot be explained by a simple, nonspecific overactivation of synaptic activity because the excitatory neurotransmitter and agonist glutamate and NMDA, respectively, were unable to elicit myoclonus in this study. Both of these compounds should have produced myoclonus if the movements resulted simply from an overactivation of neural circuits. Therefore, there appears to be some neurochemical specificity underlying the generation of the abnormal movements. Specifically, the data suggest that disinhibition of $GABA_A$ receptors has an important role in the pathogenesis of myoclonus.

If pharmacologic antagonism of $GABA_A$ receptors elicits myoclonus, one would expect that other conditions in which there is a functional impairment in $GABA_A$ function to also be associated with myoclonus. Therefore, it is noteworthy that frequent myoclonic jerks are reported in a transgenic mouse strain in which the β_3 subunit of $GABA_A$ receptors is knocked out (24). Other strains of mice in which $GABA_A$ receptor function is severely compromised have not been reported, probably because severe and widespread abnormalities in GABA-ergic function are likely to be lethal.

Effects of $GABA_A$ Antagonism in Specific Regions of the Central Nervous System

Application of $GABA_A$ antagonists into discrete regions of the central nervous system can elicit myoclonus in animals. This section summarizes the results from such injections into the cortex, caudate, putamen, nucleus reticularis of the thalamus, and spinal cord.

Cortex

The involvement of the cortex in myoclonus is well established. The pathophysiology of cortical reflex myoclonus is particularly well characterized and summarized in chapter 10. It is therefore noteworthy that several investigators have reported that disruption of GABA-ergic activity in the cortex elicits myoclonus to varying degrees in animals (25–28). Topical cortical application of the $GABA_A$ channel blocker picrotoxin has been reported to elicit myoclonus in the contralateral forelimb of virtually all animals tested

(27). The region of the cortex that is disinhibited appears to have some consequences for the localization of the myoclonus, with more posterior applications predominantly affecting the hindlimbs and progressively fewer animals exhibiting the abnormal movements (27). Therefore, antagonism of $GABA_A$ receptors in the cortex, a key region of the brain that has a well-characterized role in the pathophysiology myoclonus, may also contribute to the generation of the abnormal movements.

Caudate

The caudate is a prominent structure in the basal ganglia, having a well-documented role in motor control. Disruption of activity in the caudate can lead to a number of different movement disorders (29), one of which is myoclonus.

A number of laboratories have reported that decreasing activity at $GABA_A$ receptors in the caudate of rats elicits myoclonus. Most of the studies involve microinjection of the $GABA_A$ channel blocker picrotoxin into the caudate, but similar effects have been reported with drugs that act at least in part as $GABA_A$ antagonists (bicuculline, benzylpenicillin, d-tubocurarine) or glutamic acid decarboxylase inhibitors (dl-c-allylglycine, thiosemicarbazide) (26,28,30). The production of myoclonus that is elicited through the caudate does not appear dependent on dose, exhibiting more of an all-or-none response pattern. For example, within the active dose range for picrotoxin (0.5 to 1.5 μg), there is no difference in the latency or duration of the movements (28). The myoclonus elicited through the caudate begins in the contralateral forelimb and is rhythmic in nature. However, these localized movements can rapidly progress into focal seizures, which are evident both behaviorally and electrophysiologically (28). A GABA-ergic mechanism is inferred because the behavioral and electrophysiologic changes elicited by picrotoxin can be reversed by intracaudate microinjections of GABA (28). In contrast, the following compounds that alter other neurochemical systems are unable to modify the myoclonus produced by intracaudate injections of picrotoxin: 5-hydroxytryptophan (5-HTP, serotonin precursor), methysergide (5-HT antagonist), α-methyl-p-tyrosine (dopamine synthesis inhibitor), chlorpromazine or haloperidol (dopamine antagonists), levadopa plus carbidopa (dopamine precursor plus peripheral decarboxylase inhibitor), amphetamine (dopamine agonist), clonidine (norepinephrine agonist) (28). Thus, in the caudate, the specific disruption of GABA-ergic activity appears to be an important contributor to the pathogenesis of myoclonus.

Measurements of local cerebral glucose utilization during picrotoxin-induced myoclonus further reveals activation of the frontal cortex, thalamus, globus pallidus, and subthalamic nucleus (25,31), suggesting the potential importance of activity in these brain regions following disruption of GABA-ergic function in the caudate. In some reports, the picrotoxin-induced, intrastriatally evoked myoclonus appears to be an artifact of concurrent disruption of function in the sensorimotor cortex (26,27,31), but subsequent studies suggest otherwise. These latter studies demonstrate that the myoclonus evoked by picrotoxin through the caudate can be elicited when the cannula tract is angled to avoid the sensorimotor cortex (25). Furthermore, the picrotoxin-induced myoclonus elicited through the caudate, but not the cortex, is significantly attenuated by prior lesions to the subthalamic nucleus or pallidum, two efferents of the striatum (25,28). Thalamic lesions, on the other hand, significantly attenuate the myoclonus evoked through both the caudate and cortex (25). The data therefore indicate that although there are interactions and overlap between the neural pathways underlying myoclonus evoked through the caudate and cortex, differences also exist.

Putamen

The putamen is another structure in the basal ganglia that is closely connected to the caudate. Together, the caudate and putamen are collectively referred to as the striatum. As might be expected from the studies involving the caudate, microinjection of the GABA$_A$ antagonist bicuculline in the lateral part of the putamen of monkeys elicits myoclonus (32). The myoclonus affects the side contralateral to the injection, and the upper limb is most commonly involved (32). The data from the caudate and putamen studies indicate that disruption of GABA-ergic activity in the striatum can lead to the production of myoclonus. The underlying circuit responsible for the myoclonus is thought to involve disruption of GABA-ergic projections from the striatum to the globus pallidus (33), which in turn project to the subthalamic nucleus (34). This mechanism is consistent with the lesioning studies described above in rats (25,28) as well as with observations in patients with Huntington disease. In Huntington disease, degeneration of striatal GABA-ergic neurons are a hallmark feature (35,36), and these patients can exhibit pronounced myoclonus as part of their symptomology (37–41). Therefore, the data suggest that descending extrapyramidal pathways contribute to the pathophysiology of myoclonus, in addition to well-characterized cortical pathways involving pyramidal tracts.

Nucleus Reticularis of the Thalamus

The nucleus reticularis of the thalamus (NRT) is a prominent feature of the diencephalon of all mammals (42). It is densely populated with GABA-ergic neurons (43), and extensive neuropathologic changes are observed in this region of the brain in posthypoxic myoclonic rats (44). The NRT is thought to have an important role in coordinating and modulating the bidirectional activity that passes between the thalamus and the cortex (43,45). Neurons in this region of the brain feature prolonged, Ca^{2+}-dependent burst firing as part of their normal function (46). Under normal conditions, this neuronal firing pattern is thought to contribute to thalamocortical rhythmicity, such as that associated with slow wave sleep, and in pathologic states to abnormal rhythms, such as those associated with absence epilepsy (46) and myoclonus.

Microinjection of the GABA$_A$ antagonist bicuculline into the NRT produces spontaneous, rhythmic myoclonus in rats (23). Similar to the all-or-none effects observed after injection of picrotoxin into the caudate, the myoclonus elicited through the NRT is also not dose dependent. Almost all of the animals (more than 74%) exhibit myoclonus over the active dose range (2.5 to 10 nmol), with no significant difference in the latency, intensity or frequency of the movements between the active doses. The jerking movements affect the side of the body ipsilateral to the microinjection. Jerk-locked back-averages of electrophysiologic recordings reveal a rostral-caudal recruitment of muscles that follows a central/frontal negative cerebral potential, indicating a cortical involvement. Despite similar levels of GABA$_A$ and GABA$_B$ receptors in the NRT (47), the GABA$_B$ antagonist phaclofen (10 nmol) does not elicit myoclonus under comparable conditions, suggesting that GABA$_B$ receptors in the NRT do not have a primary role in the pathogenesis of myoclonus, although they may be involved in other pathologic states (46,48).

When taken together, the data suggest that disruption of GABA$_A$ receptor function in the NRT triggers myoclonus via a circuit involving the cortex. Given the lack of direct efferents from the NRT to the cortex and the delay before the onset of the movements, we hypothesize that following the injection of bicuculline into the NRT, other thalamic relays are activated, which in turn progressively recruit cortical neurons that are responsible for the pathogenesis of myoclonus. The ipsilateral lateralization of the movements and the long latencies observed in the electrophysiologic recordings suggest that subsequent to the cortex, extrapyramidal rather than pyramidal systems are involved in the myoclonus elicited through the NRT.

Miscellaneous Brain Regions

As part of the studies involving injections into the caudate, putamen, and NRT, additional information involving small samples sizes have been collected regarding the presence or absence of myoclonus following microinjections of GABA$_A$ antagonists or channel blockers into the brain. Microinjection of GABA$_A$ antagonists or channel blockers into the following areas produce myoclonus (number of affected animals per total tested indicated in parentheses): corona radiata (2 of 2), hippocampus (2 of 6), lateral pallidum (1 of 23), globus pallidus (3 of 8) (23,28,32). Additionally, microinjection of bicuculline into the lateral amygdala, though failing to produce spontaneous myoclonus, elicits audiogenic myoclonus in which synchronous muscle jerks can be evoked by a train of metronome clicks (3 of 3). In contrast, myoclonus was not observed when injections were made into the following regions of the brain (number of tested animals indicated in parentheses): amygdala (N = 9), central amygdala (N = 2), anterior commissure/extreme capsule (N = 6), ventral hippocampus (N = 4), ventral hippocampal commissure (N = 3), anterior hypothalamic area (N = 1), internal capsule (N = 2), globus pallidus, medial segment (N = 3), optic tract (N = 1), substantia innominata (N = 13), thalamus (N = 4), anteroventral thalamus (N = 2), ventrolateral thalamus (N = 2), septofimbrial nucleus (N = 2), septohypothalamic nucleus (N = 1), triangular nucleus (N = 3) (23,28,32).

Spinal Cord

The pathophysiology of spinal myoclonus is not well understood. However, a useful model for better understanding the circuit properties that underlie this disorder is an *in vitro* spinal cord preparation. In this preparation, robust, synchronous motoneuronal oscillations, which are augmented in the presence of glycinergic antagonists, can be recorded that are similar in frequency to myoclonic behavior in intact animals (49). As such, these oscillations in the *in vitro* preparation can be thought of as neural correlates of myoclonus. In this preparation, antagonism of GABA$_A$, but not GABA$_B$, receptors abolishes these synchronous oscillations (49), suggesting a critical role of GABA$_A$ receptors in the premotoneuronal circuitry responsible for these oscillations.

Summary

The animal studies confirm that disruption of GABA-ergic function at any number of points along the neural axis can lead to the production of myoclonus. The data further indicate an important role for GABA$_A$ receptors; there is no evidence that GABA$_B$ or GABA$_C$ receptors contribute to myoclonus, but an involvement may exist under conditions not examined to date.

The myoclonus elicited through each of the structures described herein encompasses a different spectrum of features; the movements look slightly different and appear to involve distinct, but overlapping neural pathways. The fact that myoclonus can be triggered as a result of disruption of any number of points along the neural axis, together with the lack of a consistent and specific lesion in the brain (see below), suggests that the movements may result from dysfunctions in neural circuits rather than structural abnormalities in discrete brain regions. Circuits that appear important include traditional corticospinal pathways that have been well characterized in the context of myoclonus as well as less characterized extrapyramidal pathways. In addition, neurons that feature burst firing or oscillatory activity, such as those in the NRT and spinal cord, may represent particularly vulnerable points that can trigger, and possibly sustain, the abnormal circuit activity contributing to myoclonus.

GABA AND MYOCLONUS: CLINICAL EVIDENCE

Reduced GABA Levels

Decreased GABA levels have been measured in the cerebrospinal fluid of patients with myoclonus. This data includes seven patients with postanoxic encephalopathy and three patients with progressive myoclonus epilepsy, where there was a 55% reduction in GABA in the cerebrospinal fluid (50). In another study that involved 15 patients with progressive myoclonic epilepsy, there was a significant 25% reduction in GABA compared to epileptic controls (51). Moreover, in this latter group, there was a trend for the GABA concentrations to correspond to the degree of impairment exhibited by the patients (51).

Damage to Brain Regions Associated with Myoclonus

Although decreased GABA levels have been measured in the cerebrospinal fluid of patients with myoclonus, these studies do not reveal the level in the neural axis that is affected. Insight about the anatomic localization can thus be obtained from postmortem and imaging studies, when they are considered together with other existing information.

Of the postmortem studies of patients with myoclonus that have been conducted, the pathologic changes that have been reported vary between individuals. This is related, in part, to the differing types of myoclonus studied. For example, the pathology associated with focal myoclonus can be relatively localized, predominantly to lesions and/or dysfunction of dentate-rubral-olivary pathways in palatal myoclonus (52,53). In cortical or spinal myoclonus, cases have been reported in which there are relatively localized pathologies in the expected regions of the central nervous system (54); however, there is also much evidence that even these types of myoclonus can be secondary to focal lesions in other parts of the central nervous system (55). For multifocal or generalized myoclonus, the pattern of damage, as might be expected, can be quite complex, especially when taking into account the spectrum of etiologies that lead to these abnormal movements. Thus, with perhaps the exception of palatal myoclonus, there is no circumscribed site of pathology that can be identified even when the myoclonus is well defined.

For any given type of myoclonus, the pattern of pathology tends to fall into two groups: (a) cases in which almost no pathology is observed

and (b) cases in which the abnormalities are widespread. This applies even to patients diagnosed with posthypoxic myoclonus where the movements are particularly debilitating (56,57). The most likely explanation for this peculiar all-to-none pattern of pathology is that myoclonus does not result from structural damage to a particular brain region as seen in Parkinson or Huntington disease, but rather from a functional dysregulation of critical motor circuits. Thus, the regions of damage in those individuals with identifiable pathologies can provide insight into the neural circuits that may be dysfunctional.

Although postmortem studies cannot reveal whether the damaged regions are the cause or result of the disease symptoms and it is likely that disruption of activity in any number of points along the neural axis can lead to the production of myoclonus, it is noteworthy that changes have been documented in many of the regions implicated in animal models: cortex, caudate, putamen, spinal cord (54,56,57). Although the NRT is not specifically mentioned in these studies, the thalamus is implicated (56,57), and it is likely that in at least some cases, the pathology includes the NRT. That these changes in postmortem tissue may have functional relevance to myoclonus is supported by single photon emission computed tomography studies demonstrating abnormalities in the cortex, which in at least some cases appears secondary to damage in subcortical regions of the brain in patients with myoclonus (58,59). Thus, despite the complications involved in interpreting postmortem data, there appears to be good confirming data between animal and human studies regarding some of the sites in the central nervous system that are involved in myoclonus. However, given the relatively few sites and cases that have been studied in detail to date, it is likely that other regions that are not mentioned in this review may also be involved.

GABA and Myoclonus: Pharmacotherapies

Since myoclonus is often thought to be a fragment of epilepsy and it has been associated with deficits in GABA-ergic function, it is logical that anticonvulsants with GABA-enhancing properties be tested for antimyoclonic actions. Although all of the drugs possess multiple mechanisms of action (60), only those mechanisms that alter GABA-ergic function are summarized here. Among the most effective antimyoclonic agents are clonazepam (Klonopin) and valproic acid (Depakote), both of which possess GABA-enhancing abilities.

Clonazepam

Clonazepam (Klonopin) is a benzodiazepine that enhances GABA function by increasing the frequency of opening of the $GABA_A$ receptor complex (61,62). Administration of clonazepam to humans has been reported to alleviate the symptoms of the following myoclonic disorders: infantile spasms, progressive myoclonus epilepsy, Ramsay Hunt syndrome, postencephalitic myoclonus, epilepsia partialis continua, posthypoxic myoclonus, Lennox-Gastaut syndrome, status myoclonus, juvenile myoclonic epilepsy, and photosensitive myoclonic seizures (63).

Other benzodiazepines such as lorazepam (Ativan) and nitrazepam (Mogadon) have also been tested clinically as antimyoclonic agents. They have been reported effective against the following myoclonic syndromes: myoclonic seizures of childhood, serotonin syndrome, and nocturnal myoclonus (64,65). However, in other situations, they are less efficacious than clonazepam (66,67). In addition, lorazepam and nitrazepam tend to have limiting pharmacokinetic features that make them less favored as antimyoclonic agents than clonazepam. Lorazepam is short acting, whereas nitrazepam has a long elimination half-life that enhances its potential for residual side effects.

Diazepam (Valium), another benzodiazepine that is an effective anticonvulsant, is generally not an effective antimyoclonic agent (67). The reason for this difference is not known. However, given the heterogeneity of $GABA_A$ receptor isoforms, it is possible that diazepam acts at $GABA_A$ receptors with a different subunit com-position from clonazepam, or with different efficacy at receptors containing the same subunits (7). Alternatively, diazepam may differentially affect postreceptor events, such as those contributing to its higher liability for the development of tolerance and dependence as compared to other benzodiazepines (5).

Valproic Acid

Valproic acid (Depakote) is a wide spectrum antiepileptic that possesses multiple mechanisms of action that could contribute to its anticonvulsant actions (68). Among them is the ability of valproic acid to increase the activity of an enzyme (glutamic acid decarboxylase) that is responsible for the synthesis of GABA and to inhibit enzymes (GABA transaminase, succinic semialdehyde dehydrogenase, aldehyde dehydrogenase) that are responsible for the catabolism of GABA (60,68). One consequence of increasing synthesis and/or decreasing catabolism of GABA is to allow more of it to be available for physiologic actions at the synapse. Thus, it is not surprising that with its GABA-enhancing properties, valproic acid has been reported to produce therapeutic actions against the following myoclonic disorders: progressive myoclonus epilepsy, posthypoxic myoclonus, myoclonic epilepsies of childhood, and myoclonic astatic epilepsy (67,69).

Other Drugs Targeting $GABA_A$ Receptor Complex

As mentioned earlier, the $GABA_A$ receptor complex also contains binding sites for barbiturates, the binding of which enhances GABA function by increasing the open time of the receptor complex (16,17). Many barbiturates, including primidone and phenobarbital, are effective anticonvulsants (70). However, as monotherapy, barbiturates have not been effective against myoclonic disorders, although they provide benefit when included in polytherapy (55,67,71). In addition to their limited efficacy, a practical limitation of this class of GABA-ergic drugs is their side effects, which may contribute to the preferential use of other classes of GABA-ergic drugs, such as benzodiazepines, for myoclonic disorders.

Other modulators of the GABA$_A$ receptor, such as neurosteroids, have not been reported to produce consistent and/or significant antimyoclonic effects. However, ethanol has been reported to produce benefit in at least some patients with the following types of myoclonus: posthypoxic myoclonus and progressive myoclonus epilepsy (72–74).

Other GABA-ergic Drugs

Baclofen (Lioresal), a GABA$_B$ agonist that is typically used as an antispastic agent, has been reported to attenuate myoclonus in patients with hereditary essential myoclonus (75) and in a patient with progressive encephalomyelopathy with rigidity and myoclonus (76). It has also been reported effective as part of a polytherapy for posthypoxic myoclonus in a patient unresponsive to antiepileptic drugs (77). However, baclofen has failed to provide or has had limited benefit in other cases, including posthypoxic myoclonus (67), nocturnal myoclonus (78), and a patient with spinal myoclonus.

Progabide, a GABA precursor and agonist that was developed as a potential anticonvulsant, has been of benefit in limited trials in patients with intention myoclonus (79). However, progabide had no significant effect in single patients with progressive myoclonus epilepsy, essential myoclonus, or oro-branchio-respiratory myoclonus (63,79). In addition, the development of this drug was discontinued after it was shown to produce hepatotoxicity and to have limited efficacy in controlled clinical trials for epilepsy (80).

Tiagabine (Gabitril), a GABA uptake inhibitor that enhances the availability of GABA at synapses, is approved for use as adjunctive therapy for the treatment of partial seizures. It has been reported to have antimyoclonic actions in animal models (81,82), but its effect on myoclonic disorders in humans is still largely unknown.

In contrast to all of the other GABA-ergic drugs described in this section, vigabatrin (Sabril), a GABA transaminase inhibitor, appears capable of provoking the appearance of myoclonus in both humans (83–85) and experimental animals (26,86). This compound is generally accepted as a selective inhibitor of an enzyme involved in the catabolism of GABA. As such, it can produce GABA-enhancing effects, which are thought to contribute to its effectiveness as an antiepileptic agent (60). However, there is evidence that vigabatrin, and another GABA transaminase inhibitor (+)-γ-acetylenic GABA, can also act as functional antagonists under certain conditions. When they are applied locally in the striatum or cortex of experimental animals, vigabatrin and (+)-γ-acetylenic GABA elicits myoclonus that is indistinguishable from that produced by the GABA$_A$ channel blocker picrotoxin (26,27). Moreover, the fact that the myoclonus elicited by these GABA transaminase inhibitors can be reversed by administering GABA or a GABA receptor agonist (86) suggests that the myoclonus results from functional decrements in GABA-ergic activity. This possibility is further supported by the observation that iontophoretic application of γ-acetylenic GABA can reverse the inhibitory effects of GABA on neurons (87). In addition, vigabatrin has been reported to reduce GABA-mediated inhibition in the CA1 region of the hippocampus (88) and to attenuate GABA-stimulated Cl$^-$ flux from the cerebral cortex (89), again suggesting that the compound can act as a functional GABA antagonist under certain conditions. Although further studies are needed to fully understand the dual and apparently opposing functional effects of GABA transaminase inhibitors on GABA-ergic systems, the existing data suggest that this class of compounds can produce promyoclonic actions.

INTERACTIONS WITH OTHER NEUROCHEMICAL SYSTEMS RELEVANT TO MYOCLONUS

Dysfunctions in numerous neurochemical systems have been implicated in the pathophysiology of myoclonus. Serotonin and glycine are two neurochemical systems that can contribute to myoclonus and are reviewed in other chapters contained in this book. Therefore, this section briefly summarizes data demonstrating interactions of GABA with serotonergic or glycinergic systems.

Serotonin

Animal studies suggest that subsequent to disinhibition of GABA-ergic systems, serotonergic systems are altered, which may contribute to the sustaining of the pathophysiology. This is surmised from animal models in which myoclonic movements are induced by GABA$_A$ receptor antagonists, such as the channel blocker picrotoxin. In these animals, the abnormal movements can be abated with the serotonin precursor 5-HTP, whereas pretreatment with the serotonin depletor *p*-chlorophenylalanine potentiates the myoclonus (90). That the pathogenesis of the myoclonus involves a GABA-ergic mechanism has been confirmed by the ability of the GABA transaminase inhibitor aminooxyacetic acid to attenuate the picrotoxin-induced myoclonus (90), thus suggesting that the influence of serotonergic systems occurs downstream from the initial dysfunction in GABA-ergic systems. A potential interaction between GABA-ergic and serotonergic systems in myoclonus in humans is also supported by dual changes in both GABA and the serotonin metabolite 5-HIAA in the cerebrospinal fluid of patients with myoclonus. In fact, in this group of patients with progressive myoclonus epilepsy, there was a high degree of correlation ($r = 0.88$) between concentrations of GABA and 5-HIAA in the cerebrospinal fluid; a similar relationship was not observed in the epileptic controls (51).

Glycine

Glycine is a major inhibitory neurotransmitter in the spinal cord, whereas in supraspinal structures, GABA predominates as the major inhibitory neurotransmitter. In myoclonic disorders such as an inherited form affecting Poll Hereford cows in which a glycinergic deficit has been well characterized (see chapter 27 in this book), there are numerous alterations to GABA-ergic systems at both the spinal and supraspinal levels (91,92). Specifically, there is an increase in benzodiazepine binding in the spinal cord of these animals (91). Furthermore, at the supraspinal level, there is an enhancement of cerebral cortical GABA-ergic activity, including an increase in GABA-stimulated benzodiazepine binding (92). Whether this enhancement represents a compensatory mechanism to counteract the problems caused by the glycinergic deficit or an actual contributor to the pathology is unclear. There are reports in which overactivation of GABA-ergic systems with muscimol can cause myoclonus, but it is unlikely that this effect is mediated through a GABA-ergic mechanism since it cannot be antagonized with the GABA$_A$ antagonist bicuculline, nor can it be evoked using other drugs that enhance GABA-ergic function such as the agonist THIP or GABA-transaminase inhibitors (93). Although it is conceivable that either an overactivation or underactivation of the GABA$_A$ receptor could lead to a dysregulation in GABA-ergic systems that contribute to myoclonus, the vast majority of data implicate a GABA-ergic deficit in the pathogenesis of myoclonus. Nevertheless, when there is already a dysregulation of inhibitory systems such as glycine, antagonism of GABA-ergic mechanisms may serve to normalize the circuit activity rather than to cause the pathogenesis of the disorder. The potential importance of such an interaction between glycinergic and GABA-ergic systems may be especially relevant for spinal myoclonus. In the *in vitro* spinal cord model of myoclonus mentioned earlier, in contrast to the augmentation of the oscillations caused by glycine antagonists, antagonism of GABA$_A$ receptors alone do not alter the "myoclonic" oscillations of the spinal motoneurons (49). However, GABA$_A$ antagonists greatly attenuate the augmentation of the oscillations caused by the glycine antagonists (49). Therefore, while alterations in either of the two inhibitory systems at spinal and supraspinal levels may contribute to the pathogenesis of myoclonus, they may also work in concert to normalize the abnormal circuit activity caused by the other.

CONCLUSIONS

The data demonstrate that antagonism of $GABA_A$ receptors at any number of points along the neural axis can lead to the production of myoclonus. The fact that myoclonus can be triggered from numerous regions along the neural axis, together with the lack of a consistent lesion in the brain, suggests that the movements result from dysfunctions in neural circuits rather than specific structural abnormalities. Neurons that feature burst firing or oscillatory activity as part of their normal function may represent vulnerable triggering points in these circuits. Once the myoclonic activity is triggered, corticospinal and extrapyramidal pathways are important descending systems for transducing these neural signals into muscle jerks. In addition, the thalamus appears to be an important relay in this process. Efforts to restore the functioning of GABA-ergic systems in these circuits or to target downstream neurochemical systems that become altered following initial disinhibition of $GABA_A$ receptors thus provide a logical strategy for identifying effective therapeutic agents for treating myoclonus. Hence, the GABA-enhancing properties of many clinically useful antimyoclonic agents provide a logical mechanism to explain their effectiveness.

ACKNOWLEDGMENTS

This work was supported by the Myoclonus Research Foundation.

REFERENCES

1. Nieuwenhuys R. *Chemoarchitecture of the brain.* Berlin: Springer-Verlag, 1985.
2. Johnston GAR. $GABA_C$ receptors: relatively simple transmitter-gated ion channels? *Trends Pharmacol Sci* 1996;17:319–323.
3. Barnard EA, Skolnik P, Olsen RW, et al. International Union of Pharmacology. XV. Subtypes of γ-aminobutyric acid$_A$ receptors: classification on the basis of subunit structure and receptor function. *Pharmacol Rev* 1998;50:291–313.
4. Bormann J. The "ABC" of GABA receptors. *Trends Pharmacol Sci* 2000;21:16–19.
5. Costa E. From $GABA_A$ receptor diversity emerges a unified vision of GABAergic inhibition. *Ann Rev Pharmacol Toxicol* 1998;38:321–350.
6. Macdonald RL, Olsen RW. $GABA_A$ receptor channels. *Ann Rev Neurosci* 1994;17:569–602.
7. Sieghart W. Structure and pharmacology of γ-amino butyric acid$_A$ receptor subtypes. *Pharmacol Rev* 1995;47:181–234.
8. Sinkkonen ST, Hanna MC, Kirkness EF, et al. $GABA_A$ receptor ε and θ subunits display unusual structural variation between species and are enriched in the rat locus ceruleus. *J Neurosci* 2000;20:3588–3595.
9. Fritschy JM, Benke D, Mertens S, et al. Five subunits of the type A γ-aminobutyric acid receptors identified in neurons by double and triple immunofluorescence staining with subunit-specific antibodies. *Proc Natl Acad Sci U S A* 1992;89:6726–6730.
10. Persohn E, Malherbe P, Richards JC. Comparative molecular neuroanatomy of cloned $GABA_A$ receptor subunits in the rat CNS. *J Comp Neurol* 1992;326:193–216.
11. Wisden W, Laurie DJ, Monyer H, et al. The distribution of 13 $GABA_A$ receptor subunit mRNAs in the rat brain. I: telencephalon, diencephalon, mesencephalon. *J Neurosci* 1992;12:1040–1062.
12. Bonnert, TP, McKernan RM, Farrar S, et al. θ, a novel γ-aminobutyric acid type A receptor subunit. *Proc Natl Acad Sci U S A* 1999;96:9891–9896.
13. Hedblom E, Kirkness EF. A novel class of $GABA_A$ receptor subunit in tissues of the reproductive system. *J Biol Chem* 1997;272:15346–15350.
14. Neelands TR, Macdonald RL. Incorporation of the π subunit into functional γ-aminobutyric acid$_A$ receptors. *Mol Pharmacol* 1999;56:598–610.
15. Neelands TR, Fisher JL, Bianchi M, et al. Spontaneous and γ-aminobutyric acid (GABA)-activated $GABA_A$ receptor channels formed by ε subunit-containing isoforms. *Mol Pharmacol* 1999;1:168–178.
16. Study RE, Barker JL. Diazepam and ($\pm$)pentobarbital: Fluctuation analysis reveals different mechanisms for potentiation of γ-aminobutyric acid responses in cultured central neurons. *Proc Natl Acad Sci USA* 1981;78:7180–7184.
17. Twyman RE, Rogers CJ, Macdonald RL. Differential mechanisms for enhancement of GABA by diazepam and phenobarbital: a single channel study. *Ann Neurol* 1989;25:213–220.
18. Pritchett DB, Luddens H, Seeburg P. Type I and type II $GABA_A$-benzodiazepine receptor produced in transfected cells. *Science* 1989;245:1389–1392.
19. Blair LA, Levitan ES, Marshall J, et al. Single subunits of the $GABA_A$ receptor form ion channels with properties of the native receptor. *Science* 1988;242:577–579.
20. Cestari IN, Min KT, Kulli JC, et al. Identification of an amino acid defining the distinct properties of murine β_1

and β₃ subunit-containing GABA_A receptors. *J Neurochem* 2000;74:827–838.

21. Thompson SA, Whiting PJ, Wafford KA. Barbiturate interactions at the human GABA_A receptor: dependence on receptor subunit composition. *Br J Pharmacol* 1996; 117:521–527.

22. Majewska MD. Neurosteroids: endogenous bimodal modulators of the GABA_A receptor: mechanism of action and physiological significance. *Prog Neurobiol* 1992;38:379–395.

23. Matsumoto RR, Truong DD, Nguyen KD, et al. Involvement of GABA_A receptors in myoclonus. *Mov Disord* 2000;15(Suppl 1):47–52.

24. Homanics GE, DeLorey TM, Firestone LL, et al. Mice devoid of γ-aminobutyrate type A receptor β₃ subunit have epilepsy, cleft palate, and hypersensitive behavior. *Proc Natl Acad Sci U S A* 1997;94:4143–4148.

25. Patel S, Slater P. Analysis of the brain regions involved in myoclonus produced by intrastriatal picrotoxin. *Neuroscience* 1987;20:687–693.

26. Robin MM, Palfreyman MG, Zraika MM, et al. An analysis of the cortical and striatal involvement of dyskinesia induced in rats by intracerebral injection of GABA-transaminase inhibitors and picrotoxin. *Eur J Pharmacol* 1980;62:319–327.

27. Robin MM, Palfreyman MG, Zraika MM, et al. Mapping of dyskinetic movements induced by local application of picrotoxin or (+)-γ-acetylenic GABA on the rat motor cortex. *Eur J Pharmacol* 1980;65:411–415.

28. Tarsy D, Pycock CJ, Meldrum BS, et al. Focal contralateral myoclonus produced by inhibition of GABA action in the caudate nucleus of rats. *Brain* 1978;101: 143–162.

29. Saint-Cyr JA, Taylor AE, Nicholson K. Behavior and the basal ganglia. *Adv Neurol* 1995;65:1–28.

30. McKenzie GM, Viik K. Chemically induced choreiform activity: antagonism by GABA and EEG patterns. *Exp Neurol* 1975;46:229–243.

31. Jenner P, Leigh PN, Marsden CD, et al. Cortical involvement in forepaw myoclonus induced by intrastriatal administration of picrotoxin to rats. *Proc Br Pharmacol Soc* 1980;503P–504P.

32. Crossman AR, Mitchell IJ, Sambrook MA, et al. Chorea and myoclonus in the monkey induced by gamma-aminobutyric acid antagonism in the lentiform complex: the site of drug action and a hypothesis for the neural mechanism of chorea. *Brain* 1988;111: 1211–1233.

33. Fonnum F. Gottesfeld Z, Grofova I. Disinhibition of glutamate decarboxylase, choline acetyltransferase and aromatic amino acid decarboxylase in the basal ganglia of normal and operated rats: evidence for striatopallidal, strioentopeduncular and striatonigral GABAergic fibers. *Brain Res* 1978;145:125–138.

34. Van der Kooy D, Hattori T, Shannalz K, et al. The pallidosubthalamic projection in the rat: anatomical and biochemical studies. *Brain Res* 1981;204:253–268.

35. Perry TL, Hansen S, Kloster M. Huntington's chorea: deficiency of gamma-aminobutyric acid in brain. *N Engl J Med* 1973;288:337–342.

36. Vonsattel JP, Myers RH, Stevens TJ, et al. Neuropathological classification of Huntington's disease. *J Neuropathol Exp Neurol* 1985;44:559–577.

37. Carella F, Scaioli V, Ciano C, et al. Adult onset myoclonic Huntington's disease. *Mov Disord* 1993;8: 201–205.

38. Caviness JN, Kurth M. Cortical myoclonus in Huntington's disease associated with an enlarged somatosensory evoked potential. *Mov Disord* 1997;12:1046–1051.

39. Siesling S, Vegter-van der Vlis M, Roos RA. Juvenile Huntington disease in the Netherlands. *Pediatr Neurol* 1997;17:37–43.

40. Thompson PD, Bhatia KP, Brown P, et al. Cortical myoclonus in Huntington's disease. *Mov Disord* 1994;9: 633–641.

41. Vogel CM, Drury I, Terry LC, et al. Myoclonus in adult Huntington's disease. *Ann Neurol* 1991;29:213–215.

42. Jones EG. Some aspects of the organization of the thalamic reticular complex. *J Comp Neurol* 1975;162: 285–308.

43. Houser CR, Vaughn JE, Barber RP, et al. GABA neurons are the major cell type in the nucleus reticularis thalami. *Brain Res* 1980;200:341–354.

44. Kanthasamy AG, Nguyen BQ, Truong DD. Animal model of posthypoxic myoclonus. II: neurochemical, pathologic, and pharmacologic characterization. *Mov Disord* 2000;15(Suppl 1):31–38.

45. Scheibel ME, Scheibel AB. The organization of the nucleus reticularis thalami: a golgi study. *Brain Res* 1966; 1:43–62.

46. Huguenard JP, Prince DA. A novel T-type current underlies prolonged Ca²⁺-dependent burst firing in GABAergic neurons of the rat thalamic reticular nucleus. *J Neurosci* 1992;12:3804–3817.

47. Chu DCM, Albin RL, Young AB, et al. Distribution and kinetics of GABA_B binding sites in the rat central nervous system: a quantitative autoradiographic study. *Neuroscience* 1990;34:341–357.

48. Caddick SJ, Hosford DA. The role of GABA_B mechanisms in animal models of absence seizures. *Mol Neurobiol* 1996;13:23–32.

49. Simon E. Involvement of glycine and GABA_A receptors in the pathogenesis of spinal myoclonus: in vitro studies in the isolated neonatal rodent spinal cord. *Neurology* 1995;45:1883–1892.

50. Enna SJ, Ferkany JW, Van Woert M, et al. Measurement of GABA in biological fluids: effect of GABA transaminase inhibitors. *Adv Neurol* 1979;23:741–750.

51. Airaksinen EM, Leino E. Decrease of GABA in the cerebrospinal fluid of patients with progressive myoclonus epilepsy and its correlation with the decrease of 5HIAA and HVA. *Acta Neurol Scand* 1982;66: 666–672.

52. Dubinsky R, Hallett M, Schwankhaus J. Increased metabolism of the inferior olives in palatal myoclonus. *Neurology* 1987;37(Suppl 1):125.

53. Finelli PF, McEntee WJ, Ambler M, et al. Adult celiac disease presenting as cerebellar syndrome. *Neurology* 1980;30:245–249.

54. Davis SM, Murray NM, Diengdoh JV, et al. Stimulus-sensitive spinal myoclonus. *J Neurol Neurosurg Psychiatry* 1981;44:884–888.

55. Obeso JA, Artieda J, Rothwell JC, et al. The treatment of severe action myoclonus. *Brain* 1989;112:765–777.

56. De Lean J, Richardson JC, Rewcastle NB. Pathological findings in a case of hypoxic myoclonus treated with 5-hydroxytryptophan and a decarboxylase inhibitor. *Adv Neurol* 1986;43:21–223.

57. Hauw JJ, Escourolle R, Baulac M, et al. Postmortem studies on posthypoxic and post-methyl bromide intoxication: case reports. *Adv Neurol* 1986;43:201–214.
58. Delecluse F, Waldemar G, Vestermark S, et al. Cerebral blood flow deficits in hereditary essential myoclonus. *Arch Neurol* 1992;49:179–182.
59. Tanaka K, Suga R, Yamada T, et al. Idiopathic cortical myoclonus restricted to the lower limbs: correlation between MEPs and 99mTc-ECD single photon emission computed tomography activation study. *J Neurol Sci* 1999;163:58–60.
60. Pranzatelli MR, Nadi NS. Mechanism of action of antiepileptic and antimyoclonic drugs. *Adv Neurol* 1995;67:329–360.
61. Gibbs JW III, Schroder GB, Coulter DA. GABA_A receptor function in developing rat thalamic reticular neurons: whole cell recordings of GABA-mediated currents and modulation by clonazepam. *J Neurophysiol* 1996;76:2568–2579.
62. Puia G, Vicini S, Seeburg PH, et al. Influence of recombinant gamma-aminobutyric acid-A receptor subunit composition on the action of allosteric modulators of gamma-aminobutyric acid-gated Cl- currents. *Mol Pharmacol* 1991;39:691–696.
63. Van Woert MH, Rosenbaum D, Chung E. Biochemistry and therapeutics of posthypoxic myoclonus. *Adv Neurol* 1986;43:171–181.
64. Brown TM, Skop BP, Mareth TR. Pathophysiology and management of the serotonin syndrome. *Ann Pharmacother* 1996;30:527–533.
65. Moldofsky H, Tulis C, Quance G, et al. Nitrazepam for periodic movements in sleep (sleep-related myoclonus). *Can J Neurol Sci* 1986;13:52–54.
66. Eisele JH Jr, Grigsby EJ, Dea G. Clonazepam treatment of myoclonic contractions associated with high-dose opioids: case report. *Pain* 1992;49:231–232.
67. Frucht S, Fahn S. The clinical spectrum of posthypoxic myoclonus. *Mov Disord* 2000;15(Suppl 1):2–7.
68. Loscher W. Valproate: a reappraisal of its pharmacodynamic properties and mechanisms of action. *Prog Neurobiol* 1999;58:31–59.
69. Wallace SJ. Myoclonus and epilepsy in childhood: a review of treatment with valproate, ethosuximide, lamotrigine and zonisamide. *Epilepsy Res* 1998;29:147–154.
70. Brodie MJ, Dichter MA. Established antiepileptic drugs. *Seizure* 1997;6:159–174.
71. Iivanainen M, Himberg JJ. Valproate and clonazepam in the treatment of severe progressive myoclonus epilepsy. *Arch Neurol* 1982;39:236–238.
72. Genton P, Guerrini R. Antimyoclonic effects of alcohol in progressive myoclonus epilepsy. *Neurology* 1990;40:1412–1416.
73. Jain S, Jain M. Action myoclonus (Lance-Adam syndrome) secondary to strangulation with dramatic response to alcohol. *Mov Disord* 1991;6:183.
74. Rustom R, Fisken RA. Action myoclonus after cerebral hypoxia: treatment with clonazepam. *J Royal Soc Med* 1992;85:761–762.
75. Korten JJ, Notermans SLH, Frenken CWGM, et al. Familial essential myoclonus. *Brain* 1974;97:131–138.
76. Stayer C, Tronnier V, Dressnandt J, et al. Intrathecal baclofen therapy for stiff-man syndrome and progressive encephalomyelopathy with rigidity and myoclonus. *Neurology* 1997;49:1591–1597.
77. Coletti A, Mandelli A, Minoli G, et al. Post-anoxic myoclonus (Lance-Adams syndrome) treated with levodopa and GABAergic drugs. *J Neurol* 1980;223:67–70.
78. Guilleminault C, Flagg W. Effect of baclofen on sleep-related periodic leg movements. *Ann Neurol* 1984;15:234–239.
79. Mondrup K, Dupont E, Braendgaard H. Progabide in the treatment of hyperkinetic extrapyramidal movement disorders. *Acta Neurol Scand* 1985;72:341–343.
80. Leppik IE, Dreifuss FE, Porter R, et al. A controlled study of progabide in partial seizures: methodology and results. *Neurology* 1987;37:963–968.
81. Jaw SP, Nguyen B, Vuong QT, et al. Effects of GABA uptake inhibitors on posthypoxic myoclonus in rat. *Brain Res Bull* 1996;39:189–192.
82. Suzdak PD, Jansen JA. A review of the preclinical pharmacology of tiagabine: a potent and selective anticonvulsant GABA uptake inhibitor. *Epilepsia* 1995;36:612–626.
83. Garcia Pastor A, Garcia Zarza E, Peraita Adrados R. Acute encephalopathy and myoclonic status induced by vigabatrin monotherapy. *Neurologia* 2000;15:370–374.
84. Marciani MG, Maschio M, Spanedda F, et al. Development of myoclonus in patients with partial epilepsy during treatment with vigabatrin: an electroencephalographic study. *Acta Neurol Scand* 1995;91:1–5.
85. Neufeld MY, Vishnevska S. Vigabatrin and multifocal myoclonus in adults with partial seizures. *Clin Neuropharmacol* 1995;18:280–283.
86. Robin MM, Palfreyman MG, Schechter PJ. Dyskinetic effects of intrastriatally injected GABA-transaminase inhibitors. *Life Sci* 1979;25:1101–1109.
87. Gent JP, Normanton JR. Actions of γ-acetylenic GABA on single central neurons in rat. *Br J Pharmacol* 1978;64:383P–384P.
88. Jackson MF, Dennis T, Esplin B, et al. Acute effects of γ-vinyl GABA (vigabatrin) on hippocampal GABAergic inhibition in vitro. *Brain Res* 1994;651:85–91.
89. Suzuki Y, Mimaki T, Arai H, et al. Effect of γ-vinyl γ-aminobutyric acid on the γ-aminobutyric acid receptor-coupled chloride ion channel in vesicles from the brain of the rat. *Neuropharmacology* 1991, 30:423–427.
90. Paul V, Krishnamoorthy MS. A functional interaction between GABA and 5-HT in inhibiting picrotoxin-induced myoclonus in rats. *Ind J Physiol Pharmacol* 1990;34:139–142.
91. Gundlach AL, Dodd PR, Grabara CSG, et al. Deficit of spinal cord glycine/strychnine receptors in inherited congenital myoclonus of Poll Hereford calves. *Science* 1988;241:1807–1810.
92. Lummis SC, Gundlach AL, Johnston GA, et al. Increased gamma-aminobutyric acid receptor function in the cerebral cortex of myoclonic calves with an hereditary deficit in glycine/strychnine receptors. *J Neurochem* 1990;55:421–426.
93. Menon MK. Paradoxical blockade of a muscimol response by THIP, a GABA agonist and also by GABA-transaminase inhibitors. *Neuropharmacology* 1981;20:1183–1186.

Myoclonus and Paroxysmal Dyskinesias,
Advances in Neurology, Vol. 89,
edited by S. Fahn, et al.
Lippincott Williams & Wilkins, Philadelphia © 2002.

27

The Role of Glycine and Glycine Receptors in Myoclonus and Startle Syndromes

Peter R. Schofield

Neurobiology Research Program, Garvan Institute of Medical Research, Sydney, Australia

Fast synaptic neurotransmission is mediated by receptors of the ligand-gated ion channel superfamily. The neurotransmitters glycine and γ-aminobutyric acid (GABA) activate inhibitory (chloride-conducting) ion channels, and the neurotransmitters acetylcholine and serotonin activate excitatory (sodium-conducting) ion channels (1). Each receptor comprises five homologous subunits that form a pseudosymmetric pentameric complex around a central ion channel. The subunits of the ligand-gated ion channel receptor contain an extracellular domain that forms the ligand-binding site, four hydrophobic transmembrane domains of which the second (M2) is believed to form the ion channel lumen, and an intracellular domain located between transmembrane domains 3 and 4 (1).

Glycine is a major inhibitory neurotransmitter in the spinal cord and brainstem. Its postsynaptic receptor is a pentameric molecule that shares a common structure with other members of the ligand-gated ion channel superfamily (2). The receptor consists of both ligand-binding α subunits and structural β subunits that assemble to form a glycine-gated chloride channel and are clustered in the synaptic membrane via the cytoplasmic anchoring protein, gephyrin (3). To date, there have been four α subunits (α1 to 4) and one β subunit identified as well as splicing variants in the α1, α2, and α3 subunits (4,5). Each subunit contains a large N-terminal extracellular domain followed by four membrane-spanning domains. In the adult spinal cord, the receptor assembles with α1 subunits and β subunits in a ratio of three α1 to two β subunits (6,7; reviewed in 3,8). Disruption of glycinergic transmission by the glycine receptor antagonist strychnine at subconvulsive doses leads to hyperresponsiveness to sensory stimuli, and acute poisoning results in severe generalized hypertonia (9). These symptoms bear a marked similarity to those seen in a rare inherited neurologic condition known as startle disease or hyperekplexia. Hyperekplexia is characterized by an exaggerated startle reflex in response to unexpected auditory or tactile stimuli. Similar startle syndromes are observed in a number of animal species including mouse, cattle, dog, and horse.

HUMAN HYPEREKPLEXIA (STARTLE DISEASE)

Genetic linkage analysis of a large pedigree with hyperekplexia enabled the disease locus to be mapped to the long arm of chromosome 5 at position 5q32 (10). This region of chromosome 5 had previously been characterized as possessing several neurotransmitter receptor genes, including subunits of the $GABA_A$ receptor. However, an even more attractive candidate gene was identified when the ligand-binding α1 subunit of the glycine receptor (GlyR) was also mapped to this region

(11). Direct sequence analysis of DNA from affected and normal individuals from pedigrees with inherited hyperekplexia revealed the presence of mutations within the GlyR α1 subunit (12). Specifically, missense mutations were identified that resulted in the positively charged residue, arginine-271, which is located at the extracellular mouth of the membrane-spanning M2 domain, being converted to an uncharged residue, either leucine (R271L) or glutamine (R271Q) (12) (Fig. 27.1).

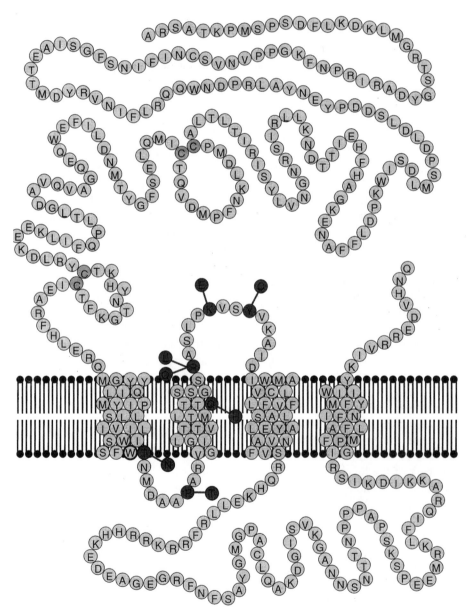

FIG. 27.1. Diagram of the human GlyR α1 subunit showing the location of known hyperekplexia missense mutations (dark gray) that flank the M2 transmembrane domain.

A number of other hyperekplexia pedigrees were screened for the presence of mutations and, to date, a total of six different disease causing mutations have been identified (reviewed in 1). Interestingly, all of the hyperekplexia mutations described to date cluster within the sequences flanking the M2 transmembrane domain (Fig. 27.1).

The GlyR subunits have been cloned and subjected to structure-function studies allowing investigation of the effects of the disease-causing mutations on receptor function. Expression of the R271L and R271Q mutations was shown to result in mutant glycine receptors with impaired glycine responses (13,14). However, the agonists β-alanine and taurine did not elicit any channel activity from the mutant GlyRs, even though the binding affinities of these ligands were unimpaired. Rather, the R271L and R271Q mutations transformed these GlyR agonists into competitive antagonists (14). The distribution of single-channel conductances is also determined by Arg-271. Mutation of this residue diminishes glycine-activated currents by a progressive decrease in the ability of the channel to conduct ions (13,14).

Additional hyperekplexia mutations K276E and Y279C result in GlyRs that have marked reductions in glycine sensitivity and "fully" transform the actions of the agonists β-alanine and taurine into competitive antagonists as seen with the Arg-271 mutations (15). The recessive startle disease mutation I244N "partially" disrupts signal transduction and converts the actions of β-alanine and taurine into partial agonists. Single-channel electrophysiological analysis of the K276E mutation reveals no change in single-channel conductances but shows a significant shortening of the open channel lifetimes, indicating that the open state of the channel has been destabilized, thus negatively affecting the gating efficacy (16). The Q266H hyperekplexia mutation, which is located in the M2 transmembrane domain, "partially" disrupts channel function also by a reduction in the open channel lifetimes (17). The P250T hyperekplexia mutation, located in the M1-M2 loop, also causes decreased glycine responses, most likely by a combination of short-ening of channel open times and decreased single-channel conductances (18).

Complementing this set of analyses of disease-causing mutations, alanine scanning mutagenesis of both the M2-M3 extracellular and the M1-M2 intracellular loops revealed that residue Val-277 "fully" disrupts, and residues Trp-243, Met-246, Leu-274, Ser-278, and Lys-281 "partially" disrupt signal transduction (15) (Fig. 27.1). Collectively, these naturally occurring and induced mutations demonstrate that residues from both the extracellular and intracellular domains form part of an "allosteric switch" responsible for inducing a conformational change in the receptor upon the binding of an agonist. Since these residues flank the ion channel lumen formed by the M2 domain, they may act as hinges, allowing the necessary conformational change required for channel gating (15,19). This mechanism may account for the M2 domain structural changes that are believed to underpin receptor activation and have been seen in the electron microscopic images of the related ligand-gated ion channel receptor, the nicotinic acetylcholine receptor (20).

MURINE STARTLE SYNDROMES

Three lines of mutant mice have been described that have a recessively inherited startle syndrome. The naturally occurring mouse mutants *spasmodic* and *spastic* are phenotypically characterized by hindlimb clenching when held suspended, arching of the body, flexion of limbs, especially the hindlimbs, and a loss of righting reflex. These symptoms are provoked by sensory stimuli. The *oscillator* mouse shows similar, but more pronounced symptoms, resulting in death at 3 weeks of age. At 3 weeks of age, there is a developmental switch in mouse GlyR subunits, with the embryonic α2 subunit being downregulated and replaced by the adult α1 subunit (3,4).

A missense mutation in the GlyR α1 subunit, resulting in the replacement of Ala-52 by Ser, is responsible for the *spasmodic* mouse (21,22) (Fig. 27.2A). Recombinant GlyRs

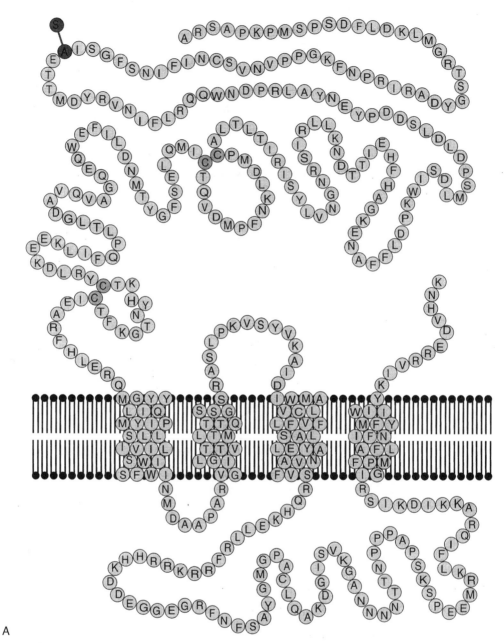

A

FIG. 27.2. Diagram of the mouse GlyR α1 and β subunits showing the location of the mutations that lead to the naturally occurring mutant mice **(A)** *spasmodic*, an α1 subunit Ala52Ser missense mutation **(B)** *oscillator*, an α1 subunit microdeletion that leads to a frameshift mutation that results in a further 147 amino acids being incorporated (illustrated in dark gray) and **(C)** *spastic*, a β subunit LINE-1 transposable element insertion in the intron *(arrows)* between exons 5 and 6. This insertion results in reduced levels of β subunit transcription, exon skipping of the unshaded exons and truncated β subunit polypeptides (dark gray).

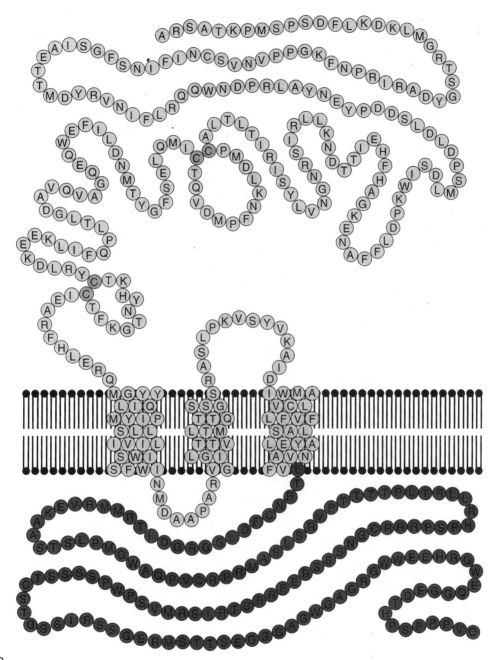

B

FIG. 27.2. *(Continued.)*

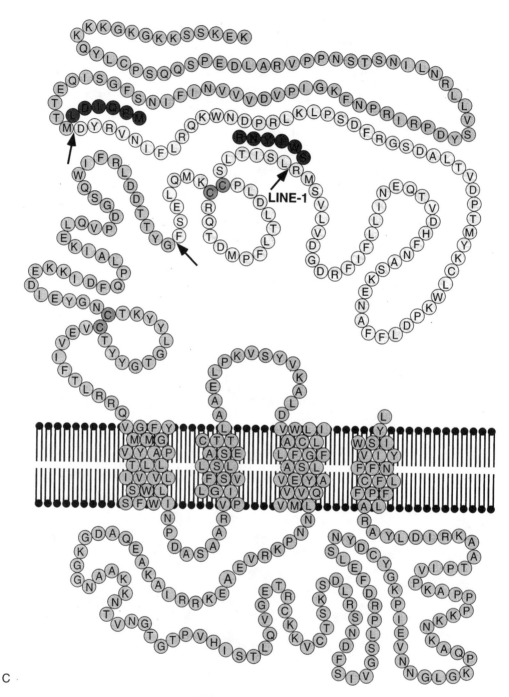

FIG. 27.2. *(Continued.)*

C

with this mutation show reduced sensitivity to glycine activation but normal ligand-binding properties. The *oscillator* mouse is caused by an α1 subunit microdeletion that results in a frameshift mutation, producing truncated proteins that are unable to assemble into functional receptors (23) (Fig. 27.2B). In *spastic* mice, an intronic insertion of a LINE-1 transposable element causes aberrant splicing of β subunit mRNAs, resulting in exon-skipping and a reduction in the levels of normal β subunit mRNA (Fig. 27.2C), thereby preventing efficient GlyR assembly (24,25). The analysis of these mutations has shed light on the molecular function of the glycine receptor and, by analogy, other members of the ligand-gated ion channel superfamily (1).

BOVINE MYOCLONUS

Bovine myoclonus is an autosomal recessive disease of Poll Hereford calves (26). The disease is characterized by hyperesthesia and myoclonic jerks of the skeletal musculature, which occur spontaneously as well as in response to tactile, visual, and auditory stimuli. Affected animals show no pathologic lesions in the central nervous system (27), and symptoms are unaltered by antiepileptic and anticonvulsive drugs (28). Bovine myoclonus has been attributed to a severe disturbance of glycine-mediated neurotransmission in the spinal cord since ligand-binding studies have shown that myoclonus is associated with specific loss of [^{3}H]-strychnine binding sites from spinal cord and brainstem in affected calves (28). In order to identify the mutation responsible for myoclonus, we examined the candidate genes, glycine receptor α1 (*Glra1*) and β (*Glrb*) subunits in affected and normal cattle.

The bovine *Glra1* and *Glrb* genes were isolated from bovine λ phage and bacterial artificial chromosome (BAC) genomic DNA libraries. Intron locations and consensus splice donor and acceptor sites were identified by comparison of the bovine genomic sequence

with sequences derived from human, rat, and mouse cDNAs and genomic DNA. Genomic DNA was isolated from a normal and an affected Poll Hereford calf with each exon and the flanking intronic regions, including the splice donor and acceptor sites and the 5' and 3' untranslated sequences of both *Glra1* and *Glrb,* being amplified by polymerase chain reaction (PCR) and sequenced. The affected calf was shown to be homozygous for a cytidine to adenine transversion at position 156 of the *Glra1* gene (156C→A) (29). Reverse transcriptase PCR (RT-PCR) was performed on mRNA from spinal cord of a normal and an affected calf, and sequence analysis confirmed that the 156C→A point mutation was present in cDNA clones derived from affected spinal cord mRNA, but not those derived from normal spinal cord. The 156A allele is predicted to substitute a termination codon for a tyrosine codon (Y24*) in exon 2 (Fig. 27.3). This substitution is predicted to result in a prematurely truncated protein that lacks ligand-binding and membrane-spanning domains (29).

The distribution of glycine receptors was examined in spinal cord sections obtained from normal and myoclonic calves by labeling with the antiglycine receptor monoclonal antibody, Mab4a (Fig. 27.4). In control animals, the immunohistochemical staining was evenly distributed within the cytoplasm of the neurons and was also clearly present on the cell membranes. However, the immunoreactivity in neurons of affected calves was confined to the cytoplasm, especially to the region surrounding the nucleus, and was absent from the cell membranes (29). Thus, the nonsense mutation in codon 24 results in a truncation of the *Glra1* polypeptide and subsequent loss of cell surface expression of the glycine receptor. This loss of cell surface expression of the glycine receptor in spinal cord suggests that the truncated polypeptide, lacking ligand-binding and membrane-spanning domains, is unable to form functional receptor complexes in the synaptic membrane.

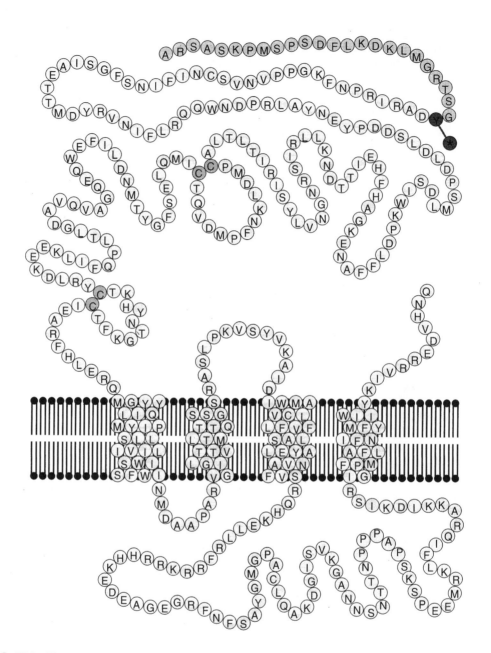

FIG. 27.3. Diagram of the bovine GlyR α1 subunit showing the location of the α1 subunit Tyr24* nonsense mutation that leads to inherited bovine myoclonus.

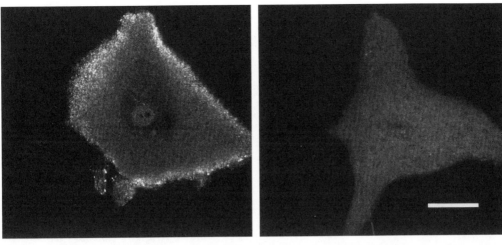

FIG. 27.4. Confocal microscopy images of individual spinal cord neurons showing glycine receptor immunoreactivity, using monoclonal antibody Mab4a, in normal and myoclonic calves. Panel **(A)** shows cell surface and intracellular labeling in a normal animal, and panel **(B)** shows intracellular labeling only in the myoclonic calf. Scale bar represents 20 μm.

CONVERGENT PHYSIOLOGY

Mutations in the glycine receptor genes have been shown to be responsible for neuromotor disorders in humans (12), mice (21–25), and cattle (29). Known molecular deficits associated with the inherited startle syndromes result in a disease phenotype through one of two mechanisms (30) (Fig. 27.5). The first mechanism occurs where α1 subunit missense mutations cause a loss of glycine receptor sensitivity, either by reduction of agonist affinity or through defective signal transduction. This mechanism underlies all dominantly and some recessively inherited human hyperekplexia mutations as well as the mouse model, *spasmodic* (21,22). The second mechanism occurs where mutations result in a reduction of glycine receptor expression levels. This mechanism underlies the mouse models *spastic*, in which a mutation in the β subunit gene causes aberrant splicing of mRNA and reduced *Glrb* expression (24,25) and *oscillator*, in which a frameshift mutation in the α1 subunit causes a loss of the third cytoplasmic loop and fourth transmembrane domain of the receptor (23). The second mechanism also underlies a hu-

man null allele in which exons 1 to 6 of the GLRA1 gene are deleted (31). The bovine myoclonus missense mutation, which results in premature termination of the α1 subunit polypeptide and subsequent lack of functional receptor expression, also fits into this latter category of mutation (29). The model may further be divided into those mutations that are lethal, including *oscillator* and bovine myoclonus, and those, including *spastic* and *spasmodic*, for which functional compensation occurs through either residual glycine receptor expression or compensatory inhibitory mechanisms. The lethality of the *Glra1* nonsense mutation in bovine myoclonus demonstrates that in cattle, despite the observed increase in GABA$_A$ receptors seen in the brain of affected calves (32), loss of the glycine receptor α1 subunit is not adequately compensated by alternative inhibitory mechanisms. Up-regulation of GABA$_A$ receptors is also seen in the *spastic* mouse (33). The recessive human *GLRA1* null mutation, however, is not lethal (31); indicating that in the human there is an alternative inhibitory compensatory mechanism.

The glycine receptor-mediated neuromotor disorders that have been defined to date have

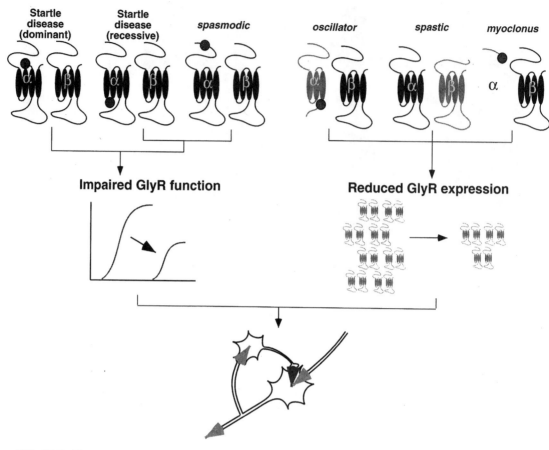

FIG. 27.5. The molecular mechanisms of the various startle disorders converge physiologically. Both dominant and recessive human startle disease mutations as well as the murine mutant *spasmodic* all lead to impaired receptor function, and the murine mutants *oscillator* and *spastic* and the bovine mutant myoclonus all lead to loss of glycine receptor expression. Phenotypically, all mutations, whether reducing glycine receptor sensitivity or reducing glycine receptor expression, diminish glycinergic inhibition and result in hypertonia, myoclonus, and an excessive startle response.

all been identified as mutations in the α1 or β subunits. As yet none have been identified in other glycine receptor subunit genes, or in gephyrin. Despite this, a gephyrin knockout mouse model shows symptoms of hyperekplexia (34). Each of these genes remain candidates for the as yet unassigned cases of human hyperekplexia and myoclonus in dogs (35) and horses (36).

CONCLUSION

The understanding of the mechanism of operation of the ligand-gated ion channel receptors has been aided by the characterization of naturally occurring genetic mutations (1). Knowledge of the structure and function of each individual receptor has given new insights into the molecular mechanisms of fast synaptic neurotransmission. Both GlyR α1 and β subunit defects can lead to impaired inhibitory neurotransmission, either by impaired glycinergic response or by reduced expression levels of the GlyR α1 subunit (30). Mutations that impair channel properties have been described for the α1 subunit in human (hyperekplexia) and mice (*spasmodic*). Mutations that result in reduced expression levels of channel proteins have been described for both the α1 subunit in mouse (*oscillator*) and in cattle (*myoclonus*) as well as for the β subunit mice (*spastic*). Functional convergence of these two phenotypic effects, namely, impaired receptor function or reduced receptor expression, which arise from the various genetic forms of startle syndrome, is seen to occur with the overall effect being the loss of inhibitory tone.

ACKNOWLEDGMENTS

I thank my numerous colleagues and collaborators who have worked on aspects of the studies presented in this overview. Supported by the Australian National Health and Medical Research Council (Block Grant 993050).

REFERENCES

1. Vafa B, Schofield PR. Heritable mutations in the glycine, GABA$_A$ and nicotinic acetylcholine receptors provide new insights into the ligand-gated ion channel receptor superfamily. *Int Rev Neurobiol* 1998;42: 285–332.
2. Grenningloh G, Reinitz A, Schmitt B, et al. The strychnine-binding subunit of the glycine receptor shows homology with nicotinic acetylcholine receptors. *Nature* 1987;328:215–220.
3. Kuhse J, Betz H, Kirsch J. The inhibitory glycine receptor: architecture, synaptic localization and molecular pathology of a postsynaptic ion-channel complex. *Curr Opin Neurobiol* 1995;5:318–323.
4. Becker C-M. Glycine receptors: molecular heterogeneity and implications for disease. *Neuroscientist* 1995;1: 130–141.
5. Nikolic Z, Laube B, Weber RG, et al. The human glycine receptor subunit α3. *GLRA3* gene structure, chromosomal localization, and functional characterization of alternative transcripts. *J Biol Chem* 1998;273: 19708–19714.
6. Grenningloh G, Pribilla I, Prior P, et al. Cloning and expression of the 58 kD β subunit of the inhibitory glycine receptor. *Neuron* 1990;4:963–970.
7. Langosch D, Thomas L, Betz H. Conserved quaternary structure of ligand-gated ion channels: the postsynaptic glycine receptor is a pentamer. *Proc Natl Acad Sci USA* 1988;85:7394–7398.
8. Rajendra S, Lynch JW, Schofield PR. The glycine receptor. *Pharmacol Ther* 1997;73:121–146.
9. Gilman AG, Rall TW, Nies AS, et al. *Goodman and Gilman's the pharmacological basis of therapeutics*, 8th ed. New York: Pergamon, 1991.
10. Ryan SG, Sherman SL, Terry JC, et al. Startle disease, or hyperekplexia: response to clonazepam and assignment of the gene (STHE) to chromosome 5q by linkage analysis. *Ann Neurol* 1992;31:663–668.
11. Baker E, Sutherland GR, Schofield PR. Localization of the glycine receptor α1 subunit gene (GLRA1) to chromosome 5q32 by FISH. *Genomics* 1994;22:491–493.
12. Shiang R, Ryan SG, Zhu Y-Z, et al. Mutations in the α1 subunit of the inhibitory glycine receptor cause the dominant neurologic disorder, hyperekplexia. *Nat Genet* 1993;5:351–357.
13. Langosch D, Laube B, Rundstrom N, et al. Decreased agonist affinity and chloride conductance of mutant glycine receptors associated with human hereditary hyperekplexia. *EMBO J* 1994;13:4223–4228.
14. Rajendra S, Lynch JW, Pierce KD, et al. Mutation of an arginine residue in the human glycine receptor transforms beta-alanine and taurine from agonists into competitive antagonists. *Neuron* 1995;14:169–175.
15. Lynch JW, Rajendra S, Pierce KD, et al. Identification of intracellular and extracellular domains mediating signal transduction in the inhibitory glycine receptor chloride channel. *EMBO J* 1997;16:110–120.
16. Lewis TM, Sivilotti LG, Colquhoun D, et al. Properties of human glycine receptors containing the hyperekplexia mutation alpha1(K276E), expressed in Xenopus oocytes. *J Physiol (Lond)* 1998;507:25–40.
17. Moorhouse AJ, Jacques P, Barry PH, et al. The startle disease mutation Q266H, in the second transmembrane domain of the human glycine receptor, impairs channel gating. *Mol Pharmacol* 1999;55:386–395.
18. Saul B, Kuner T, Sobetzko D, et al. Novel GLRA1 missense mutation (P250T) in dominant hyperekplexia defines an intracellular determinant of glycine receptor channel gating. *J Neurosci* 1999;19:869–877.
19. Lynch JW, Han N-LR, Haddrill J, et al. The surface accessibility of the glycine receptor M2-M3 loop is increased in the channel open state. *J Neurosci* 2001; 21:2589–2599.
20. Unwin N. Acetylcholine receptor channel imaged in the open state. *Nature* 1995; 373:37–43.
21. Ryan SG, Buckwalter MS, Lynch JW, et al. A missense mutation in the gene encoding the α1 subunit of the inhibitory glycine receptor in the *spasmodic* mouse. *Nat Genet* 1994;7:131–135.
22. Saul B, Volker S, Kling C, et al. Point mutation of glycine receptor α1 subunit in the *spasmodic* mouse affects agonist responses. *FEBS Lett* 1994;350:71–76.
23. Buckwalter MS, Cook SA, Davisson MT, et al. A frameshift mutation in the mouse α1 glycine receptor gene (*Glra1*) results in progressive neurological symptoms and juvenile death. *Hum Mol Genet* 1994;3: 2025–2030.
24. Mulhardt C, Fischer M, Gass P, et al. The spastic mouse: Aberrant splicing of glycine receptor β subunit mRNA caused by intronic insertion of the L1 element. *Neuron* 1994;13:1003–1015.
25. Kingsmore SF, Giros B, Suh D, et al. Glycine receptor β-subunit gene mutation in *spastic* mouse associated with LINE-1 element insertion. *Nat Genet* 1994;7:136–141.
26. Healy PJ, Harper PAW, Bowler JK. Prenatal occurrence and mode of inheritance of neuraxial oedema in Poll Hereford calves. *Res Vet Sci* 1985;38:96–98.
27. Harper PAW, Healy PJ, Dennis JA. Inherited congenital myoclonus of polled Hereford calves (so-called neuronal oedema): a clinical, pathological and biochemical study. *Vet Rec* 1986;119:59–62.
28. Gundlach AL, Dodd PR, Grabara CS, et al. Deficit of spinal cord glycine/strychnine receptor in inherited my-

oclonus of poll hereford calves. *Science* 1988;241: 1807–1809.

29. Pierce KD, Handford CA, Morris R,et al. A nonsense mutation in the α1 subunit of the inhibitory glycine receptor associated with bovine myoclonus. *Mol Cell Neurosci* 2001;17:354–363.

30. Rajendra S, Schofield PR. Molecular mechanisms of inherited startle syndromes. *Trends Neurosci* 1995;18: 80–82.

31. Brune W, Weber RG, Saul B, et al. GLRA1 null mutation in recessive hyperekplexia challenges the functional role of glycine receptors. *Am J Hum Genet* 1996; 58:989–997.

32. Lummis SC, Gundlach AL, Johnston GAR, et al. Increased γ-aminobutyric acid receptor function in the cerebral cortex of myoclonic calves with an hereditary deficit in glycine/strychnine receptors. *J Neurochem* 1990;55:421–426.

33. White WF, Heller AH. Glycine receptor alteration in the mutant mouse *spastic*. *Nature* 1982;298:655–657.

34. Feng G, Tintrup H, Kirsch J, et al. Dual requirement for gephyrin in glycine receptor clustering and molybdoenzyme activity. *Science* 1998;282:1321–1324.

35. Holland JM, Davis WC, Prieur DJ. et al. Lafora's disease in the dog: a comparative study. *Am J Pathol* 1970; 58:509–530.

36. Gundlach AL, Kortz G, Burazin TC, et al. Deficit of inhibitory glycine receptors in spinal cord from Peruvian Pasos: evidence for an equine form of inherited myoclonus. *Brain Res* 1993;628:263–270.

Myoclonus and Paroxysmal Dyskinesias,
Advances in Neurology, Vol. 89,
edited by S. Fahn, et al.
Lippincott Williams & Wilkins, Philadelphia © 2002.

28

The Isolated Rat Spinal Cord as an *In Vitro* Model to Study the Pharmacologic Control of Myoclonic-Like Activity

*Kristine C. Cowley, †Cima Cina, *Brian J. Schmidt, and ‡Shawn Hochman

*Department of Physiology, University of Manitoba, Winnipeg, Manitoba, Canada; †Department of
Pharmacology, Prescient Neuropharma Inc., Vancouver, British Columbia, Canada; and
‡Department of Physiology, Emory University School of Medicine, Atlanta, Georgia

The key feature of positive myoclonus is the production of an abrupt motor discharge. Typically, the discharge recruits synchronously more than one muscle group (1). Thus, central mechanisms must be able to simultaneously activate multiple motoneuron populations in the brainstem and/or spinal cord. Because neuronal hyperexcitability has been implicated in the genesis of myoclonus (2–4), it is not surprising that therapeutic agents known to depress cell excitability are commonly employed in the treatment of these disorders. For instance, drugs may act by (a) potentiating actions at inhibitory γ-aminobutyric acid (GABA) receptors (e.g., clonazepam, baclofen, primidone), (b) blocking actions at excitatory glutamate receptors (e.g., primidone), or (c) blocking voltage-dependent Na^+ channels (e.g., valproate). The diverse inhibitory actions of these drugs imply that therapeutic efficacy is achieved by reducing neural excitability. However, other mechanisms, resistant to the inhibitory actions of these drugs, may contribute to hyperexcitability and synchronous activation of motoneurons during myoclonic movements.

One such mechanism may involve abnormal amplification of electrotonic coupling between neurons, resulting in a widespread synchronization of interconnected neurons. In contrast to neurochemical transmission, gap junctions mediate electrical transmission from one cell to another. Gap junctions feature hemichannels, or connexins, that serve as portals for transfer of electrolytes and small messenger molecules between cells. Gap junctions are found in a variety of regions throughout the mammalian nervous system (5).

Several studies in the early 1980s provided evidence that electrotonic coupling may have a role in the production of synchronous epileptic discharge. Epileptogenic substances such as strychnine, penicillin, tetraethylammonium (TEA), and pentylenetetrazole significantly enhance electrical transmission in Aplysia (6), and synchronous epileptic discharge was observed in the hippocampal slice preparation in the absence of chemical synaptic transmission (7,8). The opening of neuronal gap junctions in the hippocampus contributes to epileptogenesis since agents that block gap junctions can abolish bursting activity (9–11). Thus, enhanced current flow through electrical synapses that are normally weak or silent may lead to the activation and synchronization of groups of neurons.

Several observations support the possibility that increased electrical coupling may contribute to the generation of at least some forms of myoclonus. First, acetazolamide, which can induce central nervous system acidosis (12), is sometimes used in the treatment of myoclonus; acidification is known to block gap junctional communication (10). Second, the serotonergic hypothesis of myoclonus originally derives from clinical and pharmacologic data suggesting a deficiency of 5-hydroxytryptamine (5-HT) actions in patients with posthypoxic myoclonus (13, 14). Therefore, it is of interest that serotonin blocks gap junctional coupling in the rat cortex (15). However, some animal models of myoclonus are consistent with a role for increased serotonin sensitivity in the production of myoclonus (16). Third, palatal myoclonus has been associated with lesions of the dentatorubral-olivary complex. The olivary nucleus is the site of abundant gap junctional neuronal interconnections and is capable of generating oscillatory activity (17,18). Finally, an increase in electrical transmission may occur following hypoxic, ischemic, or neurotoxic insults. For example, drugs that slightly prolong action potential duration greatly enhance electrical transmission (6), and *in utero* hypoxia leads to increased numbers of voltage-dependent Na^+ channels in the rat brain (19). The connection between subtle changes in Na^+ channels and enhanced electrical coupling may explain why hypoxic insults during development lead to seizures in adults even in the absence of overt differences in cell number or electrophysiologic properties (20).

The isolated *in vitro* neonatal rat spinal cord is capable of generating robust and reproducible paroxysmal synchronous motor activity following application of glycine or GABA $_A$ receptor antagonists (21–23). These observations are consistent with acquired and hereditary animal models that implicate impaired inhibitory amino acid transmission, especially at the spinal cord level, in the development of myoclonus and other paroxysmal hyperkinetic disorders such as hyperekplexia (24). Using the *in vitro* neonatal rat preparation, Simon (24) demonstrated synchronous high frequency (5 to 15 Hz) oscillations among motoneurons in the presence of glycine receptor blockade; he also highlighted

the potential value of this model for the study of myoclonic disorders. Importantly, this preparation permits precise control of the extracellular milieu including drug delivery at defined concentrations. In addition, the neonatal rat spinal cord is known to possess electrotonic coupling (25–27). The present series of experiments involved induction of synchronous motor activity in neonatal rat spinal cord to determine (a) the actions of several drugs used to treat myoclonus, (b) whether there is evidence that electrical synapses contribute to the generation of the synchronous discharge, and (c) the effects on synchronous discharge of 5-HT receptor blockade.

METHODS

Experiments were performed on 1- to 6-day-old neonatal Sprague-Dawley rats (n = 49). The experimental procedures are similar to those we have detailed previously (21). In brief, following induction of anesthesia with ether, the animals were decerebrated and placed in a 50-mL bath solution containing (in millimoles): NaCl 125, KCl 2.5, $NaH_2PO_4H_2O$ 1.25, $CaCl_2$ 2.0. $MgCl_2H_2O$ 1.0, $NaHCO_3$ 26, and D-glucose 25, equilibrated with 95% O_2/5% CO_2, pH 7.4. The spinal cord was transected at the first cervical level and then removed, bilaterally intact, with the pelvis and hindlimbs attached for experiments in which hindlimb motor nerve activity was monitored via electroneurograms. The peroneal and tibial nerves were used to monitor ankle flexor and extensor activity, respectively. In experiments involving ventral root recordings, the spinal cord was removed, bilaterally intact, without the pelvis or hindlimbs attached (Fig. 28.1). Surgery was performed with cool bath temperatures (4°C), and recordings were obtained at 25 to 27°C. Paroxysmal motor activity was evoked by applying to the bath the inhibitory amino acid receptor antagonist strychnine (a glycine receptor antagonist) or bicuculline (a GABA$_A$ receptor antagonist) in conjunction with the neuroexcitants serotonin (5-HT), dihydrokainic acid (DHK), or N-methyl-D-aspartate

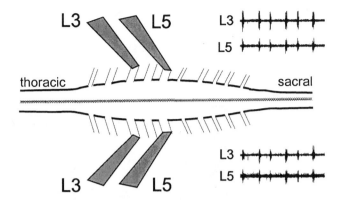

FIG. 28.1. Typical experimental arrangement to study synchronous motor activity. Suction recording electrodes are attached to lumbar ventral roots of the isolated neonatal rat spinal cord maintained in artificial cerebrospinal fluid. In some experiments, hindlimbs were left intact with the spinal cord to allow dissection of peripheral nerves for electroneurographic recordings (not illustrated). An example of synchronous motor activity recorded from four ventral roots is presented at the right. *L,* lumbar segment.

(NMDA). Records were digitized at 5.5 kHz and stored using a Vetter pulse code modulator videocassette adaptor. A continuous paper copy of the data was produced by an Astromed (model MT9500) oscillographic recorder. Further analysis and display of selected segments of taped data was performed on a Masscomp 5400 computer (sample rate 2 kHz per channel).

All neurochemicals were initially dissolved in distilled water and stored as millimolar stock solutions. Neurochemical concentrations, including ranges, specified in this report refer to the final bath concentration. Concentrations ranges were as follows: 5-HT, 10 to 60 μM; DHK, 100 μM; NMDA, 2 to 12.5 μM; strychnine, 2 to 40 μM; bicuculline methiodide, 10 to 30 μM. Concentration ranges of all other drugs tested are noted in the results section.

RESULTS

We first tested the effect, on synchronous discharge, of several drugs used to treat myoclonus and other paroxysmal motor disorders. However, neither primidone (505 to 1,400 μM; n = 3), acetazolamide (565 to 1,440 μM; n = 3), nor valproate (850 to 2,500

μM; n = 4) blocked synchronous motor activity (Fig. 28.2). In these experiments synchronous activity was evoked using 5-HT/strychnine (n = 3) or 5-HT/bicuculline (n = 7).

Gabapentin and pregabalin are GABA analogs; their full range of anticonvulsant actions remains to be determined. Gabapentin has been reported to be effective in treating an animal model of posthypoxic myoclonus (28). In the present series, both gabapentin (20 to 50 μM; n = 2) and pregabalin (50 μM; n = 1 of 2) reversibly blocked NMDA/strychnine-evoked synchronous activity when relatively low concentrations of NMDA (2 to 4 μM) and high concentrations of strychnine (20 to 40 μM) were used (Fig. 3A). However, when higher concentrations of NMDA (5 to 10 μM) were used (in combination with high strychnine concentrations), gabapentin (50 to 1,300 μM) failed to completely block the synchronous rhythm (Fig. 28.3B; n = 2).

In previous studies, octanol and heptanol have been used to block gap junctions at concentrations in the high micromolar to low millimolar range (10,29). However, because of their nonspecific actions at these concentrations (30,31), we tested their actions at relatively low concentrations (20 μM). In all cases, both octanol (n = 5) and heptanol (Fig.

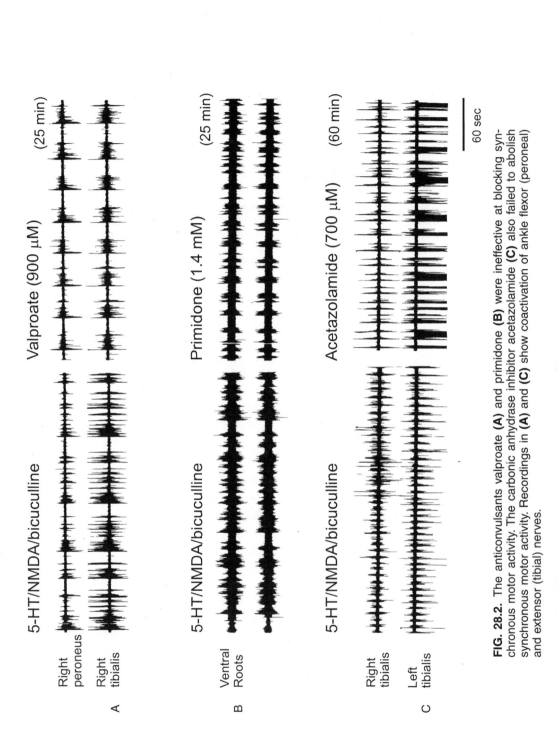

FIG. 28.2. The anticonvulsants valproate **(A)** and primidone **(B)** were ineffective at blocking synchronous motor activity. The carbonic anhydrase inhibitor acetazolamide **(C)** also failed to abolish synchronous motor activity. Recordings in **(A)** and **(C)** show coactivation of ankle flexor (peroneal) and extensor (tibial) nerves.

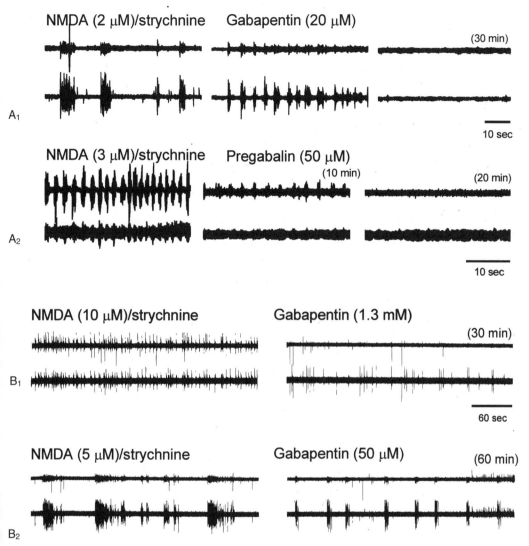

FIG. 28.3. The anticonvulsant gabapentin and its structural analogue pregabalin reduced or blocked synchronous motor activity. **A₁** and **A₂**: Synchronous motor activity induced by strychnine and low concentrations of NMDA (2 to 4 μM) were reversibly blocked by gabapentin or pregabalin. **B₁** and **B₂**: However, when synchronous motor activity was induced with strychnine and relatively high concentrations of NMDA (10 or 5 μM for **B₁** and **B₂**, respectively), gabapentin partially reduced the paroxysmal bursts but did not block bursting.

28.4A; n = 4) completely blocked neurochemically evoked synchronous motor discharge. However, dorsal root stimulation-evoked reflex discharge was also abolished (not illustrated), suggesting that the suppressive effects of the alcohols may have been due to a general nonspecific depression of chemical synaptic transmission rather than gap junction blockade alone.

Glycyrrhetinic acid and carbenoxolone are other compounds that have been reported to block gap junctional communication (27,29, 32–34). These agents were tested at concentrations ranging from 20 to 600 μM. Bath ap-

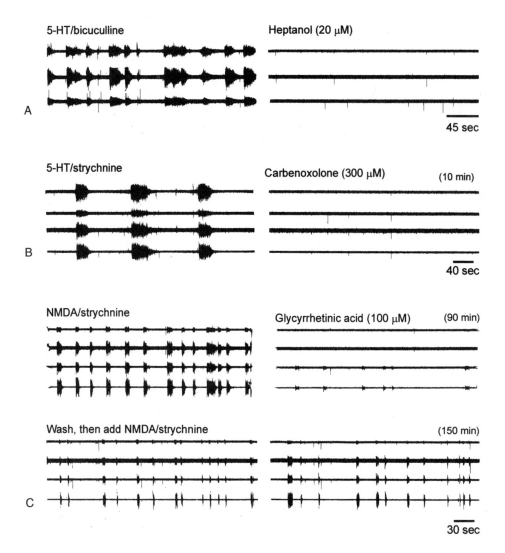

FIG. 28.4. Effect of gap junction blockers on synchronous motor activity. **A:** Heptanol and octanol consistently and potently block synchronous motor activity. In this example, heptanol blocked the synchronous motor activity recorded from three ventral roots. **B:** The gap junction blocker carbenoxolone abolished synchronous motor activity. **C:** The gap junction blocker glycyrrhetinic acid attenuated and blocked synchronous motor activity. After 90 minutes, glycyrrhetinic acid blocked synchronous motor activity in two ventral roots and strongly attenuated activity in the other two roots. Following washout of glycyrrhetinic acid and reapplication of NMDA and strychnine, synchronous motor activity returned and remained unchanged for the duration of the recording (150 minutes).

plication of carbenoxolone at 20 μM did not block convulsant activity but appeared to reduce burst duration and frequency (n = 2). In comparison, a higher concentration of carbenoxolone (300 to 330 μM) blocked or reduced synchronous motor activity (Fig. 28.4B; in two of three experiments). However, in two experiments following application of carbenoxolone, synchronous rhythm could not be reelicited after washout, raising the possibility of relatively long-term effects of these drugs on central nervous system activity. Similar effects were observed following bath application of glycyrrhetinic acid (Fig. 28.4C; n = 1; 100 µM). In two experiments in which glycyrrhetinic acid was only applied for short time periods at higher concentrations (less than 20 minutes; 200 to 600 µM) synchronous rhythm could not be reinstated after washout. The actions of these compounds required a long incubation period before inhibitory actions were observed (e.g., 90 minutes in Fig. 28.4C). Figure 28.4C demonstrates that following washout of lower concentrations of glycyrrhetinic acid (100 µM) and reapplication of the NMDA/strychnine, synchronous activity was reinstated and remained for the duration of the recording (150 minutes). Glycyrrhizic acid (20 to 300 µM), an inactive analogue of glycyrrhetinic acid, was effective at attenuating synchronous discharge in only one of the six animals.

Due to the possible involvement of serotonergic systems in the generation of paroxysmal discharges (35), serotonin receptor antagonists were also tested. NAN-190, the high affinity 5-HT$_{1A}$ receptor antagonist, did not block synchronous motor activity at concentrations that would support receptor-selective actions (< 1.0 µM). For example, 4 µM NAN-190 did not block synchronous motor activity; however, 8 µM and 10 µM were effective (Fig. 28.5A,B, respectively). Similarly, the high-affinity 5-HT$_2$ receptor antagonist mianserin failed to block synchronous motor activity at receptor-selective concentrations (1 µM; n = 2; mianserin was present in bath for 1.75 to 2.5 hours), but could attenuate the amplitude of the discharge and completely block activity after a long incubation period in one of two experiments at 2 µM (Fig. 28.6A). Much higher concentrations of mianserin (200 to 300 µM) blocked synchronous motor activity comparatively fast in all four preparations tested (Fig. 28.6B). Clozapine, an antipsychotic with very high affinity for the D$_4$ dopamine and 5-HT$_7$ receptor, was also incapable of blocking activity at submicromolar, receptor-selective concentrations, but did decrease discharge frequency at 1 µM (Fig. 28.7A). All activity

was abolished at higher (10 to 11 µM) concentrations (Fig. 7B; n = 2). In contrast, several other 5-HT receptor selective antagonists failed to block motor activity despite using relatively high micromolar concentrations. These included the 5-HT$_{1A}$ receptor antagonist WAY-100635 (n = 1, 11 µM), the 5-HT$_{1B}$ receptor antagonist CGS-12066A (n = 2, 10 to 11 µM), the 5-HT$_{2C}$ receptor antagonist normethyl-clozapine (n = 2, 1 to 10 µM), and the 5-HT$_2$ receptor antagonist ketanserin (215 µM; n = 1).

A summary of the actions of all drugs tested is provided in Table 28.1.

DISCUSSION

The *in vitro* neonatal rat spinal cord is a useful model for the study of myoclonic-like activity for the following reasons: (a) this *in vitro* preparation permits precise control of the extracellular milieu and drug delivery to an intact spinal neural apparatus, (b) epileptogenic substances, such as strychnine or biculline, consistently produce robust myoclonic-like discharge in this preparation (21, 24,36), (c) certain types of clinical myoclonus can be generated within the spinal cord itself (e.g., segmental and propriospinal myoclonus) (1,35), (d) this model may be used to reveal new agents that possess therapeutic efficacy via novel mechanisms of action, such as gap junction blockade.

The varied clinical presentations of myoclonus and the multiple animal models of myoclonus developed to date suggest multiple neural and transmitter mechanisms can produce myoclonus (3,16). Interestingly, in the isolated rat spinal cord preparation, several drugs that are used to treat myoclonus with variable clinical efficacy (i.e., acetazolamide, primidone, valproate) failed to block spinal paroxysmal activity. In part, this may be because the degree of synchronous excitation induced in this model, by coapplication of excitatory receptor agonists and inhibitory receptor antagonists, is more powerful than that which usually occurs in clinical myoclonic states.

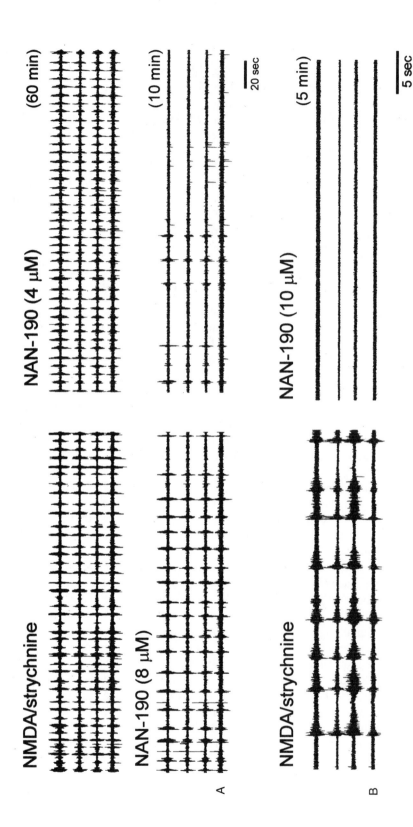

FIG. 28.5. The high affinity 5-HT$_{1A}$ receptor antagonist NAN-190 reversibly blocked synchronous motor activity at concentrations that exceed receptor-selective actions. **A:** Concentration dependence of NAN-190. NAN-190 at 4 μM was incapable of altering synchronous motor activity, even after bath incubation for 60 minutes. However NAN-190 at 8 μM first reduced frequency and then the amplitude of synchronous motor bursts before blocking activity completely. **B:** Simultaneous recordings from four lumbar ventral roots show that NAN-190 at 10 μM completely blocking synchronous motor activity within 5 minutes.

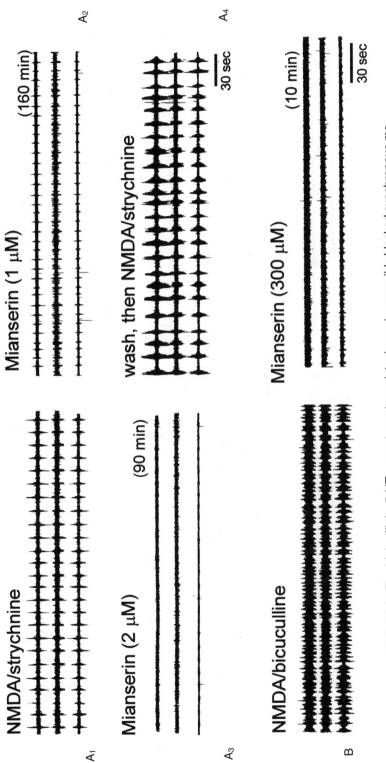

FIG. 28.6. The high affinity 5-HT$_2$ receptor antagonist mianserin reversibly blocked synchronous motor activity at concentrations that exceed receptor-selective actions. **A:** Mianserin applied at 1 μM concentration attenuated the amplitude of synchronous motor activity after a long incubation period (160 minutes; **A$_2$**). **A$_3$**: Subsequent application of an additional 1 μM (i.e., total 2 μM mianserin) blocked motor activity after a further 90 minutes of incubation. **A$_4$**: Washout of mianserin and reapplication of NMDA/strychnine reinstated synchronous motor activity demonstrating that the mianserin effect was reversible. In contrast, higher concentrations of mianserin (300 μM) blocked activity relatively faster (within 10 minutes).

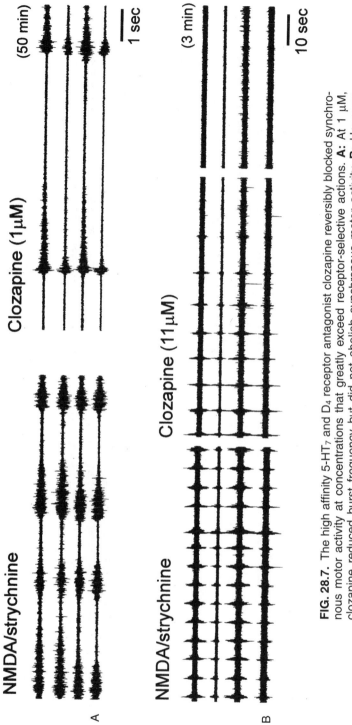

FIG. 28.7. The high affinity 5-HT$_7$ and D$_4$ receptor antagonist clozapine reversibly blocked synchronous motor activity at concentrations that greatly exceed receptor-selective actions. **A:** At 1 µM, clozapine reduced burst frequency but did not abolish synchronous motor activity. **B:** However, 11 µM clozapine completely blocked synchronous motor activity within 3 minutes.

TABLE 28.1. *Effect of various compounds on induced spinal synchronous motor activity*

Ligand	Concentration	Result
Anticonvulsants		
Valproate	850–2,500 µM (n = 4)	May slow activity
Acetazolamide	700–1,400 µM (n = 3)	No effect
Primidone	500–1,400 µM (n = 3)	No effect
GABA analogs		
Gabapentin	20–50 µM (n = 3)	Blocked or attenuated activity
Pregabalin	1,300 µM (n = 1)	Attenuated activity
	20 and 50 µM (n = 2)	Blocked only at 50 µM
Gap junction blockers		
Heptanol	20 µM (n = 4)	Complete block
Octanol	20 µM (n = 4)	Complete block
Carbenoxolone	20 µM (n = 2)	Reduced burst duration
	300 µM (n = 2)	Blocked activity
Glycyrrhetinic acid	20 µM (n = 2)	Blocked in one animal
	100 and 600 µM (n = 2)	Blocked or attenuated activity
Glycyrrhizic acid	20 µM (n = 4)	Blocked in 1 of 4 animals
	300 µM (n = 1)	Attenuated activity
Serotonergics		
NAN-190	8–10 µM (n = 2)	Blocked activity
Clozapine	10 and 11 µM (n = 2)	Blocked activity
Mianserin	1–20 µM (n = 3)	Blocked or attenuated activity
	200–300 µM (n = 4)	Blocked activity
Ketanserin	215 µM (n = 1)	Attenuated activity
WAY-100635	11 µM (n = 1)	No effect
Normethyl-clozapine	1–10 µM (n = 3)	No effect
CGS-12066A	10–11 µM (n = 2)	Decreases frequency

Sample sizes are in brackets.

Dysfunction in brain serotonergic systems has been implicated in various forms of myoclonus (16,28,37), and serotonin receptor agonists (38) and antagonists (37) have been shown to reduce posthypoxic myoclonus in animal models. While the present experiments demonstrated that 5-HT$_1$ and 5-HT$_2$ receptor antagonists can block myoclonic-like activity, the *in vitro* preparation also allowed us to determine that these drugs were effective at concentrations that exceed receptor subtype selectivity (39–41) and suggest that these drugs may be mediating their actions at currently unknown sites. This may explain the apparently inconsistent findings that high-affinity antagonists for 5-HT$_{1A}$ and 5-HT$_2$ receptors either blocked (e.g., NAN-190 and mianserin) or failed to block (e.g., WAY 100635, normethyl clozapine, or ketanserin) motor activity in these experiments. It further suggests that earlier results from *in vivo* studies using 5-HT receptor ligands should be interpreted cautiously (37,38).

The adult rat spinal cord contains many ultrastructurally identified synapses possessing gap junctions, albeit of unknown physiologic function (42). In the neonatal rat spinal cord, electrical synapses have been shown to contribute to the synchronization of motor output (27). The alcohols heptanol and octanol, conventionally used as gap junction blockers, were the most effective agents at blocking synchronous activity. However, because alcohols also blocked sensory root-evoked reflexes, it remains to be determined whether their effect on myoclonic-like discharge should be attributed specifically to actions on gap junctions versus nonspecific suppression of neural excitation (27). Carbenoxolone and glycyrrhetinic acid also appear to be able to block synchronous motor activity at concentrations similar to or lower than those concentrations previously reported effective at blocking gap junctions with some selectivity in this preparation (27). Overall, these results suggest that cell-to-cell electrical transmission via gap junctions may contribute to myoclonic-like activity in the neonatal rat spinal cord.

Future studies should be directed at using the *in vitro* neonatal rat spinal cord preparation to assess the actions of various other pharmaceuticals, applied at known concentrations, on myoclonic-like activity.

ACKNOWLEDGMENTS

Supported by the Myoclonus Research Foundation. We thank Parke-Davis for providing gabapentin and pregabalin.

REFERENCES

1. Bussel B, Roby-Brami A, Azouvi P, et al. Myoclonus in a patient with spinal cord transection. Possible involvement of the spinal stepping generator. *Brain* 1988;111 (Pt 5):1235–1245.
2. Pranzatelli MR, Nadi NS. Mechanism of action of antiepileptic and antimyoclonic drugs. *Adv Neurol* 1995;67:329–360.
3. Hallett M. Myoclonus and myoclonic syndromes. In: J Engel Jr, Pedley TA, eds. *Epilepsy: a comprehensive textbook.* Philadelphia: Lippincott-Raven, 1997:2717–2723.
4. Kanthasamy AG, Nguyen BQ, Truong DD. Animal model of posthypoxic myoclonus. II: neurochemical, pathologic, and pharmacologic characterization. *Mov Disord* 2000;15(Suppl 1):31–38.
5. Dermietzel R, Spray DC. Gap junctions in the brain: where, what type, how many and why? *Trends Neurosci* 1993;16:186–192.
6. Rayport SG, Kandel ER. Epileptogenic agents enhance transmission at an identified weak electrical synapse in Aplysia. *Science* 1981;213:462–463.
7. Taylor CP, Dudek FE. Synchronous neural afterdischarges in rat hippocampal slices without active chemical synapses. *Science* 1982;218:810–812.
8. Jefferys JG, Haas HL. Synchronized bursting of CA1 hippocampal pyramidal cells in the absence of synaptic transmission. *Nature* 1982;300:448–450.
9. Valiante TA, Perez Velazquez JL, Jahromi SS, et al. Coupling potentials in CA1 neurons during calcium-free-induced field burst activity, *J Neurosci* 1995;15: 6946–6956.
10. Perez-Velazquez JL, Valiante TA, Carlen PL. Modulation of gap junctional mechanisms during calcium-free induced field burst activity: a possible role for electrotonic coupling in epileptogenesis. *J Neurosci* 1994;14: 4308–4317.
11. Perez Velazquez JL, Carlen PL. Gap junctions, synchrony and seizures. *Trends Neurosci* 2000;23:68–74.
12. Kohshi K, Kinoshita Y, Fukata K. Brain pH responses to acetazolamide and hypercapnia in cats. *Neurol Med Chir (Tokyo)* 1997;37:313–318.
13. Pranzatelli MR. Serotonin and human myoclonus: rationale for the use of serotonin receptor agonists and antagonists. *Arch Neurol* 1994;51:605–617.
14. Hallett M. Physiology of human posthypoxic myoclonus. *Mov Disord* 2000;15(Suppl 1):8–13.
15. Rorig B, Sutor B. Serotonin regulates gap junction coupling in the developing rat somatosensory cortex. *Eur J Neurosci* 1996;8:1685–1695.
16. Nguyen BQ, Kanthasamy AG, Truong DD. Animal models of myoclonus: an overview. *Mov Disord* 2000; 15(Suppl 1):22–25.
17. Llinas R. Electronic transmission in the mammalian central nervous sytem. In: Bennett MVL, Spray DC, eds. *Gap junctions.* New York: Cold Spring Harbour Press, 1985:337–353.
18. Welsh JP, Chang B, Menaker ME, et al. Removal of the inferior olive abolishes myoclonic seizures associated with a loss of olivary serotonin. *Neuroscience* 1998;82: 879–897.
19. Xia Y, Haddad GG. Voltage-sensitive Na+ channels increase in number in newborn rat brain after in utero hypoxia. *Brain Res* 1994;635:339–344.
20. Owens J Jr, Robbins CA, Wenzel HJ, et al. Acute and chronic effects of hypoxia on the developing hippocampus. *Ann Neurol* 1997;41:187–199.
21. Cowley KC, Schmidt BJ. Effects of inhibitory amino acid antagonists on reciprocal inhibitory interactions during rhythmic motor activity in the in vitro neonatal rat spinal cord. *J Neurophysiol* 1995;74:1109–1117.
22. Bracci E, Ballerini L, Nistri A. Spontaneous rhythmic bursts induced by pharmacological block of inhibition in lumbar motoneurons of the neonatal rat spinal cord. *J Neurophysiol* 1996;75:640–647.
23. Kremer E, Lev-Tov A. Localization of the spinal network associated with generation of hindlimb locomotion in the neonatal rat and organization of its transverse coupling system. *J Neurophysiol* 1997;77: 1155–1170.
24. Simon ES. Involvement of glycine and GABA$_A$ receptors in the pathogenesis of spinal myoclonus: in vitro studies in the isolated neonatal rodent spinal cord. *Neurology* 1995;45:1883–1892.
25. Walton KD, Navarrete R. Postnatal changes in motoneurone electrotonic coupling studied in the in vitro rat lumbar spinal cord. *J Physiol (Lond)* 1991;433: 283–305.
26. Chang Q, Gonzalez M, Pinter MJ, et al. Gap junctional coupling and patterns of connexin expression among neonatal rat lumbar spinal motor neurons. *J Neurosci* 1999;19:10813–10828.
27. Tresch MC, Kiehn O. Motor coordination without action potentials in the mammalian spinal cord. *Nat Neurosci* 2000;3:593–599.
28. Kanthasamy AG, Vu TQ, Yun RJ, et al. Antimyoclonic effect of gabapentin in a posthypoxic animal model of myoclonus. *Eur J Pharmacol* 1996;297:219–224.
29. De Curtis M, Manfridi A, Biella G. Activity-dependent pH shifts and periodic recurrence of spontaneous interictal spikes in a model of focal epileptogenesis. *J Neurosci* 1998;18:7543–7551.
30. Largo C, Tombaugh GC, Aitken PG, et al. Heptanol but not fluoroacetate prevents the propagation of spreading depression in rat hippocampal slices. *J Neurophysiol* 1997;77:9–16.
31. Kim YJ, Elliott AC, Moon SJ, et al. Octanol blocks fluid secretion by inhibition of capacitative calcium entry in

rat mandibular salivary acinar cells. *Cell Calcium* 1999; 25:77–84.

32. Davidson JS, Baumgarten IM, Harley EH. Effects of 12-O-tetradecanoylphorbol-13-acetate and retinoids on intercellular junctional communication measured with a citrulline incorporation assay. *Carcinogenesis* 1985;6: 645–650.

33. Davidson JS, Baumgarten IM, Harley EH. Reversible inhibition of intercellular junctional communication by glycyrrhetinic acid *Biochem Biophys Res Commun* 1986;134:29–36.

34. Davidson JS, Baumgarten IM. Glycyrrhetinic acid derivatives: a novel class of inhibitors of gap-junctional intercellular communication: structure-activity relationships. *J Pharmacol Exp Ther* 1988;246: 1104–1107.

35. Brown P, Marsden CD. Myoclonus. In: Klawans HL, Goetz CG, Tanner CM, eds. *Textbook of clinical neuropharmacology and therapeutics*. New York: Raven Press, 1992.

36. MacLean JN, Schmidt BJ, Hochman S. NMDA receptor activation triggers voltage oscillations, plateau potentials and bursting in neonatal rat lumbar motoneurons in vitro. *Eur J Neurosci* 1997;9:2702–2711.

37. Goetz CG, Vu TQ, Carvey PM, et al. Posthypoxic myoclonus in the rat: natural history, stability, and serotonergic influences. *Mov Disord* 2000;15(Suppl 1):39–46.

38. Truong DD, Kanthasamy A, Nguyen B, et al. Animal models of posthypoxic myoclonus. I: development and validation. *Mov Disord* 2000;15(Suppl 1):26–30.

39. Connell LA, Wallis DI. 5-hydroxytryptamine depolarizes neonatal rat motoneurons through a receptor unrelated to an identified binding site. *Neuropharmacology* 1989;28:625–634.

40. Wallis DI, Wu J, Wang X. Descending inhibition in the neonate rat spinal cord is mediated by 5-hydroxytryptamine. *Neuropharmacology* 1993;32:73–83.

41. Hoyer D, Clarke DE, Fozard JR, et al. VIIth International Union of Pharmacology classification of receptors for 5-hydroxytryptamine (serotonin). *Pharmacol Rev* 1994;46:157–203.

42. Rash JE, Dillman RK, Bilhartz BL, et al. Mixed synapses discovered and mapped throughout mammalian spinal cord. *Proc Natl Acad Sci U S A* 1996;93:4235–4239.

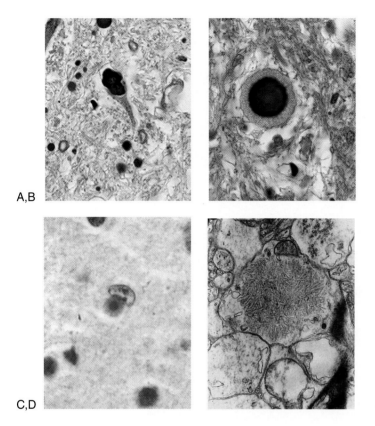

A,B

C,D

Color Plate 1 (See Figure 21.2)

COX II   FeS

Normal

KSS

MERRF

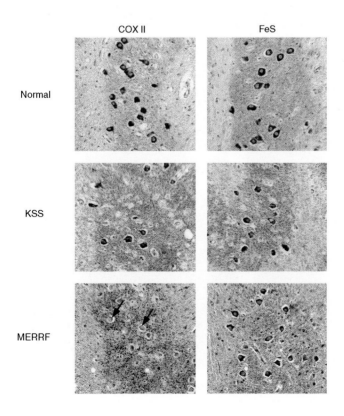

Color Plate 2 (See Figure 23.4)

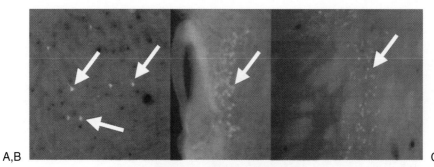

Color Plate 3 (See Figure 30.3)

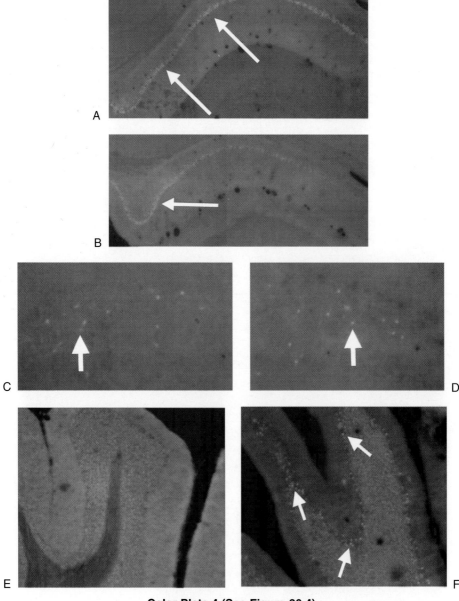

Color Plate 4 (See Figure 30.4)

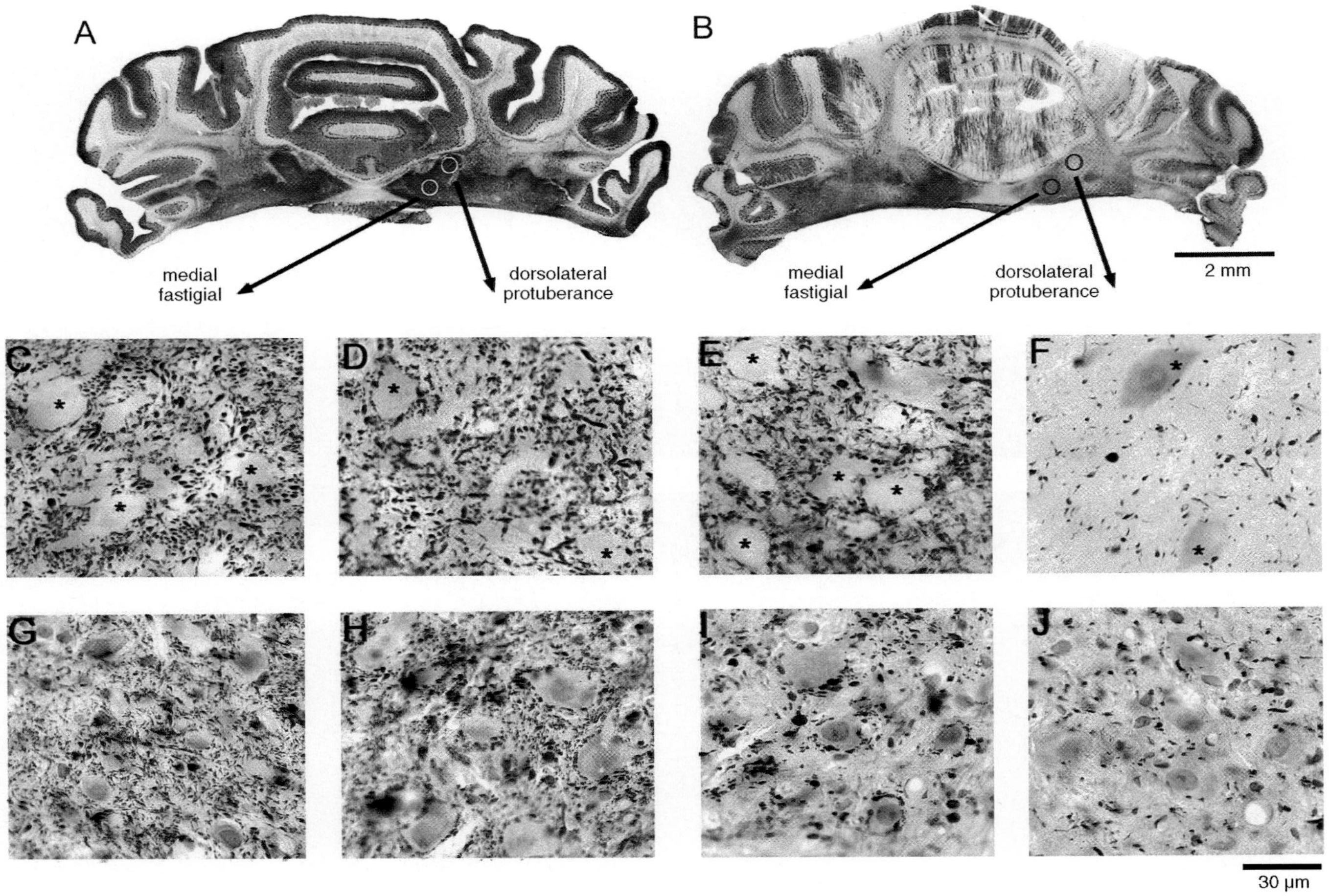

Color Plate 5 (See Figure 32.11)

aldolase C   EAAT4

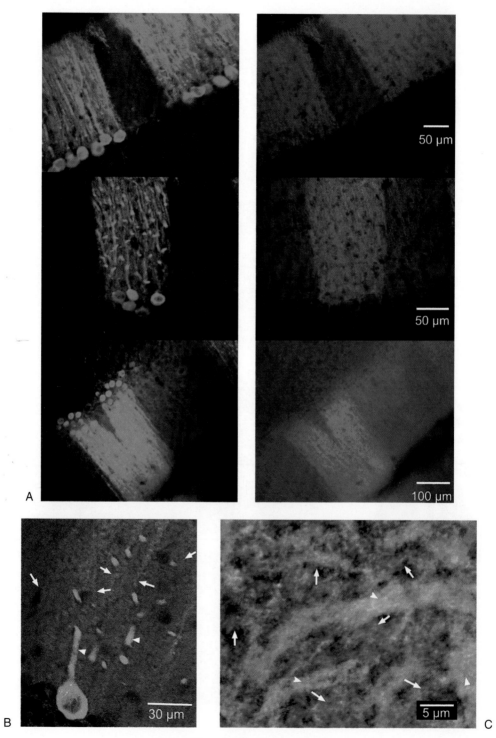

Color Plate 6 (See Figure 32.10)

Myoclonus and Paroxysmal Dyskinesias,
Advances in Neurology, Vol. 89,
edited by S. Fahn, et al.
Lippincott Williams & Wilkins, Philadelphia © 2002.

29

The Pacemaker in Posthypoxic Myoclonus: Where and What to Do About It?

William T. Thach, Jr.

Departments of Anatomy, Neurobiology and Neurology,
Washington University School of Medicine, St. Louis, Missouri

Posthypoxic myoclonus (1) has been attributed to excess excitability in cerebral cortex, thalamus, cerebellum, and most recently, the inferior olive (2). Previously, features of palatal myoclonus/tremor (PT) and essential tremor (ET) combined with results of animal experiments had been used to argue for a role for the inferior olive as the pacemaker in both palatal myoclonus and in essential tremor (3–7). More recently, posthypoxic myoclonus has been proposed to result from excessive synchronized discharge of the inferior olive. Welsh et al. (2) reported that in rats with myoclonic epilepsy, ablation of the inferior olive with 3-acetyl pyridine abolished the myoclonus. In a preliminary report, Welsh et al. found in the posthypoxic myoclonic rat a tendency for Purkinje cell complex spikes to fire rhythmically. Their interpretation was that the inferior olive climbing fiber discharged to and through the cerebellum and caused the myoclonic jerks.

The hypothesis of the inferior olive as a pacemaker of clinical movement disorders gained historic support from the harmaline studies in animals of Lamarre and Llinas and their colleagues (8–12). These studies showed that (a) harmaline produced a whole-body 8.5-second tremor in laboratory animals; (b) the tremor was time locked to a synchronous discharge in cells of the inferior olive and

other brainstem nuclei; and, most importantly, (c) the tremor was reduced by olive ablation.

It has further been proposed that the normal olive serves as the motor system "clock" necessary for initiating normal ballistic movements (10). Support came from animal studies in which no harmaline was used (13). Llinas and Yarom (14) reported tendencies for periodic discharge in guinea pig brainstem slices. Llinas and Sasaki (15) reported a tendency for synchronized discharge of climbing fiber spikes in the Purkinje cells of anesthetized rats. In ketamine anesthetized rabbits, Wylie et al. (16) found periodic discharge in Purkinje cell complex spikes in a third of the cells sampled with one or more frequency peaks (average, 8 Hz; range, 2.5 to 12.5 Hz). In awake behaving rats, Welsh et al. (17–19) and Lang et al. (20) reported that Purkinje cell climbing fiber spikes tend to fire periodically in relation to rhythmic tongue movements. Studies of human reaction-time movements had been reported to be paced by the normal human 10 per second physiologic tremor (21). Since under harmaline this tendency is dramatically increased and putatively drives the 10/sec harmaline body tremor (see above), it has been suggested that a normal periodic synchronized discharge in the olive may be the source of the normal 10/sec human physiologic tremor (3,4). As such, the inferior olive would serve as the "clock" of the motor system, triggering the onset of all movement on the beat of the 10/sec clock.

ANATOMY AND PHYSIOLOGY BASED ON THE NORMAL MACAQUE

The deep cerebellar nuclei (fastigial, globose-emboliform = interpositus, dentate) all project to and excite the Ventral Intermediate Nucleus (VIM) of the thalamus, which in turn projects to and excites cerebral cortex (areas 4, 6, 7, 8, 46). The pattern of activity in the nuclei is one of tonic maintained discharge at rest (50 to 100 per second) and phasic discharge during movement (0 to 500 per second). As to timing in relation to movement, the phasic activity leads that in motor cortex, which in turn leads electromyography and movement. As to the power of the cerebellar outflow on its targets, electrical stimulation causes movement and ablation delays (but does not abolish) movement via motor cortex and other routes. Yet certain aspects of movement *are* abolished: the automatic parts of compound movements, such as the trunk and leg muscle activity made in arm pointing movements is abolished. The inferior olive complex projects as climbing fibers exclusively to the cerebellum. A climbing fiber branches in the sagittal dimension and projects to narrow sagittal strips of ten or so Purkinje cells. The climbing fiber also has smaller collaterals to Golgi cells of the cortex and to the deep nuclear cells. Their effect is excitatory, but at least in awake monkeys is normally of very low frequency (1 to 2 per second).

CRITIQUE OF THE HYPOTHESIS OF A CAUSAL ROLE OF THE INFERIOR OLIVE IN PACING MOVEMENT

Electrical stimulation of the inferior olive does not cause quick movements. No study of single or repetitive electrical stimulation of the olive has reported prompt muscle contractions (22–25). Gibson et al. (26,27) and Nowak et al. (28) in tests specifically of this

issue say emphatically that stimulation of the inferior olive does not cause movement. Others have reported "drifting" slow eye movements (22) and changes in postural tone (29). By contrast, microstimulation of the deep cerebellar nuclei *does* cause focal bodily twitches (30,31).

Although electrical stimulation of the inferior olive does not cause quick movements, it *does* cause dramatic effects on Purkinje cell discharge. The "complex spikes" [Purkinje cell response to inferior olivary nucleus neuron (ION) climbing fiber excitation] occur at the rate of olivary stimulation. But the tonic firing of the "simple spike" (response of the Purkinje cell to mossy fibers) is reduced or stopped for periods long outlasting the stimulus (22). During this period, the simple spike response of the Purkinje cell to parallel fiber excitatory input is reduced or abolished (24).

Inactivation of the inferior olive increases Purkinje cell inhibition. By contrast, sudden inactivation of the olive (either by cooling [32] or by lesion [23]) causes within seconds a progressive *rise* in Purkinje cell simple spike discharge frequency. Since the Purkinje cell is inhibitory, a suddenly increased discharge rate would be expected to have a suppressive effect on the cerebellar nuclei, and a reduction in the cerebellar excitation of downstream targets. If these targets were themselves the source of the tremor signal, increased Purkinje cell inhibition could reduce the tremor. In this interpretation, olivary ablation would not remove the source of an excitatory pacemaker signal, but rather would augment Purkinje cell inhibition to damp the pacemaker signals originating at other downstream sites.

Harmaline does not specifically target the inferior olive. Worth mention are the clinical effects of harmaline, which is used principally as a psychedelic drug in primitive societies. Though it has widespread effects on the nervous system, it has not been reported to cause tremor in the doses used. Harmaline is one of a group of three-ringed molecules called harmala alkaloids or β-carbolines (4,9-dihydro-7-

methoxy-1-methyl-3H-pyrido-[3,4-b] indole or 7-methoxy-1-methyl-3, 4-dihydro-B-carbo-line). Stafford (33) summarizes:

> Harmaline and the other harmala alkaloids, the principle psychoactive substances in the "magical" beverage yahe, appear throughout the plant world. Although these three-ringed compounds are widespread in the plant kingdom, their use as a psychedelic is known in only two specific, geographically separate traditions: [a] scraping of the bark of *Banisteriopsis* [liana] vines to make a drink in northwestern South America and [b] ingestion of the seeds of Syrian rue *(Peganum harmala)*, a wild desert shrub, in the Near East. The Amazonian practices are better documented and colorfully illustrate purgative, healing, visual, telepathic, sexual, artistic and therapeutic potentials in psychedelics.

No mention is made of motor deficits in Stafford's review–indeed, coordination is said to have been remarkably preserved. Yet in one personal account of consuming yahe, visual hallucinations, violent vomiting, and diarrhea are said to have been accompanied by "staggering" (34). Another personal account describes the effects of consuming 500 mg of pure harmaline, which include protracted vomiting and diarrhea, "intense and annoying visual disturbances, and complete collapse of motor co-ordination...for safety's sake [I] locomoted by crawling" (35). Harmaline is virtually unknown among more sophisticated users of psychedelic drugs, presumably because of these noxious gastrointestinal side effects. Thus, its effects on humans have not been subject to scientific scrutiny. It is unclear whether personal reports of incoordination in fact constitute ataxia, rather than prostration from the concurrent gastrointestinal and psychic effects. Mention of tremor is conspicuously absent. Only at much greater doses has it been shown in laboratory animals to cause a whole body tremor (36).

Inferior olive activity is a concomitant not a direct cause of movement. As to why the inferior olive might be rhythmically active in tremor (including unit recording in harmaline animals, alert performing animals, and functional imaging in palatal and essential tremor in humans), the olive has inputs that are likely to be active in these motor activities. Olive discharge during tremor could thus be the accompaniment rather than the cause of the movements. In the alert performing rat studies (20), the periodicity of discharge was in the frequency range (8 to 15 Hz) of periodic tongue licking (and vibrissal whisking?) movements. Studies in the awake monkey also have shown the olive to fire just prior to movement, usually seen as a single complex spike in the Purkinje cell (37–39). As to whether the olive via the cerebellum *normally* generates a periodic synchronized 10-Hz signal to clock movements, unit recording studies in monkey have found no periodic signal in either in the discharge of the inferior olive inputs to Purkinje cells (38,40) or the cerebellar nuclei (41).

The ancillary evidence for synchronization and periodicity in olive discharge may also be tangential and not causal. Schweighofer et al. (42) model the electrophysiologic properties of inferior olive neurons and conclude that the gap junctions should instead serve to *desynchronize* olive discharge! In any event, the work emphasizes caution in accepting the idea that the presence of gap junctions *a priori* implies a synchronizing mechanism. The tendency for spontaneous periodic subthreshold membrane potential oscillations in guinea pig brainstem slices (14) was noted only in 10% of the preparations, was at frequencies of 4 to 6 Hz (not 10 Hz), and may have been influenced by the ketamine given previously. Finally, there is now good evidence that human reaction-time movements are not paced by the normal human 10/sec physiologic tremor (43).

Does the olive cause posthypoxic myoclonus? Human posthypoxic myoclonus is typically preceded by a period of coma and protracted seizures that have been attributed to profound malfunction of cerebral cortex (1). Because of the intentional nature of the myoclonus, the cerebellum has been suspected of somehow contributing. In both the human and in the rodent model of posthypoxic myoclonus (44,45), there is conspicuous loss of Purkinje cells. As suggested above, the consequent reduction of the tonic Purkinje cell inhibition could conceivably disinhibit downstream excitatory pacemakers.

Truong et al. (46) have recently challenged the interpretation of Welsh et al. (2) that in the posthypoxic rat the myoclonus is caused by synchronized discharge of the inferior olive to and through the cerebellum. They prepared two sets of posthypoxic myoclonic rats. One of the two sets was previously made deolivate with 3-actyl pyridine, sufficient to entirely obliterate the olive (histologically confirmed). Yet the amount and intensity of the myoclonus was equal in the two sets of animals. Truong et al. concluded that the olive could not be causing the myoclonus.

Does the olive cause palatal or essential tremor? We have reviewed elsewhere the arguments that the inferior olive serves a pacemaker roll in palatal (47) and essential tremor (48).[1] In brief, for the inferior olive to cause palatal tremor would require that it have some preferential connection through the cerebellum to muscles of branchial cleft origin. This is not the case: the inferior olive is now known to map the entire body musculature, without preferential connection to palatal, pharyngeal, facial, jaw, or diaphragmatic muscles. For the inferior olive to cause ET does not fit with evidence of pathophysiology in the reciprocal thalamocortical circuits. As with cerebellar tremor, ET has been thought possibly due to cerebellar denervation (48,49).

---

[1]A friendly critic pointed out that ET could be due to periodic inhibition of motor activity, rather than excitation. One might argue that that is how the olive might be involved, with periodic discharges going up the climbing fibers synchronously, powerfully exciting Purkinje cells synchronously, which would powerfully inhibit nuclear cells synchronously, periodically removing the excitatory cerebellar drive. However, the acid tests of the hypothesis would still be whether one could reproduce it by stimulating the olive, whether the olive is actually periodically active, or whether olive ablation removes the tremor, etc. As for palatal tremor, some recent work shows that in symptomatic palatal tremor after stroke with inferior olivary hypertrophy, over time the tremor continues but the olive atrophies to 10% or less of its normal cell count. Therefore, it further seems unlikely that the tremor comes from the olive.

What is the normal function of the inferior olive? We have reviewed elsewhere a role for the inferior olive alternative to that of pacing movements. Although there is not yet general agreement (13), the specificity of individual ION projections to individual cerebellar neurons in focal restricted areas, their unique activation patterns, their lack of participation in many overlearned movements, and reports of their participation in adapting old and acquiring new movement patterns are believed by many to be consistent with a role in motor and procedural learning (50).

Is there specific therapy for posthypoxic myoclonus? Damage of inferior the olive leads to increased discharge of Purkinje cells, increased inhibition of the tonic firing of cerebellar nuclear cells, with a likely decrease of the tonic excitation of possible downstream sources of myoclonus pacemakers. Though destruction of the olive could conceivably provide temporary relief, it would certainly lead to severe cerebellar cortical degeneration and ataxia (51). One alternative might be the chronic electrical stimulation of the cerebellar cortex, so as to increase Purkinje cell firing rates. This has been tried for control of intractable epilepsy of cerebral cortical origin, with some benefit (52). Nevertheless, in both clinical and experimental posthypoxic myoclonus, there is already severe loss of Purkinje cells (1,45), which would vitiate the effort of stimulating them. A more promising alternative is ablation or stimulation of the VIM thalamus, which is known to reduce both essential and cerebellar tremor (49,53). The rationale for this intervention is that it would prevent the cerebellothalamic tonic excitatory drive from impinging upon already hyperexcitable thalamocorticothalmic circuits. As thalamic stimulation for a variety of movement disorders proves increasingly useful—and medical treatment disappointing—thalamic stimulation seems a treatment worth trying in posthypoxic myoclonus.

ACKNOWLEDGMENTS

I thank Neal Barmack, Rodger Elble, Alan Gibson, Peter Gilbert, Walter Lewis, Mike

Mauk, John Rawson, Jerry Simpson, and Piergiorgio Strata for helpful comments.

REFERENCES

1. Lance JW, Adams RD. The syndrome of intention or action myoclonus as a sequel to hypoxic encephalopathy. *Brain* 1963;87:111.
2. Welsh JP, Chang B, Menaker ME, et al. Removal of the inferior olive abolishes myoclonic seizures associated with a loss of olivary serotonin. *Neuroscience* 1998;82: 879–97.
3. Lamarre Y. Animal models of physiological, essential, and parkinsonian-like tremors. In: Findlay LJ, Capildeo R, eds. *Movement disorders: tremor* New York: Oxford University Press, 1984:183–194.
4. Llinas R. Rebound excitation as the physiological basis for tremor: a biophysical study of the oscillatory properties of mammalian central neurones in vitro. In: Findlay LJ, Capildeo R, eds. *Movement disorders: tremor* New York: Oxford University Press, 1984:165–182.
5. Dubinsky R, Hallett M, Schwankhaus J. Increased metabolism of the inferior olives in palatal myoclonus. *Neurology* 1987;37(Suppl):125
6. Colebatch JG, Findley LJ, Frackowiak RSJ, et al. Preliminary report: activation of the cerebellum in essential tremor. *Lancet* 1990;336:1028–1030.
7. Deuschl G, Wenzelburger R, Loffler K, et al. Essential tremor and cerebellar dysfunction: clinical and kinematic analysis of intention tremor. *Brain* 2000;123:1568–1580.
8. Lamarre Y, Mercier LA. Neurophysiological studies of harmaline-induced tremor in the cat. *Can J Physiol Pharmacol* 1971;49:1049–1058.
9. Lamarre Y, de Montigny C, Dumont M, et al. Harmaline induced rhythmic activity of cerebellar and lower brain stem neurons. *Brain Res* 1971;32:246–250.
10. Montigny C de, Lamarre Y. Rhythmic activity induced by harmaline in the olivo-cerebellar-bulbar system of the cat. *Brain Res* 1973;53:81–95.
11. Llinas R, Volkind RA. The olivocerebellar system: functional properties as revealed by harmaline-induced tremor. *Exp Brain Res* 1973;18:69–87.
12. Lamarre Y, Joffroy AJ, Dumont M, et al. Central mechanisms of tremor in some feline and primate models. *Can J Neurol Sci* 1975;2:227–233.
13. Simpson JI, Wylie DR, De Zeeuw CI. On climbing fiber signals and their consequence(s). *Behav Brain Sci* 1996;1:384–398.
14. Llinas R, Yarom Y. Oscillatory properties of guinea-pig inferior olivary neurones and their pharmacological modulation: an *in vitro* study. *J Physiol Lond* 1986;376: 163–182.
15. Llinas R, Sasaki K. The functional organization of the olivo-cerebellar system as examined by multiple Purkinje cell recordings. *Eur J Neurosci* 1989;1:587–602.
16. Wylie DR, DeZeeuw CI, Simpson JI. Temporal relations of the complex spike activity of Purkinje cell pairs in the vestibulocerebellum of rabbits. *J Neurosci* 1995; 15:2875–2887
17. Welsh JP, Lang E, Sugihara I, et al. Rhythmic olivo-cerebellar control of skilled tongue movement in relation to patterned hypoglossal nerve activity. *Soc Neurosci Abstr* 1992;18:178.7.
18. Welsh JP, Lang E, Llinas R. The microstructure of coherence in the olivocerebellar system during rhythmic movement in normal and deafferented rats. *Soc Neurosci Abstr* 1993;19:529.9.
19. Welsh JP, Lang E, Llinas R. Dynamic organisation of motor control within the olivo cerebellar system. *Nature* 1995;374:453–457.
20. Lang EJ, Sugihara I, Welsh JP, et al. Patterns of spontaneous Purkinje cell complex spike activity in the awake. *Rat J Neurosci* 1999;19:2728–2739.
21. Goodman D, Kelso JAS. Exploring the functional significance of physiological tremor: a biospectroscopic approach. *Exp Brain Res* 1983;49:419–431.
22. Barmack NH. Immediate and sustained influences of visual olivo-cerebellar activity on eye movement. In: Talbot RE, Humphrey DR, ed. *Posture and movement: perspective for integrating sensory and motor research on the mammalian nervous system.* New York: Raven Press, 1979.
23. Rawson JA, Tilokskulchai K. Climbing modification of cerebellar Purkinje cell responses to parallel fiber inputs. *Brain Res* 1982;237:492–497.
24. Eckerot C-F, Kano M. Long-term depression of parallel fibre synapses following stimulation of climbing fibres. *Brain Res* 1985;342:357–360.
25. Mauk MD, Steinmetz JE, Thompson RF. Classical conditioning using stimulation of the inferior olive as the unconditioned stimulus. *Proc Natl Acad Sci USA* 1986; 83:5349–5353.
26. Gellman R, Gibson AR, Houk JC. Inferior olivary neurons in the awake cat: detection of contact and body displacement. *J Neurophysiol* 1995;54:40–60.
27. Gibson AR, Chen R. Does stimulation of the inferior olive produce movement? *Soc Neurosci* 1988;305:2.
28. Nowak AJ, Marshall-Goodell B, Kehoe EJ, et al. Elicitation, modification, and conditioning of the rabbit nictitating membrane response by electrical stimulation in the spinal trigeminal nucleus, inferior olive, interpositus nucleus, and red nucleus. *Behav Neurosci* 1997;111: 1041–1055.
29. Boylls CC. Contributions to locomotor coordination of an olivo-cerebellar projection to the vermis of the cat: experimental results and theoretical proposals. In: Courville J, ed. *The inferior olivary nucleus. Anatomy and Physiology.* New York: Raven Press, 1980:321–348.
30. Rispal-Padel L, Circirata F, Pons C. Cerebellar nuclear topography of simple and synergistic movements in the alert baboon Papio papio. *Exp Brain Res* 1982;47: 365–380.
31. Cicirata F, Angaut P, Serapide MF, et al. Multiple representation in the nucleus lateralis of the cerebellum: an electrophysiologic study in the rat. *Exp Brain Res* 1992; 89:352–362.
32. Strata P. Inferior olive: functional aspects. In: Bloedel JR, Dichgans J, Precht W, ed. *Cerebellar functions.* Berlin: Springer-Verlag, 1985:231–246.
33. Stafford P. Ayahuasca, yahe, and harmaline. In: *Psychedelics encyclopedia,* 3rd ed. Berkeley: Ronin Publishing, 1992.
34. Flores FA, Lewis WH. Drinking the South American hallucinogenic ayahuasca. *Econ Botany* 1978;32: 154–156.
35. Shulgin A, Shulgin A *TIHKAL: the continuation* Berkeley: Transform Press (Rosetta), 1977.
36. Brindlecombe RW, Pinder RM. Tremorigenic agents, In:

Tremors and tremorigenic agents. Baltimore: Williams & Wilkins, 1973:53–161.

37. Ojakangas CL, Ebner TJ. Purkinje cell complex spike activity during voluntary motor learning: relationship to kinematics. *J Neurophysiol* 1994;72:2617–2630.

38. Keating JG, Thach WT. Nonclock behavior of inferior olive neurons: interspike interval of Purkinje cell complex spike discharge in the awake behaving monkey is random. *J Neurophysiol* 1995;73:1329–1340.

39. Kitazawa S, Kimura T, Yin PB. Cerebellar complex spikes encode both destinations and errors in arm movements. *Nature* 1998;392:494–497.

40. Hakimian S, Greger B, Anderson CH , et al. Detecting periodicity in neuronal signals: have we lost "phase" in the autocorrelogram? *Abstr Soc Neurosci* 2000;26:2001.

41. Keating JG, Thach WT. No clock signal in the discharge of neurons in the deep cerebellar nuclei. *J Neurophysiol* 1997;77:2232–2234.

42. Schweighofer N, Doya K, Kawato M. Electrophysiological properties of inferior olive neurons: a compartmental model. *J Neurophysiol* 1999;82:804–817.

43. Lakie M, Combes N. There is no simple temporal relationship between the initiation of rapid reactive hand movements and the phase of an enhanced physiological tremor in man. *J Physiol* 2000;523:515–522.

44. Truong DD, Kanthasamy A, Nguyen B, et al. Animal models of post-hypoxic myoclonus. I: development and validation. *Mov Disord* 2000;15(Suppl 1):26–30.

45. Kanthasamy AG, Nguyen BQ, Truong DD. Animal model of post-hypoxic myoclonus. II: Neurochemical, pathologic, and pharmacological characterization. *Mov Disord* 2000;15(Suppl 1):31–38.

46. Truong DD, Kirby ML, Nguyen BQ, et al. The animal model of post-hypoxic myoclonus: lack of involvement of the olivo-cerebellar pathway during the acute phase. International Symposium on Myoclonus, Paroxysmal Dyskinesias and Related Disorders, Atlanta, 2000.

47. Kane SA, Thach WT: Palatal myoclonus and function of the inferior olive: are they related? *Exp Brain Res Series* 1989;17:427–460.

48. Zackowski KM, Bastian AJ, Hakimian S, et al. Thalamic stimulation reduces essential tremor but not the delayed antagonist muscle timing. *Neurology* 2001 (*in press*).

49. Jaeger CJ, Lenz FA, Seike MS, et al. Single unit analysis of thalamus in patients with cerebellar tremor. *Mov Disord* 1994;9(Suppl 1):22.

50. Thach WT, Goodkin HG, Keating JG. Cerebellum and the adaptive coordination of movement. *Ann Rev Neurosci* 1992;15:403–442.

51. Murphy MG, O'Leary JL. Neurological deficits in cats with lesions of the olivocerebellar system. *Arch Neurol* 1971;24:145–157.

52. Cooper IS, Amin I, Gilman S. The effect of chronic cerebellar stimulation upon epilepsy in man. *Trans Am Neurol Assn* 1973;98:192–196.

53. Benabid AL, Pollak P, Gao D, et al. Chronic electrical stimulation of the ventralis intermedius nucleus of the thalamus as a treatment of movement disorders. *J Neurosurg* 1996;84:203–214.

Myoclonus and Paroxysmal Dyskinesias,
Advances in Neurology, Vol. 89,
edited by S. Fahn, et al.
Lippincott Williams & Wilkins, Philadelphia © 2002.

30

Posthypoxic Myoclonus Animal Models

*Daniel D. Truong, *Michael Kirby, §Anumantha Kanthasamy,
and †Rae R. Matsumoto

*The Parkinson's and Movement Disorder Institute, Fountain Valley, California; §Department of
Biomedical Sciences, College of Veterinary Sciences, Iowa State University, Ames, Iowa;
and †Department of Pharmaceutical Sciences, University of Oklahoma Health Sciences Center,
Oklahoma City, Oklahoma

Since the classic description of posthypoxic myoclonus by Lance and Adams in 1963, more than 100 cases have been reported in the literature (1). As the term *posthypoxic* implies, this syndrome develops following cardiac arrest or anesthesia accidents. Little is known about the neuropathology of posthypoxic myoclonus because systematic studies are difficult to perform in humans and, until recently, no satisfactory animal model was available.

Early attempts to induce an animal model of myoclonus were unsuccessful, and it was initially thought that rats did not develop myoclonus following hypoxia (2). Models of myoclonus induced by pharmacologic and toxic agents have contributed to our knowledge but are less than optimal because they share neither the etiology nor the pharmacologic profile of the posthypoxic syndrome (3). A realistic animal model of myoclonus would be extremely valuable because it would permit studies of the disease pathology and testing of potential treatments. This chapter describes our efforts to develop and characterize an animal model of posthypoxic myoclonus.

METHODS

Our procedures for inducing posthypoxic myoclonus are briefly summarized here because they have been previously described in detail (4,5). Rats were anesthetized with 100 mg per kg ketamine hydrochloride and supplemented with methoxyflurane, if necessary. Succinylcholine (2 mg per kg, i.v.) was administered, and ventilator settings were adjusted to a rate of 60 strokes per mm and a volume of 7.5 mL per kg. We performed the cardiac arrest with a transthoracic intracardiac injection of KCl and cessation of ventilation. Resuscitation was begun 10 minutes after the arrest by turning on the ventilator (100% O_2), manual thoracic compressions, and i.v. injections of epinephrine hydrochloride (20 µg per kg) and sodium bicarbonate (4 mEq per kg; Lyphomed). The rat was then weaned from the ventilator over 2 to 4 hours and extubated. For some experiments, we modified the duration of cardiac arrest by initiating resuscitation at different time points (1 to 10 minutes) in order to examine the effect of duration of hypoxia. We also compared the development of myoclonus in young (180 g, approximately 6 weeks old) and adult (400 g, about 6 months old) rats.

The procedure just described was termed *chemical cardiac arrest* (4). However, because successful resuscitation and postoperative survival were the rate-limiting factors in this animal model (5–7), we have since switched to a mechanical procedure involving an L-shaped hook (8). This modification improved the survival rate and has become the standard of our techniques. Furthermore, the use of succinylcholine has been omitted to reduce peripheral complications.

In order to obtain electroencephalogram (EEG) readings, we implanted two skull screws under ketamine/xylazine anesthesia over the parietal cortex 24 hours before the procedure.

Histological Analysis

At 10 to 12 days postarrest, rats were anesthetized and perfused transcardially with saline and paraformaldehyde. Brains were stained with Flouro-Jade (9) or cresyl violet. Flouro-Jade-stained tissues were analyzed using an Olympus BH-2 fluorescence microscope with fluorescein isothiocyanate filter set connected to SPOT camera. Some brains were processed for the detection of EAAC-1 (the presynaptic neuronal glutamate transporter), glutamic acid decarboxylase, and tryptophan hydroxylase immunoreactivity.

Evaluation of Auditory-Induced Myoclonus

One day to 6 months after cardiac arrest, rats were evaluated for auditory-induced myoclonus (4,10). This testing protocol differentiates myoclonus from the startle response (5). Following at least 10 minutes of habituation to Plexiglas cages, rats were presented with 45 clicks of metronome stimulus on audiotape. Muscle jerks to each click were scored as follows: 0, no reaction; 1, ear twitch; 2, ear and head jerk; 3, ear, head, and shoulder jerk; 4, whole body jerk; and 5, whole body jerk of such severity that it caused a jump.

Pharmacologic Interventions

Because 5-hydroxytryptophan (5-HTP), valproic acid, and clonazepam are known to reduce myoclonus both clinically (11–13) and experimentally (14,15), we tested their effects in our model to validate its pharmacologic profile. The following medications were administered (all i.p.): 5-HTP (100 mg per kg in 1% hydroxypropylcellulose), valproic acid (50 and 300 mg per kg in saline), and clonazepam (0.5 and 1 mg per kg in dimethyl sulfoxide), saline, or dimethyl sulfoxide vehicle.

Following collection of a baseline myoclonus score, rats were administered one of the above drugs, then retested at 30, 60, 90, and 120 minutes. Because the myoclonus scores of the animals changed over time, only those animals that had a baseline score of 74 or higher were included in the analysis; this score is very close to the mean myoclonus score of normal, untreated rats (73 ± 16). This cutoff, which was established in preliminary studies using cluster analysis, allowed us to measure both improvement and worsening of myoclonus scores.

RESULTS

Animal Behavior after Recovery

After recovery from the arrest, rats were comatose for approximately 2 to 3 hours. They gradually reacted to painful stimuli but were unable to move themselves until 10 to 12 hours afterward. The rats were spastic with hindlimb in extensor, and they dragged the hindlimb when ambulating. Over 2 days they regained mobility. In the first 3 days after arrest, they tended to develop running seizures when exposed to loud noise. Myoclonic jerks were exhibited in all rats spontaneously, during voluntary movements, or in response to auditory stimuli. Initially, these myoclonic jerks were masked by the running seizures. When provoked by loud noise, myoclonic jerks often preceded the running seizures in the first 2 to 3 days after the arrest. With time, the incidence of noise-induced seizures declined and myoclonus alone remained. In general, after day 4, rats displayed only myoclonus when stimulated with noise. The animals needed to be fed and hydrated in the first 4 days following KCl-induced cardiac arrest and 2 to 3 days in the mechanically induced cardiac arrest. The animals continued to recover and, by 2 months after resuscitation, there was no difference in body weight between arrested animals and age-matched controls, with mechanically-induced cardiac arrested rats recovering earlier than KCl-induced rats.

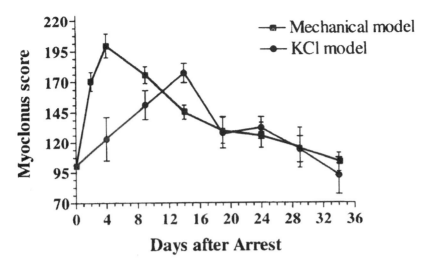

FIG. 30.1. Time course of cardiac arrest-induced posthypoxic myoclonus in rats using two different procedures, a mechanical model and a chemical (KCl) model. Each point represents mean ± SEM of 6 to 10 animals. The myoclonus score of a normal animal would be 70 to 90. (Reprinted from Wiley-Liss, Inc., a subsidiary of John Wiley & Sons, Inc., with permission.) (7)

Auditory-Induced Myoclonus

All the animals exhibited noticeable auditory-induced myoclonus after the arrest. The time course of myoclonus in KCl-induced cardiac arrest and in mechanically–induced cardiac arrest was nearly identical (Fig. 30.1). Myoclonus scores in both groups showed a steady increase followed by a more gradual decrease, with both groups returning to baseline at approximately 5 weeks after the arrest. The main difference between the two models was in the time to peak effect, which occurred at day 4 in the mechanical model and at day 14 in the KCl model. Also, animals in the KCl model were sicker. Beginning 5 to 7 days after the arrest, almost all of the animals appeared qualitatively "normal" except when exhibiting auditory-induced myoclonus; the rare exceptions were those animals with persistent hindlimb paralysis (2 of 31). In animals that had not been injected with drug or vehicle, the myoclonus scores of cardiac-arrested rats were significantly higher than those of normal, non-cardiac-arrested controls (data not shown).

The myoclonus scores of posthypoxic animals increased with the duration of hypoxia in both the KCl and mechanical models (data not shown). Myoclonus started to appear only when the duration of hypoxia reached 5 minutes, at which time 2 of 4 animals exhibited myoclonus. When the hypoxia duration was increased to 8 minutes, all rats developed myoclonus. Although the myoclonus lasted longer with increased duration of hypoxia, this increase was associated with a higher death rate during the recovery.

Adult rats (about 6 months of age) consistently showed higher myoclonus scores than

TABLE 30.1. *Myoclonus score at different postarrest days following cardiac arrest*

Rats	Day 3	Day 7	Day 14	Day 21	Day 28	Day 35
Young	210.1 ± 8.33[a]	189.6 ± 7.13[a]	142.8 + 6.68[a]	111.1 ± 5.54	92.83 ± 3.9	83.26 ± 6.48
Adult	222.0 ± 10.78[a]	202.8 ± 10.26[a]	173.0 ± 7.41[a]	140.3 ± 4.73[a]	118.4 ± 8.04[a]	102.4 ± 7.17

Adult rats consistently showed higher myoclonus scores than young rats over the 5 weeks following hypoxia. Values (mean ± SEM) are expressed as percent baseline score from 8 rats in each group.
[a]$p < 0.05$ as determined by Wilcoxon test using prism statistical program.

TABLE 30.2. *Relationship between cardiac arrest–induced mortality rate and increase in age of experimental animals*

Age	No. of animals underwent surgery	No. of survival	% Mortality
8 wk	8	8	0
6 mo	12	8	33
12 mo	4	0	100

young rats over the 5 weeks following hypoxia (Table 30.1). Adult and aged rats also showed a higher cardiac arrested mortality rate than young rats (Table 30.2) (5). In the older rats, hypoxia was more often associated with paraplegia than with myoclonus. All three of the antimyoclonic drugs tested, 5-HTP, valproate, and clonazepam, significantly

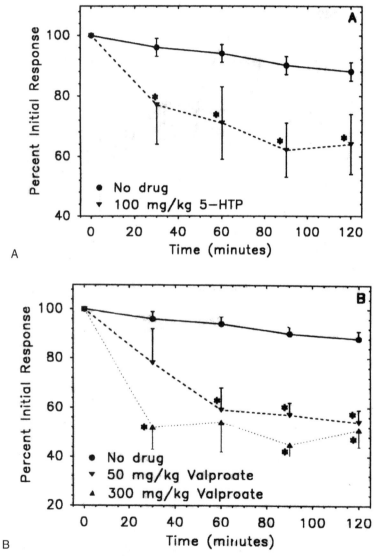

FIG. 30.2. Effects of 5-hydroxytryptophan (**A**; 100 mg per /kg, i.p), valproate (**B**; 50 and 300 mg per kg, i.p.), and clonazepam (**C**; 0.5 and 1.0 mg per kg, i.p.) on auditory-induced posthypoxic myoclonus. All three drugs significantly attenuated myoclonus scores compared to animals treated with vehicle. Scores are represented as a percentage of the initial response at time 0 (designated as 100%). (Reprinted from Wiley-Liss, Inc., a subsidiary of John Wiley & Sons, Inc., with permission.) (4)

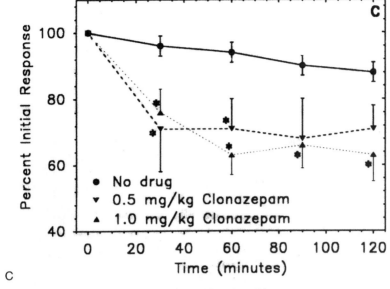

C

FIG. 30.2. *(Continued.)*

decreased myoclonus scores compared with vehicle (Fig. 30.2A–C).

Histology

Four to 6 days postsurgery, selective neuronal necrosis was observed in most posthypoxic rats as determined by Nissl staining and Fluoro-Jade histochemistry. Posthypoxic myoclonus animals sustained neuronal damage in key brain regions such as the cortex, hippocampus, thalamus, indusium griseum, and cerebellum. The damage in the cortex was lo-calized in the hindlimb representation area of the frontal cortex and parietal and temporal cortices. At the cellular level, Fluoro-Jade labeling revealed that large and small pyramidal neurons in cortical layers III to IV were damaged (Fig. 30.3A; see Color Plate 3 following page 288), as well as neurons in the indusium griseum (Fig. 30.3B). In the thalamus, the Fluoro-Jade labeling was readily discernible in the medial and lateral nucleus, including the thalamic reticular nucleus (Fig. 30.3C) Neuronal necrosis was also pronounced in the nucleus of the trapezoid body. Histologic exami-

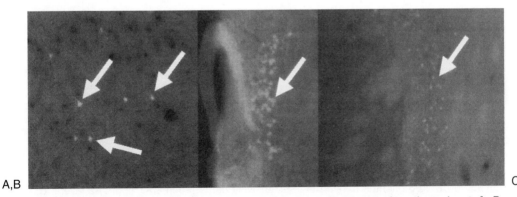

FIG. 30.3. Fluoro-Jade positive dead cells in the 8-minute cardiac arrested posthypoxic rat. **A:** Pyramidal cells in layers III and IV of cerebral cortex. **B:** Indusium griseum. **C:** Reticular thalamic nucleus (see Color Plate 3 following page 288).

nation of the hippocampus revealed bilaterally symmetrical, selective neuronal loss in the hippocampal CA1 pyramidal cell layer. Hippocampus of 8-minute hypoxic rats showed a severe loss of the pyramidal cells in CA1 and CA2 regions (Fig. 30.4A; see Color Plate 4 following page 288), with reduced damage in these areas under conditions of only 4 minutes of hypoxia (Fig. 30.4B). In the case of ischemic and nonmyoclonic rats, the neuronal injury was primarily localized to the CA1 subfield of the hippocampus. Approximately 75%

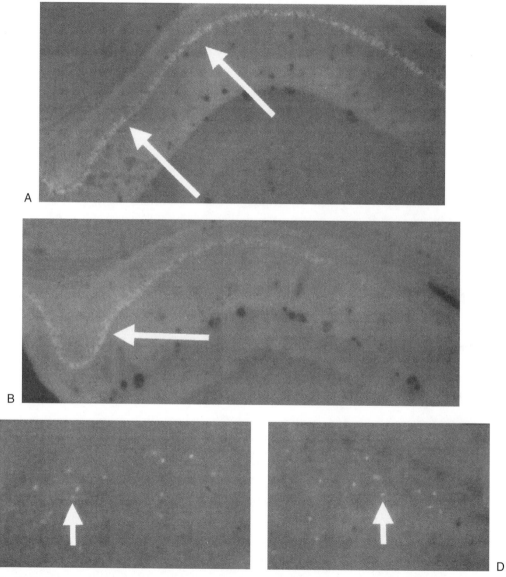

FIG. 30.4. Fluoro-Jade histology in 4- and 8-minute cardiac arrested posthypoxic rats. **A:** Hippocampus following 8 minutes of hypoxia is extensively damaged in CA1 and CA2 layers. **B:** Hippocampus following 4 minutes of hypoxia shows moderate damage in CA1 layer and no damage in CA2. **C** and **D:** Polymorphic region of the dentate gyrus following 8 or 4 minutes of hypoxia, respectively, shows similar levels of damage (see Color Plate 4 following page 288).

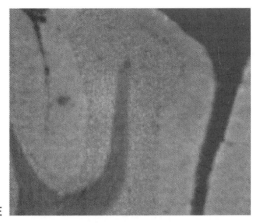

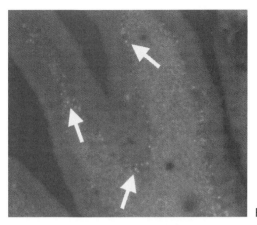

E

F

FIG. 30.4 *(Continued).* **E:** Cerebellum following 4 minutes of hypoxia shows no damage. **F:** Cerebellum following 8 minutes of hypoxia shows extensive damage in the Purkinje cell layer (see Color Plate 4 following page 288).

of hippocampal CA1 pyramidal cells were necrotic in the 8-minute cardiac arrested rats. Also, comparing 4 versus 8 minutes of hypoxia with respect to dentate granule cells, equivalent levels of moderate damage were observed (Fig. 30.4C,D). In the cerebellum, the round bipolar Purkinje cells were severely damaged only under conditions of 8-minute hypoxia (Fig. 30.4F), whereas 4 minutes of hypoxia produced no cerebellar damage (Fig. 30.4E). Approximately 30% to 40% of cerebellar Purkinje cells were necrotic in the 8-minute cardiac-arrested rats. Labeling of a few cells in the granular layer of the cerebellum of 8-minute hypoxic rats was also observed. To a lesser degree, necrotic cell was also seen in the olfactory bulbs, ventral neocortex, striatum, lateral or medial septal nuclei, dentate granule cell layer of the hippocampus, the colliculi, and substantia nigra.

Additional histologic markers for specific neuronal characterization indicated several trends toward impairment of neuronal function in key brain regions associated with modulation and coordination of motor activities. Purkinje cell loss (see above) is likely caused by AMPA receptor-mediated excitotoxicity resulting from prolonged hypoxia (16). Monoclonal antibodies to EAAC-1, the presynaptic neuronal glutamate transporter, applied to rat cerebellar tissues revealed a profound loss of EAAC-1 expression in 8-minute hypoxic rats (Fig. 30.5B) compared with normal levels of EAAC-1 expression (Fig. 30.5A).

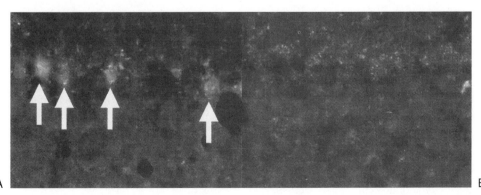

A

B

FIG. 30.5. EAAC-1 expression in Purkinje cell layer of cerebellum. **A:** EAAC-1 expression pronounced in untreated rat. **B:** EAAC-1 expression is reduced in Purkinje cell layer following 8 minutes of hypoxia.

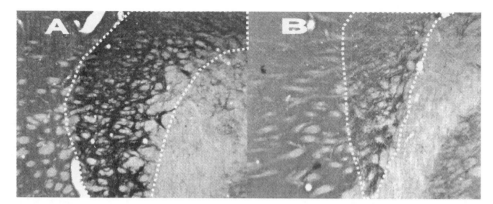

FIG. 30.6. Glutamate decarboxylase (GAD)-labeled reticular thalamic nucleus. **A:** Heavy GAD immunopositive staining in an untreated rat. **B:** Lack of immunopositive GAD staining in posthypoxic rat.

Using monoclonal antibody staining for a GABA-ergic neuronal marker, glutamate decarboxylase (GAD), we found reduced GAD expression in 8-minute hypoxic rats compared with normal rats (Fig. 30.6A,B), indicating that GABA-ergic neurons are the most vulnerable to ischemic damage.

Additionally, tryptophan hydroxylase expression was found to be severely reduced in striata of 8-minute hypoxic rats (Fig. 30.7B) compared with striatal tissues from untreated rats (Fig. 30.7A).

Electroencephalogram

The EEG became isoelectric within 15 seconds of arrest and remained isoelectric for the next 20 to 30 minutes after the insult. In the next days, periods of sharp waves and/or spikes intermixed with isoelectric periods emerged. Bursts of low voltage activity mixed with spikes and/or sharp waves appeared afterward. The EEG gradually gained in amplitude. After 2 days, the EEG showed a slow wave background with occasional sharp bursts.

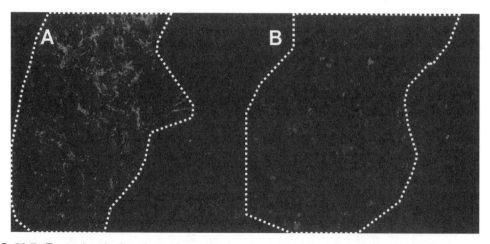

FIG. 30.7. Tryptophan hydroxylase expression in striatum. **A:** Untreated rat shows high levels of tryptophan hydroxylase expression in striatum. **B:** Tryptophan hydroxylase expression is reduced in striatum of posthypoxic rat at day 5 postsurgery.

DISCUSSION

Behavioral and Pharmacological Evaluations: Similarity to the Human Syndrome

Patients who suffer from cardiac arrest often go through a phase of deep coma lasting from days to weeks and exhibit seizures prior to the development of myoclonus. As patients slowly improve, myoclonus develops along with other neurologic sequelae. This progression of events was also seen in our model. EEG results of this model also showed a similar pattern of progression to that observed in humans who have suffered cardiac arrest. Using electromyography obtained simultaneously from the orbicularis oculi, orbicularis oris, trapezius, forepaw, and hindpaw muscles, we have previously reported a pattern similar as seen in brainstem myoclonus (5). This finding has been recently confirmed (Welsch et al. *personal communication*). The features of our model and human myoclonus are compared in Table 30.3.

Additionally, in our model, myoclonus developed only after a critical duration of hypoxia. Earlier resuscitation resulted in lower myoclonus scores as well as a shorter duration of myoclonus after recovery. A cardiac arrest time of 8 minutes represented a tradeoff at which the survival rate was acceptable and additional neurologic complications were less severe. The survival rate decreased with a longer duration of cardiac arrest, although the duration of myoclonus was also prolonged. Similar duration of myoclonus after cardiac arrest has been confirmed by others (Welsch, *personal communication*). Goetz et al. (17) also confirmed the advantages of the 8-minute cardiac arrest time.

Our data also showed that there is an advantage to using young animals for studying myoclonus. Although both young and old rats developed myoclonus, young rats seemed to develop it more consistently, whereas older rats tended to develop spasticity in addition to myoclonus. The question arose as to whether the model is more akin to acute myoclonus in humans or a mild form of chronic myoclonus. Our results showed that the myoclonus in older rats could achieve the features of the chronic model. This correlates well with the human condition, in that myoclonus tends to last longer in older patients. Additionally, because rats have much shorter life expectancy than humans (i.e., approximately 2 years), the 5-week duration of myoclonus represents a significantly greater portion of the rat's lifespan than for humans. Further investigation is needed to determine whether the difference between acute and chronic myoclonus is based primarily on the severity of damage to brain structures.

TABLE 30.3. *Comparison of the features of posthypoxic myoclonus in our animal model and in human chronic posthypoxic myoclonus*

	Human	Animal model
Improves spontaneously with time	Yes	Yes
Increased severity with age	Yes	Yes
Responsive to		
5-HTP	Yes	Yes
Valproate	Yes	Yes
Clonazepam	Yes	Yes
Piracetam	Yes	Yes
Heightened response to startling acoustic stimuli	Yes	Yes
EEG pattern	Bursts of generalized spike and polyspike activity with jerks, may be silent in between	Generalized slow waves and burst of sharp waves
Negative myoclonus	Yes	Not studied
Neuronal loss	Not studied	Yes
5-HT dysfunction	Some cases	Yes

EEG, electroencephalogram; 5-HT, 5-hydroxytryptamine; 5-HTP, 5-hydroxytryptophan.

The pharmacologic profile of our model was similar to that of human myoclonus in that it responded well to 5-HTP, valproate, and clonazepam. We have also recently found that piracetam, which has been reported to be effective in human myoclonus, was effective in our model (18).

Previous studies have implicated the 5-hydroxytryptamine (5-HT) system in the pathogenesis of posthypoxic myoclonus (19). The effectiveness of 5-HTP in treating some myoclonus patients initially raised hopes that a mechanism similar to Parkinson disease could be found. However, unlike the benefits of levodopa in Parkinson disease, which can be explained by the pathologic loss of nigral dopamine neurons, the benefits of 5-HTP in posthypoxic myoclonus cannot be explained by a parallel lack of serotonin. To date, no clear-cut, localized deficiency of 5-HT has been established in myoclonus. Nevertheless, the beneficial effects of 5-HTP and the reduced 5-HIAA levels in the cerebrospinal fluid of some patients suggest that 5-HT may somehow be involved.

In a previous study, we found that enhancement of serotonergic activity, particularly through 5-HT2 and 5-HT3 receptors, improved myoclonus scores in our model (5). High-performance liquid chromatography measurements revealed significant changes in the indole and its metabolites levels in certain brain areas. Interestingly, the changes in striatal 5-HT, cortical 5-HIAA, and mesencephalic 5-HIAA significantly correlated with the myoclonus scores of the animals (20). Matsumoto et al. (20) postulated a dysfunction in serotonergic lateral (cortical) and far lateral (extrapyramidal) ascending pathways in posthypoxic myoclonus.

The picture is more complicated, however, as shown in our previous experiments with 5-HT1A agonists. Although single injections of 5-HT1A agonists had no effect on either the intensity or time course of the disease, chronic treatments significantly attenuated the myoclonus (6). Chronic stimulation of 5-HT1A receptors in the brain may accelerate endogenous compensatory mechanisms and

shorten the time course of the disease. Methiothepin mesylate and mesulergine hydrochloride have been reported to reduce myoclonus scores in this model (21). Because methiothepin mesylate blocked 5-HT 1B, 5-HT 1D and 5-HT 2 and mesulergine hydrochloride blocked 5-HT 2A and 5-HT 2B, Pappert et al. (21) postulated that 5-HT 1B, 5-HT 2A/2B, and possibly 5-HT 1D receptor subtypes likely play a role in posthypoxic myoclonus. However, because results with high-dose antagonists are difficult to interpret, conclusions from such studies must be drawn with caution.

Histologic Observations

Several brain areas showed neuronal necrosis after ischemia in this model. These included layers III to V of the entire cortical mantle, the hippocampal CA1 pyramidal cell layer, the nucleus reticularis of the thalamus in the forebrain, and the Purkinje cell layer and the medullary reticular formation of the hindbrain. The pathologic abnormality seen in the model includes cerebellum, inferior olive, and thalamus. The role of these structures in the pathology of myoclonus is currently unclear. Although destruction of the inferior olive has been shown to protect the Purkinje cells in the cerebellum; we did not see any reduction in the myoclonus scores following this procedure.

Systematic studies using lesion techniques are needed to help clarify the neuronal pathways involved in myoclonus. It is possible that a loop starting from the brainstem to the cortex and downward again is responsible for myoclonus, which could be aggravated or modified along the axis by multiple structures such as the cortex, thalamus, and serotonin nuclei. This hypothesis may explain diverse pharmacologic agents that have seemed to have an effect on myoclonus. Drugs that have effects on one structure may not necessarily improve abnormalities related to myoclonus in another. This loop may also explain the involvement of both brainstem and cortical structures in human myoclonus. In our model, the myoclonus seems to be localized only in brainstem (5). This finding would not seem to be inconsistent with our hypothesis, and clearly, further electrophysiologic studies will be needed. This line of research is somewhat limited due to the size of our animal model and, in this context, further development of a primate model may be justified.

Additional histologic markers for specific neuronal types indicated several trends toward impairment of neuronal function in key brain regions associated with modulation and coordination of motor activities. The reticular thalamic nucleus (RTN) has been shown to be a potential center for myoclonus generation, as evidenced by studies involving direct injection of pharmacologic agents to this thalamic nucleus. Matsumoto et al. (22) injected picrotoxin, a $GABA_A$ antagonist, directly into the RTN of rats and observed a rhythmic, un-evoked myoclonus that could be synchronized to an auditory stimulus. The authors tentatively concluded that disturbance of GABA-ergic transmission could be an important component in audiogenic myoclonus resulting from hypoxia.

In a similar manner, we have shown here using monoclonal antibody staining for a GABA-ergic neuronal marker, GAD, reduced GAD expression in 8-minute hypoxic rats compared with normal rats. Loss of GAD expression is either the result of GABA neuron loss or severe impairment that results in reduced GAD gene expression. Reduced expression of this critical enzyme in the GABA biosynthetic pathway would result in reduced overall GABA-ergic tone to the RTN and would, in a general sense, produce a similar result to $GABA_A$ blockade. Long-term studies of GAD expression should be undertaken in an animal model of posthypoxic myoclonus to determine whether any recover of GAD expression in the RTN occurs, and whether this is correlated with abatement of myoclonus.

Tryptophan hydroxylase, the key enzyme that hydroxylates the amino acid tryptophan to form the neurotransmitter 5-HT, was found to be severely reduced in striata of 8-minute hypoxic rats compared with striatal tissues from untreated rats. Reduction in tryptophan hydroxylase expression, either resulting from serotonergic neuronal cell loss or metabolic impairment, would result in reduced serotonergic tone from neurons originating in the dorsal raphae nuclei projecting to target structures such as the caudate nucleus, putamen, and globus pallidus. Since loss of pontine serotonergic cell bodies was not observed here, we assume that reduced tryptophan hydroxylase expression results from metabolic impairment of serotonergic neurons projecting to the striatum. Serotonergic dysfunction is a well-established component of posthypoxic myoclonus and prophylactic reparation of reduced serotonergic tone has become a standard therapy for posthypoxic myoclonus (11, 23, 24).

Summary

The animal model presented here resembles several of the key features of human myoclonus. Further study of the neuropathology and pharmacology of this animal model will hopefully increase our knowledge of the brain structures and systems affected in this disease and permit testing of therapeutic agents for the significant number of patients who do not respond to current treatments.

ACKNOWLEDGMENTS

The authors appreciate the assistance of Bang Nguyen, Annie Tran, Brian Wyn, David Shao, and Edwin Gean in conducting these experiments and to Mary Ann Chapman for editorial assistance.

REFERENCES

1. Lance JW, Adams RD. The syndrome of intention or action myoclonus as a sequel to hypoxic encephalopathy. *Brain* 1963;86:111–136.
2. Sharma JN, Snider SR, Fahn S, et al. Anoxic myoclonus in the rat. *Adv Neurol* 1979;26:181–189.
3. Nguyen BQ, Kanthasamy AG, Truong DD. Animal models of myoclonus: an overview. *Mov Disord* 2000;15(Suppl 1):22–25.
4. Truong DD, Matsumoto RR, Schwartz PH, et al. Novel

rat cardiac arrest model of posthypoxic myoclonus. *Mov Disord* 1994;9:201–206.

5. Truong DD, Kanthasamy A, Nguyen B, et al. Animal models of posthypoxic myoclonus. I: development and validation. *Mov Disord* 2000;15(Suppl 1):26–30.

6. Jaw SP, Su DD, Truong DD. Expression of Bcl-2 and Bax in the frontoparietal cortex of the rat following cardiac arrest. *Brain Res Bull* 1995;38:577–580.

7. Kanthasamy AG, Matsumoto RR, Truong DD. Animal models of myoclonus. *Clin Neurosci* 1995–96;3: 236–245.

8. Kawai K, Penix LP, Kawahara N, et al. Development of susceptibility to audiogenic seizures following cardiac arrest cerebral ischemia in rats. *J Cereb Blood Flow Metab* 1995;15:248–258.

9. Schmued LC, Albertson C, Slikker W. Fluoro-Jade: a novel fluorochrome for the sensitive and reliable histochemical localization of neuronal degeneration. *Brain Res* 1997;751:37–46.

10. Truong DD, Garcia De Yebenes J, Pezzoli G, et al. Glycine involvement in DDT-induced myoclonus. *Mov Disord* 1988;3:222–232.

11. Fahn S. Posthypoxic action myoclonus: literature review update. *Adv Neurol* 1986;43:157–169.

12. Fahn S. Post-anoxic action myoclonus: improvement with valproic acid. *N Engi J Med* 1978;299:313–314.

13. L'hermitte F, Marteau R, Degos C-F. Analyse pharmacologique d'un nouveau cas de myoclonies d'intention et d'action post-anoxiques. *Rev Neurol Paris* 1972;126: 107–114.

14. Hwang EC, Van Woert MH. p,p-DDT-induced neurotoxic syndrome: experimental myoclonus. *Neurology* 1978;28:1020–1025.

15. Pratt JA, Rothwell J, Jenner P, et al. Myoclonus in the rat induced by p,p'-DDT and the role of altered monoamine function. *Neuropharmacology* 1985;24:361–373.

16. Brorson JR, Manzolillo PA, Gibbons SJ, et al. AMPA receptor desensitization predicts the selective vulnerability of cerebellar Purkinje cells to excitotoxicity. *J Neurosci* 1995;15:4515–4524.

17. Goetz CG, Vu TQ, Carvey PM, et al. Posthypoxic myoclonus in the rat: natural history, stability, and serotonergic influences. *Mov Disord* 2000;15(Suppl 1):39–46.

18. Nguyen BQ, Kanthasamy AG, Truong DD. Animyoclonic effect of piracetam animal model of posthypoxic myoclonus [Abstract]. *Soc Neurosci* 1999;25: 2052.

19. Chadwick D, Hallett M, Harris R, et al. Clinical, biochemical and physiological features distinguishing myoclonus responsive to 5-hydroxytryptophan, tryptophan with a monoamine oxidase inhibitor, and clonazpam. *Brain* 1977;100:455–487.

20. Matsumoto RR, Aziz N, Truong DD. Association between brain indole levels and severity of posthypoxic myoclonus in rats. *Pharm Biochem Behav* 1995;50:533–538.

21. Pappert EJ, Goetz CG. Treatment of myoclonus. In: Kurlan R, ed. *Treatment of movement disorders.* Philadelphia: JB Lippincott Co, 1995:247–356.

22. Matsumoto RR, Truong DD, Nguyen KD, et al. Involvement of GABAA receptors in myoclonus. *Mov Disord* 2000;15(Suppl 1):47–52.

23. De Lean J, Richardson JC, Hornykiewicz O. Beneficial effects of serotonin precursors in postanoxic action myoclonus. *Neurology* 1976;26:863.

24. Van Woert MH, Rosenbaum D, Howieson J, et al. Long term therapy of myoclonus and other neuorological disorders with L-5-hydroxytryptophan and carbidopa. *N Engl J Med* 1977;296:70–75.

Myoclonus and Paroxysmal Dyskinesias,
Advances in Neurology, Vol. 89,
edited by S. Fahn, et al.
Lippincott Williams & Wilkins, Philadelphia © 2002.

31

The Serotonin Hypothesis of Myoclonus from the Perspective of Neuronal Rhythmicity

*John P. Welsh, †Dimitris G. Placantonakis, ‡Sarah I. Warsetsky, †Rolando G. Marquez, §Lana Bernstein, and *Sue A. Aicher

Neurological Sciences Institute, Oregon Health and Sciences University, Beaverton, Oregon;
†Departments of Physiology and Neuroscience, New York University School of Medicine, New York,
New York; ‡Departments of Obstetrics and Gynecology, Abington Memorial Hospital, Abington,
Pennsylvania; and §Department of Internal Medicine, Harvard University and Beth Israel Deaconess
Medical Center, Boston, Massachusetts

In its most basic form, the serotonin hypothesis of myoclonus states that myoclonus results from a reduction in brain serotonin (1). It now appears clear that this strong hypothesis serves a more heuristic purpose than was envisioned at the time of its proposal, and that the global solution that it implied — enhance serotonergic neurotransmission to solve myoclonus— does not have universal application. However, with our advantage of a decade of further research, this is not surprising due to three factors. First, the actions of serotonin are among the most pleiotropic of all the neurotransmitters. This is due to the innervation of nearly all regions of the central nervous system (CNS) by serotonin fibers (2), the very large heterogeneity of serotonin receptors (14 subtypes, ref. 3), and the diversity of serotonin receptor effects on the intrinsic membrane properties of neurons. Second, the fine terminal fibers of serotonin neurons are very sensitive to neurotoxic agents (4), making them a common pathway for biasing the CNS toward a wide variety of motor and non-motor neurologic disorders. Third, serotonin is a powerful modulator of central motor function—as evidenced by its influence on neurons of the striatum (5), inferior olive (6), cerebellum (7), and even the motoneurons (8). Elucidating a clear relation between serotonin hypofunction and myoclonus

is further complicated by the fact that myoclonus is a loosely defined clinical entity. Not only is there a wide range of causal events associated with the presentation of myoclonus, in many instances there is disagreement of whether any given disorder should even be classified as myoclonus. Thus, given the breadth of myoclonic disorders and their induction, the pleiotropism and sensitivity of the serotonin system, and the powerful modulatory influence of serotonin receptors on central motor function, it would have been surprising if no myoclonic syndrome was, at least partially, ameliorated by serotonergic drugs or that no myoclonic syndrome was associated with some perturbation of the serotonin system.

Nevertheless, it is important that there have been a number of cases of human myoclonic states that were associated with reduced serotonin turnover and that responded, sometimes dramatically, to serotonergic drugs. Among the most positive examples were the beneficial response of some patients with postanoxic action myoclonus (9–12), and others with progressive myoclonic epilepsy (13,14), to the serotonin precursor 5-hydroxytryptophan (5-HTP). More recently, the essential palatal myoclonus of one patient was reversibly abolished by the specific 5-HT$_{1B/D}$ receptor agonist, sumatriptan (15). Therapeutic responses to serotonin receptor agonists, obviously, supported the serotonin hypothesis of myoclonus. On the other hand, some myoclonic cases worsened with 5-HTP (16), serotonin reuptake inhibitors (17), 5-HT$_{1A}$ receptor stimulation (18), and benefited from methysergide (16), a broad spectrum serotonin receptor antagonist—decreasing confidence in the global hypothesis. In fact, myoclonus has been induced accidentally by therapeutic doses of fluoxetine (19,20) or an overdose of sertraline (21).

Animal studies have reinforced the uncertainty surrounding the serotonin hypothesis of myoclonus. Systemic 5-HTP produced myoclonus in the guinea pig (22) through an action on the brainstem 5-HT$_1$ receptors (23). Antagonizing 5-HT$_{2A/C}$ receptors with intracerebral ketanserin attenuated pressure-induced myoclonus in rats (24). In contrast, a genetic model of myoclonic epilepsy was completely reversed by drugs that increased serotonergic transmission (25). Stimulus-sensitive myoclonus produced by anoxia in the rat was attenuated by 5-HTP (26) and also with specific agonists of the 5-HT$_{1A}$ (27) and 5-HT$_2$ and 5-HT$_3$ receptor subtypes (26,28). However, recent studies using the same preparation showed that 5-HT$_1$ and 5-HT$_2$ receptor antagonists attenuated rats' postanoxic myoclonus (29,30).

The conflicting nature of the outcomes regarding serotonergic pharmacotherapy of myoclonus may be more apparent than real. Systemically administered agents, regardless of their receptor specificity, act simultaneously at many different levels of the CNS. Moreover, the various 5-HT receptor subtypes are not uniformly distributed. Thus, different serotonergic drugs will influence different combinations of brain systems and these different brain regions may make different contributions to the final behavioral outcome. Trying to make a global conclusion about serotonin function in myoclonus is difficult, or impossible, when drugs are administered systemically, particularly when there is no clue about which brain regions may, or may not, be impaired by a disruption in serotonin neurotransmission.

A detailed analysis of the acoustic startle by Davis and associates (31) illustrated in a simple reflex system the complexity of trying to interpret systemic actions of serotonergic drugs. Raising serotonin levels with systemic 5-HTP and reducing serotonin levels with raphe lesions both enhanced the acoustic startle reflex of rats—apparently conflicting outcomes not unlike effects of such manipulations on some forms of myoclonus. To localize anatomic sites of action, serotonin delivered to the forebrain inhibited startle but delivery to the spinal cord enhanced startle. This indicated that systemic 5-HTP enhanced startle by an action at the spinal cord but that raphe lesions acted by removing supraspinal inhibition to override reduced excitation at the spinal level. To study receptor specificity, a systemically administered 5-HT$_{1A}$ agonist enhanced startle, an effect that was localized to the spinal cord. However, a systemically administered 5-HT$_{1B}$ agonist depressed startle, an action that could be strongly reproduced after delivery to the forebrain but also weakly reproduced after delivery to the spinal cord. Thus, the behavioral effect of systemically administered serotonergic agents depends upon an interaction of: (a) the relative influence of the various receptors at any given CNS level and their degree of activation; (b) the neuronal types that they influence; and (c) the specific contributions that the pharmacologically stimulated brain structures make to the final behavioral outcome. Yet, even this simple analysis does not consider possible compensatory changes in receptor function.

Because the circuits that generate the many forms of myoclonus vary, are complex, and involve many CNS levels, it may be completely unpredictable, *a priori*, which patients or experimental preparations will benefit from a serotonergic agent and whether the response will be due to activation or antagonism of a serotonin receptor subtype. Further complicating the situation is the recent understanding that many serotonin receptor antagonists are not neutral, but act as inverse agonists to reduce the constitutive activity of 5-HT receptors, induce compensatory increases in 5-HT receptor density and responsiveness, and affect receptor systems that are not direct targets of the ligands through second messenger actions (3). Amidst this complexity, what is left is a trial-and-error approach to the study of myoclonus with systemically administered serotonin drugs, an approach that may be unavoidable from a clinical management perspective but that is suboptimal from an experimental point of view. Lastly, beneficial effects of serotonergic drugs on myoclonus do not prove that a dysfunction of the serotonin system underlies the disorder. It is this experimental question that we have attempted to address using quantitative analysis of behavior, quantitative immunohistochemistry, and intracellular neurophysiology in two well-defined experimental models of myoclonus.

TWO RAT MODELS OF MYOCLONUS MODELING MYOCLONIC EPILEPSY AND POSTANOXIC MYOCLONUS INVOLVE DIFFERENT BRAINSTEM CIRCUITS

We studied two, very different myoclonic syndromes to determine the contribution and specificity of serotonergic system malfunction to the presentation of myoclonus. The first preparation is the genetically epilepsy prone rat, type 3 (GEPR3), which has a genetic form of myoclonic epilepsy (25,32,33). The second preparation is a model of posthypoxic myoclonus that is produced by sudden cardiac arrest for at least 7.5 minutes (34). Importantly, each myoclonic preparation models a form of human myoclonus that responds best to serotonin therapy—progressive myoclonic epilepsy and postanoxic myoclonus. In fact, both preparations respond beneficially to serotonin agents (25-30), as in the clinical cases (9–14). Thus, our experiments were designed to determine the breadth of serotonergic disturbance in the two preparations, to distinguish differences between the two, and to use such information to localize sites of dysfunction that may underlie the disorders.

Figure 31.1 shows general features of the myoclonus of the two rat models. The only common feature of the two myoclonias is that they are both triggered by auditory stimulation. The GEPR3 rat is genetically predisposed to exhibit a myoclonic seizure that is triggered by prolonged, loud auditory stimulation (Fig. 1A). While any long and loud wide-band stimulus will trigger the myoclonic seizure, we have used a 105 dB (re: 2×10^{-4} dynes/cm^2), ascending frequency ramp that sweeps from 1 to 14 kHz every second. The GEPR3 rat exhibits a bout of violent running and jumping beginning approximately 10 seconds after stimulus onset. The running increases in intensity over about 20 seconds, after which the rat falls to the ground in tonic flexion. The rat typically lays on its ventral surface with all four limbs remaining tonically flexed, and accompanied by dorsiflexion of the neck and back. During tonic flexion, the rat exhibits a profound, low-amplitude tremor in all of its limbs that is nearly precisely 10 Hz (33). After approximately 10 to 15 seconds of tremor, the rat exhibits very large flexion-extension clonus in its limbs and back at a frequency close to 3 Hz, which persists for about 20 seconds. The clonus gradually abates and the GEPR3 rat remains in an apparent catatonic state for a few minutes thereafter. Within 1 hour after the event the rat shows complete recovery. The GEPR3 rats' sensitivity to the auditory stimulus is permanent and the temporal details of its myoclonic seizure are completely replicable from day to day. There are no apparent motor abnormalities upon casual inspection and the rat shows a normal startle reflex to brief stimuli that is indistinguishable from that of normal inbred control rats and does not trigger the myoclonic seizure.

The myoclonus of the cardiac-arrested rat can be superficially described as a whole-body jerk to an auditory stimulus that does not habituate (Fig. 31.1B). The eliciting stimulus that we use is a 90-dB, 40-msec burst of white noise generated from a digital function generator. We have quantified the dynamics of the myoclonic response, measured its amplitude, and evaluated its stability over days. By measuring whole-body momentum with a calibrated ca-

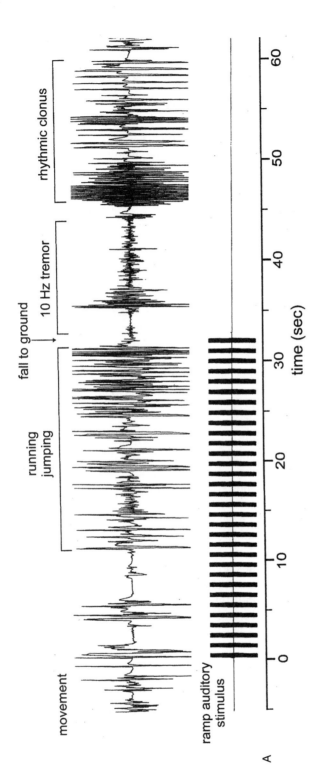

FIG. 31.1. Behavioral characterization of two forms of rodent myoclonus. Movements were recorded by a capacative sensor (Profile, Stoelting Inc., IL) that transduced body momentum into voltage. **A:** Rhythmic myoclonic seizure of a GEPR3 rat. Time 0 represents onset of a 105 dB, 1 to 14 kHz auditory ramp stimulus at 1 Hz. At 12 seconds after stimulus onset, the rat runs and jumps wildly. At 32 seconds the rat falls to the ground and shows a 10 Hz tremor that precedes large amplitude 2 to 5 Hz clonus. (Data from Welsh JP, Chang B, Menaker ME, et al. Removal of the inferior olive abolishes myoclonic seizure associated with loss of olivary serotonin. *Neuroscience* 1998;82:892–897.)

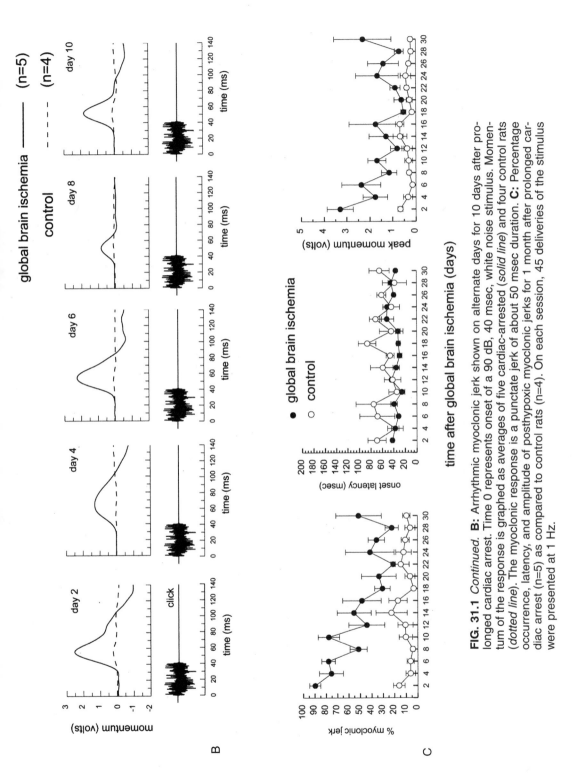

FIG. 31.1 *Continued.* **B:** Arrhythmic myoclonic jerk shown on alternate days for 10 days after prolonged cardiac arrest. Time 0 represents onset of a 90 dB, 40 msec, white noise stimulus. Momentum of the response is graphed as averages of five cardiac-arrested (*solid line*) and four control rats (*dotted line*). The myoclonic response is a punctate jerk of about 50 msec duration. **C:** Percentage occurrence, latency, and amplitude of posthypoxic myoclonic jerks for 1 month after prolonged cardiac arrest (n=5) as compared to control rats (n=4). On each session, 45 deliveries of the stimulus were presented at 1 Hz.

311

pacitive sensor, we determined that the jerk has a latency of approximately 35 msec and duration of approximately 50 msec. Peak momentum of the jerk occurs 60 msec after stimulus onset. The myoclonic jerk occurs to nearly 100% of stimuli in the first few days after the cardiac arrest, but spontaneously regresses both in amplitude and frequency with alternate-day testing over 1 month (Fig. 31.1C). The myoclonic condition produced by cardiac arrest occurs against a background of other neurologic deficits such as generalized seizures and profound ataxia. Although transient, the myoclonic jerk outlasts the spontaneous seizures but not always the ataxia.

Electromyographic analysis, using multiple, simultaneous intramuscular recordings, highlights differences between the two myoclonias and provides clues into their neural origins (Fig. 31.2). The GEPR3 myoclonus is extremely rhythmic, is synchronized across the midline, and is regenerative (Fig. 31.2A). The tremor that precedes the clonus has an upper bound of 12 Hz and is characterized by more powerful electromyographic bursts than those that occur during the clonus phase of the seizure. The data indicate that a supraspinal rhythm generator with regenerative oscillatory output and bilateral synchronization produces the tremor and myoclonus in the GEPR3 rat. As we shall see, experimental evidence indicates that a probable candidate for generating the tremor and clonus is the inferior olive.

In contrast, the posthypoxic myoclonic jerk is a markedly punctate event that is generated by a single activation wave up and down the neuraxis. Figure 31.2B shows simultaneous electromyographic recordings from six muscles, 2 days after cardiac arrest, aligned to stimulus onset. Electrodes were inserted to determine the earliest latency of activation at every CNS level from the rostral pons to the sacral spinal cord. The earliest activation occurred in the trapezius muscle, 11 msec after stimulus onset. Thereafter, the cranial nerve muscles were recruited in an upward fashion while spinal levels were recruited in a more complicated manner. At spinal levels, midline

motoneurons were recruited earliest while motoneurons innervating distal muscles were recruited later but still in a downward activation wave. The dynamics of the muscle recruitment indicated an origin of the activation wave in the medulla and resembled reticular reflex myoclonus (35), which occurs in the most severely affected humans manifesting posthypoxic myoclonus. The dynamics of muscle recruitment of rats' posthypoxic jerk were different from the underlying rats' normal acoustic startle, which had an earliest activation in the caudal pons and orderly recruitment of descending levels (Fig. 31.2C). More importantly, the duration of any muscle activation in the posthypoxic jerk was as short as 15 msec, indicating a single activation wave generated by a medullary center lacking regenerative and oscillatory properties.

RETROGRADE AMNESIA, IMPAIRED RELEARNING, AND BRAINSTEM DYSFUNCTION ARE ASSOCIATED WITH POSTHYPOXIC MYOCLONUS IN THE RAT

Patients with posthypoxic myoclonus may often retain intellect despite the devastation to their central motor system. We tested two sets of posthypoxic myoclonic rats' cognitive function using two associative learning tasks. The first task was a classical conditioning paradigm in which restrained rats acquired a tongue protrusion response to both a 2-kHz tone and 7-Hz flashing light conditioned stimulus, each 1.5 sec in duration, that was paired with injection of water into the mouth in a classical delay procedure (Fig. 31.3A; see ref. 36 for technical details). The second task was a free operant task in which identically restrained rats pressed a lever on a fixed-ratio 10 (FR-10) schedule to obtain water reinforcement (Fig. 31.3B). Both experiments were designed to test rats' memory retention after the prolonged cardiac arrest that produced posthypoxic myoclonus. The two paradigms were specifically designed to be sensitive tests of posthypoxic myoclonic rats' sensory and motor function, independent of their myoclonus. In the classical conditioning

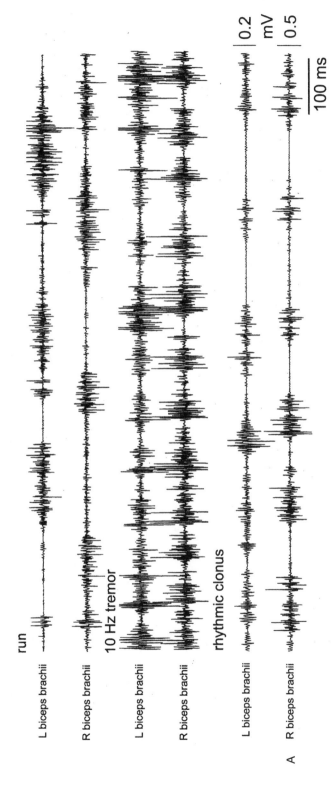

FIG. 31.2. Electromyographic analysis of a rhythmic myoclonic seizure and posthypoxic myoclonic jerk in rats. **A:** Raw EMG records obtained bilaterally from the biceps brachii during running, tremor, and clonus components of the myoclonic seizure of a GEPR3 rat. Note the alternate activity during running, the synchronized 10 Hz activity during tremor, and slower activity during rhythmic clonus.

313

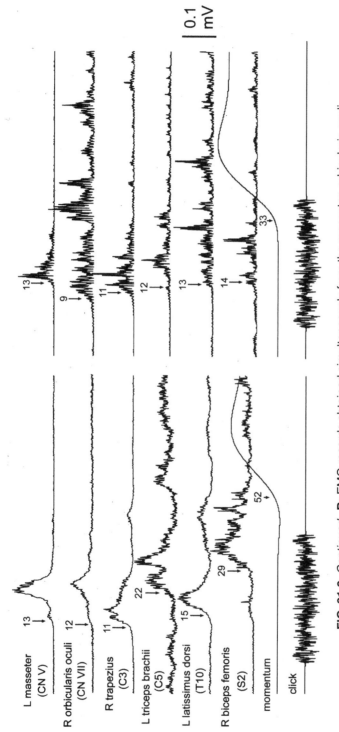

FIG. 31.2. *Continued.* **B:** EMG records obtained simultaneously from the masseter, orbicularis oculi, trapezius, triceps brachii, latissimus dorsi, and biceps femoris muscles documenting the segmental progression of a rat's posthypoxic myoclonic jerk. Traces of whole-body momentum and the stimulus are presented below the muscle records. The traces represent the rectified average of 45 myoclonic responses and show earliest activation in the trapezius muscle (11 msec) and disorganized activation of spinal levels. **C:** Identical analysis of the normal acoustic startle of a control rat. The data were presented for the first startle only, due to the rapid habituation that occurs thereafter. Note the earliest onset in the orbicularis oculi and orderly temporal progression down the neuraxis. Records were differentially recorded and band-pass filtered between 0.1 and 5 kHz.

paradigm, both visual and auditory conditioned stimuli were used to test for possible modality-specific impairments in memory after global brain ischemia. The free operant task was designed to test for changes in the rhythmicity and kinematics of a skilled movement, as an initial attempt to determine whether the reticular reflex myoclonus was accompanied by an action-induced component.

Figure 31.3A shows that six rats acquired conditioned tongue protrusion responses to both an auditory and visual conditioned stimulus to about 90% conditioned responses after six sessions of conditioning. Cardiac arrest and resuscitation were induced on the day after the tenth conditioning session and retention testing began the next day for 10 additional days. All rats showed the posthypoxic myoclonic jerk shown in Figure 31.1B, and most showed severe ataxia and spontaneous seizures for 2 to 5 days after the arrest. On the first day after cardiac arrest, the rats responded on $39 \pm 10\%$ of trials with conditioned responses, a value that was significantly lower than the performance on the day before the cardiac arrest ($p < 0.05$) and equal to the percentage conditioned responses on the very first day of conditioning, when the rats were naïve. Global brain ischemia abolished the previously acquired memory. With ten sessions of postarrest conditioning, the rats reacquired their conditioned responses to both the flashing light and auditory conditioned stimuli. However, the reacquisition was slower than the initial learning ($p < 0.01$) and showed a modality-specific impairment with relearning to the auditory stimulus being slower than to the visual stimulus ($p < 0.05$). Thus, the posthypoxic myoclonus was accompanied by a profound loss of associative memory, but those memories could be reacquired with retraining. However, the rate of learning after the global brain ischemia was slower than normal and the degree of impairment was related to sensory modality. This may have been related to a global hypersensitivity to auditory stimuli induced by the cardiac arrest.

Figure 31.3B shows performance data for five rats conditioned under the FR-10 operant schedule before and after cardiac arrest that produced posthypoxic myoclonus. In this task, restrained rats freely pressed a lever through a 90-minute session to receive water as a reinforcer. Because it was a FR-10 schedule, one drop of water was presented into the mouth after every tenth press as a reinforcer. The number and frequency of arm and tongue movements were measured by a computer. The behavior is manifested as sequences of ten lever presses at 2 to 4 Hz, after which the water reinforcer triggers a bout of faster 7 to 8 Hz rhythmic licking. On the fourteenth operant session before cardiac arrest, rats pressed the lever $1,273 \pm 470$ times and made more than 2,000 tongue movements in a single 90-minute session. Global brain ischemia impaired responsiveness in the paradigm, by bringing the number of lever presses per session down to 510 ± 204 ($p < 0.01$). Over 14 further sessions of operant conditioning, lever pressing returned to its pre-arrest levels.

More interestingly, posthypoxic myoclonus was associated with a significant reduction in maximal movement frequency. Figure 31.1C shows power spectra of conditioned tongue movements in two groups of rats, both of which underwent cardiac arrest. Five of these rats showed a profound myoclonic jerk (Fig. 31.1B), while three showed no responsiveness to the white-noise stimulus greater than the normal acoustic startle. The power spectra reveal that non-myoclonic rats performed tongue protrusions at a dominant frequency of 6.8 Hz, replicating previous results in normal rats (36). Before cardiac arrest, the second group of rats also showed a dominant movement frequency close to 7 Hz (downward arrows in Fig. 31.2C). However, beginning 4 days after cardiac arrest, the myoclonic rats showed a significant slowing in their dominant movement frequency with a peak rhythm of only 5.4 Hz. This is a very significant finding and indicates a powerful disruption of the brainstem, as the frequency of rats' rhythmic licking is specifically determined by circuits within the pons and medulla (37). The data indicated that the neuropathology that produces posthypoxic myoclonus in the rat is global and impairs brainstem motor systems.

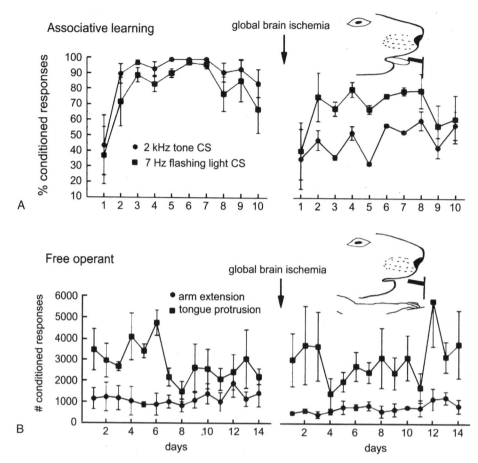

FIG. 31.3. Cognitive and motoric capabilities of posthypoxic myoclonic rats as measured with classical and operant conditioning. **A:** Percentage conditioned tongue protrusion responses on 10 daily sessions of classical conditioning before and after global brain ischemia that produced posthypoxic myoclonus. Before ischemia, rats learned to both an auditory and visual conditioned stimulus (CS). Global brain ischemia abolished the previously acquired memory and the rats showed moderate relearning of their conditioned response. **B:** Operant performance on a fixed-ratio 10 schedule in which 10 lever presses delivered a water reinforcer. Brain ischemia producing myoclonus reduced overall responsiveness in the paradigm that gradually reversed over 14 conditioning sessions after surgery.

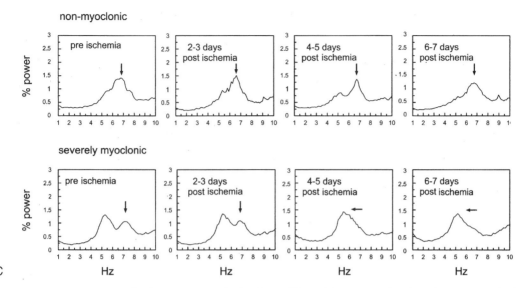

FIG. 31.3. *Continued.* **C:** Frequency analysis of conditioned tongue protrusions in non-myoclonic (n=3, **top**) and severely myoclonic rats (n=5, **bottom**) before and after cardiac arrest. Before ischemia, all rats showed an ability to lick rapidly at 7 Hz. At 4 days after ischemia, the most severely myoclonic rats showed a maximal lick rhythm of only 5.5 Hz, indicating a disruption of brainstem circuits mediating this centrally patterned movement.

LOSS OF SEROTONIN IS RELATED TO RHYTHMIC MYOCLONUS BUT NOT THE ARRHYTHMIC MYOCLONIC JERK

We performed quantitative immunohistochemical analysis of serotonin content of nearly the entire brain of posthypoxic myoclonic rats and compared them to neurochemical and immunohistochemical data that we and others have obtained for the GEPR3 rat. Figure 31.4A shows group data of serotonin content in 14 different brain regions from nine GEPR3 rats and inbred controls (32) analyzed with high-performance liquid chromatography and electrochemical detection. Figure 31.4B shows our analysis of 19 different brain regions for posthypoxic myoclonic brains analyzed by quantitative immunohistochemistry. The quantitative immunohistochemistry was performed with techniques that we have described in detail (33). Briefly, the subjects were five matched pairs of posthypoxic myoclonic and control

rats that were perfused with fixative and sectioned in 40 μm transverse slices. A polyclonal antiserum raised in rabbits against serotonin (IncStar, Stillwater MN), a biotinylated goat anti-rabbit secondary antibody (Vector Labs, Burlingame, CA), and the avidin-biotin-peroxidase method for labeling were used (38). All tissue was handled in matched pairs of myoclonic and control sections. To ensure uniform conditions for quantitative comparison, rats to be compared directly were perfused and sectioned as a pair and their tissues were processed collectively in the same containers throughout the immunostaining procedure. The amount of serotonin was quantified in optical density units using NIH-Image with an optical scale that was precisely calibrated to be a linear representation of actual transillumination. For each brain region analyzed, the data were calculated as a change in optical density for each matched pair and then expressed as averages of the full set.

The GEPR3 rat, which displays a rhythmic myoclonic seizure, is notable for the nearly

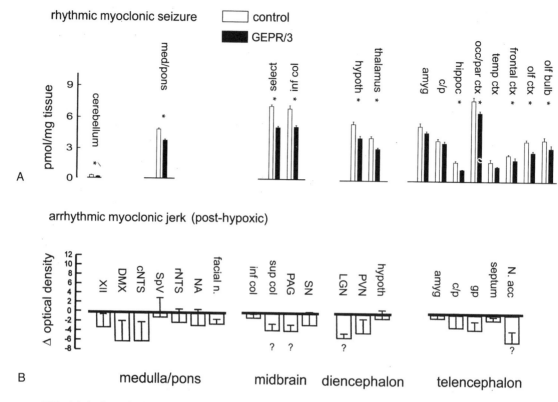

FIG. 31.4. Quantitative analysis of serotonin content in GEPR3 (**A**) and posthypoxic myoclonic (**B**) rats. Data in **A** were taken from Dailey and associates (32) and were determined by HPLC with electrochemical detection (*asterisks* determine statistically significant change). Data in **B** were determined by quantitative immunohistochemistry and optical densitometry. Question marks in **B** indicate questionable statistical significance (*p* < 0.05) of the normalized data that could only be found by multiple *t*-tests of means different than 0 without Bonferroni correction. The widespread reductions in serotonin content of the GEPR3 rat do not occur after brain ischemia leading to posthypoxic myoclonus.

global reduction of serotonin in its brain (Fig. 31.4A). Significant reductions in serotonin content were measured in the cerebellum, medulla and pons, inferior colliculus and midbrain tegmentum, hypothalamus, thalamus, hippocampus, occipital, parietal, olfactory, and frontal cortices, and olfactory bulb (32), without significant reduction in the striatum. It is notable that drugs that increase serotonin levels are effective anti-myoclonic agents in the GEPR3 rat (25), supporting the view that the global serotonin deficit is causally related to the generation of the myoclonic seizure.

In sharp contrast, there is not a global deficit of serotonin in the brain of the posthypoxic myoclonic rat (Fig. 31.4B). None of seven nuclei within the medulla and pons showed a significant change in serotonin levels after global brain ischemia. In the midbrain and thalamus, a trend toward a reduction in serotonin content occurred in the superior colliculus, periaqueductal gray, and lateral geniculate (question marked columns in Fig. 31.4B). Of five subcortical regions analyzed in the telencephalon, only the shell of the nucleus accumbens showed a trend toward a reduction in serotonin content. The significance of these trends must be accepted very cautiously because the statistical tests were very liberal. For this data set, statistical significance of p less than 0.05 could only be achieved with multiple t-tests normalized means different from 0 without Bonferroni correction, which is required to ensure that multiple comparisons do not lead to erroneous assignment of significance due to chance (39). Analysis of variance of the normalized data or any type of statistical analysis of the raw optical density values did not detect a significant difference for any region of the posthypoxic myoclonic brain. Even with the most liberal method of analysis, no change in serotonin level was detected in the structures of the nigrostriatal system. Thus, the only common feature of the GEPR3 and posthypoxic myoclonic brains was normal serotonin content in the basal ganglia. This is compelling, in as much as the striatum was the only system in the entire brain of the GEPR3 rat that did not exhibit reduced serotonin content. The converging evidence indicates that neither form of myoclonus is associated with reduced serotonin in the basal ganglia.

Figure 31.5 demonstrates the severity of the loss of serotonin in the medulla and caudal pons of the GEPR3 rat with high resolution photomicrographs. This figure shows immunostained tissue from a GEPR3 and an inbred control rat. The tissue compared in this figure was processed simultaneously and identically by collective processing during immunohistochemistry and with identical photomicrographic settings. In the caudal medulla, it is clear that serotonin is reduced in the dorsal reticular nucleus, nucleus of the solitary tract, hypoglossal nucleus, and the outer layer of the nucleus of the spinal trigeminal tract. The loss is even more prominent in the rostral medulla, with the nucleus of the solitary tract, rostroventrolateral medulla, dorsal subnucleus of the spinal trigeminal tract, and lateral posterior gigantocellular nucleus of the reticular formation showing profound losses of serotonin associated with the myoclonic seizure. In the caudal pons, the fa-

cial nucleus and ventromedial reticular formation also showed a loss of serotonin. From the photomicrographs, it is clear that the GEPR3 rat possesses a number of abnormalities in serotonergic modulation of autonomic, sensory, and cranial motor function, in addition to its predisposition to myoclonic seizure.

Figure 31.6 shows an identical analysis of serotonin content for a severely posthypoxic myoclonic rat and a simultaneously processed control rat. This set of tissue was chosen to show the changes in serotonin content that occurred in a severely myoclonic rat, 5 days after cardiac arrest. The most important point from the photomicrographs is that the myoclonic state produced by global brain ischemia was not associated with a global reduction in serotonin as occurred in the GEPR3 rat. In the medulla and pons, serotonin levels in the solitary tract nucleus, gigantocellular reticular nucleus, and facial nucleus were not reduced by global brain ischemia that induced myoclonus. In the midbrain, the dorsal and median raphe nuclei showed normal dimensions and serotonin density and the pontine nuclei and lateral tegmentum showed normal serotonin content. In the forebrain, the caudate, putamen, claustrum, and ventral pallidum showed normal serotonin content. The shell of accumbens nucleus showed a slight loss of serotonin in this matched pair, of questionable significance. The inability to detect a significant change in serotonin levels was not due to a lack of sensitivity of the immunostaining method, because the identical method revealed profound losses throughout the GEPR3 brain, confirming the decreases demonstrated with high-performance liquid chromatography and electrochemical detection (32).

INFERIOR OLIVE: AN OSCILLATOR SUPPRESSED BY SEROTONIN AND NECESSARY FOR ONE TYPE OF RHYTHMIC MYOCLONUS

The GEPR3 rat demonstrates a profound and highly replicable loss of serotonin in the inferior olive (33). This is significant because

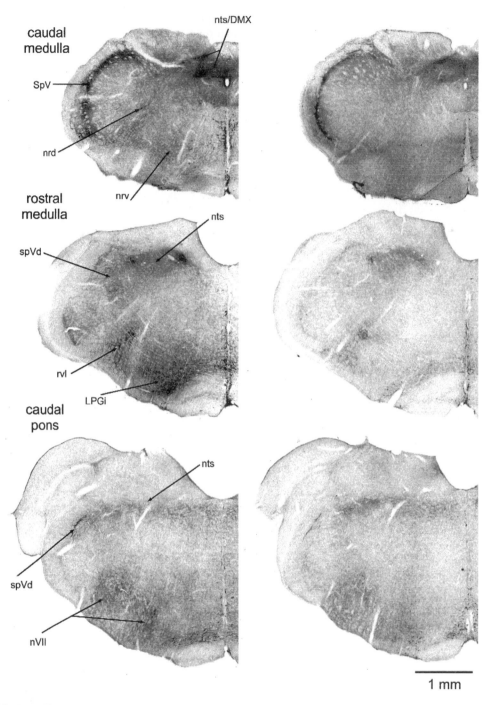

FIG. 31.5. The regional reduction of serotonin in the brainstem of the GEPR3 rat (**right**) as compared to a non-myoclonic inbred control rat (**left**). The tissue in this figure was immunoprocessed collectively and photographed under identical conditions. Serotonin is profoundly reduced at every location in the rhythmically myoclonic brain stem, most notably in the ventrolateral reticular formation of the rostral medulla. Abbreviations: LPGi, lateral posterior gigantocellular nucleus; nrd, nucleus reticularis dorsalis; nrv, nucleus reticularis ventralis; nts, nucleus tractus solitarius; nVII, facial nucleus; rvl, rostroventrolateral medulla; SpV, spinal trigeminal nucleus.

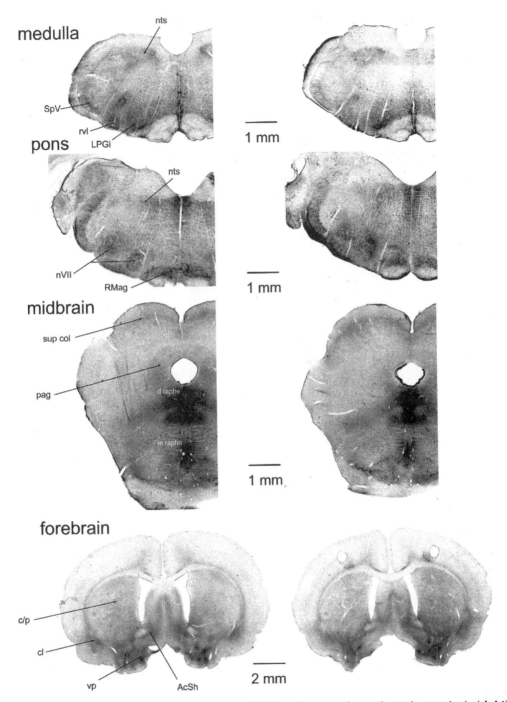

FIG. 31.6. Serotonin immunostaining in a normal (**left**) and a severely posthypoxic myoclonic (**right**) rat for four levels of the brain. The tissue was immunoprocessed collectively and photographed under identical conditions. No significant difference can be detected. Abbreviations: AcSh, shell of nucleus accumbens; c/p, caudate and putamen; cl, claustrum; LPGi, lateral posterior gigantocellular nucleus; nrd, nucleus reticularis dorsalis; nrv, nucleus reticularis ventralis; nts, nucleus tractus solitarius; nVII, facial nucleus; PAG, periaquaductal gray; Rmag, raphe magnus; rvl, rostroventrolateral medulla; sup col, superior colliculus; SpV, spinal trigeminal nucleus; vp, ventral pallidum. Survival time was 5 days after cardiac arrest.

the inferior olive is the source of climbing fibers to the cerebellum (40). By virtue of this anatomic relation, the inferior olive can drive 10-Hz whole-body tremor upon systemic (41,42) or local (43) pharmacologic activation. Moreover, neurons of the inferior olive are single-cell oscillators (44) that can synchronize their output and drive a rhythmic signal through the cerebellum to rhythmically modulate motor behavior (45).

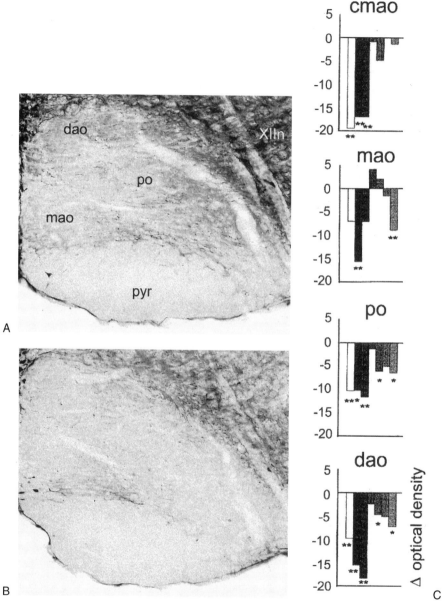

FIG. 31.7. Serotonin and 5-HT$_2$ receptor immunostaining in the inferior olive and its relation to rhythmic myoclonus in the GEPR3 rat. **A,B:** Serotonin immunostaining reveals plexa of fibers coursing through the inferior olive of a normal (A) but not GEPR3 (B) rat. **C:** Quantitative analysis of the decrease in serotonin immunostaining through 4 subnuclei of the inferior olive for seven matched sets of GEPR3 and inbred control tissue. Asterisks represent $p < 0.05$ (·) and $p < 0.01$ (··).

Unlike all other brain areas of the rhythmically myoclonic GEPR3 rat, which show a subtotal reduction of serotonin (Figs. 31.4A, 31.5), the inferior olive of the GEPR3 is virtually completely deafferented from the nuclei that provide its serotonergic innervation. This results in a virtual absence of serotonin in the inferior olive. Figure 31.7 shows the inferior olive of a non-myoclonic control rat (Fig. 31.7A) and a rhythmically myoclonic GEPR3 rat (Fig. 31.7B) collectively immunostained for the presence of serotonin. Serotonin fibers that innervate the inferior olive emanate from the midline raphe pallidus and obscurus as well as from the parapyramidal cell group in the paragigantocellular nucleus (46). Serotonin fibers make *en passant* synapses with olivary neurons as they course mediolaterally through the nucleus (47). The serotonergic innervation of the inferior olive

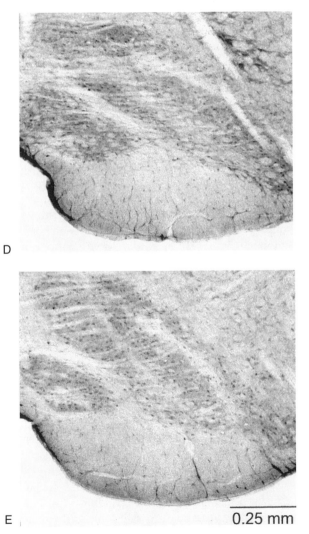

D

E   0.25 mm

FIG. 31.7. *Continued.* **D,E:** 5-HT$_2$ receptors are present in neurons of the normal and GEPR3 inferior olive, despite the lack of serotonin fibers in the latter. Antibody against the 5-HT$_2$ receptor was a gift of Dr. S. Garlow (50). Abbreviations: dao, dorsal accessory olive; mao, medial accessory olive; po, principal olive; pyr, pyramidal tract; XIIn, hypoglossal nerve.

is greatest in the dorsal accessory subnucleus, the lateral part of the principal subnucleus, and in the caudal aspect of the medial accessory subnucleus. Figure 31.7 shows sections through the rostral half of the inferior olive. At this level, the non-myoclonic rat shows plexa of very fine serotonin fibers in the medial and dorsal aspect of the dorsal accessory subnucleus, the lateral principal subnucleus, and the lateral aspect of the medial accessory subnucleus (Fig. 31.7A). In contrast, the GEPR3 inferior olive shows virtually no serotonin fibers in any of these subnuclei (Fig. 31.7B). Quantitative analysis of seven matched pairs of GEPR3 and inbred control tissue revealed significant ($p < 0.05$) reductions in serotonin content in all subnuclei (33), effects that were most replicable in the principal and dorsal accessory subnuclei (Fig. 31.7C). The loss of serotonin in the inferior olive in rhythmically myoclonic rats is contrasted by the normal complement and density of postsynaptic 5-HT$_2$ receptors on olivary neurons within all subnuclei in the same tissue (compare Fig. 31.7D and E).

We examined the effect of serotonin on the electrical properties of olivary neurons to understand how olivary neurons might behave in the absence of serotonin (6). It is well known that olivary neurons maintained *in vitro* exhibit oscillations in membrane potential that are subthreshold for spiking (44,48). The frequency of such subthreshold oscillations is strictly limited to a range of 3 to 10 Hz. and serves as a carrier rhythm that entrains the rhythmic output of the olivary nucleus. When studied in parasagittally cut sections of the brainstem maintained *in vitro*, olivary neurons are deafferented from their serotonergic input and can be presumed to behave as they would in the absence of serotonin. Replacement of serotonin under the highly controlled conditions of *in vitro* physiology allowed a biophysical analysis of serotonin's effects on the rhythmicity and ionic currents of olivary neurons with intracellular recording.

Figure 31.8A shows that serotonin blocks the subthreshold oscillations and the rhythmicity of firing of olivary neurons via an ac-

tion at the 5-HT$_2$ receptor. Application of serotonin in concentrations as low as 5 µM depolarized olivary neurons and blocked their subthreshold oscillations. The ability of serotonin to suppress olivary rhythmicity is mediated by the 5-HT$_2$ receptor, because it was blocked with the 5-HT$_2$ receptor antagonist ketanserin (Fig. 31.8B) and reproduced with the 5-HT$_2$ receptor agonist dimethoxy-4-iodoamphetamine (DOI, Fig. 31.8C). The effect of serotonin was not mimicked by 8-hydroxy-2-(di-N-propylamino)-tetralin (8-OH-DPAT), indicating that 5-HT$_{1A}$ receptors did not mediate the effect. Moreover, all effects of serotonin were replicated in the presence of the sodium channel blocker tetrodotoxin, indicating a postsynaptic action on olivary neurons.

Serotonin's ability to block the rhythmic output of olivary neurons is due to inhibition of the low-threshold calcium conductance, I$_T$. This conductance is responsible both for the rising phase of the subthreshold oscillation and rebound excitation after the firing of an action potential, and is essential for olivary rhythmicity. The role of I$_T$ in mediating rhythmic spiking is demonstrated in Figure 31.8D in which an olivary neuron is depolarizing from a hyperpolarized potential. Such depolarization triggers a robust low-threshold calcium spike (filled arrow, Fig. 31.8D) that, in turn, recruits a sodium spike (open arrow, Fig. 31.8D). Decay of the subsequent afterhyperpolarization triggers following rebound spikes, also mediated by I$_T$, which are responsible for regenerative spiking. Serotonin significantly attenuates I$_T$, thereby reducing the slope of the rebound spikes and preventing regenerative oscillatory spiking (Fig. 31.8D, right). Although these observations were made in neonatal tissue (6), we have recently replicated them in the adult inferior olive (Placantonakis, unpublished observation). The findings indicate that serotonin constrains olivary rhythmicity due to its ability to inhibit I$_T$. The implication of the intracellular physiology is that a lack of serotonin should predispose olivary neurons to pathologically rhythmic firing, a state that should be mani-

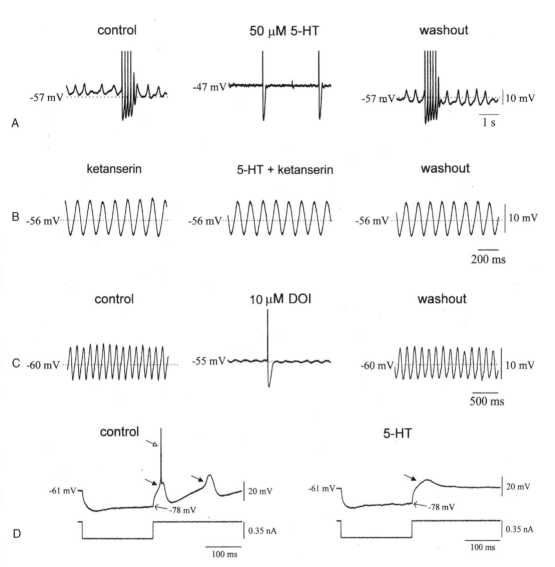

FIG. 31.8. Serotonin abolishes subthreshold oscillations in membrane potential and spike rhythmicity of inferior olivary neurons via the 5-HT$_2$ receptor and inhibiting I$_T$. **A:** Serotonin abolishes subthreshold oscillations in membrane potential of an olivary neuron and its rhythmic bursts of spikes. **B:** Effect of serotonin on subthreshold oscillations is prevented by ketanserin, an antagonist of the 5-HT$_2$ receptor. **C:** Effect of serotonin on subthreshold oscillations is replicated by DOI, an agonist of the 5-HT$_2$ receptor. **D:** Serotonin inhibits the low-threshold calcium conductance, I$_T$, and prevents regenerative firing from hyperpolarized holding potentials. Action potentials were truncated in **A** and **C**. (Data from Placantonakis DJ, Schwarz C, Welsh JP. Serotonin suppresses subthreshold oscillatory activity of rat inferior olivary neurones in vitro. *J Physiol (London)* 2000;524:833–851.)

fested in behavior as rhythmic myoclonus or tremor within the frequency range of 3 to 12 Hz.

The foregoing evidence predicts that removing the inferior olive of the GEPR3 rat should prevent its audiogenic tremor and rhythmic myoclonus. To test this hypothesis, we chemically removed the inferior olives of five GEPR3 rats with 3-acetylpyridine and studied the effect of the lesion on the myoclonic seizure for 3 months (Fig. 31.9). With their inferior olives intact, all five of these GEPR3 rats exhibited a rhythmic myoclonic seizure with both a 10 Hz tremor component and slower frequency clonus on every occasion they were tested with prolonged, frequency-ramp auditory stimulation. Complete destruction of the inferior olive (greater than 98% neurons degenerated) permanently abolished the tremor and clonus components of the GEPR3 myoclonic seizure, as determined by multiple testing over 3 months (33). The GEPR3 rats without the inferior olive would sometimes exhibit the initial running and jumping component of the seizure, but this would stop spontaneously and never progress into falling, tremor, and clonus. Subtotal destruction of the inferior olive abolished the rhythmic myoclonus for 1 month, after which the tremor and clonus returned. The contrast produced by the complete olivary lesion was extraordinary, because 10 Hz tremor and rhythmic clonus occurred in 100% of trials with the inferior olive intact, but in 0% of trials with the inferior olive removed. Taken together, the experimental evidence strongly indicated that the GEPR3 rats' lack of serotonin in its inferior olive predisposed their olivary

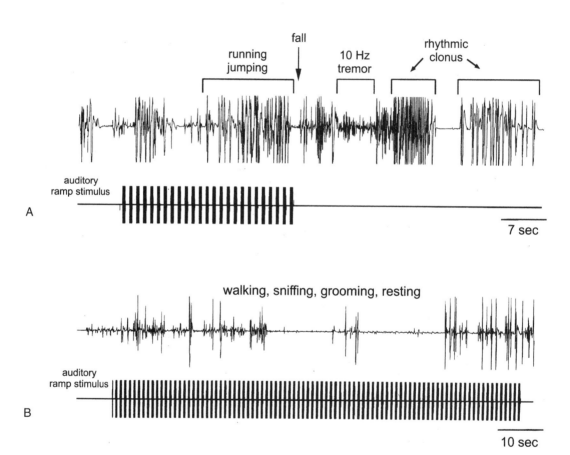

FIG. 31.9. Removing the inferior olive prevents the rhythmic myoclonic seizure of the GEPR3 rat. **A:** Rhythmic myoclonus of a GEPR3 rat with the inferior olive intact. The running, tremor, and clonus components can be identified. **B:** Same rat 72 days after inferior olive lesion. The stimulus does not trigger the seizure. Instead, the GEPR3 rat shows normal exploratory movement during 90 seconds of the stimulus. (Data from Welsh JP, Chang B, Menaker ME, Aicher SA. Removal of the inferior olive abolishes myoclonic seizures associated with a loss of olivary serotonin. *Neuroscience* 1998; 82:879–897.)

neurons to fire rhythmically in an uncontrolled manner and drive the tremor and clonus components of its rhythmic myoclonic seizure.

SUMMARY AND CONCLUSIONS

A quantitative analysis of two rat syndromes of myoclonus are presented, modeling myoclonic epilepsy and postanoxic myoclonus. Like the human conditions, both of the models benefit therapeutically from drugs that act on the serotonin system. The rat model of myoclonic epilepsy is associated with a profound loss of serotonin throughout the brain (except in the striatum) and is generated by an oscillator that is synchronized around the midline. The rat model of posthypoxic myoclonus does not demonstrate a significant reduction in serotonin in any location of its brain and is generated by a non-oscillating circuit in the medulla. Although some forms of myoclonic epilepsy may benefit from serotonin drugs because they are caused by a decrease in brain serotonin, our data indicate that posthypoxic myoclonus is not caused by a decrease in the serotonergic innervation of any region of the brain. That the raphe nuclei do not degenerate after global brain ischemia was noted by C. David Marsden in a discussion of the histologic findings of three of his human cases of posthypoxic myoclonus (page 117 of reference 10) and led him to question the hypothesis that posthypoxic myoclonus was due to a loss of serotonin neurons. Our data confirm his observation in the rat, but also indicate that density of serotonin fibers and terminals throughout the brain is not reduced by the brain ischemia that produces posthypoxic myoclonus. It remains to be determined whether the physiologic responsiveness of serotonin neurons is altered by global brain ischemia and whether changes in serotonin release or serotonin receptor properties are associated with posthypoxic myoclonus.

The stability of the serotonin system in posthypoxic myoclonic rats is remarkable when one considers the wide range of disorders that is produced by the prolonged brain ischemia. The inability of the most severely posthypoxic myoclonic rats to perform 7-Hz tongue protrusions indicates substantial physiologic disruption of brainstem motor function. Moreover, the posthypoxic myoclonic rat suffers from ataxia, seizures, retrograde amnesia, and impaired ability to learn. The wide spectrum of these deficits is sharply contrasted by its apparently intact serotonin system.

We have identified the inferior olive as a locus that may generate the rhythmic components of tremor and myoclonus in syndromes that are truly associated with a dramatic loss of brainstem serotonin. Serotonin acts within the inferior olive to constrain its rhythmic firing. Without intraolivary serotonin, olivary neurons are predisposed to oscillate continuously, providing a substrate upon which sustained rhythmic spiking may be superimposed. It is clear that such unconstrained rhythmicity produces synchronized whole-body tremor at 10 Hz (33,41–43). The effects of serotonin to suppress olivocerebellar rhythmicity are mediated by postsynaptic 5-HT$_2$ receptors that reduce the magnitude of the low-threshold calcium conductance, I$_T$. It is notable that dysregulation of this conductance has been associated with hyper–rhythmic states in the thalamus underlying cognitive disorders ranging from depression to tinnitus (49), indicating a common mechanism underlying a variety of neurologic conditions. The identification of a specific brainstem locus (inferior olive), serotonin receptor 5-HT$_2$, and ionic current I$_T$ involved in a form of rhythmic myoclonus may provide multiple clues toward which future pharmacotherapies can be directed.

ACKNOWLEDGMENTS

Supported by grant R01 NS31224 from the National Institute for Neurological Disorders and Stroke and the Myoclonus Research Foundation. D.P., S.S., R.M., and L.B. were supported by student research fellowships from the Myoclonus Research Foundation during their time at NYU Medical Center.

REFERENCES

1. Pranzatelli MR. Serotonin and human myoclonus. *Arch Neurol* 1994;51:605–614.
2. Steinbusch HWM. Distribution of serotonin-immunoreactivity in the central nervous system of the rat – cell bodies and terminals. *Neuroscience* 1981;6:557–618.
3. Pauwels PJ. Diverse signalling by 5-hydroxytrayptamine (5-HT) receptors. *Biochem Pharmacol* 2000;60:1743–1750.
4. Wilson MA, Ricaurte GA, Molliver ME. Distinct morphological classes of serotonergic axons in primate exhibit differential vulnerability to the psychotropic drug 3,4-methylenedioxymethamphetamine. *Neuroscience* 1989;28:121–137.
5. Stefani A, Surmeier DJ, Kitai ST. Serotonin enhances excitability in neostriatal neurons by reducing voltage-dependent potassium currents. *Brain Res* 1990;529:354–357.
6. Placantonakis DG, Schwarz C, Welsh JP. Serotonin suppresses subthreshold and suprathreshold oscillatory activity of rat inferior olivary neurones *in vitro*. *J Physiol (London)* 2000;524:833–851.
7. Bishop GA, Kerr CW. The physiological effects of peptides and serotonin on Purkinje cell activity. *Prog Neurobiol* 1992;39:475–492.
8. Kiehn O, Kjaerulff O, Tresch MC., et al. Contributions of intrinsic motor neuron properties to the production of rhythmic motor output in the mammalian spinal cord. *Brain Res Bull* 2000;53:649–659.
9. Magnussen I, Dupont E, Engbaek R., et al. Posthypoxic intention myoclonus treated with 5-hydroxy-tryptophan and an extracerebral decarboxylase inhibitor. *Acta Neurol Scand* 1978;57:289–294.
10. Van Woert MH, Rosenbaum D. L-5-hydroxytryptophan therapy in myoclonus. In: Fahn S., Davis J. N., Rowland L. P., eds. *Advances in Neurology, Vol. 26*. New York: Raven Press, 1979:107–122.
11. Beretta E, Regli F, de Crousaz G, et al. Postanoxic myoclonus. Treatment of a case with 5-hydroxytryptophane and a decarboxylase inhibitor. *Journal of Neurology* 1981;225: 57–62.
12. Chadwick D, Hallett M, Jenner P, et al. Treatment of posthypoxic action myoclonus: Implications for the pathophysiology of the disorder. In: Fahn S, Marsden CD, Van Woert MH, eds. *Advances in neurology, vol. 43.* New York: Raven Press, 1986:183–190.
13. Leino E, MacDonald E, Airaksinen MM, et al. L-Tryptophan-carbidopa trial in patients with long-standing progressive myoclonus epilepsy. *Acta Neurol Scand* 1981;64:130–141.
14. Pranzatelli MR, Tate E, Huang Y, et al. Neuropharmacology of progressive myoclonus epilepsy: Response to 5-hydroxy-L-tryptophan. *Epilepsia* 1995;36:783–791.
15. Scott BL, Evans RW, Jankovic J. Treatment of palatal myoclonus with sumatriptan. *Mov Disord* 1996;11:748–751.
16. Snodgrass SR. Myoclonus: analysis of monoamine, GABA, and other systems. *FASEB J* 1990;4:2775–2788.
17. Deahl M, Trimble M. Serotonin reuptake inhibitors, epilepsy and myoclonus. *Br J Psychiatry* 1991;159:433–435.
18. Pranzatelli MR, Franz D, Tat, E, et al. Buspirone in progressive myoclonus epilepsy. *J Neurol Neurosurg Psychiatry* 1993;56:114–115.
19. Lauterbach EC. Reversible intermittent rhythmic myoclonus with fluoxetine in presumed Pick's disease. *Mov Disord* 1994;9:343–346.
20. Ghika-Schmid F, Ghika J, Vuadens P, et al. Acute reversible myoclonic encephalopathy associated with fluoxetine therapy. *Mov Disord* 1997;12:622–623.
21. Rendel DH, Bodkin JA, Yang JM. Massive sertraline overdose. *Ann Emerg Med* 2000;36:524–526.
22. Klawans HL, Goetz G, Weiner WJ. 5-Hydroxytryptophan-induced myoclonus in guinea pigs and the possible role of serotonin in infantile myoclonus. *Neurology* 1973;23,1234–1240.
23. Luscombe G, Jenner P, Marsden CD. 5-Hydroxytrptophan (5-HT)-dependent myoclonus in guinea pigs is induced through brainstem 5-HT-1 receptors. *Neurosci Lett* 1984;44:241–246.
24. Kriem B, Rostain JC, Abraini JH. Contribution of central 5-HT2 receptors in the occurrence of locomotor activity and myoclonia in freely moving rats exposed to high pressure. *Neuroreport* 1996;7:2687–2690.
25. Reigel CE, Dailey JW, Jobe PCI. The genetically epilepsy prone rat: an overview of seizure-prone characteristics and responsiveness to anticonvulsive drugs. *Life Sci* 1986;39:763–774.
26. Matsumoto RR, Hussong MJ, Truong DD. Effects of selective serotonergic ligands on posthypoxic audiogenic myoclonus. *Mov Disord* 1995;10:615–621.
27. Jaw SP, Dang T, Truong DD. Chronic treatments with 5-HT1A agonists attenuate posthypoxic myoclonus in rats. *Pharmacol Biochem Behav* 1995;52:577–580.
28. Jaw SP, Hussong MJ, Matsumoto RR, et al. Involvement of 5-HT2 receptors in posthypoxic stimulus-sensitive myoclonus in rats. *Pharmacol Biochem Behav* 1994;49:129–131.
29. Pappert EJ, Goetz CG, Vu TQ, et al. Animal model of posthypoxic myoclonus. Effects of serotonergic antagonists. *Neurology* 1999;52:16–21.
30. Goetz CG, Vu TQ, Charvey PM., et al. Posthypoxic myoclonus in the rat: natural history, stability, and serotonergic influences. *Mov Disord* 2000;15(suppl. 1):39–46.
31. Davis M, Cassella JV, Wrean WH, et al. Serotonin receptor subtype agonists: different effects on sensorimotor reactivity measured with acoustic startle. *Psychopharmacol Bull* 1986;22:837–843.
32. Dailey JW, Mishra PK, Ko KH, et al. Serotonergic abnormalities in the central nervous system of seizure naïve genetically epilepsy-prone rats. *Life Sci* 1991;50:319–326.
33. Welsh JP, Chang B, Menaker ME, et al. Removal of the inferior olive abolishes myoclonic seizures associated with a loss of olivary serotonin. *Neuroscience* 1998;82:879–897.
34. Truong DD, Matsumoto RR, Schwartz PH, et al. Novel rat cardiac arrest model of posthypoxic myoclonus. *Mov Disord* 1994;9:201–206.
35. Hallett M, Chadwick D, Adam J, et al. Reticular reflex myoclonus: a physiological type of human posthypoxic myoclonus. *J Neurol Neurosurg Psychiatry* 1977;40:253–264.
36. Welsh JP. Systemic harmaline blocks associative and motor learning by the actions of the inferior olive. *Eur J Neurosci* 1998;10:3307–3320.

37. Brozek G, Zhuravin IA, Megirian D, et al. Localization of the central rhythm generator involved in spontaneous consummatory licking in rats: functional ablation and electrical brain stimulation studies. *Proc Natl Acad Sci USA* 1996;93:3325–3329.

38. Hsu SM, Raine L, Fanger H. Use of avidin-biotin-peroxidase complex (ABC) in immunoperoxidase techniques: a comparison between ABC and unlabeled antibody (PAP procedures). *J Histochem Cytochem* 1981; 29:557–580.

39. Winer BJ. *Statistical principles in experimental design.* New York: McGraw-Hill, 1971.

40. Desclin JC. Histological evidence supporting the inferior olive as the major source of cerebellar climbing fibers in rat. *Brain Res* 1974;77:365–384.

41. Lamarre Y, deMontigny C, Dumont M, et al. Harmaline-induced rhythmic activity of cerebellar and lower brain stem neurons. *Brain Res* 1971;32:246–250.

42. Llinás R, Volkind RA. The olivocerebellar system: functional properties as revealed by harmaline-induced tremor. *Exp Brain Res* 1973;18:69–87.

43. DeMontigny C, Lamarre Y. Effects produced by local applications of harmaline in the inferior olive. *Can J Physiol Pharmacol* 1975;53:845–849.

44. Llinás R, Yarom Y. Oscillatory properties of guinea-pig inferior olivary neurones and their pharmacological modulation: an in vitro study. *J Physiol (London)* 1986; 376:163–182.

45. Welsh JP, Lang EJ, Sugihara I, et al. Dynamic organization of motor control within the olivocerebellar system. *Nature* 1995;374:453–457.

46. Bishop GA, Ho RH. Cell bodies of origin of serotonin-immunoreactive afferents to the inferior olivary complex of the rat. *Brain Res* 1986;399:369–373.

47. King JS, Ho RH, Burry RW. The distribution and synaptic organization of serotonergic elements in the inferior olivary complex of the oppossum. *J Comp Neurol* 1984; 227:357–368.

48. Bernardo L, Foster E. Oscillatory behavior in inferior olive neurons: mechanism, modulation, cell aggregates. *Brain Res Bull* 1986;17:773–784.

49. Llinás RR, Ribary U, Jeanmonod D, et al. Thalamocortical dysrhythmia: a neurological and neuropsychiatric syndrome characterized by magnetoencephalography. *Proc Natl Acad Sci USA* 1991;96:15222–15227.

50. Garlow SJ, Morilak DA, Dean RR, et al. Production and characterization of a specific 5-HT2 receptor antibody. *Brain Res* 1993;615:113–120.

Myoclonus and Paroxysmal Dyskinesias,
Advances in Neurology, Vol. 89,
edited by S. Fahn, et al.
Lippincott Williams & Wilkins, Philadelphia © 2002.

32

Why Do Purkinje Cells Die So Easily After Global Brain Ischemia? Aldolase C, EAAT4, and the Cerebellar Contribution to Posthypoxic Myoclonus

*John P. Welsh, †Genevieve Yuen, *‡Dimitris G. Placantonakis, §Toan Q. Vu, ‖Florent Haiss, ¶Elizabeth O'Hearn, ¶Mark E. Molliver, and *Sue A. Aicher

Neurological Sciences Institute, Oregon Health and Sciences University, Beaverton, Oregon; †Department of Neuroendocrinology, Weill Medical College of Cornell University and Rockefeller University, New York, New York; ‡Department of Physiology and Neuroscience, New York University School of Medicine, New York, New York; §Department of Neurology, University of Missouri Health Care, Columbia, Missouri; ‖Institute of Anatomy, University of Tübingen, Tübingen, Germany; ¶Departments of Neurology and Neuroscience, Johns Hopkins School of Medicine, Baltimore, Maryland

In 1995, C. David Marsden and colleagues published an important paper entitled "Progressive myoclonic ataxia associated with coeliac disease: the myoclonus is of cortical origin but the pathology is in the cerebellum" (1). In that paper, Marsden and his colleagues described four patients with coeliac disease, an autoimmune disorder of the intestine that is sometimes associated with neurologic deficits. All four of Marsden's patients showed debilitating action-induced myoclonus of cerebral cortical origin, as confirmed by grossly exaggerated cortical field potentials evoked by stimuli and that preceded the myoclonic jerks. Postmortem histologic studies, unexpectedly, did not detect any abnormality of the cerebral cortex, thalamus, or basal ganglia. However, there was a massive loss of Purkinje cells in the cerebellum.

Surprisingly, Marsden and associates did not address the conspicuous mismatch between the anatomic and physiologic pathoses underlying the coeliac variant of action-induced myoclonus. The coeliac cases were unique for their highly specific cell loss, and sharply contrasted with the widespread brain damage of similarly myoclonic patients whose symptoms are produced by global ischemia. This raises the question: What, exactly, was the functional relation of cerebellar damage to cortical myoclonus in the coeliac patients? The subtitle of this article was cryptic, and can be read either as a warning that the loss of Purkinje cells is unrelated to myoclonus or as a bold proposal that myoclonus of "cortical origin" might be produced by neuronal loss far away in the cerebellum. To decide between the two possibilities, we conducted research to determine the functional contribution of Purkinje cell loss to myoclonus, in particular that produced by prolonged cardiac arrest, and to elucidate the reasons why Purkinje cells are so susceptible to early death by global brain ischemia.

Is there a cerebellar contribution to posthypoxic myoclonus? Death of Purkinje cells is among the most reliably reported neuropathosis associated with posthypoxic myoclonus (2–4) (Fig. 32.1). However, the functional re-

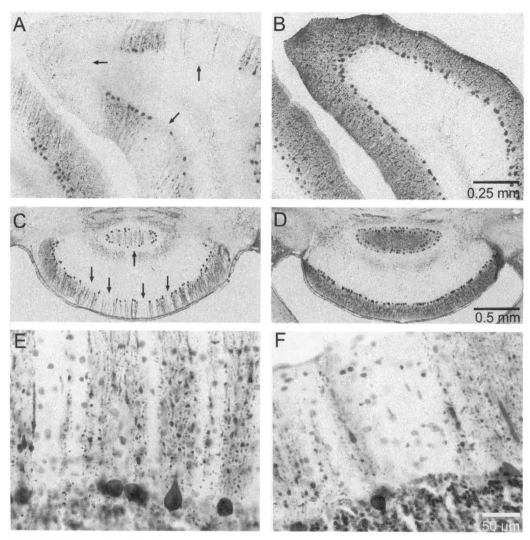

FIG. 32.1. Examples of Purkinje cell loss after 8 minutes of global brain ischemia in the rat. Purkinje cells were immunostained with an antibody against calbindin, a protein present only in Purkinje cells in the cerebellar cortex. **A,B:** Matched sections of the dorsal aspect of the paravermal cerebellar cortex of an ischemic and normal cerebellum. In the normal folium (**B**), Purkinje cell somata are uniformly distributed in a monolayer with their dendrites extending toward the pia. After ischemia (**A**), the uniform staining is disrupted due to the death of Purkinje cells (arrows). **C,D:** Matched sections of the lingula. The normal example shows a uniform distribution of Purkinje cells (**D**) while the ischemic example shows discrete regions of Purkinje cell death (*arrows*). **E,F:** Higher power photomicrographs of tissue counterstained with thionin shows that the loss of calbindin immunoreactivity after ischemia reflects the loss of the Purkinje cells. Moreover, granule cell density was not affected by ischemia. Sections were cut in the transverse plane.

lationship between this conspicuous loss and the syndrome remains unknown. Although Lance and Adams (5) hypothesized that posthypoxic myoclonus was a cerebellar syndrome produced by pathologic activation of the dentate nucleus, more recent work has deemphasized a role for the cerebellum. The recent trend of minimizing a possible cerebellar contribution to posthypoxic myoclonus is due to a strict adherence to localized neurophysiology experiments in the clinic, which have found that activation of the motor cortex (6) or medullary reticular formation (7) are the shortest latency activities that precede myoclonic events. It is then assumed that neuropathosis should be found in the thalamocortical system or brainstem. Such experiments have tended to rule out the cerebellum on the basis that the conduction time of the polysynaptic pathways through which the cerebellum influences the descending motor systems would be too long to allow it to be an origin for the jerk. Almost no experiments have examined the possibility that diaschisis produced by Purkinje cell loss is a major factor underlying posthypoxic myoclonus. Indeed, this possibility was favorably considered by Lance and Adams in their original description of posthypoxic myoclonus (5) and would be consistent with Marsden's coeliac cases. However, it must be recognized that not all syndromes of cerebellar damage produce myoclonus. Thus, if the cerebellar-diaschisis hypothesis of myoclonus is correct, then it must be the case that only *particular patterns* of Purkinje cell loss produce myoclonus. This is the first issue that our experiments have addressed.

A second issue that we have addressed is: Why do cerebellar Purkinje cells die so easily after global brain ischemia? The selective early death of Purkinje cells in the cerebellum by global brain ischemia is an extraordinary example of a "laminar lesion" that has been recognized for over 30 years (8,9) but remains unexplained. Much work has focused on the role of excitotoxicity in mediating Purkinje cell death. Indeed, Purkinje cells have two well-known predisposing features for rapid excitotoxic death: a very high degree of excitatory amino acid–mediated synaptic transmission (10) and a very high density of receptor- and voltage-gated calcium channels in their plasma membranes (11,12). Both climbing and parallel fiber inputs to Purkinje cells trigger calcium influx, the former producing a massive burst of calcium spikes that is synchronized throughout the dendritic tree (12). Recent experiments have demonstrated that

reduced ability to desensitize 2-(aminomethyl) phenylacetic acid (AMPA) receptors may account for Purkinje cells' sensitivity to excitotoxicity (13,14); this is supported by the finding that AMPA receptor blockade protects against ischemia-induced loss of Purkinje cells (15). However, current views assume that the profound calcium influx is the necessary and sufficient event that leads to Purkinje cells' early susceptibility to ischemia. Almost no attention has been directed toward the possibility that an unusually low anaerobic capacity to maintain ionic homeostasis during anoxia may account for Purkinje cells' rapid death by ischemia or that different populations of Purkinje cells may be differentially sensitive to global ischemia. The following experiments addressed this possibility.

METHODS

Induction of Global Brain Ischemia

Global brain ischemia was induced in anesthetized (200 mg/kg ketamine, 0.4 mg/kg atropine) rats weighing 200 to 300 g according to the method of Kawai and associates (16). Rats were prepared by loosely attaching their limbs to the table in the supine position and ventilating with 100% oxygen via a tracheal catheter (18G, Terumo Medical, SR-OX1832CA) at 60 strokes/min (2.5-mL tidal volume). Venous and arterial catheters (24G, Terumo Medical, SR-OX2419CA) were sewn into the right femoral vessels, to allow drug injections and blood pressure measurement, respectively. Before ischemia onset, 0.2 mL of heparinized 0.9% saline (10 U/mL) was injected via the femoral vein. A 1-mm diameter wire probe, with 1 cm of its distal end bent into a U, was inserted into the mediastinum at the level of the second intercostal segment. The distal end of the device was gently manipulated along the dorsal wall of the thorax and was twisted 45 degrees to be positioned under the bundle of major cardiac blood vessels. The device was lifted while finger pressure was placed on the chest in order to rapidly and completely interrupt the circulation, which was verified by blood pressure measurement from the femoral artery. Artificial ventilation was stopped at the time that blood pressure dropped below 10 mm Hg. The wire probe could be removed from the chest 3 to 5 minutes after ischemia onset without spontaneous return of mean arterial blood pressure. Five to ten minutes after ischemia onset, the rat was injected with 5 µg of epinephrine (0.1 mL, 1:50,000) via the femoral vein, ventilated (120 strokes/min, 2.5-mL tidal volume), and given sternal chest compression (180/min). Successful resuscita-

tion was identified by an abrupt increase in arterial blood pressure after an initial plateau at approximately 30 mm Hg (Fig. 32.2A). Spontaneous breathing usually resumed within 30 minutes after restoring mean arterial blood pressure, at which time mechanical respiration was gradually withdrawn. Following successful resuscitation, the catheters were removed, the wounds were sewn, and the rat was placed back into its cage. Core body temperature was maintained between 36 and 38° C throughout the procedure by a rectal thermistor and servo-controlled warm water

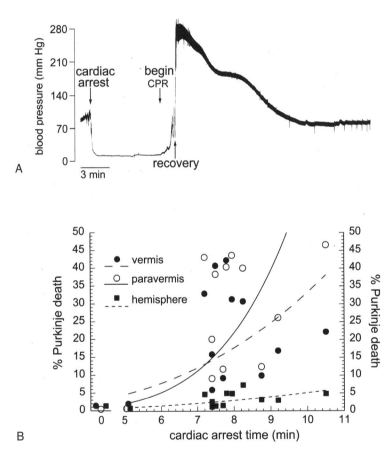

FIG. 32.2. Relation of the duration of global brain ischemia to the magnitude of Purkinje cell death. **A:** Arterial blood pressure during the cardiac arrest procedure and its reinstatement by cardiopulmonary resuscitation. **B:** Purkinje cell death 5 days after various durations of ischemia for 12 rats. Significance is determined by comparison with the mean of 4 normal rats (0 minutes ischemia; 1 SEM of the control mean was less than the symbol height). Correlation coefficients of power regression fits equaled 0.54, 0.74, and 0.61 for vermis, paravermis, and hemisphere, respectively (all $p < 0.06$).

heating pad (Gaymar, T-Pump). The duration of global brain ischemia was determined to be the time between the initial, rapid fall in arterial pressure and when the heart could maintain pressure on its own after resuscitation (Fig. 32.2A).

On the second day after surgery, rats were tested for audiogenic myoclonic jerks using the method of Truong and associates (17) with the quantitative techniques that we described in this volume (see Chapter 31). Briefly, myoclonic jerks were measured in response to 45 presentations of a 40-msec, 95-dB auditory white noise at 1 Hz. Measurements of myoclonic jerks were accomplished with a capacitive sensor that transduced whole-body momentum into voltage. The voltage response was digitized at DC-2.5 kHz bandpass and parameters of the response were analyzed with Datapac 2000 (Run Technologies, Laguna Hills, CA) and software that we wrote for the application (ASYST, v. 4.01).

Immunohistochemistry

Five days after cardiac arrest, rats were anesthetized (150 mg/kg pentobarbital) and sequentially perfused transcardially with heparinized saline (10 mL), 3.8% acrolein in 2% paraformaldehyde (50 mL), and 2% paraformaldehyde (200 mL). The brain was placed in 2% paraformaldehyde for 30 minutes. The brainstem and cerebellum were sectioned (40 μm), placed in 0.1 M phosphate buffer, in 0.1% sodium borohydride for 30 minutes, in 0.5% bovine serum albumin for 30 minutes, and were processed for immunoperoxidase labeling using the avidin-biotin-peroxidase method (18). Alternate sections were placed in an antibody solution against calbindin-D28 (1:200) for 18 hours at room temperature. The antibody was raised in mouse and was visualized using a biotinylated antibody directed against mouse IgG raised in horse (Vector Laboratories, 1:400). The biotin was visualized by 30 minutes incubation in avidin-biotin complex followed by 1 to 3 minutes incubation in 3', 3'-diaminobenzidine and hydrogen peroxide (0.003%). Zebrin II

monoclonal antibody raised in mouse (1:200, gracious gift of Dr. R. Hawkes) was used to detect aldolase C using the same procedure. Sequence analysis of the antigen recognized by the zebrin II antibody indicated 98% homology with aldolase C (19). To verify that the antibody recognized aldolase C, dot-blot immunochemistry was performed using 98% pure aldolase C obtained from human brain (20) (Biogenesis, Brentwood, NH). Two-μL aliquots of aldolase C dissolved in 1 M tris buffer (pH 7.4) ranging from 0 to 10 mM were placed onto filter paper via a manifold (Scheiber and Schvell, SRC-96/0) that constrained each aliquot to a 5-mm diameter well. The paper was dried, exposed to paraformaldehyde vapor for 1 hour at 80° C, and immunostained with zebrin II antibody as described above.

Double-label immunofluorescence histochemistry was performed on three cerebella to determine the co-localization of aldolase C/zebrin II and excitatory amino acid transporter — type 4 (EAAT4) within parasagittal zones of the cerebellum and within single Purkinje cells. Anesthetized rats were perfused with 4% paraformaldehyde (600 mL), the brains were removed and the cerebellum was blocked and placed into fixative for 30 minutes. Sections (40 μm) were cut on a vibrating microtome and placed in 0.1 M phosphate buffer and then rinsed in tris-saline and placed in 0.5% bovine serum albumin for 30 minutes to reduce nonspecific antibody binding. Sections were again rinsed and placed in a cocktail containing both mouse anti-zebrin II (1:100) and rabbit anti-rat EAAT4 (1:500; Alpha Diagnostic, San Antonio, TX) antibodies at 4° C for two nights. Sections were rinsed again in tris buffer and placed into a cocktail of secondary antibodies containing a mixture of goat-anti-mouse IgG-conjugated to Alexa 488 and goat-anti-rabbit IgG conjugated to Alexa 546 (Molecular Probes, Eugene, OR) for 2 hours at room temperature. Sections were thoroughly rinsed in tris buffer followed by successive rinses in 0.1 M and 0.05 M phosphate-buffer before they were mounted onto gelatin-coated slides, dried, and coverslipped with Prolong antifade mounting medium (Molecular Probes). Slides were sealed with nail polish and stored in the dark. The immunostaining was visualized with epifluorescence (Zeiss Axioskop, Thornwood, NY) and confocal (Zeiss LSM-510) microscopes.

Quantification of Purkinje Cell Death

Measurements were made from digital images captured with a Spot-2 camera (1.4×10^6 pixels, Diagnostics Instruments, Sterling Heights, MI) attached to a light microscope fitted with a 1.25X objective (Zeiss Axioskop). The images were shade-corrected to ensure uniform background, interpolated by two, thresholded so that background illumination was white, smoothed with 3×3 pixel averaging, and converted to binary format to produce images of only black and white pixels having values of 1 and 0, respectively. Optical density profiles were obtained from linear samples taken from cerebellar molecular layer oriented parallel to the folial surfaces (Scion Image, Frederick, MD). The profiles represented the presence or absence of Purkinje cell dendrites with 4 µm resolution. Multiple profiles were obtained to cover the perimeter of each folium unilaterally from every second or third section. Purkinje cell death was calculated as the percentage length of molecular layer that did not possess calbindin immunostaining, as determined from sums of optical density profiles. This was appropriate because, after image adjustment, the width of the thin axis of the Purkinje cell dendritic signal reflected the loss of the soma (Fig. 32.1). Examination of tissue counterstained with thionin confirmed that the loss of dendritic signal represented the loss of the Purkinje cell soma (Fig. 32.1E,F). The ability of the method to detect the full complement of Purkinje cells was determined in four control rats in which $98.95 \pm 0.18\%$ of 2,362 mm of molecular layer contained calbindin immunostaining, reflecting the ubiquitous presence of Purkinje cells throughout cerebellar cortex. For 12 ischemia cases, 9,670 mm of tissue was analyzed.

Inferior Cerebellar Pedunculotomy

Twelve weeks prior to cardiac arrest, rats were anesthetized (150 mg/kg ketamine, 10 mg/kg xylazine), the occipital bone was removed, and the cerebellum was lifted at the obex to look into the rhomboid fossa using a surgical microscope. A probe was inserted into the fourth ventricle to transect the right inferior cerebellar peduncle. The craniotomy was covered with Gelfoam and the incision was closed.

Multielectrode Recording of the Inferior Olive During Global Brain Ischemia

Multisite recordings from the inferior olive were obtained using specially fabricated microelectrode arrays that we have described in detail (21,22). Arrays of microelectrodes were constructed in our laboratory from electrolytically etched, 100 µm diameter, tungsten rod producing tip profiles of 5 to 7 degrees. The electrodes were insulated with varnish to generate tip impedance between 2 and 6 MΩ. The arrays were fabricated to have 16 electrodes, organized in two rows of eight, with interelectrode distances of 260 µm. Extracellular recordings were obtained with the MNAP multichannel recording system (Plexon, Dallas TX) allowing simultaneous recording of single neurons and field potentials from all of the 16 electrodes. Field potentials were obtained by band-pass filtering the signals between 3 and 90 Hz and sampling at 1 kHz, while recordings of neuronal spikes were obtained by filtering the same signals between 0.15 and 9 kHz and sampling at 40 kHz. A skull screw electrode was placed in the frontal cortex to allow simultaneous monitoring of the frontal electroencephalogram (EEG).

After preparing the rats for induction of global brain ischemia as previously described in a stereotaxic frame, access to the inferior olive was obtained from the retropharyngeal approach under ketamine (100 mg/kg) and xylazine (10 mg/kg) anesthesia. After cutting the dura and visualizing the basilar artery and pyramids, the microelectrode array was positioned 0.5 mm lateral to the median fissure and slowly lowered 600 μm below the surface with a hydraulic microdrive (FHC Inc, Bowdoinham, ME). The inferior olive was identified by the shift from electrical quiescence in the pyramidal tract to the characteristic rhythmic field potentials of the inferior olive that sound like a "slow freight-train" when played through an audio speaker. After the electrodes were properly positioned in the inferior olive, cardiac arrest and resuscitation were accomplished as previously described. Recordings were obtained for 15 minutes prior to cardiac arrest and for 60 minutes thereafter.

Ibogaine Induction of Purkinje Cell Death

To induce Purkinje cell death pharmacologically, a single dose of 100 mg/kg of ibogaine HCl was given intragastrically to six normal Sprague-Dawley rats (200–250 g). The drug was dissolved in a 25% solution of 2-hyrdoxypropyl-beta-cyclodextrin to a final concentration of 20 mg/mL. Five rats showed a prominent 10 Hz tremor within a few minutes after ibogaine. Rats were tested for an audiogenic myoclonic jerk for the 5 days after ibogaine delivery, using the method previously described. At the end of behavioral testing, the rats were killed and their cerebella were processed for calbindin immunohistochemistry to visualize Purkinje cells using the methods previously described.

Intracellular Recordings of Inferior Olivary Neurons

Intracellular recordings were obtained from inferior olivary neurons in brainstem slices of postnatal day 12 to 21 Sprague-Dawley rats with methods we have described (23,24). Rats were anesthetized with 15 to 20 mg ketamine and decapitated. A vibratome was used to cut 400 μm parasagittal sections of the brainstem in artificial cerebrospinal fluid (ACSF) at 4° C. After sectioning, the sections were transferred to a chamber containing ACSF at room temperature and allowed to sit for at least 1 hour. Individual sections were moved subsequently to a submersion recording chamber

where the temperature was increased to 33 to 35° C over 10 minutes. ACSF flow rates of at least 5 mL/min were used to perfuse the slices in the recording chamber and pass 100 μM ibogaine. Intracellular recordings were performed in current-clamp mode with borosilicate glass microelectrodes filled with 3 M potassium acetate, whose direct current resistance ranged from 60 to 100 MΩ. Only neurons with membrane potentials negative to -50 mV, showing dendritic and somatic calcium currents, fast sodium spikes, and slow inward rectification were analyzed. Recordings were amplified with an Axoclamp2B amplifier, digitized at 5 kHz, and stored on the hard drive of a computer with pCLAMP 6 acquisition software (Axon Instruments, Foster City, CA).

RESULTS

Why do cerebellar Purkinje cells die so easily after global brain ischemia? Twelve rats were subjected to cardiac arrest to induce global brain ischemia for a duration of 5.1 to 10.5 min (Fig. 32.2A). After recovery, many rats showed profound ataxia, seizures, and audiogenic myoclonus, resembling human anoxic encephalopathy (5), as we described in Chapter 31 of this volume. The duration of cardiac arrest determined the severity of the syndrome such that ischemia greater than 7 minutes produced myoclonus while ischemia for less than 6 minutes did not.

Global brain ischemia killed between 18,000 and 107,100 Purkinje cells (mean ± SEM = 64,702 ± 10,096, n = 11, Fig. 32.2B), depending on the duration of ischemia, as calculated from a total of 340,000 Purkinje cells in the rat (25). Granule cell density was unaffected as indicated by inspection of sections counterstained with thionin. Purkinje cell death was greatest in the midline, where up to 47% were killed by 10.5 minutes of ischemia, but was modest in the hemisphere (Fig. 32.2B). Although no Purkinje cell death occurred with 5.1 minutes of ischemia, 7.2 to 7.5 minutes of ischemia resulted in a loss of 28 ± 8% and 24 ± 8% of paravermal and ver-

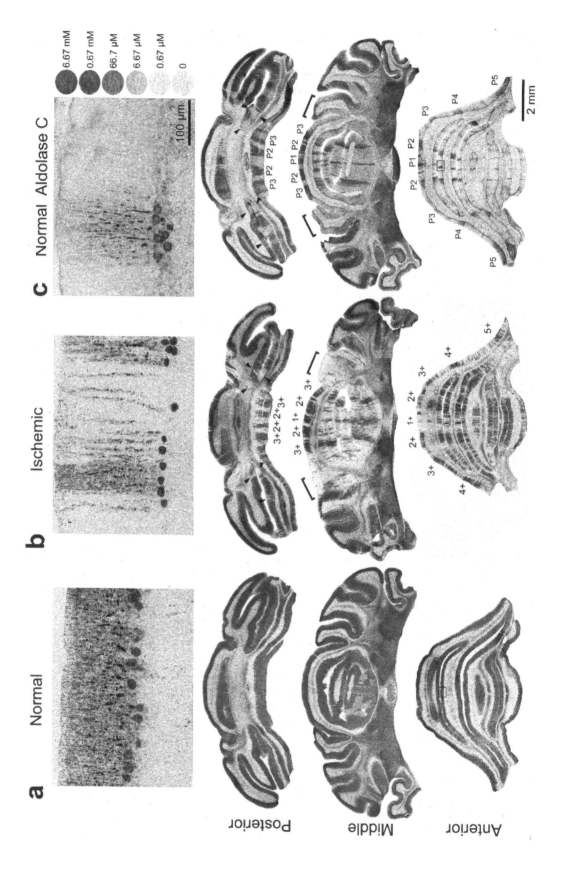

c   Normal   Ischemic   Normal Aldolase C

6.67 mM

0.67 mM

66.7 µM

6.67 µM

0.67 µM

0

100 µm

a   **b**

Posterior

Middle

Anterior

P3 P2 P2 P3

P3 P2 P1 P2 P3

P3 P2 P1 P2 P3

P5 P4 P3 P2 P1 P2 P3 P4 P5

2 mm

3+ 2+ 2+ 3+

3+ 2+ 1+ 2+ 3+

2+ 1+ 2+ 3+ 4+ 5+

3+ 4+

mal Purkinje cells, respectively (n = 5). Thus, the threshold duration of ischemia for Purkinje cell loss resided between 5.1 and 7.2 minutes, a range remarkably similar to the 5- to 7-minute time in which adenylate charge falls to near zero in brain following sudden ischemia (26). The uneven distribution of neuronal death was unexpected given the uniformity of Purkinje cells' synaptic density and tendency to accumulate calcium (10–12). The major questions to be resolved were: what spared the Purkinje cells that survived ischemia and what, if any, synaptic input killed the ones that did not survive?

Closer examination revealed that global brain ischemia killed Purkinje cells in sharply demarcated zones. The sharpness of the death zones had the effect of sculpting out bands of ischemia-resistance that could be followed through the cerebellum. The bands of ischemia resistance were numbered by their spatial relation to a midline band of surviving Purkinje cells (*1+* in Fig. 32.3B, middle). Second (*2+*) and third (*3+*) bands of ischemia-resistant Purkinje cells were symmetrically positioned around the *1+* band at all levels of the vermis and the *3+* band was flanked by massive loss of Purkinje cells in paravermis (brackets in Fig. 32.3B, middle), as well as by patches of Purkinje death in the hemisphere (arrowheads in Fig. 32.3B, posterior). Anteriorly, the *1+*, *2+*, and *3+* bands were flanked

by fourth (*4+*) and fifth (*5+*) bands of ischemia-resistant Purkinje cells (Fig. 32.3B, anterior). The nearly identical pattern occurred among the most severely affected cases.

The distribution of Purkinje cells that survived ischemia was essentially identical to the distribution of aldolase C, a glycolytic enzyme (27) that is localized to subpopulations of Purkinje cells (19,28) whose ordered distribution is highly conserved among individuals and species (29). In our quantitative cell-count analysis of the normal rat cerebellum, 66%, 70%, and 90% of vermal, paravermal, and hemispheral neurons expressed aldolase C, respectively (n = 35,320 Purkinje cells counted). The prevalence of aldolase C corresponded closely to the proportion of Purkinje cells that survived ischemia in each region (vermis, 76 ± 4%; paravermis, 70 ± 5%; hemisphere, 96 ± 1%, n = 11). Aldolase C was localized to a midline band of Purkinje cells (P1) that was flanked by symmetric bands of enzyme positivity (29) (P2, P3, Fig. 32.3C, middle). The P1, P2, and P3 bands of aldolase C positivity corresponded to the *1+*, *2+*, and *3+* bands of ischemia-resistant Purkinje cells. The paravermal region where Purkinje cell death was most severe corresponded to a region of aldolase C negativity (brackets, Fig. 32.3B and C, middle) and the patches of death in the hemisphere corresponded to patches of aldolase C negativity (arrowheads in Fig.

FIG. 32.3. Organization of Purkinje cell death following global ischemia and the distribution of aldolase C. **A:** Normal cerebellum, calbindin immunohistochemistry. At high magnification (*top*), the monolayer of Purkinje cell somata and their overlying dendrites are uniformly present. At low magnification (*below*), Purkinje cells are uniformly present in all cerebellar folia. **B:** Cerebellum after ischemia, calbindin immunohistochemistry. At high magnification (*top*), some Purkinje cell somata have dropped out of the monolayer, leaving discontinuities in the dendritic staining. At low magnification (*below*), Purkinje cell loss is organized in zones oriented in the parasagittal plane that can be followed through the cerebellum. **C:** Normal cerebellum, aldolase C immunohistochemistry. At high magnification (*top*), a cluster of Purkinje cell somata and dendrites is selectively stained. At low magnification (*bottom*), aldolase C distribution resembles the pattern of Purkinje cell survival after ischemia. Zones of aldolase C positivity are numbered using the nomenclature of Hawkes and associates (29). Dot-blot immunochemistry (*top right*) indicated a significant logarithmic relation between aldolase C concentration and density of immunostaining (optical density=175.9–19.1*ln[μM aldolase C]; r=0.95, *p* < 0.01), indicating recognition of aldolase C by the zebrin II antibody. The boxed regions in the anterior sections are shown in the high magnification micrographs (*top*).

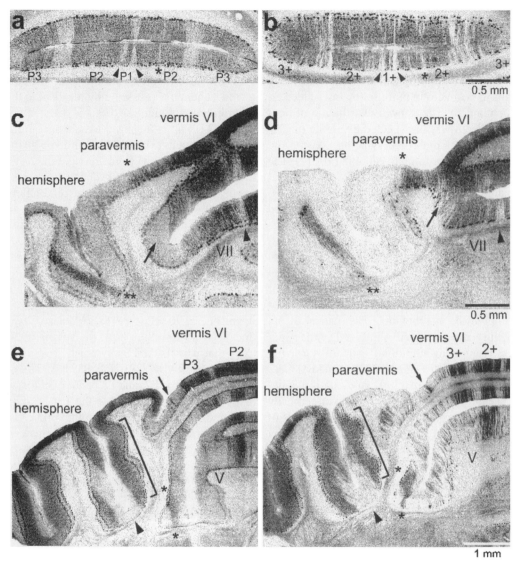

FIG. 32.4. Correspondence between the presence of aldolase C in Purkinje cells of normal cerebella (**A,C,E**) and the pattern of Purkinje cell survival after ischemia (**B,D,F**). **A,B:** Vermal lobule VIII. Aldolase C was expressed in symmetric zones of Purkinje cells separated by regions of enzyme negativity. The enzyme negative zones nearly perfectly mirrored zones of ischemic death of Purkinje cells, including a 20 μm wide band of enzyme negativity (*asterisk*). **C,D:** Vermal lobules VI, VII, and hemisphere. Nearly all Purkinje cells in the dorsal vermis expressed aldolase C, except for a 90 μm strip of Purkinje cells whose dendrites ran along the margin of the vermis (*arrowhead*). Vermal Purkinje cells here survived ischemia, except within the strip where aldolase C was absent (*arrowhead*). Abrupt transitions between Purkinje cell survival and death mirrored the transitions between aldolase C positivity and negativity, as seen at the fissures between vermis and paravermis (*arrow*), between paravermis and hemisphere (*double asterisk*), and on the surface (*asterisk*). **E,F:** Vermal lobules V, VI, and hemisphere 800 μm anterior to **C** and **D**. P2 and P3 bands of aldolase C positivity corresponded to bands of ischemia-resistant Purkinje cells, including a 30 μm band of enzyme positivity (*arrow*). Aldolase C positivity in the paravermis and hemisphere was interrupted by a strip of enzyme negativity (*arrowhead*) that corresponded to a strip of ischemic death.

32.3B and C, posterior). Analysis of variance indicated that the percentage of aldolase C positive Purkinje cells in ischemic rats was abnormally high ($p < 0.001$), verifying that most surviving Purkinje cells contained aldolase C. For instance, in normal rats, 68 ± 3% and 72 ± 4% of Purkinje cells in vermal and paravermal lobule VI were aldolase C positive, whereas after ischemia 90 ± 2% and 86 ± 3% of the remaining Purkinje cells in those folia expressed aldolase C.

Figure 32.4 documents the congruity between the pattern of aldolase C expression in normal cerebella and resistance to ischemia of cardiac-arrested rats. The first example was taken from vermal lobule VIII in which the P1 aldolase C band was only two to three Purkinje cells wide and was bordered by two regions of enzyme negativity, each four neurons wide (*arrowheads*, Fig. 32.4A). In ischemic lobules, the midline 1+ band of ischemia resistance was also three Purkinje cells wide and was bordered by bands of ischemic death, each two to five neurons wide (*arrowheads*, Fig. 32.4B). In addition, vermal lobule VIII showed a satellite band of enzyme negativity only two Purkinje cells wide (*asterisk*, Fig. 32.4A) which corresponded to a two-neuron wide death zone in the middle of the *2+* ischemia-resistant band (*asterisk*, Fig. 32.4B).

Another example was taken from the posterior lobe where the vermis joined the paravermis. Here, the normal vermis was completely aldolase C positive, except for a narrow band of enzyme negativity (*arrowhead*, Fig. 32.4C) that corresponded to a narrow band of Purkinje death after ischemia (*arrowhead*, Fig. 32.4D). Moreover, the transition from vermis to paravermis was characterized by a region of enzyme negativity in the fissure (*arrow*, Fig. 32.4C) and a sharp transition from enzyme positivity to negativity on the surface (*asterisk*, Fig. 32.4C). These regions corresponded to a region of death along the fissure (*arrow*, Fig. 32.4D) and to a sharp transition from resistance to ischemia to profound death on the surface (*asterisk*, Fig. 32.4D). Further, a thin strip of enzyme positivity ran from the paravermis to the hemisphere (*double aster-*

isk, Fig. 32.4C), corresponding to a strip of survival (*double asterisk*, Fig. 32.4D).

More anteriorly, a corrugated pattern of aldolase C positivity and negativity corresponded to regions of ischemia-resistance and ischemic death, respectively (compare P2, P3 with *2+*, *3+* in Fig. 32.4E and F). In lateral vermis, a satellite band of aldolase C positivity, only one Purkinje cell wide, corresponded to one to two ischemia-resistant neurons (arrows, Fig. 32.4E and F). At this level, the lateral paravermis was aldolase C positive, corresponding to an expansive region of ischemia resistance (*brackets*, Fig. 32.4E and F). Likewise, a narrow region of aldolase C positivity, along the fissure separating two vermal lobules, was resistant to ischemia (*asterisks*, Fig. 32.4E and F) and a band of aldolase C negativity separating the paravermis from the hemispheres corresponded exactly to a region of Purkinje cell death (*arrowheads*, Fig. 32.4E and F).

The extremely tight correspondence between aldolase C positivity and resistance to ischemia suggested that aldolase C allowed Purkinje cells to survive up to 10 minutes of ischemia. By cleaving fructose 1,6-diphosphate into dihydroxyacetone phosphate and glyceraldehyde 3-phosphate, aldolase catalyzes an essential metabolic step within the glycolytic pathway that allows adenosine triphosphate (ATP) and pyruvate to be generated from glucose (27). During aerobisis, pyruvate provides substrate for the citric acid cycle and, thereafter, oxidative phosphorylation. However, during ischemia, neither the citric acid cycle nor oxidative phosphorylation are operant and ATP production is limited to 6% of its capacity due to glycolysis alone (30). Aldolase occurs in three isoforms (27), two of which – A and C – are expressed by neurons. Purkinje cells have a repressed expression of aldolase A (31), but instead express high levels of aldolase C within a subset of neurons in parasagittal compartments (19,28,29). The absence of aldolase C in ischemia-sensitive Purkinje cells indicates that the most important metabolic pathway for producing ATP during anaerobisis is impaired in these cells.

We hypothesized that Purkinje cell death by global ischemia was triggered by synaptic excitation, which drove aldolase C-negative Purkinje cells into energy deficiency and death. If true, deafferenting Purkinje cells from excitatory input should attenuate their death. In two rats, the Purkinje cells on one side of the cerebellum were deprived of monosynaptic excitation from the inferior olive by transecting the inferior cerebellar peduncle 12 weeks prior to cardiac arrest. Such deafferentation relieves Purkinje cells from the prolonged depolarization (32) and sustained barrages of calcium influx that are triggered by the climbing fiber input from inferior olivary neurons (11,12). Moreover, the transection would have further reduced excitation by removing a subset of mossy fiber input to the cerebellum, largely originating from the spinal cord. Because all ascending fibers contained within the inferior cerebellar peduncle synapse ipsilaterally in the cerebellum, unilateral transection ensured that Purkinje cells on only one side of the cerebellum were deafferented from the inferior olive.

Transecting the inferior cerebellar peduncle completely protected Purkinje cells from death by ischemia (Fig. 32.5). After transecting the right inferior cerebellar peduncle (*arrowhead*, Fig. 32.5B), ischemia failed to kill Purkinje cells on the right while patterned death occurred on the left. The lateralized death was again organized in discrete zones corresponding to the aldolase C-negative regions of normal cerebella. Figure 32.6 shows sections through the entire anterior-posterior extent of the cerebellum of a pedunculotomized rat that experienced global brain ischemia. Here it can be seen that the striped Purkinje cell loss was nearly completely restricted to the side opposite of the pedunculotomy and was sharply bounded precisely on the midline throughout the cerebellum. The data strongly indicated that synaptic excitation from climbing fibers, issued from the inferior olive, killed Purkinje cells after global brain ischemia.

Multielectrode recordings were used to determine the early electrophysiologic changes in the inferior olive during recovery from global brain ischemia (Fig. 32.7). Prior to cardiac arrest, field potentials from the inferior olive showed highly regular, synchronized oscillations at 1 Hz (Fig. 32.7A). Simultaneous recording of the frontal cortex EEG showed that the activities of the cerebrum and the inferior olive were not synchronized. At this time, the frontal EEG showed low-amplitude, high frequency activity within the range of 30 to 70 Hz upon which larger, slower frequency burst potentials were superimposed (Fig. 32.7A). Cardiac arrest induced a gradual transition to isoelectricity at all sites, which was maintained for the duration of the arrest, and which persisted for 10 to 12 minutes after restoration of the heart beat and mean arterial pressure (Fig. 32.7B).

By 14 minutes after resuscitation, isoelectric potentials were replaced by spike-like fields in both the inferior olive and frontal cortex (Fig. 32.7C). The amplitude of the spike-fields in the frontal EEG were normal compared to the pre-ischemia values, but did not occur against a background of low-amplitude, high-frequency activity as before ischemia. Moreover, during emergence from isoelectricity, the spike fields were again synchronized within the inferior olive but not between the inferior olive and frontal cortex.

A dramatically different picture emerged at 45 minutes after recovery from cardiac arrest (Fig. 32.7D). At this time, the inferior olive showed a storm of very large amplitude, irregular bursting that was nearly completely synchronized with the frontal EEG. The spike bursts in the frontal EEG occurred more frequently at this time, but still against an absence of higher-frequency background activity, as previously shown (33). Similar outcomes were observed in three rats studied. The characteristics of the pathologic olivary fields indicated that olivary neurons manifested high-frequency bursts of highly synchronized firing during recovery from ischemia. The pathologic bursting showed no signs of abatement at 60 minutes after resuscitation, at which time the recordings were stopped. Sustained, synchronized bursting of olivary neurons would be expected to cause

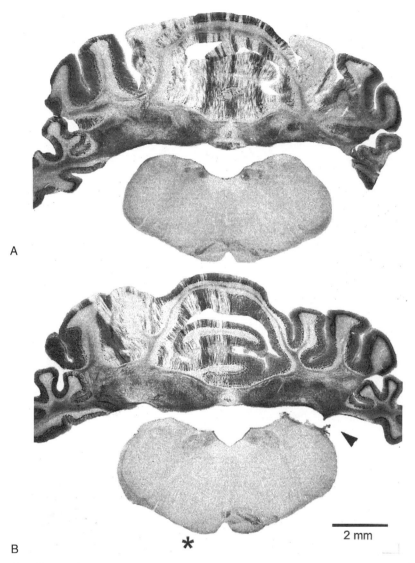

FIG. 32.5. Deafferentation prevents patterned cerebellar death by global ischemia. **A:** Normal pattern of Purkinje cell death produced by ischemia (calbindin immunohistochemistry). **B:** Pattern of Purkinje cell death induced by ischemia after the right inferior cerebellar peduncle was surgically transected (*arrowhead*). The transection caused retrograde degeneration of the left inferior olive (*asterisk*) but protected Purkinje cells on the right from death by ischemia.

sustained depolarization of Purkinje cells in the cerebellum, possibly leading to excitotoxicity and death.

The fact that Purkinje cell death after global brain ischemia was associated with unusually intense burst activity in the inferior olive in the acute postischemic state and was prevented by removing climbing fiber innervation, led us to hypothesize that ischemia-driven glutamate release induces the inferior olive to fire high-frequency bursts of action potentials and drive Purkinje cells into excitotoxicity. Indeed, excessive glutamate release occurs in the acute postischemic state (34) and glutamatergic *N*-

Posterior

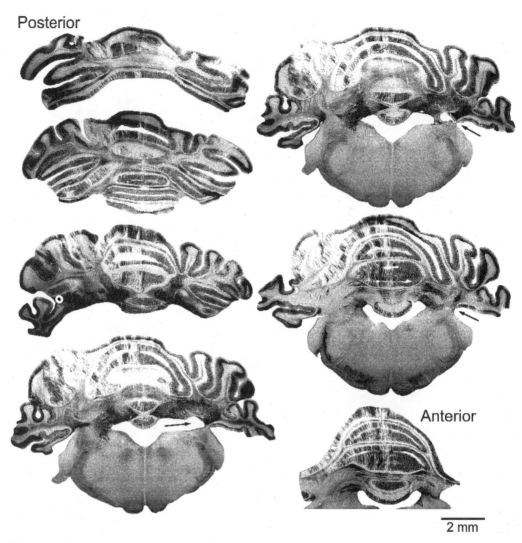

Anterior

2 mm

FIG. 32.6. Coronal sections of the cerebellum of a pedunculotomized rat subjected to global brain ischemia (calbindin immunostaining). Note the transection of the inferior cerebellar peduncle on the right (*arrows*) which leaves the middle cerebellar peduncle and underlying brainstem intact. Purkinje cell death is nearly totally localized to the left.

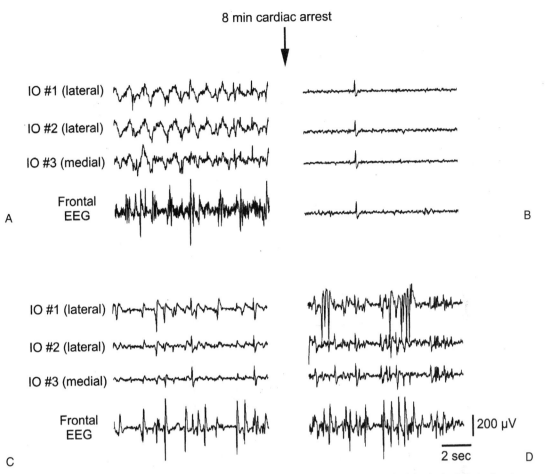

FIG. 32.7. Early electrophysiological changes in the inferior olive after global brain ischemia *in vivo*. Records were obtained simultaneously from three sites within the inferior olive and are shown in registration with the EEG taken from the frontal cortex. **A.** Before Cardiac Arrest. **B.** 10 minutes after resuscitation. **C.** 14 minutes after resuscitation. **D.** 49 minutes after resuscitation.

methyl-D-aspartate (NMDA) receptor activation induces neuronal oscillatory activity in many areas of the CNS (35–39). Although it is well known that olivary neurons have intrinsic oscillatory activity (40,41), whether NMDA receptors played a role in olivary neuronal oscillation was unknown. We found that NMDA receptor activation depolarizes olivary neurons and induces high-amplitude subthreshold oscillations at 4 Hz (Fig. 32.8A, ref. 24). Such oscillations are functionally important within the context of recovery from global brain ischemia for two reasons. First, the NMDA oscillations occur at depolarized potentials close to the threshold for action potential firing. Second, the oscillations are large in amplitude (approximately 15 mV), thus achieving large depolarization during their peak and ensuring a high probability that sodium channels will be activated and trigger axonal spikes. The result is that NMDA oscillations in olivary neurons can reliably trigger bursts of action potentials (Fig. 32.8B), and lead to Purkinje cell activation *in vivo*. Our pharmacologic experiments have indicated that the glutamatergic induction of olivary oscillations is specifically due to activation of the NMDA receptor, because it is blocked by the NMDA receptor an-

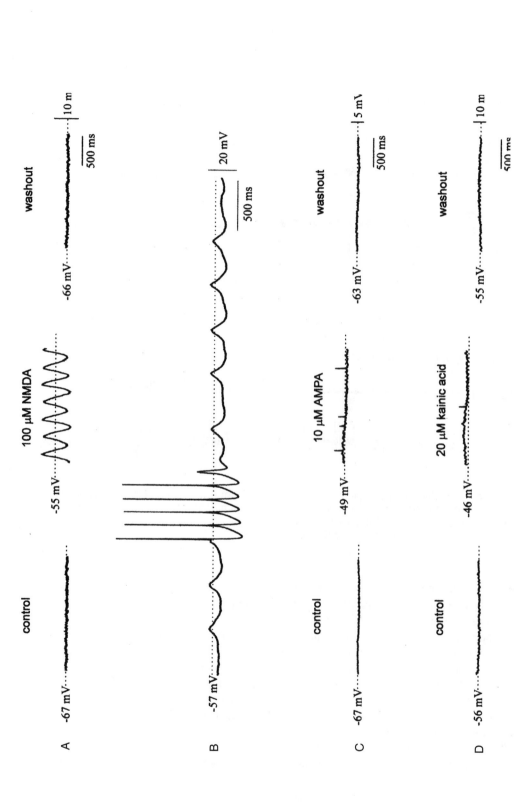

tagonists MK-801 and ketamine (24) and because activation of non-NMDA glutamate receptors with AMPA (Fig. 32.8C) or kainic acid (Fig. 32.8D) does not produce oscillations, even though they both depolarize the membrane (24). Moreover, high-threshold NMDA oscillations are blocked by antagonists of the L- and P-type high threshold calcium channel (e.g., nifedipine and ω-agatoxin IVA, respectively).

Although extremely reliable, the relation between the regional expression of aldolase C and resistance to ischemia was only a correlation (with nearly 100% congruence to zones as small as one to two neurons wide), leaving open the possibility that biochemical factors other than the patterned distribution of aldolase C led to the same pattern of Purkinje cell death after global brain ischemia. It is known that EAAT4 is concentrated in parasagittal zones that resemble those that express aldolase C (42). EAAT4 is one of a family of glutamate-transporter proteins that functions to reduce the extracellular concentration of glutamate (43). Moreover, EAAT4 is a glutamate-gated chloride channel (44) that is located extrasynaptically on Purkinje cell spines (42,45), close to the climbing fiber–Purkinje cell synapses (46). Thus, EAAT4 is presumed to play an important role in limiting the temporal duration of the excitation produced by climbing fibers on Purkinje cell dendrites, to reduce glutamate spillover, and to prevent excitotoxicity.

Double immunofluorescence histochemistry revealed perfect congruity of aldolase C and EAAT4 compartmentation in the rat cerebellum. Figure 32.9 shows low-power fluorescent images of posterior-lobe cerebellar cortex doubly immunostained for aldolase C and EAAT4. The section shown in Fig. 32.7 was chosen to demonstrate a complex pattern of aldolase C compartmentation in the vermis as well as an oblique aldolase C negative zone in the medial hemisphere. Note that the EAAT4 immunostaining reflects the precise details of the aldolase C compartmentation in every folium, without exception. Identical 100% correspondence was seen through all anterior-posterior levels of the cerebellum in each of three cases studied. Control experiments were performed in which tissue was doubly immunoreacted with both aldolase C and EAAT4 primary antibodies but with only one of the two fluorescent-probe tagged secondary antibodies. The control experiments indicated that there was no bleed-through of the fluorescent signals or cross-labeling, indicating excellent detection and discrimination of the two antigens by our procedure.

Higher power epifluorescence microscopy of doubly immunostained tissue (Fig. 32.10A) (see Color Plate 6 following page 288) indicated that EAAT4 immunostaining respected the borders of aldolase C immunostaining within Purkinje cell clusters. However, confocal microscopy revealed that aldolase C and EAAT4 were not co-localized within the same subcellular compartments. Aldolase C was most prominently expressed in the soma and thick dendrites of Purkinje cells, while EAAT4 was present as fine puncta within the dendritic tree (Fig. 32.10B). High-power confocal microscopy (Fig. 32.10C) detected aldolase C in tertiary dendrites and revealed that EAAT4 puncta showed their highest density along the circumference of these fine processes (*arrows*, Fig. 32.10C). In contrast, EAAT4 expression was significantly lower around the thicker secondary dendrites of the Purkinje cell (*arrowheads*, Fig. 32.10C). The data were consistent

---

FIG. 32.8. Effect of glutamate receptor activation on olivary neuron oscillation as determined by intracellular recording *in vitro*. **A:** NMDA at 100 μM reversibly depolarized olivary neurons and induced high-amplitude oscillations in membrane potential that were subthreshold for spiking. **B:** Such subthreshold oscillations at depolarized potentials entrained bursts of rhythmic action potentials at 7 Hz. **C,D:** In contrast, neither AMPA (10 μM) nor kainic acid (20 μM) induced oscillations, even though both depolarized the membrane. (Data from Placantonakis DG, Welsh JP. Two distinct oscillatory states determined by the NMPA receptor in rat inferior olive. *J Physiol* (*London*) 2001;534:123–140.)

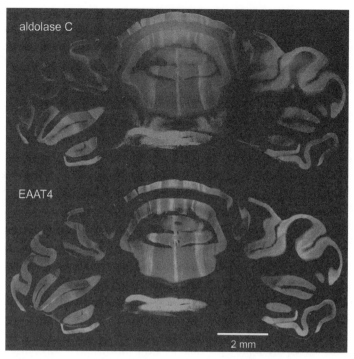

FIG. 32.9. Double-label immunofluorescence detection of aldolase C and EAAT4 in the same cerebellar section. EAAT4 is expressed in parasagittal stripes that correspond precisely to the aldolase C positive zones in the same tissue section.

with localization of EAAT4 to Purkinje cell spines and verified the differential subcellular localization of the two proteins revealed with the electron microscope (47).

Taken together, the data strongly suggest that the reason why Purkinje cells are so easily killed by global brain ischemia is due to the convergence of three factors: (a) enhanced synaptic excitation by the inferior olivary climbing fibers in the acute posthypoxic state; (b) a reduced level of aldolase, which attenuates ability for anaerobic metabolism during anoxia;

and (c) absence of EAAT4, which functions to minimize glutamate overexcitation. The entire process may be initiated by glutamatergic stimulation of the NMDA receptor of olivary neurons, leading to sustained burst activity in the acute postischemic period.

Does Patterned Death of Purkinje Cells Contribute to PostHypoxic Myoclonus? The detailed patterning of Purkinje cell death after ischemia is critically important for understanding posthypoxic myoclonus, because it has the consequence of disinhibiting discrete

FIG. 32.10. Photomicrographs of aldolase C and EAAT4 localization in Purkinje cells. **A:** Epifluorescence photomicrographs of three clusters of Purkinje cells showing that the two antigens respect the same zonal borders. In all three examples, EAAT4 distribution follows the fine details of aldolase C expression within a Purkinje cell cluster. **B:** Confocal image 0.4 µm of a single Purkinje cell showing aldolase C in the soma and thick dendrites and localization of EAAT4 to finer processes. **C:** High power confocal image showing distribution of EAAT4 puncta along the circumference of the thinnest aldolase C positive Purkinje cell dendrites (*arrows*). Thicker, secondary dendrites (*arrowheads*) show a relative paucity of EAAT4 puncta. (See Color Plate 6 following page 288.)

adolase C   EAAT4

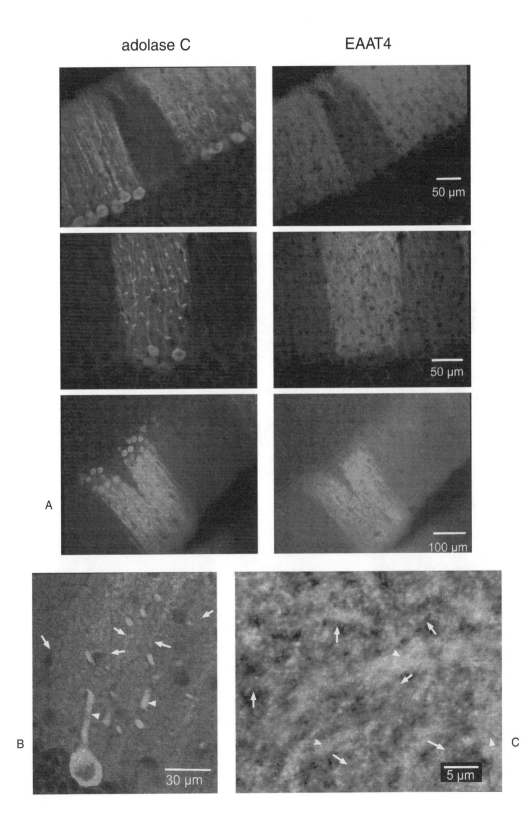

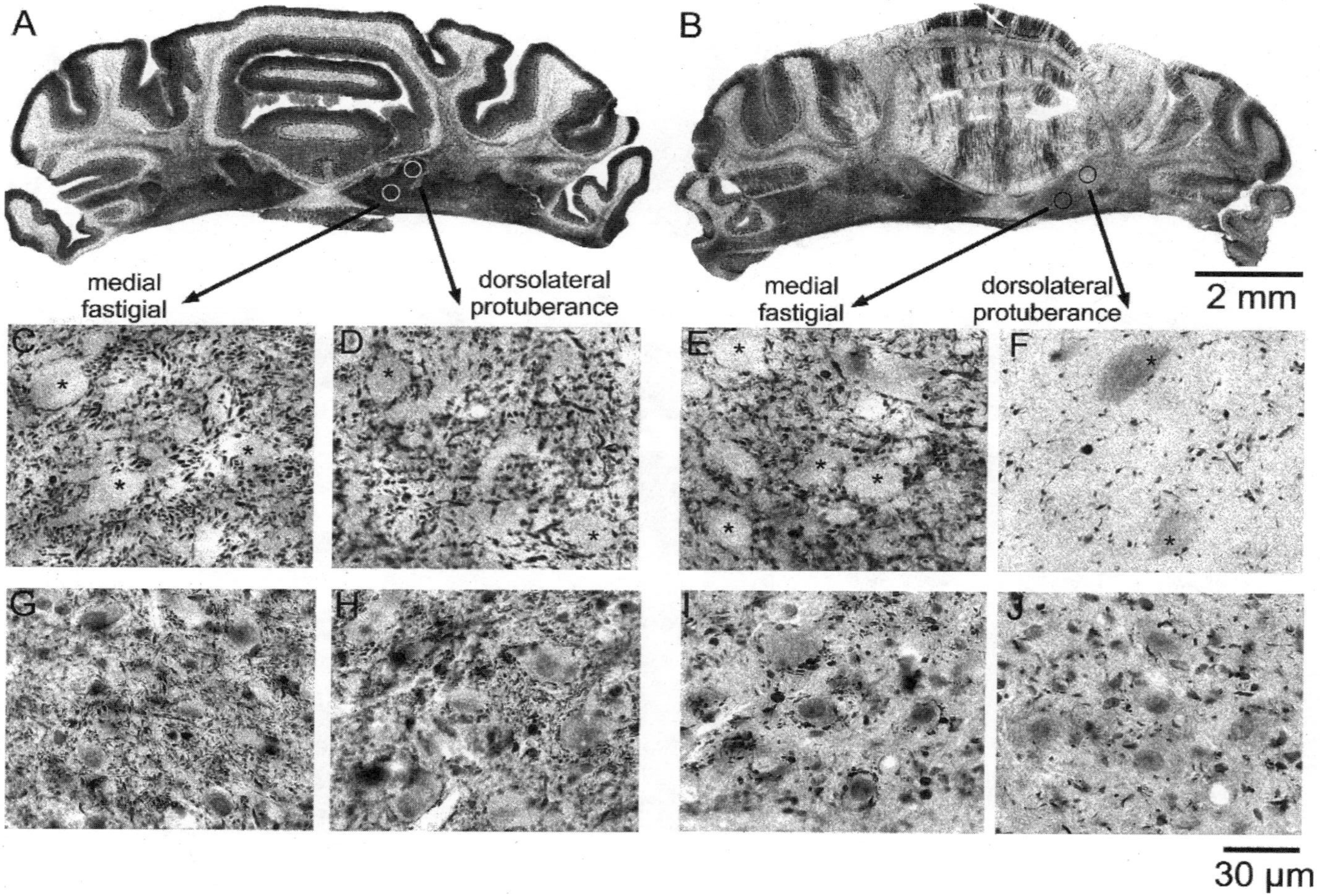

B

dorsolateral
protuberance

medial
fastigial

2 mm

A

dorsolateral
protuberance

medial
fastigial

30 μm

regions of the deep cerebellar nuclei. This is due to the fact that the compartmentation of the cortico-deep nuclear projections (48) is identical to the aldolase C compartmentation (28), and is physiologically significant because Purkinje cells are the sole output neuron of the cerebellar cortex and are GABAergic. Thus, the effect of losing an entire population of Purkinje cells within a parasagittal compartment could be predicted to enhance the excitability of discrete collections of neurons within the deep nuclei. The result would be increased excitatory drive upon regions of the brainstem and thalamus innervated by the deafferented regions of the deep nuclei.

Figure 32.11 (see Color Plate 5 following page 288) illustrates the effect of parasagittally organized Purkinje cell death on the deep cerebellar nuclei. The uniform distribution of Purkinje cells in the normal cerebellar cortex leads to a uniformly dense innervation of the deep cerebellar nuclei by Purkinje cell terminals (Fig. 32.11A). With calbindin immunostaining, the Purkinje cell terminals can be identified as stained puncta that surround the somata of deep nuclear neurons (Fig. 32.11C,D,G,H). In the ischemic cerebellum (Fig. 32.11B), Purkinje cells are lost discretely in parasagittal zones, in turn, producing a loss of Purkinje cell terminals within defined zones of the deep nuclei. To illustrate this effect, high-magnification photomicrographs are shown from the medial aspect (Fig. 32.11E,I) and the dorsolateral protuberance (Fig. 32.11F,J) of the fastigial nucleus of an ischemic rat. Here, it can be easily

seen that the neurons within dorsolateral protuberance of the fastigial nucleus are deafferented from the cerebellar cortex after ischemia (compare Fig. 32.11F,J with Fig. 32.11D,H) while the medial fastigial nucleus' innervation is undisturbed (compare Fig. 32.11C,G with Fig. 32.11E,I). This is very significant, because the deafferented regions of fastigial nucleus identified in Figure 32.11 provide excitatory innervation to the nucleus reticularis gigantocellularis (49) and ventrolateral thalamic nucleus (50–52)—regions where excitability changes occur in reticular and cortical myoclonus after anoxia (6,7).

To test whether patterned death of Purkinje cells contributes to posthypoxic myoclonus, we induced Purkinje cell death with ibogaine in normal rats. Ibogaine induces patterned Purkinje cell death that is also organized in parasagittal zones (53–56). Moreover, the neurotoxic effect of ibogaine is highly specific to Purkinje cells, and is not observed in any other region of the CNS with the exception of the posterior cingulate gyrus (O'-Hearn and Molliver, unpublished observation). The mechanism of ibogaine's destruction of Purkinje cells is well understood and is due to excitotoxicity at the climbing fiber-Purkinje cell synapse resulting from ibogaine's prolonged activation of the inferior olive for 18 hours after a single 100 mg/kg dose (55). We verified ibogaine's ability to induce burst-firing in olivary neurons and identified its mechanism of action with intracellular recording *in vitro* (Fig. 32.12). Ibogaine hyperpolarized olivary neu-

FIG. 32.11. Ischemia-induced death of parasagittal zones of Purkinje cells deafferented subregions of the fastigial nucleus from descending GABAergic input. All photomicrographs are of calbindin immunostaining, which selectively stains Purkinje cell somata, dendrites, and terminals within the cerebellum and which are known to be GABAergic. **A:** Normal cerebellum. **B:** Ischemic cerebellum. **C,D:** High-power photomicrographs showing the normal density of Purkinje cell terminals in the medial aspect (**C**) and dorsolateral protuberance (**D**) of the fastigial nucleus. **E,F:** Photomicrographs from identical regions of the ischemic fastigial nucleus. Asterisks in **C–F** indicate deep nuclear neurons which are not significantly stained with calbindin immunohistochemistry. **G–J:** Photomicrographs of the regions shown above in Nissl counterstained tissue to show the relationship between fastigial neurons and Purkinje cell terminals. After ischemia, fastigial neurons in the dorsolateral protuberance are no longer innervated by Purkinje cells (**F,J**). (See Color Plate 5 following page 288.)

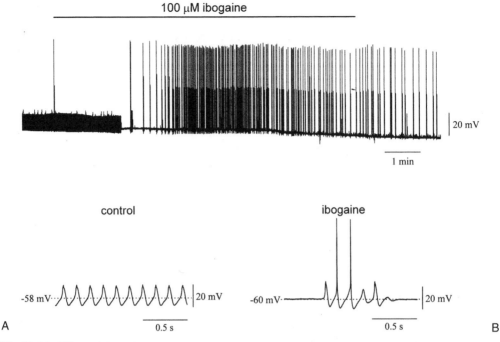

FIG. 32.12. Effect of ibogaine HCl on olivary neuron firing as determined by intracellular recording *in vitro*. **A:** Ibogaine (100 μM) hyperpolarized the membrane and increase action potential firing. **B:** High sweep speed traces from the recording shown in **A**. Before ibogaine (*left*), spontaneous oscillations failed to trigger action potentials. After ibogaine (*right*), the slope of the subthreshold oscillation increased, triggering rhythmic bursts of action potentials (*arrowheads*) at the characteristic 7 Hz intrinsic frequency of olivary neurons.

rons, thereby increasing the recruitment of the low-threshold calcium current (I_T) and triggering bursts of action potentials from a hyperpolarized potential (Fig. 32.12B). In this way, ibogaine's mechanism of action was identical to harmaline, another β-carboline, which acts on the inferior olive to accentuate burst firing and generate 10 Hz tremor (40,57–59).

The pattern of Purkinje cell degeneration produced by ibogaine is strikingly similar to that produced by global brain ischemia (Fig. 32.13), and thus provides a good model to test the contribution of patterned Purkinje cell death to myoclonus in isolation from other brain damage. Ibogaine-induced Purkinje cell death is most prominent in the vermis and posterior paravermis and is symmetrically organized about the midline. After ibogaine, two stripes of Purkinje cell death surround the midline at all levels of the cerebellum. These stripes of Purkinje cell death are identical to the ischemia death zones that neighbor the P1 aldolase C positive zone (Fig. 32.3). Purkinje cell death after ibogaine is also severe in the posterior lobe vermis lateral to the midline (Fig. 32.13B) and is similar to that produced by ischemia. In the anterior lobe (Fig. 32.13D), Purkinje cell death after ibogaine is restricted to the two midline zones and does not show the more widespread lateral damage that occurs after ischemia. Thus, ibogaine neurotoxicity reproduces many of the details of the patterned Purkinje cell death after ischemia, particularly in the posterior lobe, although the damage is not as great quantitatively.

Ibogaine-induced death of Purkinje cells induced a form of audiogenic myoclonus that mimicked that produced by global brain is-

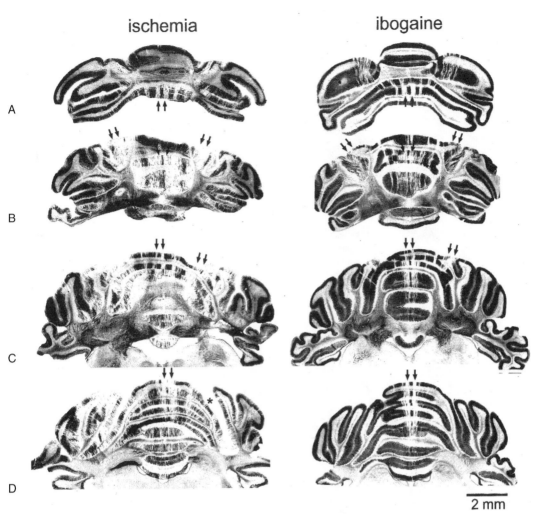

FIG. 32.13. Correspondence of ischemia- and ibogaine-induced Purkinje cell death in the cerebellum (calbindin immunohistochemistry). Ibogaine-induced degeneration, like that produced by ischemia, is concentrated in parasagittal zones in the vermis and the paravermis. Regions of precise correspondence are indicated by arrows. Although less intense than ischemia-induced degeneration, patterned Purkinje cell death produced by ibogaine demonstrates many of the spatial features of that induced by ischemia, especially in the posterior lobe.

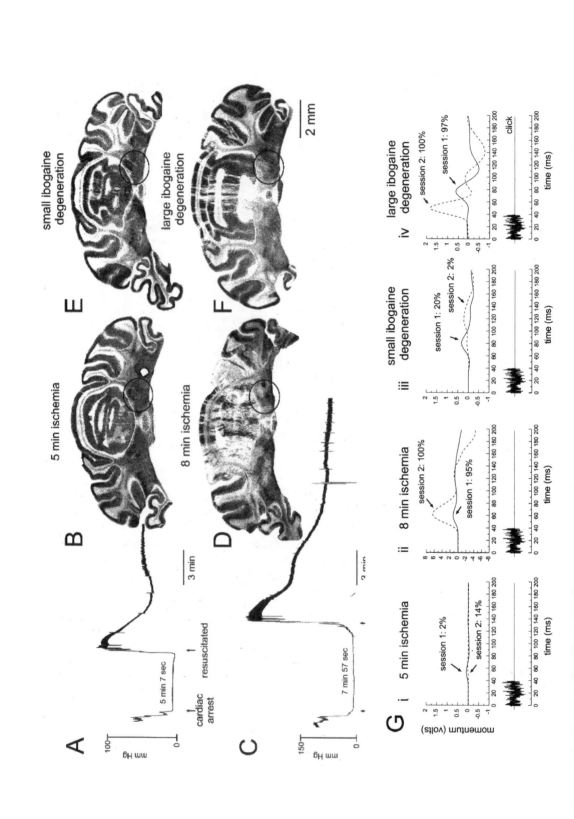

A

100 - mm Hg - 0

5 min 7 sec

cardiac arrest

resuscitated

3 min

B   5 min ischemia

C

150 - mm Hg - 0

7 min 57 sec

2 min

D   8 min ischemia

E   small ibogaine degeneration

F   large ibogaine degeneration

2 mm

G   momentum (volts)

i   5 min ischemia

session 1: 2%
session 2: 14%

20 40 60 80 100 120 140 160 180 200
time (ms)

0 20 40 60 80 100 120 140 160 180 200

ii   8 min ischemia

session 2: 100%
session 1: 95%

0 20 40 60 80 100 120 140 160 180 200
time (ms)

0 20 40 60 80 100 120 140 160 180 200

iii   small ibogaine degeneration

session 1: 20%
session 2: 2%

20 40 60 80 100 120 140 160 180 200
time (ms)

0 20 40 60 80 100 120 140 160 180 200

iv   large ibogaine degeneration

session 2: 100%
session 1: 97%

20 40 60 80 100 120 140 160 180 200
time (ms)

click

0 20 40 60 80 100 120 140 160 180 200

chemia in rats. Figure 32.14 contrasts four rats with different degrees of patterned cerebellar damage produced by ischemia or ibogaine. The first rat was subjected to 5 minutes, 7 seconds of global brain ischemia (Fig. 32.14A) and suffered no detectable loss of Purkinje cells (Fig. 32.14B). This rat showed a normal startle response to a loud click that rapidly habituated (Fig. 32.14G,i). The frequency of startle responses was 2% and 14% on the second and fourth days after the ischemia. The second rat received 7 minutes, 57 seconds of global brain ischemia (Fig. 32.14C) and exhibited profound loss of Purkinje cells within parasagittal zones (Fig. 32.14D). This rat showed an intense audiogenic myoclonic jerk on nearly 100% of the trials on the second and fourth days after ischemia (Fig. 32.14G,ii). A third rat received 100 mg/kg ibogaine that produced mild tremor and a detectable but relatively small degree of Purkinje cell death within the medial aspect of the posterior lobe vermis (Fig. 32.14E). This case showed 20% startle responses to the auditory stimulus on the day after the ibogaine; however, the rat quickly habituated such that it only showed 2% responses on the second day of testing and 7% thereafter (Fig 32.14G,iii). The fourth rat also received 100 mg/kg ibogaine, but had a sustained, severe tremor after the drug and a much larger loss of Purkinje cells in parasagittal zones (Fig. 32.14F). This rat showed nearly 100% myoclonic responses to the auditory stimulus on the first two days after ibogaine (Fig. 32.14G,iv). On the third day

of testing the percentage responses was 31%, and the response habituated by the fifth session (5%), at which time it was processed for immunohistochemistry. Close inspection of the deep cerebellar nuclei of the two ibogaine-treated rats (circled regions in Fig. 32.14) revealed that the ibogaine-induced myoclonus was underlain by a loss of Purkinje cell terminals in the dorsolateral protuberance of the fastigial nucleus—nearly identical to the denervation after ischemia. However, the Purkinje cell innervation of the posterior interpositus nucleus was less affected by ibogaine than by ischemia. Thus, at the level of the deep cerebellar nuclei, ibogaine-induced degeneration reproduced most of the midline degeneration but not the full breadth of the lateral loss seen after ischemia. The experiment demonstrated that the induction of patterned Purkinje cell death in isolation induced a myoclonic state that resembled that produced after global brain ischemia in the rat, although less severe in terms of duration and amplitude. This may be due to the larger contingent of Purkinje cells killed by ischemia and due to additional effects of ischemia on non-cerebellar systems.

SUMMARY AND CONCLUSIONS

The experiments strongly suggested that the reason why Purkinje cells die so easily after global brain ischemia relates to deficiencies in aldolase C and EAAT4 that allow them to survive pathologically intense synaptic input from the inferior olive after the restoration

---

FIG. 32.14. Comparison of audiogenic myoclonus induced by global brain ischemia and ibogaine. **A,B:** Mean arterial blood pressure during 5-minute cardiac arrest (**A**) leading to no Purkinje cell degeneration (**B**). **C,D:** Mean arterial blood pressure during 8-minute cardiac arrest (**C**) leading to substantial Purkinje cell loss (**D**). **E,F:** Purkinje cell degeneration produced by 100 mg/kg ibogaine. The case shown in **E** showed mild Purkinje cell loss in the medial vermis. The case shown in **F** showed significant Purkinje cell loss in vermal parasagittal zones. Cases **D** and **F** showed substantially less Purkinje cell terminals in the fastigial nucleus as compared to cases **B** and **E** (*circled regions*). **G:** Records of audiogenic myoclonus in the 4 cases shown in **B–F**. Responses to the auditory stimulus were larger and more frequent in cases that showed Purkinje cell loss (cases D and F) as compared to cases with little (case E) or no (case B) cerebellar damage. Patterned death of vermal Purkinje cells, on its own, induces a form of audiogenic myoclonus.

of blood flow. This conclusion is based on: (a) the remarkably tight correspondence between the regional absence of aldolase C and EAAT4 in Purkinje cells and the patterned loss of Purkinje cells after a bout of global brain ischemia; (b) the necessity of the olivo-cerebellar pathway for the ischemic death of Purkinje cells; and (c) the build-up of pathologically synchronous and high-frequency burst activity within the inferior olive during recovery from ischemia. Indeed, the correspondence between the absence of aldolase C and EAAT4 to sensitivity to ischemia could be demonstrated for zones of Purkinje cells as small as two neurons. A second finding was that Purkinje cells are not uniformly sensitive to transient ischemia, since they die most frequently in zones where aldolase C and EAAT4 are absent. One implication of the experiment is that factors beyond the unique synaptic and membrane properties of Purkinje cells play an important role in determining this neuron's high sensitivity to ischemia. The data strongly imply that two properties of Purkinje cells that make them susceptible to ischemic death are their reduced capability to sequester glutamate and reduced ability to generate energy during anoxia.

The patterned death of Purkinje cells is sufficient to induce a form of audiogenic myoclonus, as determined with a neurotoxic dose of ibogaine. Ibogaine-induced myoclonus is recognized behaviorally as a reduced ability to habituate to a startle stimulus and resembles the myoclonic jerk of rats during recovery from a prolonged bout of global brain ischemia. Commonalities of ischemia and ibogaine-induced neurodegeneration are the intricately striped Purkinje cell loss in the posterior lobe and a nearly complete deafferentation of the lateral aspect of the fastigial nucleus from the cerebellar cortex, in particular the dorsolateral protuberance. Thus, the data point strongly to a cerebellar contribution to audiogenic myoclonus.

Single-neuron electrophysiology experiments in monkeys have demonstrated that the evoked activity in the deep cerebellar nuclei occurs too late to initiate the startle response

(60) and electromyography of the postischemic myoclonus of rats corroborates this view (see Chapter 31) (20). However, the nearly complete loss of GABAergic terminals in the dorsolateral protuberance after Purkinje cell death would be expected to dramatically increase its tonic firing and the background excitation of the brain-stem structures that it innervates. The fastigial nucleus innervates a large number of autonomic and motor structures in the brain-stem and diencephalon, including the ventro-lateral nucleus of the thalamus and the gigantocellular reticular nucleus in the medulla—structures that have been implicated in human posthypoxic myoclonus (6,7).

We propose that the posthypoxic myoclonic jerk of rats is, at least in part, due to disinhibition of the fastigial nucleus produced by patterned Purkinje cell death in the vermis. The argument is as follows: the loss of GABAergic inhibition in the fastigial nucleus after ischemia leads to diaschisis of the motor thalamus and reticular formation which, in turn, is responsible for enhanced motor excitability and myoclonus. That the audiogenic myoclonus after global brain ischemia in the rat gradually resolves over a period of 2 to 3 weeks is consistent with this view, as restoration of background excitability after CNS damage in rats has been documented to occur within this time-frame (61). Our view brings together the physiologic finding that posthypoxic myoclonus appears to originate in the sensory-motor cortices and/or reticular formation with the consistent anatomical finding of Purkinje cell loss after ischemia, and explains the puzzle of Marsden's unique cases of myoclonus associated with coeliac disease (1). Moreover, our argument is consistent with findings both in rats (62,63) and humans (64) that damage to the vermis impairs the long-term habituation of the startle reflex. It remains to be determined whether the pathologically enhanced startle responses after vermal damage resemble brain-stem reticular or cortical myoclonus at the electrophysiologic level of analysis.

What is the purpose of the regional expression of aldolase C and EAAT4 in Purkinje cells? The close correspondence between the spatial distribution of aldolase C and the parasagittal anatomy of the cerebellum (48) has led to the view that aldolase C may help specify connectivity during development. While the present experiments do not address this issue, they underscore the fact that aldolase plays a fundamental role in metabolism. Because Purkinje cells have a repressed expression of aldolase A (31), whatever role the absence of aldolase C may play during development comes at the price of metabolic frailty later in adulthood.

From another point of view, aldolase C and EAAT4 appear to confer upon Purkinje cells the ability to survive their own climbing fiber. Indeed, climbing fibers form a distributed synapse that synchronously releases glutamate (or aspartate) at all levels of the dendritic tree simultaneously (65,66). Such synchronous activation triggers calcium influx throughout the Purkinje cell dendrites at a magnitude that is unparalleled in the nervous system (12), and, thus, places an extraordinarily high metabolic demand on the Purkinje cell. The apparently reduced level of aldolase in a subpopulation of Purkinje cells provides the condition for energy failure and death during anoxia so long as the climbing fibers are intact or when climbing fiber activation is pharmacologically enhanced under normoxic conditions, such as after ibogaine (53–56).

Lastly, the argument that diaschisis produced by patterned cerebellar degeneration leads to thalamo-cortical and reticular hyperexcitability agrees with C. David Marsden and his colleagues' bold demonstration of an inhibitory influence of cerebellar cortex on motor cortex in humans (67). Our anatomic data indicate that the spatially distinct zones of Purkinje cells, which are killed by global brain ischemia, may be the origin of such inhibition.

ACKNOWLEDGMENTS

Supported by grant R01 NS31224 from the National Institute for Neurological Disorders and Stroke and the Myoclonus Research Foundation. G.Y., D.P., and F.H. were supported by student research fellowships from the Myoclonus Research Foundation during their time at NYU Medical Center. We thank Dr. Dean Hillman for valuable surgical assistance and Sarita Sharma and Jennifer Mitchell for excellent technical assistance.

REFERENCES

1. Bhatia KP, Brown P, Gregory R, et al. Progressive myoclonic ataxia associated with coeliac disease. The myoclonus is of cortical origin, but the pathology is in the cerebellum. *Brain* 1995;118:1087–1093.
2. Richardson JC, Rewcastle NB, De Lean J. Hypoxic myoclonus: clinical and pathological observations. In: Rose FC, ed. *Physiological aspects of clinical neurology*. Oxford: Blackwell, 1977:231–245.
3. Hauw JJ, Escourolle R, Baulac M, et al. Postmortem studies on posthypoxic and postmethyl bromide intoxication: case reports. In: Fahn S, Marsden CD, Van Woert MH, eds. *Advances in neurology. Vol. 43.* New York: Raven, 1986:201–214,.
4. Castaigne P, Cambier J, Escourolle R, et al. Observation anatomo-clinique d'un syndrome myoclonique postanoxique. *Rev Neurol (Paris)* 1964;111:60–73.
5. Lance JW, Adams RD. The syndrome of intention or action myoclonus as a sequel to hypoxic encephalopathy. *Brain* 1963;86:111–136.
6. Hallett M, Chadwick D, Marsden CD. Cortical reflex myoclonus. *Neurology* 1979;29:1107–1125.
7. Hallett M, Chadwick D, Marsden CD, et al. Reticular reflex myoclonus: a physiological type of human posthypoxic myoclonus. *J Neurol Neurosurg Psychiatry* 1977;40:253–264.
8. Schadé, JP, McMenemey WH. *Selective vulnerability of the brain in hypoxaemia.* Philadelphia: FA Davis, 1963.
9. Cervos-Navarro J, Diemer NH. Selective vulnerability in brain hypoxia. *Crit Rev Neurobiol* 1991;6:149–182.
10. Ottersen OP, Chaudhry FA, Danbolt NC, et al. Molecular organization of cerebellar glutamate synapses. In: DeZeeuw CI, Strata P, Voogd J, eds. *Progress in brain research. Vol 114. The cerebellum: from structure to control.* Amsterdam: Elsevier, 1997:97–107.
11. Llinás R, Sugimori M. Electrophysiological properties of *in vitro* Purkinje cell dendrites in mammalian cerebellar slices. *J Physiol (London)* 1980;305:197–213.
12. Sugimori M, Llinás RR. Real-time imaging of calcium influx in mammalian cerebellar Purkinje cells in vitro. *Proc Natl Acad Sci USA* 1990;87:5084–5088.
13. Brorson JR, Manzolillo PA, Gibbons SJ, et al. AMPA receptor desensitization predicts the selective vulnerability of cerebellar Purkinje cells to excitotoxicity. *J Neurosci* 1995;15:4515–4524.
14. Tomiyama M, Palacios JM, Cortes R, et al. Flip and flop variants of AMPA receptor subunits in the human cerebellum: implication for the selective vulnerability of Purkinje cells. *Synapse* 1999;31:163–167.
15. Balchen T, Diemer NH. The AMPA antagonist, NBQX, protects against ischemia-induced loss of cerebellar Purkinje cells. *Neuroreport* 1992;3:785–788.
16. Kawai K, Nitecka L, Ruetzler CA, et al. Global cerebral

ischemia associated with cardiac arrest in the rat: I. Dynamics of early neuronal changes. *J Cerebral Blood Flow Metab* 1992;12:238–249.

17. Truong DD, Matsumoto RR, Schwartz PH, et al. Novel rat cardiac arrest model of posthypoxic myoclonus. *Mov Disord* 1994;9:201–206.

18. Hsu SM, Raine L, Fanger H. Use of avidin-biotin-peroxidase complex (ABC) in immunoperoxidase techniques: a comparison between ABC and unlabeled antibody (PAP procedures). *J Histochem Cytochem* 1981;29:557–580.

19. Ahn A, Dziennis S, Hawkes R, et al. The cloning of zebrin II reveals its identity with aldolase C. *Development* 1994;120:2081–2090.

20. Willson VJC, Thompson RJ. Human brain aldolase C_4 isozyme: purification, radioimmunoassay, and distribution in human tissues. *Ann Clin Biochem* 1980;17:114–121.

21. Welsh JP, Schwarz C. Multielectrode recording from the cerebellum. In: Nicolelis MAL, ed. *Methods for neural ensemble recordings*. Boca Raton: CRC Press, 1990;79–100.

22. Schwarz C, Welsh JP. Dynamic modulation of mossy fiber system throughput by inferior olive synchrony: a multielectrode study of cerebellar cortex activated by motor cortex. *J Neurophysiol* 2001;86(5):2489-2504.

23. Placantonakis DG, Schwarz C, Welsh JP. Serotonin suppresses subthreshold and suprathreshold oscillatory activity of rat inferior olivary neurones *in vitro*. *J Physiol (London)* 2000;524: 833–851.

24. Placantonakis DG, Welsh JP. Two distinct oscillatory states determined by the NMDA receptor in rat inferior olive. *J Physiol (London)* 2001;534:123–140.

25. Armstrong DM, Schild R. A quantitative study of the Purkinje cells in the cerebellum of the albino rat. *J Comp Neurol* 1970;139:449–456.

26. Siesjö BK. Cerebral circulation and metabolism. *J Neurosurg* 1984;60:883–908.

27. Horecker BL, Tsolas O, Lai CY. Aldolases. In: Boyer PD, ed. *The enzymes. 3rd ed, vol 7*. New York: Academic, 1980:213–258.

28. Brochu G, Maler L, Hawkes R. Zebrin II: a polypeptide antigen expressed selectively by Purkinje cells reveals compartments in rat and fish cerebellum. *J Comp Neurol* 1990;291:538–552.

29. Hawkes R, Brochu G, Doré L, et al. Zebrins: molecular markers of compartmentation in the cerebellum. In: Llinás R, Sotelo C, eds. *The cerebellum revisited*. New York: Springer-Verlag, 1992:22–55.

30. Erecinska M, Silver IA. Ions and energy in mammalian brain. *Prog Neurobiol* 1994;43:37–71.

31. Mukai T, Yatsuki H, Hasuko S, et al. The structure of the brain-specific rat aldolase C gene and its regional expression. *Biochem Biophys Res Commun* 1991;174:1035–1042.

32. Eccles J, Llinás R, Sasaki, K. The action of antidromic impulses on the cerebellar Purkinje cells. *J Physiol (London)* 1996;182:316–343.

33. Geocadin RG, Muthuswamy J, Sherman DL, et al. Early electrophysiological and histologic changes after global ischemia in rats. *Mov Disord* 2000;15(suppl 1):14–21.

34. Rossi DJ, Oshima T, Attwell D. Glutamate release in severe brain ischaemia is mainly by reversed uptake. *Nature* 2000;403:316–321.

35. Hochman S, Jordan LM, MacDonald JF. N-methyl-D-aspartate receptor mediated voltage oscillations in neurons surrounding the central canal in slices of rat spinal cord. *J Neurophysiol* 1994;72:565–577.

36. Hochman S, Jordan LM, Schmidt BJ. TTX-resistant NMDA receptor-mediated voltage oscillations in mammalian lumbar motorneurons. *J Neurophysiol* 1994;72:2559–2562.

37. Kim YI, Chandler SH. NMDA-induced burst discharge in guinea pig trigeminal motorneurons in vitro. *J Neurophysiol* 1995;74:334–346.

38. Guertin PA, Hounsgaard J. NMDA-induced intrinsic voltage oscillations depend on L-type calcium channels in spinal motorneurons of adult turtles. *J Neurophysiol* 1998;80:3380–3382.

39. Prime L, Pichon Y, Moore LE. N-methyl-D-aspartate-induced oscillations in whole cell clamped neurons from the isolated spinal cord of *Xenopus laevis* embryos. *J Neurophysiol* 1999;82:1069–1073.

40. Llinás R, Yarom Y. Oscillatory properties of guinea-pig inferior olivary neurones and their pharmacological modulation: an in vitro study. *J Physiol (London)* 1986; 376:163–182.

41. Bernardo L, Foster E. Oscillatory behavior in inferior olive neurons: mechanism, modulation, cell aggregates. *Brain Res Bull* 1986;17:773–784.

42. Nagao S, Kwak S, Kanazawa I. EAAT4, a glutamate transporter with properties of a chloride channel, is predominantly localized in Purkinje cell dendrites, and forms parasagittal compartments in rat cerebellum. *Neuroscience* 1997;78:929–933.

43. Danbolt NC. The high affinity uptake system for excitatory amino acid neurotransmitters in the brain. *Prog Neurobiol* 1994;44:377–396.

44. Fairman WA, Vandenberg RJ, Arriza JL, et al. An excitatory amino-acid transporter with properties of a ligand-gated chloride channel. *Nature* 1995;375:599–603.

45. Tanaka J, Ichikawa R, Watanabe M, et al. Extra-junctional localization of glutamate transporter EAAT4 at excitatory Purkinje cell synapses. *Neuroreport* 1997;8:2461–2464.

46. Otis TS, Kavanaugh MP, Jahr CE. Postsynaptic glutamate transport at the climbing fiber-Purkinje cell synapse. *Science* 1997;277:1515–1518.

47. Dehnes Y, Chaudhry FA, Ullensvang K, et al. The glutamate transporter EAAT4 in rat cerebellar Purkinje cells: a glutamate-gated chloride channel concentrated near the synapse in parts of the dendritic membrane facing astroglia. *J Neurosci* 1998;18:3606–3619.

48. Voogd J, Ruigrok TJ. Transverse and longitudinal patterns in the mammalian cerebellum. In: DeZeeuw CI, Strata P, Voogd J, eds.*Progress in brain research, vol 114.The cerebellum: from structure to control*. Amsterdam: Elsevier, 1997:21–37.

49. Homma Y, Nonaka S, Matsuyama K, et al. Fastigiofugal projection to the brainstem nuclei in the cat: an anterograde PHA-L tracing study. *Neurosci Res* 1995;23:89–102.

50. Angaut P, Bowsher D. Ascending projections of the medial cerebellar (fastigial) nucleus: an experimental study in the cat. *Brain Res* 1970;24:49–68.

51. Batton RR, Jayaraman A, Ruggiero D, Carpenter MB. Fastigial efferent projections in the monkey: an autoradiographic study. *J Comp Neurol* 1977;174:281–306.

52. Bava A, Cicirata F, Licciardello S, et al. Fastigial nuclei projections on the ventralis lateralis (VL) thalamic nucleus neurons. *Brain Res* 1979;168:169–175.

53. O'Hearn E, Molliver ME. Degeneration of Purkinje cells in parasagittal zones of the cerebellar vermis after treatment with ibogaine or harmaline. *Neuroscience* 1993;55:303–310.

54. O'Hearn E, Long DB, Molliver ME. Ibogaine induces glial activation in parasagittal zones of the cerebellum. *Neuroreport* 1993;4:299–302.

55. O'Hearn E, Molliver ME. The olivocerebellar projection mediates ibogaine-induced degeneration of Purkinje cells: a model of indirect, trans-synaptic excitotoxicity. *J Neurosci* 1997;7:8828–8841.

56. Xu Z, Chang LW, Slikker W, et al. A dose-response study of ibogaine-induced neuropathology in the rat cerebellum. *Toxicol Sci* 2000;57:95–101.

57. Lamarre Y, deMontigny C, Dumont M, et al. Harmaline-induced rhythmic activity of cerebellar and lower brainstem neurons. *Brain Res* 1971;32:246–250.

58. Llinás R, Volkind RA. The olivocerebellar system: functional properties as revealed by harmaline-induced tremor. *Exp Brain Res* 1973;18:69–87.

59. DeMontigny C, Lamarre Y. Effects produced by local applications of harmaline in the inferior olive. *Can J Physiol Pharmacol* 1975;53:845–849.

60. Mortimer JA. Temporal sequence of cerebellar Purkinje and nuclear activity in relation to the acoustic startle response. *Brain Res* 1973;50:457–462.

61. Benedetti F, Montarolo PG, Rabacchi S. Inferior olive lesion induces long-lasting functional modification in the Purkinje cells. *Exp Brain Res* 1984;55:368–371.

62. Leaton RN, Supple WF. Cerebellar vermis: essential for long-term habituation of the acoustic startle response. *Science* 1986;232:513–515.

63. Lopiano L, De'Sperati C, Montarolo PG. Long-term habituation of the acoustic startle response: Role of the cerebellar vermis. *Neuroscience* 1990;35:79–84.

64. Maschke M, Drepper J, Kindsvater K, et al. Involvement of the human medial cerebellum in long-term habituation of the acoustic startle response. *Exp Brain Res* 2000;133:359–367.

65. Llinás R, Nicholson C. Reversal properties of climbing fiber potential in cat Purkinje cells: an example of a dis.

66. Kreitzer AC, Gee KR, Archer EA, et al. Monitoring presynaptic calcium dynamics in projection fibers by in vivo loading of a novel calcium indicator. *Neuron* 2000; 27:25–32.

67. Ugawa Y, Day BL, Rothwell JC, et al. Modulation of motor cortical excitability by electrical stimulation over the cerebellum in man. *J Physiol (London)* 1991;441:57–72.

Myoclonus and Paroxysmal Dyskinesias,
Advances in Neurology, Vol. 89,
edited by S. Fahn, et al.
Published by Lippincott Williams & Wilkins, Philadelphia, 2002.

33

The Unified Myoclonus Rating Scale

*Steven J. Frucht, †Sue E. Leurgans, ‡Mark Hallett, and *Stanley Fahn

*Department of Neurology, Columbia University, Columbia-Presbyterian Medical Center, The
Neurological Institute, New York, New York; †Departments of Neurological Sciences and Preventive
Medicine, Rush University Medical College, Chicago, Illinois; ‡National Institute of Neurological
Disorders And Stroke, National Institutes of Health, Bethesda, Maryland

In 1988, Truong and Fahn developed a clinical rating scale to evaluate patients with myoclonus. The Truong-Fahn scale was used in several clinical trials of anti-myoclonic agents and is currently the most comprehensive tool for rating patients with myoclonus. However it became clear over time that some elements of the scale needed to be revised, and new sections added to better reflect patients' functional performance. In response to these needs, members of the Myoclonus Study Group met in April of 1998 to revise and approve a final version of the scale. The result was the Unified Myoclonus Rating Scale (UMRS), a quantitative 73-item clinical rating instrument designed to evaluate the response of patients with myoclonus to anti-myoclonic therapies. This chapter will summarize the planning and execution of a collaborative effort to statistically validate the scale, and discuss how the scale may best be used in future trials of myoclonus therapies.

BACKGROUND: RATING SCALE DEVELOPMENT

Contrary to popular belief, myoclonus is not a rare movement disorder. It is four times as common as Huntington's disease and nearly half as common as dystonia (1). Unfortunately the application of experimental therapeutics to myoclonus has significantly lagged behind other movement disorders. A literature search of Medline performed in October 2000 revealed 134 double-blind placebo-controlled clinical trials in patients with Parkinson's disease, 24 trials in patients with dystonia, 23 trials in patients with tics, 22 trials for essential tremor, and 17 trials for Huntington's disease, but only one double-blind placebo-controlled trial for patients with myoclonus (2). There are only three other placebo-controlled clinical trials of anti-myoclonic agents even published (3–5), and clonazepam and valproic acid, the two most commonly used drugs to treat myoclonus, have never been systematically studied. Statistically validated clinical rating scales are currently available to evaluate treatments for Parkinson's disease (6), dystonia (7), tremor (8), tics (9), and Huntington's disease (10), but not myoclonus. A reliable rating scale would encourage the development and testing of new anti-myoclonic therapies.

What are the features of an ideal clinical rating instrument for myoclonus? It should be simple to use, with detailed instructions for performing the examination and scoring the patient. It should include a videotape protocol, allowing patient examinations to be filmed and rated in blinded fashion at a later date. It should measure both patient's and physician's assessment of disability. It should be comprehensive enough to capture all elements of the myoclonus examination, including myoclonus at rest, stimulus-sensitivity, myoclonus with action, and negative myoclonus. It should also include simple tests of functional performance that reflect the patient's ability to live independently. Finally the scale should not be too cumbersome, or researchers and patients will simply not use it. Most neurologists in clinical practice do not have time to use movement disorder ratings scales, and with the exception of the Unified Parkinson's Disease Rating Scale, even academic movement disorder neurologists may only use rating scales if they are conducting clinical trials.

COMPONENTS OF UNIFIED MYOCLONUS RATING SCALE

The UMRS appears in the Appendix to this chapter. The scale contains a patient questionnaire, a handwriting and spiral sheet, rating instructions, a score sheet and a videotape protocol. A videotape of the entire scale can be included on 13 minutes of Hi-8 videotape.

The scale consists of eight sections: section 1, patient questionnaire (11 items); section 2, myoclonus at rest (frequency and amplitude, 16 items); section 3, stimulus sensitivity of myoclonus (17 items); section 4, severity of myoclonus with action (frequency and amplitude, 20 items); section 5, performance on functional tests (five items); section 6, physician rating of patient's global disability (one item); section 7, presence of negative myoclonus (one item); section 8, severity of negative myoclonus (one item). Each item is rated on a scale of 0 to 4, with the exception of section 3 (where stimulus sensitivity is either present [score: 1] or absent [score: 0]), section 7 (negative myoclonus present [score: 1] or absent [score: 0]) and section 8 (scores: 0–3).

VALIDATION OF THE UNIFIED MYOCLONUS RATING SCALE

Statistical validation of the UMRS was performed in a collaborative effort by members of the Myoclonus Study Group. Twenty patients with chronic myoclonus (i.e., present for more than 1 year) were identified and videotaped while the UMRS was performed. We recruited patients with various intensities and etiologies of myoclonus (posthypoxic, Ramsey-Hunt, myoclonus-dystonia, cortical and spinal segmental myoclonus). Videotapes were returned to the first author (SJF), and using a pseudo-random number generator, the second author (SL) randomized the videotapes to create four master tapes, each with five patients. An attempt was made to balance the tapes, so that each contained one patient with focal myoclonus and each included patients with myoclonus of varying severity. Eighteen neurologists with movement disorder expertise were asked to review and score two tapes (ten patients per neurologist). The completed rating sheets were returned and the data were entered into a standardized database.

A Cronbach's α-score was calculated for each section of the UMRS. Cronbach's α-score is a measure of reliability, in this setting measuring the interrater reliability of the scale. Cronbach's α values for sections 1 to 5 of the UMRS were: section 1, 0.92; section 2, frequency 0.80, amplitude 0.74; section 3, 0.90; section 4, frequency 0.85, amplitude 0.86; section 5, 0.89. This confirmed that the UMRS possesses excellent interrater reliability.

USING THE UNIFIED MYOCLONUS RATING SCALE

Two projects that involved use of the UMRS have been completed. The first, described previously, involved videotaping 20 patients with various etiologies and severities of myoclonus for the purpose of validation of the scale. Frucht has also used the UMRS in a pilot tolerability and efficacy study of levetiracetam in eight patients with chronic myoclonus. The comments that follow are based on his experience using the scale.

The UMRS is indeed easy to use and can be completed in less than 15 minutes. One can eliminate bias by videotaping patients and having a blinded observer score videotapes at a later date. The UMRS appears to be sensitive to changes in myoclonus of all severities.

For the purpose of clinical trials, the most useful primary endpoints are the change in scores of action myoclonus (section 4) and functional performance (section 5). Although some treatments may also improve myoclonus at rest (section 2) and stimulus sensitivity (section 3), these parameters may be less important contributors to global disability. The UMRS also provides an indirect measure of the placebo effect. Two patients enrolled in the pilot trial of levetiracetam claimed to be better as measured by section 1 (patient self-assessment), but blinded videotape review of action myoclonus and functional performance scores demonstrated no appreciable change.

Total scores for sections 1, 3, 5, 6, 7, and 8 of the UMRS can be calculated by simple addition. The maximum scores for these sections are 40, 17, 20, 4, 1, and 3 respectively. Sections 2 and 4 include ratings of frequency and amplitude of myoclonic jerks affecting each body region. We recommend calculating myoclonus subscores by multiplying frequency by amplitude for each body region. In this way, the rated disability of a small amplitude jerk (rating 1) of high frequency (rating 4) would be equivalent to that of a moderate amplitude jerk (rating 2) of moderate frequency (rating 2). The maximum score for sections 2 and 4 are 128 and 160 when calculated in this manner.

How should improvements in myoclonus be quantified? Patients with severe, generalized myoclonus typically have scores between 90 and 120 on section 4, and 15 to 18 on section 5. A treatment that might reduce the score on section 4 from 100 to 60, for example, would represent a significant improvement. We recommend measuring the effect of anti-myoclonic therapies as a percentage change relative to the patient's original score. In this manner, a change of identical amplitude (from 50 to 10) would represent the same raw change in section 4 score, but a greater improvement in functional disability.

It is our hope that the availability of this simple, user-friendly, reliable clinical rating instrument will encourage investigators to explore new treatments for patients with myoclonus.

ACKNOWLEDGMENTS

We thank members of the Myoclonus Study Group, including Drs. Arnold Gold, Daniel Truong, Christopher Goetz, Hiroshi Shibasaki, and Joseph Jankovic for their help in revising the UMRS and videotaping patients. We also thank UCB Pharma for allowing us to publish their computer template of the scale. Dr. Frucht was supported by generous grants from the Myoclonus Research Foundation as a postdoctoral fellow and young investigator. We also thank Norman Seiden and Theodora Mason of the Myoclonus Research Foundation for their guidance and support.

APPENDIX 33.1

The Unified Myoclonus Rating Scale

Videotape Instructions for the Unified Myoclonus Rating Scale

The following comments serve as general guidelines for obtaining videotapes of the performance of the UMRS.

Space and Equipment

Use a high-8 camcorder mounted on a tripod for recording. Avoid taping in front of a window or in poor lighting. It is recommended to play back a sample tape in a high-8 tape deck, as the quality of the image in the viewfinder of the camera is sometimes better than the recorded image. Use a room large enough to record the patient walking 15 feet. Alternatively, the tripod can be moved into a hallway for taping the patient's gait. Avoid including any identifying information in the tape which would reveal the patient's identity, date or location. Always tape patients in the same room on each visit.

Procedures

Ask the patient to sign a standard consent form at taping, giving permission to use the tape and the information contained in it for research, including publication in scientific journals. Patients will not be identified by name. The patient's name, diagnosis, medications and date of taping can be filmed for several seconds to permanently record the information on the tape (this will later be edited out).

All recordings should have the whole body in the picture unless otherwise specified. Position the tripod approximately 10 feet from the patient.

Patients should be videotaped wearing a standard hospital gown, which allows visualization of their arms and legs. Patients will sit in a hard-backed chair, lacking arm supports if possible. For performance of the functional tests, a portable table of comfortable height should be used. Plastic, clear glasses with an easily visible 8-ounce mark, and a soupspoon should be used.

TABLE 33.1. *Videotape Protocol*

Section 2: Myoclonus at rest		
	Focus on face	30 seconds
	Full front	30 seconds
	Focus on hands	30 seconds
Section 3: Stimulus sensitivity		
Threat	Full front	15 seconds
Clap hands	Full front	15 seconds
Tap nose	Upper body	15 seconds
Jaw jerk	Upper body	15 seconds
Pin prick: Cheek	Face	15 seconds
Pin prick: Right forearm	Upper body	15 seconds
Pin prick: Left forearm	Upper body	15 seconds
Pin prick: Right foot	Lower body	15 seconds
Pin prick: Left foot	Lower body	15 seconds
Finger flick: right index	Focus on right arm	15 seconds
Finger flick: left index	Focus on left arm	15 seconds
Toe flick: right great toe	Focus on right foot	15 seconds
Toe flick: left great toe	Focus on left foot	15 seconds
Reflexes: right bicep	Upper body	15 seconds
Reflexes: left bicep	Upper body	15 seconds
Reflexes: right knee	Lower body	15 seconds
Reflexes: left knee	Lower body	15 seconds
Section 4: Myoclonus with action		
Close eyelids	Focus on face	15 seconds
Neck movements	Upper body	15 seconds
Trunk	Full front	15 seconds
Arms extended, palms down	Upper body	30 seconds
Arms extended, palms down, wrists extended	Focus on hands	30 seconds
Right finger-to-nose	Upper body	30 seconds
Left finger-to-nose	Upper body	30 seconds
Right leg heel-to-shin	Lower body	30 seconds
Left leg heel-to-shin	Lower body	30 seconds
Arising	Full front	15 seconds
Standing	Full front	30 seconds
Walking	Full front	30 seconds
Section 5: Functional performance		
Handwriting	Focus on hand and table	30 seconds
Right spiral	As above	30 seconds
Left spiral	As above	30 seconds
Pouring water	Upper body	30 seconds
Soup spoon	Upper body	30 seconds

Total Time: **13:15**

SECTION 1: MYOCLONUS PATIENT QUESTIONAIRE

A. Speech

- ☐ 0 My speech is normal.
- ☐ 1 My speech is slightly affected, but I am easily understood.
- ☐ 2 People have moderate difficulty understanding me.
- ☐ 3 I can communicate but only with great difficulty.
- ☐ 4 I cannot communicate verbally.

B. Reading (silently)

- ☐ 0 My ability to read is normal
- ☐ 1 I have slight difficulty reading.
- ☐ 2 I have moderate difficulty reading.
- ☐ 3 I have great difficulty reading.
- ☐ 4 I cannot read.

C. Handwriting

- ☐ 0 My handwriting is normal.
- ☐ 1 Writing is more difficult but I can write legibly.
- ☐ 2 It is difficult to read my writing.
- ☐ 3 My writing is illegible.
- ☐ 4 I cannot hold or control the pen to write.

D. Eating

- ☐ 0 I eat normally.
- ☐ 1 I can eat by myself, but with effort.
- ☐ 2 I can feed myself but others must cut my food.
- ☐ 3 I can only feed myself finger food.
- ☐ 4 I am dependent on others to feed me.

E. Drinking

- ☐ 0 I drink normally.
- ☐ 1 I can drink from a cup but I need to be careful.
- ☐ 2 I need a special cup to drink, or I use two hands.
- ☐ 3 I must use a straw to drink.
- ☐ 4 I cannot drink by myself.

F. Swallowing

- ☐ 0 I swallow without difficulty.
- ☐ 1 I choke occasionally.
- ☐ 2 I choke frequently and have difficulty swallowing.
- ☐ 3 I am unable to swallow firm foods.
- ☐ 4 I cannot swallow soft food or liquids.

MYOCLONUS PATIENT QUESTIONAIRE (continued)

G. Hygiene

- ☐ 0   I bathe (or shower), brush my teeth and comb my hair normally.
- ☐ 1   I can perform all of these activities but I am clumsy.
- ☐ 2   I need help with some activities but can do most on my own.
- ☐ 3   I need help with most activities.
- ☐ 4   I am dependent on others to perform these activities.

H. Dressing

- ☐ 0   I can get dressed without a problem.
- ☐ 1   I can dress myself but I am clumsy.
- ☐ 2   I can dress myself but I need help with certain activities, for example buttons.
- ☐ 3   I need significant assistance in order to get dressed.
- ☐ 4   I am dependent on others to dress me.

I. Arising

- ☐ 0   I arise from a chair without difficulty.
- ☐ 1   I arise from a chair with slight difficulty.
- ☐ 2   I arise from a chair with significant difficulty, but I do not require assistance.
- ☐ 3   I need help to arise from a chair.
- ☐ 4   I cannot arise from a chair unless I am pulled up.

J. Standing

- ☐ 0   I can stand by myself without difficulty.
- ☐ 1   I can stand by myself but I am a little unsteady.
- ☐ 2   I can stand by myself but I am quite unsteady.
- ☐ 3   I can stand only if someone holds on to me.
- ☐ 4   I cannot stand even if I am assisted.

K. Walking

- ☐ 0   I walk normally.
- ☐ 1   I can walk without difficulty but I am a little unsteady.
- ☐ 2   I can walk with difficulty but I don't need help.
- ☐ 3   I can walk if someone holds on to me.
- ☐ 4   I cannot walk

PATIENT GLOBAL ASSESSMENT

- ☐ 0   I have no disability.
- ☐ 1   I have mild disability but I function independently.
- ☐ 2   I have moderate disability. I depend on others to help me.
- ☐ 3   I have marked disability. There are many things I cannot do even with help.
- ☐ 4   I am completely disabled. I am totally dependent on others.

SECTION 2: MYOCLONUS AT REST

A. Upper face

FREQUENCY AT REST	AMPLITUDE AT REST
☐ 0 No jerks.	☐ 0 Zero.
☐ 1 ≤jerk per 10 seconds.	☐ 1 Trace movement only.
☐ 2 2 or 3 jerks per 10 seconds.	☐ 2 Small amplitude jerks, easily visible (<25% of possible maximum movement).
☐ 3 4 to 9 jerks per 10 seconds.	☐ 3 Moderate amplitude jerks (25%-75% of possible maximum movement).
☐ 4 ≥10 jerks per 10 seconds.	☐ 4 Large amplitude jerks (near maximum movement).

B. Lower face

FREQUENCY AT REST	AMPLITUDE AT REST
☐ 0 No jerks.	☐ 0 Zero.
☐ 1 ≤jerk per 10 seconds.	☐ 1 Trace movement only.
☐ 2 2 or 3 jerks per 10 seconds.	☐ 2 Small amplitude jerks, easily visible (<25% of possible maximum movement).
☐ 3 4 to 9 jerks per 10 seconds.	☐ 3 Moderate amplitude jerks (25%-75% of possible maximum movement).
☐ 4 ≥10 jerks per 10 seconds.	☐ 4 Large amplitude jerks (near maximum movement).

C. Neck

FREQUENCY AT REST	AMPLITUDE AT REST
☐ 0 No jerks.	☐ 0 Zero.
☐ 1 ≤jerk per 10 seconds.	☐ 1 Trace movement only.
☐ 2 2 or 3 jerks per 10 seconds.	☐ 2 Small amplitude jerks, easily visible (<25% of possible maximum movement).
☐ 3 4 to 9 jerks per 10 seconds.	☐ 3 Moderate amplitude jerks (25%-75% of possible maximum movement).
☐ 4 ≥10 jerks per 10 seconds.	☐ 4 Large amplitude jerks (near maximum movement).

D. Trunk

FREQUENCY AT REST	AMPLITUDE AT REST
☐ 0 No jerks.	☐ 0 Zero.
☐ 1 ≤jerk per 10 seconds.	☐ 1 Trace movement only.
☐ 2 2 or 3 jerks per 10 seconds.	☐ 2 Small amplitude jerks, easily visible (<25% of possible maximum movement).
☐ 3 4 to 9 jerks per 10 seconds.	☐ 3 Moderate amplitude jerks (25%-75% of possible maximum movement).
☐ 4 ≥10 jerks per 10 seconds.	☐ 4 Large amplitude jerks (near maximum movement).

MYOCLONUS AT REST (continued)

E. R arm

FREQUENCY AT REST		AMPLITUDE AT REST	
☐ 0	No jerks.	☐ 0	Zero.
☐ 1	≤jerk per 10 seconds.	☐ 1	Trace movement only.
☐ 2	2 or 3 jerks per 10 seconds.	☐ 2	Small amplitude jerks, easily visible (<25% of possible maximum movement).
☐ 3	4 to 9 jerks per 10 seconds.	☐ 3	Moderate amplitude jerks (25%-75% of possible maximum movement).
☐ 4	≥10 jerks per 10 seconds.	☐ 4	Large amplitude jerks (near maximum movement).

F. L arm

FREQUENCY AT REST		AMPLITUDE AT REST	
☐ 0	No jerks.	☐ 0	Zero.
☐ 1	≤jerk per 10 seconds.	☐ 1	Trace movement only.
☐ 2	2 or 3 jerks per 10 seconds.	☐ 2	Small amplitude jerks, easily visible (<25% of possible maximum movement).
☐ 3	4 to 9 jerks per 10 seconds.	☐ 3	Moderate amplitude jerks (25%-75% of possible maximum movement).
☐ 4	≥10 jerks per 10 seconds.	☐ 4	Large amplitude jerks (near maximum movement).

G. R leg

FREQUENCY AT REST		AMPLITUDE AT REST	
☐ 0	No jerks.	☐ 0	Zero.
☐ 1	≤jerk per 10 seconds.	☐ 1	Trace movement only.
☐ 2	2 or 3 jerks per 10 seconds.	☐ 2	Small amplitude jerks, easily visible (<25% of possible maximum movement).
☐ 3	4 to 9 jerks per 10 seconds.	☐ 3	Moderate amplitude jerks (25%-75% of possible maximum movement).
☐ 4	≥10 jerks per 10 seconds.	☐ 4	Large amplitude jerks (near maximum movement).

H. L leg

FREQUENCY AT REST		AMPLITUDE AT REST	
☐ 0	No jerks.	☐ 0	Zero.
☐ 1	≤jerk per 10 seconds.	☐ 1	Trace movement only.
☐ 2	2 or 3 jerks per 10 seconds.	☐ 2	Small amplitude jerks, easily visible (<25% of possible maximum movement).
☐ 3	4 to 9 jerks per 10 seconds.	☐ 3	Moderate amplitude jerks (25%-75% of possible maximum movement).
☐ 4	≥10 jerks per 10 seconds.	☐ 4	Large amplitude jerks (near maximum movement).

SECTION 3: STIMULUS SENSITIVITY

Instructions on performing this section are included in the score sheet. Each stimulus is performed only once.

SECTION 4: MYOCLONUS WITH ACTION

A. Close Eyelids

FREQUENCY WITH ACTION		AMPLITUDE WITH ACTION: Ask the patient to close his eyes:	
☐	0 No jerks.	☐	0 No jerks
☐	1 ≤jerk per 10 seconds.	☐	1. Trace blinking.
☐	2 2 or 3 jerks per 10 seconds.	☐	2. Blinks are easily visible; eyelid closure only.
☐	3 4 to 9 jerks per 10 seconds.	☐	3. Moderate orbicularis closure.
☐	4 ≥10 jerks per 10 seconds.	☐	4. Severe orbicularis closure.

B. Neck

FREQUENCY WITH ACTION		AMPLITUDE WITH ACTION: Ask the patient to move his head in flexion-extension and side to side rotation:	
☐	0 No jerks.	☐	0 No jerks.
☐	1 ≤jerk per 10 seconds.	☐	1. Trace movement only.
☐	2 2 or 3 jerks per 10 seconds.	☐	2. Small amplitude jerks, easily visible (<25% of possible maximum movement).
☐	3 4 to 9 jerks per 10 seconds.	☐	3. Moderate amplitude jerks (25-75% of possible maximum movement).
☐	4 ≥10 jerks per 10 seconds.	☐	4. Large amplitude jerks (near maximum movement).

C. Trunk

FREQUENCY WITH ACTION		AMPLITUDE WITH ACTION: Ask the patient to flex his trunk when sitting or lying down:	
☐	0 No jerks.	☐	0 No jerks.
☐	1 ≤jerk per 10 seconds.	☐	1. Trace movement only.
☐	2 2 or 3 jerks per 10 seconds.	☐	2. Small amplitude jerks, easily visible (<25% of possible maximum movement).
☐	3 4 to 9 jerks per 10 seconds.	☐	3. Moderate amplitude jerks (25-75% of possible maximum movement).
☐	4 ≥10 jerks per 10 seconds.	☐	4. Large amplitude jerks (near maximum movement).

MYOCLONUS WITH ACTION (continued)

D. R arm

FREQUENCY WITH ACTION		AMPLITUDE WITH ACTION: Ask the patient to hold both arms forward with palms down for 10 seconds. Then ask the patient to extend both wrists for 10 seconds. Then perform the finger to nose test four times. Ask the patient to finish by leaving his finger on his nose for 10 seconds. Score the worst myoclonus seen on finger to nose testing.	
☐ 0	No jerks.	☐ 0	Zero.
☐ 1	≤jerk per 10 seconds.	☐ 1	Trace movement only.
☐ 2	2 or 3 jerks per 10 seconds.	☐ 2	Small amplitude jerks, easily visible (<25% of possible maximum movement).
☐ 3	4 to 9 jerks per 10 seconds.	☐ 3	Moderate amplitude jerks (25%-75% of possible maximum movement).
☐ 4	≥10 jerks per 10 seconds.	☐ 4	Large amplitude jerks (near maximum movement).

E. L arm

FREQUENCY WITH ACTION		AMPLITUDE WITH ACTION: Ask the patient to hold both arms forward with palms down for 10 seconds. Then ask the patient to extend both wrists for 10 seconds. Then perform the finger to nose test four times. Ask the patient to finish by leaving his finger on his nose for 10 seconds. Score the worst myoclonus seen on finger to nose testing.	
☐ 0	No jerks.	☐ 0	Zero.
☐ 1	≤jerk per 10 seconds.	☐ 1	Trace movement only.
☐ 2	2 or 3 jerks per 10 seconds.	☐ 2	Small amplitude jerks, easily visible (<25% of possible maximum movement).
☐ 3	4 to 9 jerks per 10 seconds.	☐ 3	Moderate amplitude jerks (25%-75% of possible maximum movement).
☐ 4	≥10 jerks per 10 seconds.	☐ 4	Large amplitude jerks (near maximum movement).

F. R leg

FREQUENCY WITH ACTION		AMPLITUDE WITH ACTION: Ask the patient to perform the heel to toe shin 4 times. Score the worst myoclonus seen.	
☐ 0	No jerks.	☐ 0.	No jerks.
☐ 1	≤jerk per 10 seconds.	☐ 1.	Trace movement only (heel always remains on knee and shin).
☐ 2	2 or 3 jerks per 10 seconds.	☐ 2.	Small amplitude jerks, easily visible (heel leaves the shin at times but can complete the slide).
☐ 3	4 to 9 jerks per 10 seconds.	☐ 3.	Moderate amplitude jerks (heel is unable to complete the slide).
☐ 4	≥10 jerks per 10 seconds.	☐ 4.	Cannot even initiate the task (cannot place the heel on the knee).

G. L leg

FREQUENCY WITH ACTION	AMPLITUDE WITH ACTION: Ask the patient to perform the heel to toe shin 4 times. Score the worst myoclonus seen.
☐ 0 No jerks.	☐ 0. No jerks.
☐ 1 ≤jerk per 10 seconds.	☐ 1. Trace movement only (heel always remains on knee and shin).
☐ 2 2 or 3 jerks per 10 seconds.	☐ 2. Small amplitude jerks, easily visible (heel leaves the shin at times but can complete the slide).
☐ 3 4 to 9 jerks per 10 seconds.	☐ 3. Moderate amplitude jerks (heel is unable to complete the slide).
☐ 4 ≥10 jerks per 10 seconds.	☐ 4. Cannot even initiate the task (cannot place the heel on the knee).

H. Arising

FREQUENCY WITH ACTION	AMPLITUDE WITH ACTION: Ask the patient to arise from the chair without the use of his arms. If the patient cannot, ask them to arise using arm assist. If still unable, the examiner attempts to help the patient arise.
☐ 0 No jerks.	☐ 0 Patient arises without difficulty.
☐ 1 ≤jerk per 10 seconds.	☐ 1. Patient arises with slight difficulty but does not need arm assist.
☐ 2 2 or 3 jerks per 10 seconds.	☐ 2. Patient arises only by pushing off with his arms, or requires several trials to arise.
☐ 3 4 to 9 jerks per 10 seconds.	☐ 3. Patient cannot arise without the help of the examiner.
☐ 4 ≥10 jerks per 10 seconds.	☐ 4. Patient cannot arise unless pulled to their feet by the examiner.

I. Standing

FREQUENCY WITH ACTION	AMPLITUDE WITH ACTION: Ask the patient to stand with his feet one foot apart. If necessary, the examiner helps the patient into a standing document. If the patient cannot stand unassisted, the examiner stands by the patient or supports the patient.
☐ 0 No jerks.	☐ 0. No jerks.
☐ 1 ≤jerk per 10 seconds.	☐ 1. Trace movement, does not interfere with standing.
☐ 2 2 or 3 jerks per 10 seconds.	☐ 2. Small amplitude jerks, mildly interferes with standing.
☐ 3 4 to 9 jerks per 10 seconds.	☐ 3. Moderate amplitude jerks, definitely interferes with ability to stand without assistance.
☐ 4 ≥10 jerks per 10 seconds.	☐ 4. Large amplitude jerks prevent standing.

MYOCLONUS WITH ACTION (continued)	
J. Walking	

FREQUENCY WITH ACTION	AMPLITUDE WITH ACTION: Ask the patient to walk down the a corridor for 15 seconds, turn, then walk back and sit down. Patients who are unsteady or at risk for falling will walk with the examiner at their side, holding one arm if necessary.
☐ 0 No jerks.	☐ 0 Zero.
☐ 1 ≤jerk per 10 seconds.	☐ 1 Trace movement only.
☐ 2 2 or 3 jerks per 10 seconds.	☐ 2 Small amplitude jerks, easily visible (<25% of possible maximum movement).
☐ 3 4 to 9 jerks per 10 seconds.	☐ 3 Moderate amplitude jerks (25%-75% of possible maximum movement).
☐ 4 ≥10 jerks per 10 seconds.	☐ 4 Large amplitude jerks (near maximum movement).

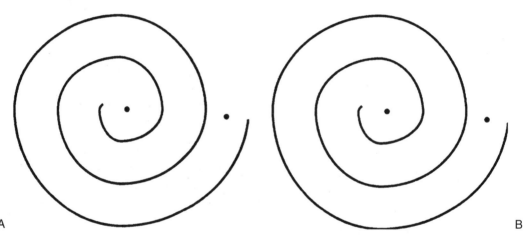

A   B

FIG. 33.1. Myoclonus Rating Scale: Handwriting/Drawing Sample. Step 1: Write "London, England." Dominant hand (right/left) rests on desk. Step 2: Complete the spiral by connecting the dots with your right hand. Keep your arm off of the desk (**A**). Step 3: Complete the spiral by connecting the dots with your left hand. Keep your arm off of the desk (**B**)

SECTION 5: FUNCTIONAL TESTS

A. Writing

Ask the patient to write "London, England", in script with their hand resting on the desk. Patients who do not write in script may print. Circle the hand used to write.

☐ 0. Normal.

☐ 1. Mild sloppiness but easily legible.

☐ 2. Illegible.

☐ 3. Cannot complete the words.

☐ 4. Cannot hold the pen or keep the pen on the paper.

B. R hand spiral

Ask the patient to complete the spiral connecting the dots with the right hand in one continuous motion. The hand remains off the desk during the task.

☐ 0. Normal.

☐ 1. Completes the spiral but crosses lines ≤ 2 times.

☐ 2. Completes the spiral but crosses lines 3-10 times.

☐ 3. Completes the spiral but crosses lines> 10 times.

☐ 4. Cannot complete the spiral, or cannot hold the pen or keep it on the paper.

C. L hand spiral

Ask the patient to complete the spiral connecting the dots with the left hand in one continuous motion. The hand remains off the desk during the task.

☐ 0. Normal.

☐ 1. Completes the spiral but crosses lines ≤ 2 times.

☐ 2. Completes the spiral but crosses lines 3-10 times.

☐ 3. Completes the spiral but crosses lines > 10 times.

☐ 4. Cannot complete the spiral, or cannot hold the pen or keep it on the paper.

D. Pouring water

Ask the patient to pour an eight-ounce glass of water into an empty eight-ounce glass with his dominant hand, without touching the two glasses. Use clear plastic glasses.

☐ 0. Normal, no spill.

☐ 1. Clumsy but does not spill.

☐ 2. Spills < half of the water.

☐ 3. Spills ≥ half the water.

☐ 4. Cannot hold the glass or refuses to try secondary to fear of spilling water.

FUNCTIONAL TESTS (continued)

E. Soup spoon

Ask the patient to use a soupspoon to bring water from a cup to his mouth with his dominant hand.

- ☐ 0. Normal, no spill.
- ☐ 1. Clumsy but does not spill.
- ☐ 2. Spoon reaches the mouth but spills at least some water.
- ☐ 3. Cannot reach his mouth with the spoon.
- ☐ 4. Cannot hold the spoon or refuses to try secondary to inability to hold the spoon.

SECTION 6: SCORE GLOBAL DISABILITY

- ☐ 0. Normal.
- ☐ 1. Mild disability. Completely independent.
- ☐ 2. Moderate disability. Depends on others for moderate assistance.
- ☐ 3. Marked disability; many tasks impossible even with assistance.
- ☐ 4. Severe disability. Invalid.

SECTION 7: IS NEGATIVE MYOCLONUS PRESENT?

- ☐ 0. No (less than 50% likely).
- ☐ 1. Yes (more than 50% likely).

SECTION 8: IF NEGATIVE MYOCLONUS IS PRESENT, HOW SEVERE IS IT?

- ☐ 0. Not present.
- ☐ 1. Mild.
- ☐ 2. Moderate.
- ☐ 3. Severe.

UMRS SCORE SHEET

1. PATIENT QUESTIONNAIRE	2. MYOCLONUS AT REST		
A. (Speech) _____	**Body Part**	**Frequency**	**Amplitude**
B. (Reading) _____	Upper Face	_____ X	_____
C. (Handwriting) _____	Lower Face	_____ X	_____
D. (Eating) _____	Neck	_____ X	_____
E. (Drinking) _____	Trunk	_____ X	_____
F. (Swallowing) _____	R Arm	_____ X	_____
G. (Hygiene) _____	L Arm	_____ X	_____
H. (Dressing) _____	R Leg	_____ X	_____
I. (Arising) _____	L Leg	_____ X	_____
J. (Standing) _____		**TOTAL**	
K. (Walking) _____			
TOTAL ____			
PT. GLOBAL ASSESSMENT ____			

3. STIMULUS SENSTIVITY. Score 1 if a stimulus produces a jerk in any body part; score 0 if no jerk is elicited. Each stimulus is performed only once.

Threat: thrust hands towards patient's face unexpectedly:		_____
Claps hands unexpectedly:		_____
Tap patient's nose with patient's eyes closed:		_____
Elicit jaw jerk:		_____
Pin prick:	On cheek	_____
	R arm (flexor surface of wrist)	_____
	L arm (flexor surface of wrist)	_____
	R leg (bottom of foot)	_____
	L leg (bottom of foot)	_____
Finger flick:	R index finger	_____
	L index finger	_____
Toe flick:	R great toe	_____
	L great toe	_____
Reflexes:	R bicep	_____
	L bicep	_____
	R knee jerk	_____
	L knee jerk	_____
Stimulus Sensitivity Total:		_____

4. MYOCLONUS WITH ACTION				5. FUNCTIONAL TESTS	
Action	**Frequency**		**Amplitude**		
A. Close Eyelids		X		A. Writing	
B. Neck		X		B. R hand spiral	
C. Trunk		X		C. L hand spiral	
D. R arm		X		D. Pouring water	
E. L arm		X		E. Soup spoon	
F. R leg		X		**TOTAL**	
G. L leg		X			
H. Arising		X			
I. Standing		X			
J. Walking		X			
			TOTAL		

6. GLOBAL DISABILITY SCORE	
7. NEGATIVE MYOCLONUS SCORE	
8. NEGATIVE MYOCLONUS SEVERITY SCORE	

REFERENCES

1. Caviness JN, Alving LI, Maraganore DM, et al. The incidence and prevalence of myoclonus in Olmstead County, Minnesota. *Mayo Clin Proc* 1999;74:565–569.
2. Koskiniemi M, Van Vleymen B, Hakamies L, et al. Piracetam relieves symptoms in progressive myoclonus epilepsy: a multicentre, randomized, double blind, crossover study comparing the efficacy and safety of three dosages of oral piracetam with placebo. *J Neurol Neurosurg Psychiatry* 1998;64:344–388.
3. Pranzatelli MR, Tate E, Galvan I, et al. A controlled trial of 5-hydroxy-L-tryptophan for ataxia in progressive myoclonus epilepsy. *Clin Neurol Neurosurg* 1996;98: 161–164.
4. Brown P, Steiger MJ, Thompson PD, et al. Effectiveness of piracetam in cortical myoclonus. *Mov Disord* 1993;8: 63–68.
5. Truong DD, Fahn S. Therapeutic trial with glycine in myoclonus. *Mov Disord* 1998;3:222–232.
6. Martinez-Martin P, Gil-Nagel A, Gracia LM, et al. Unified Parkinson's Disease Rating Scale characteristics and structure. The cooperative multicentric group. *Mov Disord* 1994;9:76–83.
7. Burke RE, Fahn S, Marsden CD, et al. Validity and reliability of a rating scale for the primary torsion dystonias. *Neurology* 1985;35:73–77.
8. Bain PG, Findley LJ, Atchison P, et al. Assessing tremor severity. *J Neurol Neurosurg Psychiatry* 1993;56: 868–873.
9. Goetz CG, Tanner CM, Wilson RS, et al. A rating scale for Gilles de la Tourette's syndrome: description, reliability and validity data. *Neurology* 1987;37:1542–1544.
10. Huntington Study Group. Unified Huntington's Disease Rating Scale: reliability and consistency. *Mov Disord* 1996;11:136–142.

Myoclonus and Paroxysmal Dyskinesias,
Advances in Neurology, Vol. 89,
edited by S. Fahn, et al.
Published by Lippincott Williams & Wilkins, Philadelphia, 2002.

34

The Early History of Paroxysmal Dyskinesias

Stanley Fahn

Department of Neurology, Columbia University, Columbia-Presbyterian Medical Center,
The Neurological Institute, New York, New York

Although there are many paroxysmal disorders in neurology, the most common being migraine and epilepsy, paroxysmal movement disorders are relatively uncommon. Some movement disorders, particularly tics that occur in bursts, are not even considered in the category of paroxysmal disorders. Placed in this specific category are those conditions designated as paroxysmal dyskinesias (chorea, dystonia, athetosis, ballism), hypnogenic dyskinesias, episodic ataxias, and transient dyskinesias of infancy. The paroxysmal dyskinesias were the first reported and have an interesting evolution.

EARLIEST DESCRIPTIONS: RELATIONSHIP TO EPILEPSY

The earliest descriptions of the paroxysmal dyskinesias were reported as epilepsy. It is likely that some of the cases in the first report of movement-induced seizures by Gowers (1) were actually what today we would call paroxysmal dyskinesias. One was a girl whose attacks started at the age of 11 and whose attacks occurred on suddenly arising after prolonged sitting. Subsequently many reports by other authors published under the designation of reflex epilepsy and tonic seizures induced by movement were possibly paroxysmal dyskinesias. Such cases had no loss of consciousness, and the movements were described as tonic contraction, namely sustained twisting, or athetosis and chorea. Sometimes the cerebral site of these "seizures" was suspected as originating in the basal ganglia. Spiller (2) called two of his patients with brief tonic spasms brought on by voluntary movement of the involved limbs as subcortical epilepsy.

Sterling (3) used the term "extrapyramidal epilepsy" to describe a series of patients with encephalitis lethargica who had brief or prolonged (up to 6 hours) painful sustained spasms that occurred intermittently. Consciousness was unimpaired. He used the term tetanoid to depict the postures of the hands and feet. Years later, Lance (4) questioned the use of the term extrapyramidal epilepsy because of the long duration of some of the attacks, as well as the origin of the attacks.

Wimmer (5) used the term "striatal epilepsy" to describe a boy who had attacks of torticollis and unilateral tonic limb spasms, lasting a few seconds without loss of consciousness. Because these attacks subsequently became one of athetoid or torsion spasms, Wimmer labeled them as striatal epilepsy, based on a previous report by Stertz (6). According to Wilson (7), Stertz had reported a patient who developed seizures and then dystonia, with postmortem evidence of postencephalitic lesions in the striatum.

The first report of movement-induced paroxysmal movements appears to be in 1927 in a report by Spiller (2), who described two patients with brief tonic spasms brought on by voluntary movement of the involved limbs. In one of them, the attacks were also induced by passive manipulation of the limbs. The contractions were painful and accompanied by sensations of heat or burning. No autopsy was performed. Spiller preferred the term "subcortical epilepsy" rather than striatal epilepsy because of the pain associated with the attacks. Wilson (7) subsequently considered subcortical epilepsy in his description of a 5-year-old boy who had brief attacks of unilateral torsion and tonic spasms that lasted up to 3 minutes and were precipitated by fright or excitement. There was no loss of consciousness. The attacks could be preceded by pain. Wilson considered this to be a subcortical origin of reflex tonic epilepsy.

The concept that attacks of tonic, often twisting, contractions without loss of consciousness are seizure disorders has persisted in more modern times. For example, Lishman and associates (8) described seven patients with tonic and athetoid spasms induced by movement while remaining conscious. Abnormal sensations of numbness, vibration and tightness, but not pain, were noted in the affected limbs before the attacks. These authors considered that the movement-induced attacks were a form of reflex epilepsy and discussed other idiopathic cases in the literature, such as one case each by Pitha, (9) and Michaux and Granier (10). Two years later, in 1964, Whitty and associates (11) and Burger and associates (12) described two patients with movement-induced "seizures". Japanese neurologists (13) and others (14) have also referred to these "seizures" as some form of epilepsy. Today, these movement-induced involuntary movements would be considered paroxysmal choreoathetosis/dystonia rather than convulsive movements of the reflex epilepsy type.

The best evidence that at least some paroxysmal dystonias are cortical epilepsies has come from studies on hypnogenic paroxysmal dystonias. Many of these derive from the frontal lobe, especially the supplementary sensorimotor area (15).

REPORTED AS A PAROXYSMAL DISORDER OF INVOLUNTARY MOVEMENTS

In 1940, a new concept was introduced by Mount and Reback (16). They called attacks of tonic spasms plus choreic and athetotic movements as a paroxysmal type of movement disorder, rather than reflex epilepsy. They described a 23-year-old man who had such "spells" since infancy, preceded by a sensory aura of tightness in parts of the body or by a feeling of tiredness. Sometimes the attacks lasted for as long as 2 hours. There was never a loss of consciousness or clonic convulsive movements, biting of the tongue, or loss of sphincter control. Drinking alcohol, coffee, tea, or cola would usually precipitate an attack. Fatigue, smoking, and concentrating were other precipitating factors. The attacks would clear more rapidly if the patient lay down and would be aborted by asleep. Between attacks, the neurologic examination was normal. Phenytoin and phenobarbital were without effect, and scopolamine was the only drug found to reduce the frequency, severity, and duration of the attacks. The family history revealed 27 other members who had similar attacks, with the pedigree showing autosomal dominant inheritance with what appears to be complete penetrance. Mount and Reback called this disorder "familial paroxysmal choreoathetosis." Today, the paper by Mount and Reback is recognized as the seminal paper in the field of paroxysmal dyskinesias. The Mount-Reback syndrome has undergone different name changes, first paroxysmal dystonic choreoathetosis (17) and most recently paroxysmal nonkinesigenic dyskinesias.

The next two reports of this syndrome were also reports of large families with similar attacks of muscle spasms (4,18). However, neither referred to Mount and Reback's paper. Later, Lance (17) was to write one of the definitive papers in this field, containing a useful classification scheme, in which he related his family to those of Mount and Reback (16), Forssman (18), and Richards and Barnett (19).

REPORTING KINESIGENIC FORMS OF PAROXYSMAL DYSKINESIAS

In 1941, the year following Mount and Reback's paper, Smith and Heersema (20) reported three similar cases (two of them familial) seen at the Mayo Clinic that they labeled as "periodic dystonia." The ages at onset were 7, 8, and 14. These authors thought that their cases were similar to the family of Mount and Reback. Their first patient was described as being able to induce the involuntary movements by shaking a leg. In reporting a family with three members affected by brief attacks of torsion movements of the torso and choreoathetosis of the limbs precipitated by initiation of sudden movement seen at the Mayo Clinic, Hudgins and Corbin (21) also provided a follow-up report of the three individuals reported by Smith and Heersema (20). From a review of the Mayo Clinic records, Hudgins and Corbin recognized that the initiation of movement was the principal factor in the provocation of the daily dystonic attacks in the three cases reported by Smith and Heersema. Thus, it appears that the first report of paroxysmal kinesigenic choreoathetosis/dystonia was that of Smith and Heersema, although these authors did not particularly recognize this phenomenon as a critical factor.

Kertesz (22) introduced the term *paroxysmal kinesigenic choreoathetosis*. The kinesigenic labeling has been used in subsequent classification schemes. Kertesz reported ten new cases of paroxysmal dyskinesia and reviewed the literature. Among the important features of his paper, Kertesz differentiated the kinesigenic variety (induced by sudden movement) from that described by Mount and Reback and by Lance, which were not aggravated by movement but by alcohol, caffeine, and fatigue. Kertesz failed to mention the paper by Forssman. Prior to the introduction of the new terminology, papers simply used paroxysmal choreoathetosis (23–25), the same as used by Mount and Reback. There were a large number of kinesigenic cases reported after the introduction of the kinesigenic terminology by Kertesz (22).

NOMENCLATURE FOR THE NON-KINESIGENIC FORM

After the 1963 paper by Lance (4), Weber (26) reported a family with four affected members with non-kinesigenic paroxysmal dystonia and used the term *familial paroxysmal dystonia*. Richards and Barnett (19) reported the next big family with the same type of paroxysmal dyskinesia as Mount and Reback's case, and thought that Lance's family (4) represented a variant because there were only tonic spasms and no movements in that family. The family of Richards and Barnett consisted of nine affected members with the trait inherited in an autosomal dominant pattern. They emphasized the non-kinesigenic nature of the attacks and thought that a wide array of terms could describe the attacks, depending on severity of each one. They considered that the terms rigidity, tremor, dystonia, torsions, spasm, athetosis, chorea, and hemiballism could all be used for such movements, often blending into each other. To emphasize the postural and increased tone, they added dystonic to the label. They recommended avoiding the term epilepsy until pathophysiology is better known. Richards and Barnett coined the term *paroxysmal dystonic choreoathetosis* (PDC), which was later adopted by Lance (17), and was then widely adopted for those paroxysmal dyskinesias not induced by sudden movement. The terms paroxysmal non-kinesigenic choreoathetosis and paroxysmal dystonia were then proposed instead of PDC (27,28). The most recent suggestion by Demirkiran and Jankovic (29) was to substitute the word dyskinesia for choreoathetosis because it is more broadly appropriate. Thus, the term *paroxysmal nonkinesigenic dyskinesia* (PNKD) is the one being adopted.

SECONDARY CAUSES OF THE PAROXYSMAL DYSKINESIAS

The original reports of paroxysmal non-kinesigenic dyskinesias were of unknown etiology and usually familial. Symptomatic cases began to appear in the 1960s, but earlier similar attacks occurring in patients with multiple sclerosis had been described and considered as a form of epilepsy. A listing of the secondary causes was provided in the review of the paroxysmal dyskinesias by Fahn (28). Psychogenicity as a cause of many sporadic non-kinesigenic cases was described and may be more common than appreciated (27,30).

GENETICS OF PAROXYSMAL DYSKINESIAS

Today, many genes have been mapped for the various paroxysmal dyskinesias. The first descriptions were for the episodic ataxias (31–40). Recognizing that the episodic ataxias are due to mutations of ion channel genes has led to the realization that probably most, if not all, of the primary paroxysmal dyskinesias are also channelopathies. The genes for the paroxysmal dyskinesias are now being unraveled (41–49).

TREATMENT OF PAROXYSMAL DYSKINESIAS

Although phenytoin was recognized earlier as a very useful agent for paroxysmal kinesigenic choreoathetosis/dystonia, carbamazepine was later found to be as useful and was introduced as a treatment by Kato and Araki (50). This drug currently appears to be the one most commonly used for this disorder. Although PNKD is not usually successfully treated, clonazepam was introduced for this disorder by Lance (17).

PAROXYSMAL EXERTION DYSKINESIA

Lance (17) was the first to describe what he called an intermediate form of PDC (this term is now called PNKD). Today, this family would appear to have PED. The family had attacks that were briefer than classical PNKD, lasting from 5 to 30 minutes, and in which the attacks are precipitated by prolonged exercise and not by cold, heat, stress, ethanol, excitement, or anxiety. The spasms affected mainly the legs. A second family was reported by Plant and associates (51). In both families, the inheritance pattern was autosomal dominant transmission. In neither family did anyone derive any benefit from barbiturate, levodopa, or clonazepam. A sporadic case was reported by Nardocci and colleagues (52) (case 3). This patient also had interictal chorea without any family history of a similar condition. This patient was helped by clonazepam. Another sporadic case was reported by Wali (53); this was an 18-year-old man in whom attacks of right hemidystonia lasting about 10 minutes were precipitated by prolonged running (about 10 minutes) or by cold. The electroencephalogram (EEG) and computed tomography (CT) results were normal; anticonvulsants were not helpful. Demirkiran and Jankovic (29) mentioned seeing five patients, three being females. The largest series of sporadic cases is that by Bhatia and asscoiates (54). Familial cases appear to be autosomal dominant (55). A large family with PED with four affected members had onset of 9 to 15 years and a male: female ratio of 3:1 (56).

PAROXYSMAL HYPNOGENIC DYSKINESIA

In an odd reverse of history, many of the hypnogenic variety of paroxysmal dyskinesias are today being recognized as epileptic in origin. The initial report of hypnogenic paroxysmal dyskinesias was by Horner and Jackson (57). Lugaresi and his colleagues (58,59) independently rediscovered and eventually popularized the syndrome of hypnogenic paroxysmal dyskinesias.

There has long been considerable speculation as to whether the short-duration hypnogenic attacks could be a manifestation of epilepsy because they respond so well to anticonvulsants. The lack of abnormal EEG findings during the attack has been used to argue against this concept. However, there is accumulating evidence that many hypnogenic paroxysmal dyskinesias are, indeed, due to seizures. Tinuper and associates (60) described three patients with this disorder who had EEG evidence for frontal lobe seizures as a cause of these attacks. Sellal and colleagues (61) and Meierkord and associates (62) studied a series of patients with hypnogenic dystonia and have concluded that these represent seizure disorders, particularly of frontal lobe epilepsy because repeated nocturnal EEG recordings often reveal epileptic patterns of abnormalities. Seizures arising near the mesial posterior frontal supplementary sensorimotor area (SSMA) may be a particular culprit in inducing paroxysmal hypnogenic dyskinesias in children (63). These types of seizures tend to be brief, frequent, and with bilateral tonic posturing, gross proximal limb movements, and preserved consciousness. Dystonic and other dyskinetic features may result from spread of epileptic activity from the mesial frontal region to the basal ganglia because there are close anatomic connections between them. It appears that the short-lasting attacks of paroxysmal hypnogenic dyskinesias are most likely due to seizures, but the question remains whether those patients without abnormal EEGs and more prolonged hypnogenic attacks could be more akin to the paroxysmal dyskinesias.

The genetics of hypnogenic dyskinesias/seizures is being explored. A large autosomal dominant Australian family (64) and Norwegian family (65) have been described with mutations in the nicotinic acetylcholine receptor alpha 4 subunit (CHRNA4) gene, located on chromosome 20q13.2-q13.3.

TRANSIENT PAROXYSMAL DYSKINESIA IN INFANCY

Snyder (66) introduced a new type of paroxysmal dyskinesia that he called "paroxysmal torticollis in infancy." He described 12 cases of intermittent head tilting in young infants. The age at onset was between 2 and 8 months of age, except for three cases whose first attacks occurred at 14, 17, and 30 months. The attacks would occur about two to three times a month and last from 10 minutes to 14 days, usually 2 to 3 days. The head would tilt to either side and often rotate slightly to the opposite side. There is no distress unless a parent attempts to straighten the head, upon which the baby cries. In some cases the head tilting is associated with vomiting, pallor, and agitation for a short period. The infant is normal between attacks, and they disappear after months or years, usually around age 2 or 3 years. Subsequently, a number of similar cases have been described (67–69), including familial cases (70). Sanner and Bergstrom (68) reported a patient whose father had a similar condition in early infancy, suggesting that this disorder is hereditary.

In 1988, the clinical spectrum expanded with the report by Angelini and associates (71) under the title of "transient paroxysmal dystonia in infancy." They described nine patients; eight who had onset of the paroxysmal dyskinesias between 3 and 5 months of age, and one patient with an onset at 1 month. Three of the patients had a history of perinatal brain damage. The attacks consisted of opisthotonus, increased muscle tone with twisting of the limbs; and in three, with neck and trunk twisting, thereby linking this with "paroxysmal torticollis in infancy." The attacks last several minutes, with a maximum of 2 hours in one patient. They would occur from several attacks per day to once a month. Remission occurred between the ages of 8 to 22 months, with two not yet having reached a remission.

EPISODIC ATAXIAS

In 1946, Parker (72) described six patients in four families with idiopathic familial paroxysmal ataxia, which he labeled as periodic ataxia. The age at onset ranged from 21 to 32 years. The attacks affected gait and speech and lasted from 30 seconds to 30 minutes. There could be several attacks per day, or there could be interval-free periods of several weeks. Vestibular symptoms occurred in some of the patients. Progressive cerebellar ataxia developed in some members.

In 1963, Farmer and Mustian (73) reported a family from rural North Carolina with idiopathic paroxysmal ataxia. The major clinical difference from Parker's cases were the high frequency of accompanying vestibular symptoms of vertigo, diplopia, and oscillopsia, and the lack of speech involvement. They labeled their family as vestibulo-cerebellar ataxia. The age at onset ranged from 23 to 42 years. The attacks ranged from a few minutes to 2 months. The brief episodes may occur daily, but free intervals could last a year or more. Progressive ataxia also developed in some affected family members.

A second family from the same region in North Carolina also had ocular motility problems. These were abnormal smooth pursuit with normal saccades, dampened opticokinetic nystagmus, inability to suppress the vestibulo-ocular reflex, gaze-evoked nystagmus, with episodic attacks of horizontal diplopia, oscillopsia, ataxia, nausea, vertigo, and tinnitus (74). This family was considered part of the same neurologic disorder referred to as periodic vestibulo-cerebellar ataxia, just as in Farmer and Mustian's family. Of special clinical significance is the lack of dysarthria. Genetic studies showed that this family is distinct from the two types of episodic ataxias already characterized genetically (see below).

Hill and Sherman (75) described another family, but with onset in childhood in many of the affected patients and no development of progressive ataxia. Another family of childhood onset and benign course was described by White (76). All the families showed inheritance as autosomal dominant.

An important advance was the discovery by Griggs and associates (77) that acetazolamide can effectively prevent attacks. These authors showed this benefit in one kindred with familial paroxysmal ataxia. Donat and Auger (78) the following year had similar results in another kindred. Fahn (79,80) reported a woman who had paroxysmal tremor, both intention and resting, associated with ataxia and postural instability during the attack; acetazolamide eliminated the attacks.

Mayeux and Fahn (81) reported a patient with PNKD in a background of hereditary ataxia. Onset of PNKD was at age 10; onset of ataxia was age 19. During an attack, which could last 10 minutes to 4 hours, there was also an accompanying increase of ataxia. Initially there was an 8-month response to acetazolamide. After the drug was no longer effective, the patient's PNKD responded to clonazepam. It is possible that this patient might be a link between familial PNKD and paroxysmal ataxia.

Families with a combination of periodic ataxia and persistent, continuous electrical activity in several muscles, reported as either myokymia (82–85) or as neuromyotonia (86), have been described. Description of the attacks, which are of brief duration and are sometimes preceded by sudden movement, include dyskinetic movements and sustained posturing, as well as ataxia, dysarthria, and vertigo. This type of paroxysmal ataxia is now called episodic ataxia 1 (EA-1).

In 1986, Gancher and Nutt (84) classified the hereditary episodic ataxias into three syndromes. In one group are those cases associated with persistent myokymia or neuromyotonia (now called EA-1). They described the attacks being precipitated by fatigue, excitement, stress, and physical trauma, but the family reported by Vaamonde and associates (86) had attacks triggered by sudden movement, and kinesigenicity is now recognized as a feature. There is neither dizziness nor vertigo. The attacks last 2 minutes or less. Acetazolamide and anticonvulsants are usually ineffective. The gene for this type of paroxysmal ataxia has been located at chromosome 12p13 (33).

The second group (now known as EA-2) is featured by attacks of ataxia (with or without interictal nystagmus, and with or without persistent ataxia), responding to acetazolamide or amphetamines. The attacks are precipitated by exercise, fatigue, and stress and occasionally by carbohydrate or alcohol ingestion. In addition to ataxia, the attacks are accompanied by vertigo, headache, nausea, and malaise. The attacks last for several hours or until the patient falls asleep. In recent years additional families have been reported with these features (87–89). The siblings reported by Bain and associates (88) had persistent diplopia due to superior oblique paresis as part of the syndrome. Using ^{31}P nuclear magnetic resonance spectroscopy, Bain and his colleagues (90) found the pH levels in the cerebellum to be increased in untreated subjects with acetazolamide-responsive paroxysmal ataxia; the pH dropped to normal with treatment. The gene for this type of paroxysmal ataxia has been mapped to chromosome 19p13 (37,38).

Gancher and Nutt (84) listed a third group, which is kinesigenic. Typical PKD can occur in some members of the family. The attacks of ataxia last minutes to hours, while the PKD lasts seconds. The disorder can resolve with time. Acetazolamide appears to be ineffective, but phenytoin is effective for both the kinesigenic ataxia and the PKD. In their review, Griggs and Nutt (91) place this third type with associated PKD in the first group of paroxysmal ataxias. Genotyping has now definitively placed this as EA-1.

A case was reported in which a young girl had attacks of ataxia associated with fevers and accompanied by vertical supranuclear ophthalmoplegia (92). The ataxia and eye findings can last days.

Secondary cases of intermittent ataxia have also been reported, such as those due to metabolic defects such as Hartnup disease (93), pyruvate decarboxylase deficiency (94–96), and maple syrup urine disease (97). Paroxysmal ataxia and dysarthria has also been reported to occur in multiple sclerosis (98–102), which is a disorder that also can cause paroxysmal choreoathetosis/dystonia.

REFERENCES

1. Gowers WR. *Epilepsy and other chronic convulsive diseases. Their causes, symptoms and treatment.* New York: Dover (Reprint of 1885 edition); 1964:75–76.
2. Spiller WG. Subcortical epilepsy. *Brain* 1927;50:171–187.
3. Sterling W. Le type spasmodique tetanoide et tetaniforme de l'encephalite epidemique remarques sur l'epilepsie "extra-pyramidale." *Rev Neurol (Paris)* 1924;2:484–492.
4. Lance JW. Sporadic and familial varieties of tonic seizures. *J Neurol Neurosurg Psychiatry* 1963;26:51–59.
5. Wimmer A. Efudes sur les syndromes extra-pyramidaux spasm detorsion infantile debutant par crises d'hemi-

6. spasms tonique (epilepsie strice). *Rev Neurol (Paris)* 1925;32:281–295.
6. Stertz. Der Extrapyramidale Symptomenkomplex. 1924; as reported by Wilson.
7. Wilson SAK. The Morrison Lectures on nervous semeiology, with special reference to epilepsy. Lecture III. Symptoms indicating increase of neural function. *BMJ* 1930;2:90–94.
8. Lishman WA, Symonds CD, Whitty CW, et al. Seizures induced by movement. *Brain* 1962;85:93–108.
9. Pitha V. Epilepsie reflexe. *Rev Neurol (Paris)* 1938;70:178–181.
10. Michaux M, Granier M. Epilepsie bravais-jacksonienne reflexe: debut crural des crises: intervention constante dans leur declanchement de contractions musculaires du membre inferieur du meme cote. *Ann Medicopsychol (Paris)*1945;103:172–177.
11. Whitty CWM, Lishman WA, FitzGibbon JP. Seizures induced by movement: a form of reflex epilepsy. *Lancet* 1964;1:1403–1406.
12. Burger LJ, Lopez RI, Elliott FA. Tonic seizures induced by movement. *Neurology* 1972;22:656–659.
13. Fukuyama S, Okada R. Hereditary kinesthetic reflex epilepsy. Report of five families of peculiar seizures induced by sudden movements. *Adv Neurol Sci (Tokyo)* 1967;11:168–197.
14. Hishikawa Y, Furuya E, Yamamoto J, et al. Dystonic seizures induced by movement. *Arch Psychiatry Nervenkr* 1973;217:113–138.
15. Lüders HO. Paroxysmal choreoathetosis. *Eur Neurol* 1996;36:20–23.
16. Mount LA, Reback S. Familial paroxysmal choreoathetosis. *Arch Neurol Psychiatry* 1940;44:841–847.
17. Lance JW. Familial paroxysmal dystonic choreoathetosis and its differentiation from related syndromes. *Ann Neurol* 1977;2:285–293.
18. Forssman H. Hereditary disorder characterized by attacks of muscular contractions, induced by alcohol amongst other factors. *Acta Med Scand* 1961;170:517–533.
19. Richards RN, Barnett HJ. Paroxysmal dystonic choreoathetosis. A family study and review of the literature. *Neurology* 1968;18:461–469.
20. Smith LA, Heersema PH. Periodic dystonia. *Staff Meet Mayo Clin* 1941;16:842–846.
21. Hudgins RL, Corbin KB. An uncommon seizure disorder: familial paroxysmal choreoathetosis. *Brain* 1966;89:199–204.
22. Kertesz A. Paroxysmal kinesigenic choreoathetosis. An entity within the paroxysmal choreoathetosis syndrome. Description of 10 cases, including 1 autopsied. *Neurology* 1967;17:680–690.
23. Williams J, Stevens H. Familial paroxysmal choreaathetosis. *Pediatrics* 1963;31:656–659.
24. Rosen JA. Paroxysmal choreoathetosis. Associated with perinatal hypoxic encephalopathy. *Arch Neurol* 1964;11:385–387.
25. Stevens H. Paroxysmal choreo-athetosis. *Arch Neurol* 1966;14:415–420.
26. Weber MB. Familial paroxysmal dystonia. *J Nerv Ment Dis*1967;145:221–226.
27. Bressman SB, Fahn S, Burke RE. Paroxysmal nonkinesigenic dystonia. *Adv Neurol*1988;50:403–413.
28. Fahn S. Paroxysmal dyskinesias. In: Marsden CD, Fahn S, eds. *Movement disorders 3.* Oxford: Butterworth-Heinemann, 1994:310–345.

29. Demirkiran M, Jankovic J. Paroxysmal dyskinesias: clinical features and classification. *Ann Neurol* 1995; 38:571–579.

30. Fahn S, Williams DT. Psychogenic dystonia. *Adv Neurol* 1988;50:431–455.

31. Browne DL, Gancher ST, Nutt TG, et al. Episodic ataxia/myokymia syndrome is associated with point mutations in the human potassium channel gene, KCNA1. *Nat Genet* 1994;8:136–140.

32. Comu S, Giuliani M, Narayanan V. Episodic ataxia and myokymia syndrome: a new mutation of potassium channel gene Kv1.1. *Ann Neurol* 1996;40:684–687.

33. Litt M, Kramer P, Browne D, et al. A gene for episodic ataxia/myokymia maps to chromosome 12p13. *Am J Hum Genet* 1994;55:702–709.

34. D'Adamo MC, Liu ZP, Adelman JP, et al. Episodic ataxia type-1 mutations in the hKv1.1 cytoplasmic pore region alter the gating properties of the channel. *EMBO J* 1998;17:1200–1207.

35. Zerr P, Adelman JP, Maylie J. Episodic ataxia mutations in Kv1.1 alter potassium channel function by dominant negative effects or haploinsufficiency. *J Neurosci* 1998; 18:2842–2848.

36. Eunson LH, Rea R, Zuberi SM, et al. Clinical, genetic, and expression studies of mutations in the potassium channel gene KCNA1 reveal new phenotypic variability. *Ann Neurol* 2000;48:647–656.

37. Vahedi K, Joutel A, van Bogaert P, et al. A gene for hereditary paroxysmal cerebellar ataxia maps to chromosome 19p. *Ann Neurol* 1995;37:289–293.

38. Von Brederlow B, Hahn A, Koopman WJ, et al. Mapping the gene for acetazolamide responsive hereditary paryoxysmal cerebellar ataxia to chromosome 19p. *Hum Mol Genet* 1995;4:279–284.

39. Yue Q, Jen JC, Nelson SF, et al. Progressive ataxia due to a missense mutation in a calcium-channel gene. *Am J Hum Genet* 1997;61:1078–1087.

40. Yue Q, Jen JC, Thwe MM, et al. De novo mutation in CACNA1A caused acetazolamide-responsive episodic ataxia. *Am J Med Genet* 1998;77:298–301.

41. Tomita H, Nagamitsu S, Wakui K, et al. Paroxysmal kinesigenic choreoathetosis locus maps to chromosome 16p11.2-q12.1. *Am J Hum Genet* 1999;65:1688–1697.

42. Bennett LB, Roach ES, Bowcock AM. A locus for paroxysmal kinesigenic dyskinesia maps to human chromosome 16. *Neurology* 2000;54:125–130.

43. Swoboda KJ, Soong BW, McKenna C, et al. Paroxysmal kinesigenic dyskinesia and infantile convulsions—Clinical and linkage studies. *Neurology* 2000;55:224–230.

44. Valente EM, Spacey SD, Wali GM, et al. A second paroxysmal kinesigenic choreoathetosis locus (EKD2) mapping on 16q13-q22.1 indicates a family of genes which give rise to paroxysmal disorders on human chromosome 16. *Brain* 2000;123:2040–2045.

45. Fouad GT, Servidei S, Durcan S, et al. A gene for familial paroxysmal dyskinesia (FPD1) maps to chromosome 2q. *Am J Hum Genet* 1996;59:135–139.

46. Fink JK, Rainier S, Wilkowski J, et al. Paroxysmal dystonic choreoathetosis: tight linkage to chromosome 2q. *Am J Hum Genet* 1996;59:140–145.

47. Fink JK, Hedera P, Mathay JG, et al. Paroxysmal dystonic choreoathetosis linked to chromosome 2q: clinical analysis and proposed pathophysiology. *Neurology* 1997;49:177–183.

48. Jarman PR, Davis MB, Hodgson SV, et al. Paroxysmal

dystonic choreoathetosis - Genetic linkage studies in a British family. *Brain* 1997;120:2125–2130.

49. Auburger G, Ratzlaff T, Lunkes A, et al. A gene for autosomal dominant paroxysmal choreoathetosis spasticity (CSE) maps to the vicinity of a potassium channel gene cluster on chromosome 1p, probably within 2 cM between D1S443 and D1S197. *Genomics* 1996;31:90–94.

50. Kato M, Araki S. Paroxysmal kinesigenic choreoathetosis. Report of a case relieved by carbamazepine. *Arch Neurol* 1969;20:508–513.

51. Plant GT, Williams AC, Marsden CD, et al. Familial paroxysmal dystonia induced by exercise. *J Neurol Neurosurg Psychiatry* 1984;47:275–279.

52. Nardocci N, Lamperti E, Rumi V, et al. Typical and atypical forms of paroxysmal choreoathetosis. *Dev Med Child Neurol* 1989;31:670–674.

53. Wali GM. Paroxysmal hemidystonia induced by prolonged exercise and cold. *J Neurol Neurosurg Psychiatry* 1992;55:236–237.

54. Bhatia KP, Soland VL, Marsden CD, et al. Paroxysmal exercise-induced dystonia: Eight new sporadic cases and a review of the literature. *Mov Disord* 1997;12: 1007–1012.

55. Kluge A, Kettner B, Zschenderlein R, et al. Changes in perfusion pattern using ECD-SPECT indicate frontal lobe and cerebellar involvement in exercise-induced paroxysmal dystonia. *Mov Disord* 1998; 13:125–134.

56. Munchau A, Valente EM, Shahidi GA, et al. A new family with paroxysmal exercise induced dystonia and migraine: a clinical and genetic study. *J Neurol Neurosurg Psychiatry* 2000;68:609–614.

57. Horner FH, Jackson LC. Familial paroxysmal choreoathetosis. In: Barbeau A, Brunette JR, eds. *Progress in Neuro-Genetics*. Amsterdam: Excerpta Medica Foundation;1969:745–751.

58. Lugaresi E, Cirignotta F. Hypnogenic paroxysmal dystonia: epileptic seizure or a new syndrome? *Sleep* 1981; 4:129–138.

59. Lugaresi E, Cirignotta F, Montagna P. Nocturnal paroxysmal dystonia. *J Neurol Neurosurg Psychiatry* 1986; 49:375–380.

60. Tinuper P, Cerullo A, Cirignotta F, et al. Nocturnal paroxysmal dystonia with short-lasting attacks: three cases with evidence for an epileptic frontal lobe origin of seizures.*Epilepsia*1990;31:549–556.

61. Sellal F, Hirsch E, Maquet P, et al. Postures et mouvements anormaux paroxystiques au cours du sommeil: dystonie paroxystique hypnogenique ou epilepsie partielle? (Abnormal paroxysmal movements during sleep: hypnogenic paroxysmal dystonia or focal epilepsy?) *Rev Neurol* 1991;147:121–128.

62. Meierkord H, Fish DR, Marsden CD, et al. Is nocturnal paroxysmal dystonia a form of frontal lobe epilepsy? *Mov Disord* 1992;7:38–42.

63. Bass N, Wyllie E, Comair Y, et al. Supplementary sensorimotor area seizures in children and adolescents. *J Pediatr* 1995;126:537–544.

64. Oldani A, Zucconi M, Asselta R, et al. Autosomal dominant nocturnal frontal lobe epilepsy—A video-polysomnographic and genetic appraisal of 40 patients and delineation of the epileptic syndrome. *Brain* 1998; 121:205–223.

65. Nakken KO, Magnusson A, Steinlein OK. Autosomal dominant nocturnal frontal lobe epilepsy: An electro-

clinical study of a Norwegian family with ten affected members. *Epilepsia* 1999;40:88–92.

66. Snyder CH. Paroxysmal torticollis in infancy. *Am J Dis Child* 1969;117:458–460.

67. Gourley IM. Paroxysmal torticellis in infancy. *Can Med Assoc J* 1971;105:504–505.

68. Sanner G, Bergstrom B. Benign paroxysmal torticollis in infancy. *Acta Paediatr Scand* 1979;68:219–223.

69. Bratt HD, Menelaus MB. Benign paroxysmal torticollis of infancy. *J Bone Joint Surg [Br]* 1992;74:449–451.

70. Lipson EH, Robertson WC Jr. Paroxysmal torticollis of infancy: familial occurrence. *Am J Dis Child* 1978;132: 422–423.

71. Angelini L, Rumi V, Lamperti E, et al. Transient paroxysmal dystonia in infancy. *Neuropediatrics* 1988;19: 171–174.

72. Parker HL. Periodic ataxia. *Mayo Clin Proc* 1946;38: 642–645.

73. Farmer TW, Mustian VM. Vestibulocerebellar ataxia. *Arch Neurol* 1963;8:471–480.

74. Damji KF, Allingham RR, Pollock SC, et al. Periodic vestibulocerebellar ataxia, an autosomal dominant ataxia with defective smooth pursuit, is genetically distinct from other autosomal dominant ataxias. *Arch Neurol* 1996;53:338–344.

75. Hill W, Sherman H. Acute intermittent familial cerebellar ataxia. *Arch Neurol* 1968;18:350–357.

76. White JC. Familial periodic nystagmus, vertigo, and ataxia. *Arch Neurol* 1969;20:276–280.

77. Griggs RC, Moxley RT III, Lafrance RA, et al. Hereditary paroxysmal ataxia: Response to acetazolamide. *Neurology* 1978;28:1259–1264.

78. Donat JR, Auger R. Familial periodic ataxia. *Arch Neurol* 1979;36:568–569.

79. Fahn S. Paroxysmal tremor. *Neurology* 1983;33(suppl 2):131.

80. Fahn S. Atypical tremors, rare tremors, and unclassified tremors. In: Findley LJ, Capildeo R, eds. *Movement Disorders: Tremor.* New York: Oxford University; 1984: 431–443.

81. Mayeux R, Fahn S. Paroxysmal dystonic choreoathetosis in a patient with familial ataxia. *Neurology* 1982;32: 1184–1186.

82. Van Dyke DH, Griggs RC, Murphy MJ, et al. Hereditary myokymia and periodic ataxia. *J Neurol Sci* 1975; 25:109–118.

83. Hanson PA, Martinez LB, Cassidy R. Contractures, continuous muscle discharges, and titubation. *Ann Neurol* 1977;1:120–124.

84. Gancher ST, Nutt JG. Autosomal dominant episodic ataxia: a heterogeneous syndrome. *Mov Disord* 1986;1: 239–253.

85. Brunt ERP, Van Weerden TW. Familial paroxysmal ki-

nesigenic ataxia and continuous myokymia. *Brain* 1990;113:1361–1382.

86. Vaamonde J, Artieda J, Obeso JA. Hereditary paroxysmal ataxia with neuromyotonia. *Mov Disord* 1991;6: 180–182.

87. Baloh RW, Winder A. Acetazolamide-responsive vestibulocerebellar syndrome: clinical and oculographic features. *Neurology* 1991;41:429–433.

88. Bain PG, Larkin GBR, Calver DM, et al. Persistent superior oblique paresis as a manifestation of familial periodic cerebellar ataxia. *Br J Ophthalmol* 1991;75: 619–621.

89. Hawkes CH. Familial paroxysmal ataxia: report of a family. *J Neurol Neurosurg Psychiatry* 1992;55:212–213.

90. Bain PG, O'Brien MD, Keevil SF, et al. Familial periodic cerebellar ataxia: a problem of cerebellar intracellular pH homeostasis. *Ann Neurol* 1992;31:147–154.

91. Griggs RC, Nutt JG. Episodic ataxias as channelopathies. *Ann Neurol* 1995;37:285–287.

92. Nightingale S, Barton ME. Intermittent vertical supranuclear ophthalmoplegia and ataxia. *Mov Disord* 1991; 6:76-78.

93. Baron DN, Dent CE, Harris H, et al. Hereditary pellagra-like skin rash with temporary cerebellar ataxia, constant renal amino-aciduria and other bizarre biochemical features. *Lancet* 1956;2:421–428.

94. Blass JP, Avigan J, Uhlendorf BW. A defect in pyruvate decarboxyalase in a child with an intermittent movement disorder. *J Clin Invest* 1970;49:423–432.

95. Blass JP, Kark RAP, Engel WK. Clinical studies of a patient with pyruvate decarboxylase deficiency. *Arch Neurol* 1971;25:449–460.

96. Lonsdale D, Faulkner WR, Price JW, et al. Intermittent cerebellar ataxia associated with hyperpyruvic acidemia, hyperalaninemia, and hyperalaninuria. *Pediatrics* 1969;43:1025–1034.

97. Dancis J, Hutzler J, Rokkones T. Intermittent branched-chain ketonuria: variant of maple-syrup-urine disease. *N Engl J Med* 1967;276:84–80.

98. Andermann F, Cosgrove JBR, Lloyd-Smith D, et al. Paroxysmal dysarthria and ataxia in multiple sclerosis. *Neurology* 1959;9:211–215.

99. Espir MLE, Watkins SM, Smith HV. Paroxysmal dysarthria and other transient neurological disturbances in disseminated sclerosis. *J Neurol Neurosurg Psychiatry* 1966;29:323–330.

100. DeCastro W, Campbell J. Periodic ataxia. *JAMA* 1967; 200:892–894.

101. Miley CE, Forster FM. Paroxysmal signs and symptoms in multiple sclerosis. *Neurology* 1974;24:458–461.

102. Gorard DA, Gibberd FB. Paroxysmal dysarthria and ataxia-associated MRI abnormality. *J Neurol Neurosurg Psychiatry* 1989;52:1444–1445.

Myoclonus and Paroxysmal Dyskinesias,
Advances in Neurology, Vol. 89,
edited by S. Fahn, et al.
Published by Lippincott Williams & Wilkins, Philadelphia, 2002.

35

Classification of Paroxysmal Dyskinesias and Ataxias

Joseph Jankovic and *Meltem Demirkiran

Department of Neurology, Parkinson's Disease Center and Movement Disorders Clinic,
*Baylor College of Medicine, Houston, Texas; *Department of Neurology,*
Çukurova University School of Medicine, Adana, Turkey

Paroxysmal dyskinesias are involuntary, intermittent movements consisting of dystonia, chorea, athetosis, ballismus, or any combination of these hyperkinetic disorders. Paroxysmal dyskinesias may occur spontaneously or they may be precipitated by sudden voluntary movement, prolonged exertion, sleep, stress, or several other factors including alcohol, coffee, tea, fatigue, heat, and cold (1). We prefer the generic term "paroxysmal dyskinesia" because the phenomenology of the movement disorder is often mixed or complex and the attacks are not always witnessed by the examiner.

Initially, paroxysmal dyskinesias were classified into three categories primarily according to the duration of the attack, and secondarily according to the precipitant (2). Recently, we proposed a modification of this classification based mainly on precipitating factors, phenomenology, duration of attacks, and etiology: (a) paroxysmal kinesigenic dyskinesia (PKD) induced by sudden movement, (b) paroxysmal non-kinesigenic dyskinesia (PNKD) occurring spontaneously, (c) paroxysmal exertion-induced dyskinesia (PED) induced after prolonged exercise, and

(d) paroxysmal hypnogenic dyskinesia (PHD) occurring during sleep (Table 35.1) (1). We further subdivided the groups according to the duration of attacks as either short-lasting (≤ 5 minutes) or long-lasting (> 5 minutes) attacks and classified the paroxysmal dyskinesias according to possible etiologies into idiopathic (familial or sporadic) or secondary.

PAROXYSMAL KINESIGENIC DYSKINESIA

Paroxysmal kinesigenic dyskinesia (PKD) consists of sudden attacks of involuntary movements precipitated by voluntary movement. This paroxysmal hyperkinetic movement disorder was initially regarded as a form of epilepsy and several terms such as subcortical epilepsy reflex epilepsy, seizures induced by movement, tonic seizures, kinesthetic reflex epilepsy, kinesigenic seizure, and dystonic seizure induced by movement, have drawn attention to the overlap in clinical phenomenology between epilepsy and PKD (3–13). On the other hand, some authors recognized the possible involvement of the extrapyramidal system and used terms such as periodic dystonia, paroxysmal choreoathetosis, and kinesigenic choreoathetosis to describe PKD (8,14–22). In 1967, Kertesz introduced the widely accepted term *paroxysmal*

Modified and reproduced with permission from *Ann Med Sci 2001*;10:92–103.

TABLE 35.1. *Clinical features of paroxysmal dyskinesias*

	PKD	PNKD	PED	PHD	EA	
					EA-1	EA-2
Precipitant	Sudden movement, startle, hyperventilation, photic stimulation	None	Prolonged exertion, passive movements	Sleep	Sometimes sudden movement	None
Duration	Short: sec to 5 min Long: >5 min to hr	Short: sec to 5 min Long: >5 min to days	Short: sec to 5 min Long: >5 min	Short: sec to 5 min Long: >5 min	Sec to min	15 min to days
Frequency	1/mo–100/day	2/mo–20/day	1/day–5/mo	5/day–few/yr	1/day–few/yr	1/day–few/yr
Gender	Male > females	Male ≥ female	Familial: female > male Sporadic: male = female	Male > female	Male = female	Male = female
Exacerbating factors	Stress, menses, heat, cold	Stress, alcohol, caffeine, cold, menses, heat fatigue, fasting, chocolate, smoking	Cold, menses, stress, alcohol, heat	Stress, menses, fatigue	Startle, stress	Stress, fatigue, alcohol, coffee, carbohydrate
Onset age	Childhood, adoloscense (4 mo–57 yr)	Childhood, adoloscense (2 mo–50 yr)	Childhood (2–30 yr)	Childhood (2–47 yr)	Childhood, adoloscence	Childhood, adoloscence (1–30 yr)
Etiology	AD, AR, sporadic, secondary (MS, trauma, hypoxia, stroke, endocrine, encephalitis)	AD, sporadic, secondary (MS, hypoxia, encephalitis, stroke, endocrine, trauma, psychogenic)	AD, sporadic, secondary (trauma)	AD, sporadic, secondary (trauma, MS)	AD, sporadic, secondary (metabolic diseases)	AD, sporadic, secondary (metabolic diseases)
Treatment	Anticonvulsants, acetazolamide, levodopa, flunarizine, tetrabenazine	Anticonvulsants? acetazolamide, levodopa, tetrabenazine, antimuscarinics	Not satisfactory, anticonvulsants? levodopa, acetazolamide	Anticonvulsants, acetazolamide	Acetazolamide, anticonvulsants?	Acetazolamide

AD, autosomal dominant; AR, autosomal recessive; EA, episodic ataxia; PED, paroxysmal exertion-induced dyskinesia; PHD, paroxysmal hypnogenic dyskinesia; PKD, paroxysmal kinesigenic dyskinesia; PNKD, paroxysmal nonkinesigenic dyskinesia; MS, multiple sclerosis.

kinesigenic choreoathetosis for attacks induced by sudden movement (2,23–27).

PKD is characterized by paroxysmal attacks of dystonia, chorea, athetosis, ballism, or any combination of these hyperkinetic movement disorders. By definition, the attacks are always triggered by voluntary movement. Some attacks can be precipitated also by talking, yawning, startle, photic stimulation, hyperventilation, stress, menses, heat, and cold. The frequency may be as high as 100 per day. The attacks usually occur daily, but sometimes they can occur only once a month or less frequently. (1,5,6,13,23,25,28,29). The duration of attacks is generally seconds to 5 minutes, but rarely the attacks last longer than 5 minutes, up to hours (1,30) (Table 35.1). Attacks of PKD are usually unilateral or asymmetrical (1,23,25,29,31). Extremities are affected most often, but facial, neck, and trunk muscles can be affected as well. Facial muscle involvement can cause facial grimacing and sometimes dysarthria. Some patients report inability to speak, but this is never due to loss of or alteration of consciousness. The attacks may be disabling, interfering with walking, working, and daily activities (1,28,29). Prior to the onset of the attacks some patients experience variable sensations, termed sensory aura, such as muscle tension, crawling sensation, tingling, and paraesthesia in the affected limb or body part, and dizziness (1,2,5,15,21,23,25,28,29).

The age at onset is generally younger than 20 years, usually in childhood, especially in idiopathic familial and sporadic cases. However, it can range from 4 months to 57 years (1,2,13,23,28,32). Although in our studies we found equal gender representation, PKD has been reported to be a more common in males, with a ratio ranging from 2:1 to 4:1 (2,13,23, 28) (Table 35.1).

PKD can be sporadic; however, the familial occurrence is one of its characteristic features (13,28,29). In most of the reported families there was an autosomal dominant inheritance (6,11,16,20,21,23,29). The disorder, however, may be inherited either as an autosomal dominant trait with incomplete penetrance or as an autosomal recessive trait (2,21,29). In some

families with autosomal dominant PKD, a locus has been mapped to pericentromeric region of chromosome 16, 16p11.2-q12.1 between D16S3093 and D16S416 in 8 Japanese families and to 16p11.2-q11.2 between D16S3100 and D16S771 in an African American kindred (33, 34). The PKD region in both Japanese families and African American kindred overlaps with the region responsible for infantile convulsions and paroxysmal choreoathetosis (ICCA) that was mapped to chromosome 16p12-q12 (35, 36). Because of the overlap, some investigators have suggested that one gene is responsible for both PKD and infantile convulsions with paroxysmal choreoathetosis (ICCA). However, the paroxysmal dyskinesia in the ICCA family described by Szepetowski and associates (35) was not kinesigenic (35). On the other hand, the Chinese family with ICCA reported by Lee and colleagues seemed to have PKD (36). Recently, Swoboda and associates reported linkage to chromosome 16 locus (a 26-cM region between markers D16S3131 and D16S3396) in 11 families with PKD and IC having a diverse ethnic background (37). This finding narrowed the critical region for ICCA to a 3.2cM region spanning the centromere, but locus heterogeneity may clearly exist for this phenotype. Valente and colleagues reported another locus on the long arm of chromosome 16, 16q13-q22.1, in a large Indian family with PKD distinct from the previous regions, not overlapping with the ICCA locus or the locus identified in Japanese families with PKD, again highlighting the genetic heterogeneity of PKD and virtually excluding the possibility of only one gene being responsible for both PKD and ICCA (38). They suggested that there could be a cluster of genes on human chromosome 16 that is responsible for paroxysmal movement disorders (Table 35.2).

In several families with autosomal dominant PKD, an analysis of possible linkage to loci involving chromosome 2q33-35 of PNKD, chromosome 1p of paroxysmal choreoathetosis/spasticity (CSE), chromosome 12p13 of episodic ataxia/myokymia (EA-1), chromosome 10q23.3-q24 of partial epilepsy and chromosome 20q13.2-q13.3 of benign

TABLE 35.2. *Paroxysmal dykinesias: genetics*

Type	Chromosome	Gene	Channelopathy	Reference
PKD	16p11.2-q12.1	?	?	33,34
	16q13-q22.1	?	?	38
ICCA?	16p11.2-q12.1	?	?	37
	16p12-q12			36
PNKD	2q33-35	SLC2C	Anion exchanger?	96–101
CSE?	1p	?	?	95
ICCA?	16p12-q12	?	?	35
PED (+ rolandic epilepsy + writer's cramp)	16p12-11.2	?	?	109
CSE?	1p	?	?	95
PHD	?	?	?	
(ADNFLE)	20q13.2-13.3	CHRNA4	Nicotinic acetylcholine receptor	128
EA-1	12p13	KCNA1	K channel	139–151,153
EA-2	19p13	CACNL1A4	Ca Channel	154–166

ADNFLE, autosomal-dominant nocturnal frontal lobe epilepsy; CSE, choreoathetosis/spasticity; EA, episodic ataxia; ICCA, infantile convulsions with paroxysmal choreoathetosis; PED, paroxysmal exertion-induced dyskinesia; PHD, paroxysmal hypnogenic dyskinesia; PKD, paroxysmal kinesigenic dyskinesia; PNKD, paroxysmal non-kinesigenic dyskinesia.

neonatal convulsions excluded these candidate genes for PKD (39,40).

There are many causes of secondary PKD, including multiple sclerosis (MS) (9,41–47), head trauma (6,48,49), peripheric trauma (1), stroke (1,50–52), encephalitis (1), perinatal hypoxia (19), hypoparathyroidism (22,53,54), pseudohypoparathyroidism (55), hyperthyroidism (56), progressive supranuclear palsy (57), nonketotic hyperglycemia (58,59), and diabetes mellitus (60) (Table 35.1) (see Chapter 36).

The frequency of the PKD attacks tends to diminish with age, and occasionally there may be spontaneous remissions. This disorder responds to anticonvulsant drugs such as phenytoin (1,5,10,23,24,27,32), phenobarbital (5–7,13,21,48), primidone (5,6,10), clonazepam (61), valproic acid (27), and carbamazepine (1,13,32,44,61,62). In addition to anticonvulsants, PKD has been reported to improve with acetazolamide (45) levodopa (24,63), flunarizine (64), and tetrabenazine (1) (Table 35.1).

PAROXYSMAL NON-KINESIGENIC DYSKINESIA

In 1940 Mount and Reback (65) described choreoathetoid attacks involving limbs occur-

ring spontaneously, sometimes precipitated by alcohol, coffee, tea, fatigue, and smoking in a patient with a family history of similar episodes. The attacks occurred two to three times a day and lasted 5 minutes to hours. In this report they introduced the term *familial paroxysmal choreoathetosis* for the first time. Later, familial, sporadic or symptomatic cases similar to this case followed with terms such as "tonic seizures" (9,10,66), "paroxysmal dyskinesia" (67,68), "paroxysmal choreoathetosis" (8,69), and "paroxysmal dystonic choreoathetosis" (70). After Lance's 1977 publication of his classification (2), paroxysmal dystonic choreoathetosis (PDC) became the most preferred term for this type of paroxysmal dyskinesia. In 1988, Bressman and associates (71) reported sporadic cases with paroxysmal dystonic choreoathetosis, and used the term *paroxysmal non-kinesigenic dystonia*, emphasizing the absence of precipitating movement in the attacks. In our classification, we modified this term as paroxysmal non-kinesigenic dyskinesia, because the phenomenology of the attacks was not limited to choreoathetosis.

The phenomenology of the attacks of PNKD, just like PKD, consists of paroxysmal attacks of any combination of dystonia, chorea, athetosis, and ballism. These attacks occur spontaneously without any specific precipitant. However, they can be exacerbated by stress, excitement, fatigue, alcohol, coffee, tea, cold, heat, and chocolate. The frequency of the attacks is lower and more variable as compared to PKD ranging from 2 to 3 per month to 20 per day (1,36,51) and they tend to diminish with age (2,71–73). The attacks of PNKD usually last minutes to hours, but there have been several reports of non-kinesigenic attacks lasting seconds or days (1,71,74) (Table 35.1). Similar to PKD, the attacks of PNKD are usually unilateral or asymmetrical, but may be bilateral. Extremities are generally affected more than the other body parts, but face, neck, and trunk may be also involved. Dysarthria or muteness can be present during the attacks. If the attack is severe enough, it can cause falls and it may interfere with daily activities. Prior to the onset of the attacks some patients report variable sensations, sensory aura, such as muscle tension or paresthesias in the involved limb (1,25,28).

There is a wide range of age at onset of PNKD from 2 months to 50 years, but most of the cases have their onset in childhood or adolescence (1,3,25,28,32,75–93). The male gender preponderance is not as striking in PNKD as it is in PKD. However, in familial cases males are affected more than females (2,25, 28,32) (Table 35.1).

By definition, attacks of PNKD are unpredictable, but their occurrence may be influenced by various environmental and endogenous factors. Jarman and associates (94) reported a sleep benefit and diurnal variations in attack frequency, with the highest frequency in the afternoon or evening. In another family with autosomal dominant PNKD, initially presenting as paroxysmal dyskinesia, the involuntary movements became more continuous in some members of the family (95).

Although sporadic cases have been reported, PNKD is often familial with an autosomal dominant pattern of inheritance (2,25, 28,62,65,70–72,75–77,95). Auburger and associates (96) initially reported a gene for paroxysmal choreoathetosis and spasticity, a disorder clinically similar to PNKD and PED

but with persistent spasticity, which they mapped to a potassium channel gene cluster, 12 cM region, on chromosome 1p. Later, Fink and colleagues (97) mapped PNKD to the long arm of chromosome 2, 2q33-35, in a family from Poland assigning the locus to 15 cM interval between the flanking markers D2S164 and D2S159. Fouad and colleagues (98) then mapped an Italian family with PNKD to the same chromosome and narrowed interval of interest to 10 cM, between D2S128 and D2S126. Following this report, Hofele and associates (99) detected the same gene marker in German kindred, refining the candidate region to 3.6 cM, between markers D2S164 and D2S2359. In a study of a British kindred with PNKD, Jarman and colleagues (100) narrowed the region further to 4 cM between flanking markers D2S295 and D2S377. Raskind and associates (101) confined the PNKD gene to a 5 cM region bounded by the markers D2S164 and D2S377. Matsuo and associates (102) reported that the PNKD gene is located in 15.3 cM interval lying between D2S371 and D2S339 in a Japanese family. Taking into consideration the previous reports they suggested the probable location to be 2.5 cM interval between D2S295 and D2S2359. All these reports draw attention to the possibility that PNKD may be a channelopathy because of a cluster of ion-channel genes existing on chromosome 2q, near the PNKD locus. Sodium channel genes (on choromosome 2q21-24) and potassium channel genes (on chromosome 2q21) are mapped proximal to the PNKD locus (2q33-35), and the anion exchanger gene SLC2C is located on chromosome 2q36 between D2S128 and D2S126 (98,103) (Table 35.2). This SLC2C gene controls the exchange of bicarbonate for chloride and is thought to modulate GABA-A receptor. This receptor contains a benzodiazepine binding site and that diazepam drugs are the preferred drugs for PNKD.

MS is one of the leading causes of secondary cases of PNKD as it is in PKD (1,9, 10,41,66). Although psychogenic PKD is rare, there have been several cases of PNKD with psychogenic etiology (1,71,79). Other causes include perinatal hypoxia (10,71,80), encephalitis (1,67,71), cystinuria (68), hypoparathyroidism (69,81), pseudohypoparathyroidism (55), thyrotoxicosis (91), transient ischemic attacks (82,83), head injury (1,49, 74), hypoglycemia (84,90,92), basal ganglia calcification (89), acquired immune deficiency (85), diabetes (86), meningioma (71), ischemia or stroke (1,71), Leigh syndrome (93), and dopamine blockers (87) (Table 35.1).

Similar to PKD, the attacks of PNKD may diminish in frequency and intensity with age (2,3,71–73). PNKD, however, is more difficult to treat than PKD and does not respond to anticonvulsant drugs, as does PKD. While clonazepam appears to be the drug of choice (2,3, 28,71,73), phenobarbital and valproic acid (62) may also be effective in this type of paroxysmal dyskinesia. Other drugs such as antimuscarinics, benztropin mesylate (65), sometimes in combination with phenytoin (67), have been found to be effective. Carbamazepine (45,60, 88), chlordiazepoxide (8), acetazolamide (71), trihexyphenidyl (87), and haloperidol (62,88) have been tried with variable results. Although levodopa has been reported to worsen the attacks (62), three of our patients had moderate benefit with levodopa. One of our patients had relief with tetrabenazine while another reported worsening of the symptoms with haloperidol (1) (Table 35.1).

PAROXYSMAL EXERTION-INDUCED DYSKINESIA

This form of paroxysmal dyskinesia induced by prolonged exertion was first labeled according to the duration of attacks as intermediate form (2). PED consists mainly of attacks of dystonia, sometimes combined with chorea and athetosis. The attacks of PED are triggered by prolonged exertion, such as walking or running for 5 to 15 minutes before the onset of the attack. There can be other precipitants such as passive movement of the limb, talking, chewing gum, cold, heat, menses, alcohol, and stress (1,3,104–107). The frequency of attacks ranges from one to two per day to one to five per month. Although PED attacks usually last 5 to 30 minutes (2), long-lasting attacks have also been reported (1,105–107). The attacks involve the lower limbs and the distribution is often bilateral, but it can also be unilateral. The involvement of the upper limb, trunk, neck and face is rare (1,106, 107). Münchau and associates (107) described a family with PED in which some members reported premonitory aura as a tingling sensation prior to the onset of the attacks. The onset of PED is generally in childhood ranging from 2 to 30 years (1–3,104–109). While the familial cases of PED seem to have a female preponderance, the sporadic cases have equal gender representation (Table 35.1).

There are both familial and sporadic few cases of PED described in the literature (1–3,104–109) and only one secondary PED (1). All families have an autosomal dominant pattern of transmission—a gene for paroxysmal (CSE) is reported on chromosome 1p. Although the paroxysmal choreoathetosis/spasticity reported by Auburger and associates (96), with a locus on chromosome 1p, was referred to as a PNKD, it is clinically similar to PED because the attacks are triggered by physical exercise. Recently, a syndrome of PED with rolandic epilepsy and writer's cramp has been reported to be linked to chromosome 16 (16p12-11.2) between markers D16S3133 and D16S3131 in an autosomal recessive family (110) (Table 35.2). The authors pointed out that because it overlapped with the region responsible for ICCA these two disorders could be phenotypic variations of different mutations in the same gene. However, Münchau and colleagues (107) described a family with PED and migraine in which they excluded linkage to PNKD locus on chromosome 2, the familial hemiplegic maigraine/EA2 locus on chromosome 19p, and the ICCA locus on chromosome 16. They also drew attention to the co-occurrence of migraine in several members of their family. There are other reports suggesting a link between PED and hemiplegic migraines (106,111).

PED appears to be frequently associated with other paroxysmal disorders, such as mi-

TABLE 35.3. *Association with other paroxysmal disorders*

PKD	Infantile convulsions, epilepsy, migraine, PxD, EA
PNKD	Migraine, PxD
PED	Rolandic epilepsy, seizure, migraine
PHD	Epilepsy, PxD
EA-1	Epilesy, PKD
EA-2	Familial hemiplegic migraine, PxD

EA, episodic ataxia; PED, paroxysmal exertion-induced dyskinesia; PHD, paroxysmal hypnogenic dyskinesia; PKD, paroxysmal kinesigenic dyskinesia; PNKD, paroxysmal nonkinesigenic dyskinesia; PxD, paroxysmal dyskinesia.

graine and epilepsy (106,107,111) (Table 35.3). As in other paroxysmal dyskinesias and ataxias, it is likely that this is another ion-channel disorder. Further genetic studies will undoubtedly clarify the question whether PED is a phenotype of one of the other paroxysmal dyskinesias or a different paroxysmal disorder with a unique genetic defect.

A satisfactory treatment has not been yet established for this type of paroxysmal dyskinesia. Spontaneous remission has been reported in one case (2). Phenytoin, carbamazepine, clonazepam, phenobarbital were tried with no effect (2,107). Benzodiazepines (particularly clonazepam), levodopa, tryptophan, acetazolamide, and steroids have been reported to provide benefits in some patients (1,3,104–106,111) (Table 35.1).

PAROXYSMAL HYPNOGENIC DYSKINESIA

This sleep-related disorder has been regarded as a specific type of paroxysmal dyskinesia (66,112,113). PHD consists of attacks of ballistic, dystonic, or choreoathetoid movements occurring in NREM sleep. The attacks occur generally in the second stage of NREM sleep and they are often preceded by clinical and EEG signs of arousal. The patients may open their eyes and move their limbs and trunk in a disordered, violent manner with ballistic movements and dystonic posturing. Distal limbs may show choreoathetosis. After the attacks, the patients often fall asleep, but

can recall the episodes in the morning. Stress, increased activity, and menses have been reported to aggravate PHD (114,115). Rarely, prodromal symptoms, such as painful sensations may precede the attacks (116). The attacks may be accompanied by irregular breathing, involuntary vocalizations, or tachycardia (113,114,116). The attacks may occur a few times a year to (117) to four to five times per night (41,113,115,118). The attacks of PHD usually last 20 to 50 seconds. Lugaressi and associates (118) have subgrouped the attacks into short- and long-lasting types. Several cases have been described with attacks lasting more than 5 minutes (41,113,119) (Table 35.1).

The coexistence of other types of paroxysmal dyskinesias is strikingly frequent in patients with PHD. In some of the cases, daytime kinesigenic or non-kinesigenic attacks have been also described along with hypnogenic attacks (1,3,10,112,113,116,118,120, 121) (Table 35.3). Different types of familial paroxysmal dyskinesias in the different members of the same family have been noted (122). PHD usually starts during childhood. There is a marked male preponderance among familial cases of PHD (ratio: 4:1).

Only a few families, usually with autosomal dominant inheritance, with PHD have been described (1,114,122). Sporadic cases are more frequent than the familial cases (112,113,115–118,120,121,123, 124). Only three secondary cases, two with MS (41,66) and one following head injury (119) have been reported.

In contrast to other paroxysmal dyskinesias, PHD attacks usually do not diminish with age. However, a few familial cases with spontaneous remission of PHD have been reported (125). Carbamazepine seems to be the drug of choice for most of the short-lasting cases (113,115,117,118,120,123). Some cases have been reported to respond to phenytoin (114), a combination of phenobarbital and phenytoin (125), and acetazolamide (119) (Table 35.1).

A growing body of evidence has led to the conclusion that short lasting PHD should be regarded as a form of mesiofrontal epilepsy in most patients (120,123,124,126–128). An eponym autosomal-dominant nocturnal frontal lobe epilepsy (ADNFLE) has been used to describe this disorder in six families (127,128). The gene for one of these families has been mapped to 20q13.2 and is a mutation in the alfa4 subunit of the neuronal acetylcholine receptor (CHRNA4) (129) (Table 35.2).

PAROXYSMAL ATAXIAS

Ataxias are another group of motor disorder that can occur episodically. Paroxysmal ataxias have been classified into two clinically distinct forms: episodic ataxia-type 1 (EA-1) associated with myokymia, and episodic ataxia-type 2 (EA-2) associated with nystagmus. EA-1 is an autosomal dominant disorder involving both central and peripheric nervous system. Patients have episodes of sudden onset cerebellar ataxia lasting from seconds to minutes that are provoked by startle, exercise, sudden movement, and stress. It is associated with persistent, interictal, facial myokymia, and rarely with PKD. Nystagmus is not present. Sporadic cases have also been reported. Age at onset is usually during childhood. It may respond to acetazolamide, phenytoin and valproic acid. EA-2 associated with nystagmus is an autosomal dominant disorder, but sporadic cases have also been reported. Patients display paroxysmal attacks of ataxia lasting for 15 minutes to hours or days, usually precipitated by emotional or physical stress, alcohol, carbohydrate, or coffee. This disorder is associated with interictal nystagmus and, rarely, with vertigo, nausea, diplopia, headache, confusion, oscillopsia, and sweating. Mild progressive cerebellar ataxia, dysmetria, and dysarthria develop in some patients. Age at onset is usually during childhood or adolescence, ranging from 1 to 30 years. The frequency of attacks is variable and sometimes decreases with age. It usually responds to acetazolamide. Cerebellar atrophy may be seen in MRI (130–137) (Table 35.1).

Van Dyke and associates (138) and subsequently others (132,135,139) described kindred in which multiple generations manifested features of EA-1. In 1994, Kramer and colleagues (138) localized the gene for EA-1 to chromosome 12p in three families. As a result of subsequent genetic studies, EA-1 became the first ionic channel disease to be associated with defects in a potassium channel. Missense point mutations in the voltage-gated potassium channel gene (KCNA1/Kv1.1) on chromosome 12p13 have been shown to be associated with EA1 (140,141) (Table 35.2). Up to now, ten different point mutations in the KCNA1-gene have been reported in association with the EA1 phenotype. A different missense point mutation was present in heterozygous state in each. All affected individuals are heterozygous. Expression studies have identified two broad mechanisms by which such mutations induce channel dysfunction: the first group of mutations causes homomeric channels with altered gating properties; the second group of mutations may induce a dominant negative effect with reduced channel expression (142–147).

There is increasing evidence from animal studies that dysfunctional ion channels are responsible for the commonest episodic neurological disorder, epilepsy (148). Zuberi reported the eleventh family with EA-1 (132, 139,140,149–152) and tenth mutation and pointed out the co-occurrence of EA1 and epilepsy in their group and in two other families previously reported (135,138), concluding that epilepsy was ten times more likely to develop in patients with EA1 than in normal individuals (145) (Table 35.3). To explain this phenotypic heterogeneity they suggested that other genetic factors or environmental causes could be important in influencing the phenotype. In other ion channel disorders it was recognized that the same point mutation could be associated with phenotypic heterogeneity (153). Recently Eunson and associates (154) reported three new point mutations in the voltage-gated potassium channel gene KCNA1 on chromosome 12p. Their results showed that the dysfunction of this channel did not always associate with EA, but also epilepsy or isolated myokymia could be the only manifestations. They concluded that the degree and nature of the potassium channel dysfunction might be relevant to these new phenotypic variations.

Vahedi and associates (155) noted that cerebellar signs developed in many patients with familial hemiplegic migraine (FHM). Although they did not see any patients with both hereditary paroxysmal cerebellar ataxia (HPCA) and FHM, they hypothesized that these two could be allelic disorders. Following on the observation that FHM was mapped to chromosome 19p (156) they studied a family with paroxysmal ataxia and interictal nystagmus and concluded that HPCA and EA-2 share the same gene locus (Table 35.2). Later, Kramer and associates (157) also mapped another family with HPCA (EA2) to chromosome 19p. In 1996, Ophoff and colleagues (158) showed that both FHM and EA2 had mutations within CACNA1A, a gene coding for the α1A subunit of a neuronal P/Q type calcium channel expressed throughout the central nervous system, but mostly in the cerebellum. Molecular analysis led to the finding that these two clinically distinct diseases could be due to distinct mutations within the same gene. So far, four different missense mutations in FHM and two different truncating mutations in EA2 were identified. Several reports confirming the same gene have followed (159,160). Callandriello and associates mapped an Italian family with EA-2 to chromosome 19p13 between markers D19S221 and D19S226 (159) (Table 35.2). Baloh reported migraine headaches in half of the affected members (160). Later, Yue and colleagues (162) found a nonsense mutation in a sporadic case (161) and yet other missense mutation in another EA2 family. Denier and associates (163) identified seven new mutations in four families of EA2 and 3 sporadic cases. These findings were confirmed by Battistini and associates (164) and Carrera and associates (165), who identified new missense mutations within the CACNA1A gene in two additional families with FHM. Moreover, Jen and colleagues (166) identified a novel truncating mutation in an EA2 family

with one member having also attacks of hemiplegic migraine (Table 35.3). Some authors have suggested that, because there is a great variability in the phenotype and a strict genotype-phenotype correlation cannot be established, environmental or genetic factors other than CACNA1A mutations account for this variability (163,166,167).

Although most cases of episodic ataxias are idiopathic or autosomal dominant (130–135), several autosomal recessive metabolic diseases such as Hartnup disease (168), maple syrup disease (169), and pyruvate carboxylase deficiency (170) have been reported to cause paroxysmal ataxias (Table 35.1).

Occasionally paroxysmal ataxias are accompanied by paroxysmal dyskinesias, further supporting a link between paroxysmal dyskinesias and paroxysmal ataxias (171) (Table 35.3).

Association with other Paroxysmal Disorders

The pathophysiology of paroxysmal dyskinesias is still unknown. Earliest descriptions classified this disorder as a form of epilepsy. The paroxysmal nature of the attacks, response to anticonvulsive medication, sensory prodromata preceding the attacks, and the frequent association with epilepsy were the chief reasons for linking the paroxysmal dyskinesias with seizure disorders. However, the dystonic, choreic, athetoid or ballistic nature of the attacks, absence of EEG abnormalities during the attacks, preservation of consciousness, and, lack of postictal state argues against the hypothesis that paroxysmal dyskinesias represent a form of epilepsy. Nevertheless, there is some evidence linking paroxysmal dyskinesias to epilepsy, especially PKD and more clearly PHD (3,13,25,73,120,123,124, 126,172).

Other than the similarities, frequent association with epilepsy and paroxysmal dyskinesias, more than in the general population and more in the autosomal dominant types, have been reported in several previous reports (13, 17,19,21,33,35–37,173). Furthermore, family history of seizures similar to that reported in epileptics have been noted in several reports (1,5,11,13,17,21,23,173).

Besides epilepsy, migraines appear to occur at a higher rate than expected in families with paroxysmal dyskinesia, especially in patients and family members with EA-2 and PED, but also with PNKD and PKD (107, 155,156,174) (Table 35.3).

CONCLUSION

Abnormal metabolism in the basal ganglia demonstrated by a PET scan during an attack of paroxysmal posttraumatic hemidystonia (73), and occasional reports of response to levodopa and tetrabenazine in some patients with paroxysmal dyskinesias (1,24,63), suggest possible alteration in the dopaminergic system in certain forms of paroxysmal dyskinesia. Kim and associates (175), based on proton MR spectroscopic studies in patients with PKD, suggested at least a partial dysfunction of cholinergic system in basal ganglia with decreased choline content of unilateral basal ganglia. Recently, Jarman and colleagues (94) reported no abnormalities in MR spectroscopy or PET during attacks of PNKD and PET.

There are no animal models that accurately reflect the paroxysmal dyskinesias. Neuropathologic studies in humans and mutant hamster model of paroxysmal dystonia revealed no abnormalities in the brain or the spinal cord (2,176). In two patients with PKD, autopsy showed a slight asymmetry of substantia nigra in one (15) and melanin pigment in macrophages of locus ceruleus in the other (23). Therefore, few pathologic and imaging studies failed to provide any structural abnormality, and sufficient clue as to the underlying pathophysiology in paroxysmal dyskinesias.

Although the clinical and pharmacologic data in humans and in animals suggest different pathophysiologies for each type of paroxysmal dyskinesia, overlapping clinical features and the simultaneous occurrence of different types of paroxysmal dyskinesias in the same individual or the same family suggest a possible common mechanism. Furthermore association with other paroxysmal disorders such as migraine, and epilepsy may suggest a common pathophysiological basis shared by these paroxysmal disorders. The genes identified up to now for some of the paroxysmal dyskinesias, FHM, IC, are either ion channel genes or are located in the vicinity of different ion channel genes. Most paroxysmal disorders seem to result either from mutations in the ion channels or mutations in the genes that encode proteins modulating ion channel function. Future genetic studies should provide clues to the genetic mechanisms underlying this disorder.

REFERENCES

1. Demirkiran M, Jankovic J. Paroxysmal dyskinesias: clinical features and a new classification. *Ann Neurol* 1995;38:571–579.
2. Lance JW. Familial paroxysmal dystonic choreoathetosis and its differentiation from related syndromes. *Ann Neurol* 1977;2:285–293.
3. Demirkiran M, Jankovic J. Paroxysmal dyskinesias. In: Appel S, ed. *Current neurology. Vol 16.* Chicago: Mosby–Year Book, 1996:213–251.
4. Spiller WG. Subcortical epilepsy. *Brain* 1927;50: 171–187.
5. Lishman WA, Symonds CP, Witty CMW, et al. Seizures induced by movement *Brain* 1962;85:93-108.
6. Whitty CWM, Lishman WA, FitzGibbon JP. Seizures induced by movement: a form of reflex epilepsy. *Lancet* 1964;1:1403–1406.
7. Burger LJ, Lopez RI, Elliott FA. Tonic seizures induced by movement. *Neurology* 1972;22:656–659.
8. Perez-Borja C, Tassinari AC, Swanson AG. Paroxysmal choreoathetosis and seizure induced by movement (reflex epilepsy). *Epilepsia* 1967;8:260–270.
9. Mathews WB. Tonic seizures in disseminated sclerosis. *Brain* 1958;81:193–206.
10. Lance JW. Sporadic and familial varieties of tonic seizures. *J Neurol Neurosurg Psychiatry* 1963;26: 51–59.
11. Fukuyama S, Okada R. Hereditary kinesthetic reflex epilepsy. Report of five families of peculiar seizures induced by sudden movements. *Adv Neurol Sci* 1967; 11:168–197.
12. DeBolt WL. Movement epilepsy: two case reports with photographs of typical movements. *Bull Los Angeles Neurol Soc* 1967;32:1–5.
13. Hishikawa Y, Furuya E, Yamamato J, et al. Dystonic seizures induced by movement. *Arch Psychiatr Nervenkr* 1973;217:113–138.
14. Smith LA, Heersema PH. Periodic dystonia. *Staff Meet Mayo Clin* 1941;16:842–846.
15. Stevens H. Paroxysmal choreoathetosis. *Arch Neurol* 1966;14:415–420.
16. Kato M, Araki S. Paroxysmal kinesigenic choreo-

athetosis. Report of a case relieved by carbamazepine. *Arch Neurol* 1969;20:508–513.

17. Pryles CV, Livingston S, Ford FR. Familial paroxysmal choreoathetosis of Mount and Reback. *Pediatrics* 1952;9:44–47.

18. William J, Stevens H. Familial paroxysmal choreoathetosis. *Pediatrics* 1963;31:656–659.

19. Rosen JA. Paroxysmal choreoathetosis. Associated with perinatal hypoxic encephalopathy. *Arch Neurol* 1964;11:385–387.

20. Wagner GS, Mclees BD, Hatcher MA. Familial paroxysmal choreoathetosis. *Neurology* 1966;16:307.

21. Jung SS, Chen KM, Brody JA. Paroxysmal choreoathetosis: report of Chinese cases. *Neurology* 1973;23: 749–755.

22. Tabaee-Zadeh MJ, Frame B, Kapphahn K. Kinesigenic choreoathetosis and idiopathic hypoparathyroidism. *J Neurol Neurosurg Psychiatry* 1972;286:762–763.

23. Kertesz A. Paroxysmal kinesigenic choreoathetosis. An entity within the paroxysmal choreoathetosis syndrome. Description of 10 cases, including 1 autopsied. *Neurology* 1967;17:680–690.

24. Loong SC, Ong YY. Paroxysmal kinesigenic choreoathetosis: report of a case relieved by L-dopa. *J Neurol Neurosurg Psychiatry* 1973;36:921–924.

25. Goodenough DJ, Fariello RG, Annis BL, et al. Familial and acquired paroxysmal dyskinesias. A proposed classification with delineation of clinical features. *Arch Neurol* 1978;35:827–831.

26. Homan RW, Vasko MR, Blaw M. Phenytoin plasma concentrations in paroxysmal kinesigenic choreoathetosis. *Neurology* 1980;30:673–676.

27. Suber DA, Riley TL. Valproic acid and normal computerized tomographic scan in kinesigenic paroxysmal choreoathetosis. *Arch Neurol* 1980;37:327.

28. Fahn S. The paroxysmal dyskinesias. In: Marsden CD, Fahn S, eds. *Movement disorders 3*. Oxford: Butterworth-Heinemann, 1994:310–345.

29. Houser MK, Soland VL, Marsden CD, et al. Paroxysmal kinesigenic choreoathetosis: a report of 26 patients. *J Neurol* 1999;246:120–126.

30. Shintani S, Shiozawa Z, Tsunoda S, et al. Paroxysmal choreoathetosis precipitated by movement, sound and photic stimulation in a case of arterio-venous malformation in the parietal lobe. *Clin Neurol Neurosurg* 1991;93:237–239.

31. Plant G. Focal paroxysmal kinesigenic choreoathetosis. *J Neurol Neurosurg Psychiatry* 1983;46:345–348.

32. Nagamitsu S, Matsuishi T, Hashimoto K, et al. Multicenter study of paroxysmal dyskinesias in Japan-Clinical and pedigree analysis. *Mov Disord* 1999;14: 658–663.

33. Tomita HA, Nagamitsu S, Wakui K, et al. Paroxysmal kinesigenic choreoathetosis locus maps to chromosome 16p11.2-q12.1. *Am J Hum Genet* 1999;65: 1688–1697.

34. Bennett LB, Roach ES, Bowcock AM. A locus for paroxysmal kinesigenic dyskinesia maps to human chromosome 16. *Neurology* 2000;54:125–130.

35. Szepetowski P, Rochette J, Berquin P, et al. Familial infantile convulsions and paroxysmal choreoathetosis: a new neurological syndrome linked to the pericentromeric region of human chromosome 16. *Am J Hum Genet* 1997;61:889–898.

36. Lee WL, Tay A, Ong HT, et al. Association of infantile convulsions with paroxysmal dyskinesias (ICCA syndrome): confirmation of linkage to human chromosome 16p12-q12 in a Chinese family. *Hum Genet* 1998;103:608–612.

37. Swoboda KJ, Soong BW, McKenna C, et al. Paroxysmal kinesigenic dyskinesia and infantile convulsions: clinical and linkage studies. *Neurology* 2000;55:224–230.

38. Valente EM, Spacey SD, Wali GM, et al. A second paroxysmal kinesigenic choreoathetosis locus (EKD2) mapping on 16q13-q22.1 indicates a family of genes which give rise to paroxysmal disorders on human chromosome 16. *Brain* 2000;123:2040–2045.

39. Picard F, Tassin J, Vidailhet M, et al, Brice A. Autosomal dominant paroxysmal kinesigenic choreoathetosis: a clinical and genetic study of two families. *J Neurol Neurosurg Psychiatry* 1998;65:955–956.

40. Sadamatsu M, Masui A, Sakai T, et al. Familial paroxysmal kinesigenic choreoathetosis: an electrophysiologic and genotypic analysis. *Epilepsia* 1999;40: 942–949.

41. Berger JR, Sheremata WA, Melamed E. Paroxysmal dystonia as the initial manifestation of multiple sclerosis. *Arch Neurol* 1984;41:747–750.

42. Verheul GAM, Tyssen CC. Multiple sclerosis occurring with paroxysmal dystonia. *Mov Disord* 1990;6: 180–182.

43. Roos R, Wintzen AR, Vielvoye G. Paroxysmal kinesigenic choreoathetosis as presenting symptom of multiple sclerosis. *J Neurol Neurosurg Psychiatry* 1991; 54:657–658.

44. Burguera JA, Catala J, Casanova B. Thalamic demyelination and paroxysmal dystonia in multiple sclerosis. *Mov Disord* 1991;6:379–381.

45. Sethi KD, Hess DC, Huffnagle VH, et al. Acetazolamide treatment of paroxysmal dystonia in central demyelinating disease. *Neurology* 1992;42:919–921.

46. Tranchant C, Bhatia KP, Marsden CD. Movement disorders in multiple sclerosis. *Mov Disord* 1995;10: 418–423.

47. Blakeley J, Jankovic J. Secondary paroxysmal dyskinesias. *Mov Disord* (in press).

48. Robin JJ. Paroxysmal choreoathetosis following head injury. *Ann Neurol* 1977;2:447–448.

49. Drake ME Jr, Jackson RD, Miller CA. Paroxysmal choreoathetosis after head injury. *J Neurol Neurosurg Psychiatry* 1986;49:837–843.

50. Camac A, Greene P, Khandji A. Paroxysmal kinesigenic dystonic choreoathetosis associated with a thalamic infarct. *Mov Disord* 1990;5:235–238.

51. Nijssen PCG, Tijssen CC. Stimulus sensitive paroxysmal dyskinesias associated with a thalamic infarct. *Mov Disord* 1992;7:364–366.

52. Merchut MP, Brumlik J. Painful tonic spasms caused by putaminal infarction. *Stroke* 1986;17:1319–1321.

53. Arden F. Idiopathic hypoparathyroidism. *Med J Aust* 1953;2:217–219.

54. Barabas G, Tucker SM. Idiopathic hypoparathyroidism and paroxysmal dystonic choreoathetosis. *Ann Neurol* 1988;24:585.

55. Dure LS, Mussell HG. Paroxysmal dyskinesia in a patient with pseudohypoparathyroidism. *Mov Disord* 1998;13:746–748.

56. Yen DJ, Shan DE, Lu SR. Hypothyroidism presenting as recurrent short paroxysmal kinesigenic dyskinesia. *Mov Disord* 1998;13:361–363.

57. Adam AM, Orinda D. Focal paroxysmal kinesigenic choreoathetosis preceding the development of Steele-Richardson-Olszewski syndrome. *J Neurol Neurosurg Psychiatry* 1986;49:957–968.

58. Hennis A, Corbin D, Fraser H. Focal seizures and non-ketotic hyperglycemia. *J Neurol Neurosurg Psychiatry* 1992;55:195–197.

59. Aquino A Gabor AJ. Movement induced seizures in non-ketotic hyperglycemia. *Neurology* 1980;30:600–604.

60. Clark JD, Pahwa R, Koller WC. Diabetes mellitus presenting as paroxysmal kinesigenic dystonic choreoathetosis. *Mov Disord* 1995;10:354–355.

61. Hirata K, Katayama S, Saito T, et al. Paroxysmal kinesigenic choreoathetosis with abnormal electroencephalogram during attacks. *Epilepsia* 1991;32:492–494.

62. Przuntek H, Monninger P. Therapeutic aspects of kinesigenic paroxysmal choreoathetosis and familial paroxysmal choreoathetosis of the Mount and Reback type. *J Neurol* 1983;230:163–169.

63. Reitter B, Weisser J. Familial paroxysmal choreoathetosis. Clinical course, L-dopa effect. *Monatsschr Kinderheilkd* 1978;126:405–407.

64. Lou HC. Flunarizine in paroxysmal choreoathetosis (letter). *Neuropediatrics* 1989;20:112.

65. Mount LA, Reback S. Familial paroxysmal choreoathetosis. *Arch Neurol Psychiatry* 1940;44:841–847.

66. Joynt RJ, Green D. Tonic seizures as a manifestation in multiple sclerosis. *Arch Neurol* 1962;6:293–299.

67. Mushet GR, Dreifuss FE. Paroxysmal dyskinesia. A case responsive to benzotropin mesylate. *Arch Dis Child* 1967;42:654–656.

68. Cavanagh NP, Bickell J, Howard F. Cystinuria with mental retardation and paroxysmal dyskinesia in two brothers. *Arch Dis Child* 1974;49:662–664.

69. Soffer D, Licht A, Yaar I, et al. Paroxysmal choreoathetosis as a presenting symptom in idiopathic hypoparathyroidism. *J Neurol Neurosurg Psychiatry* 1977;40:692–694.

70. Richards RN, Barnett HJ. Paroxysmal dystonic choreoathetosis. A family study and review of the literature. *Neurology* 1968;18:461–469.

71. Bressman SB, Fahn S, Burke RE. Paroxysmal non-kinesigenic dystonia. In: Fahn S, Marsden CD, Calne DB, eds. *Dystonia 2. Advances in Neurology.* Vol. 50. New York: Raven Press, 1988:403–413.

72. Kinast M, Erenberg G, Rothner AD. Paroxysmal choreoathetosis: report of five cases and review of the literature. *Pediatrics* 1980;65:74–77.

73. Bhatia KP. The paroxysmal dyskinesias. *J Neurol* 1999:246:149–155.

74. Perlmutter JS, Raichle ME. Pure hemidystonia with basal ganglion abnormalities on positron emission tomography. *Ann Neurol* 1984;15:228–233.

75. Tibbles JA, Barnes SE. Paroxysmal dystonic choreoathetosis of Mount and Reback. *Pediatrics* 1980;65: 149–151.

76. Byrne E, White O, Cook M. Familial dystonic choreoathetosis with myokymia; a sleep responsive disorder. *J Neurol Neurosurg Psychiatry* 1991;54:1090–1092.

77. Bird TD, Carlson CB, Horning M. Ten year follow-up of paroxysmal choreoathetosis: a sporadic case becomes familial. *Epilepsia* 1978;19:129–132.

78. Kurlan R, Shoulson I. Familial paroxysmal dystonic choreoathetosis response to alternate-day oxazepam therapy. *Ann Neurol* 1983;13:456–457.

79. Fahn S, Williams DT. Psychogenic dystonia. *Adv Neurol* 1988;50:431–455.

80. Erickson GR, Chun RW. Acquired paroxysmal movement disorders. *Pediatr Neurol* 1987;3:226–229.

81. Yamamoto K, Kawazawa S. Basal ganglia calcification in paroxysmal dystonic choreoathetosis. *Ann Neurol* 1987;22:556.

82. Margolin D, Marsden CD. Transient dyskinesia and cerebral ischemia. *Neurology* 1982;32:1379–1380.

83. Bennett DA, Fox J. Paroxysmal dyskinesia secondary to cerebral vascular disease-reversal with aspirin. *Clin Neuropharmacol* 1989;12:215–216.

84. Winer JB, Fish Dr, Marsden CD, et al. A movement disorder as a presenting feature of recurrent hypoglycemia. *Mov Disord* 1990;5:176–177.

85. Nath A, Jankovic J, Pettigrew LC. Movement disorders and AIDS. *Neurology* 1987;37:37–41.

86. Haan J, Kremer HPH, Padberg G. Paroxysmal choreoathetosis as a presenting symptom of diabetes mellitus. *J Neurol Neurosurg Psychiatry* 1988;52:133.

87. Micheli F, Fernandez Pardal M, de Arbelaiz R, et al. Paroxysmal dystonia responsive to anticholinergic drugs. *Clin Neuropharmacol* 1987;10:365–369.

88. Coulter DL, Donofrio P. Haloperidol for nonkinesigenic paroxysmal dyskinesia. *Arch Neurol* 1980;37: 325–326.

89. Micheli F, Frenandez Pardal M, Casas Parera I, et al. Sporadic paroxysmal dystonic choreoathetosis associated with basal ganglia calcifications. *Ann Neurol* 1986;20:750.

90. Newman R., Kinkel WR. Paroxysmal choreoathetosis due to hypoglycemia. *Arch Neurol* 1984;41:341–342.

91. Fischbeck KH, Layzer RB. Paroxysmal choreoathetosis associated with thyrotoxicosis. *Ann Neurol* 1979; 6:453–454.

92. Schmidt BJ, Pillay N. Paroxysmal dyskinesia associated with hypoglycemia. *Can J Neurol Sci* 1993;20: 151–153.

93. Lera G, Bhatia K, Marsden CD. Dystonia as the major manifestation of Leigh's syndrome. *Mov Disord* 1994; 9:642–649.

94. Jarman PR, Bhatia KP, Davie C, et al. Paroxysmal dystonic choreoathetosis: clinical features and investigation of pathophysiology in a large family. *Mov Disord* 2000;15(4):648–657.

95. Fernandez M, Raskind W, Wolff J, et al. Familial dyskinesia and facial myokymia (FDFM): a novel movement disorder. *Ann Neurol* 2001;49:486–492.

96. Auburger G, Ratzlaff T, Lunkes A, et al. A gene for autosomal dominant paroxysmal choreoathetosis/spasticity (CSE) maps to the vicinity of a potassium channel gene cluster on chromosome 1p, probably within 2 cM between D1S443 and D1S197. *Genomics* 1996; 31:90–94.

97. Fink JK, Rainier S, Wilkowski J, et al. Paroxysmal dystonic choreoathetosis: tight linkage to chromosome 2q. *Am J Hum Genet* 1996;59:140–145.

98. Fouad GT, Servidei S, Durcan S, et al. A gene for familial paroxysmal dyskinesia (FPD1) maps top chromosome 2q. *Am J Hum Genet* 1996;59:135–139.

99. Hofele K, Benecke R, Auburger G. Gene locus FPD1 of the dystonic Mount-Reback type of autosomal-

dominant paroxysmal choreoathetosis. *Neurology* 1997;49:1252–1256.

100. Jarman PR, Davis MB, Marsden CD, et al. Paroxysmal dystonic choreoathetosis: genetic linkage studies in a British family. *Brain* 1997;120:2125–2130.

101. Raskind WH, Bolin T, Wolf J, et al. Further localization of a gene for paroxysmal dystonic choreoathetosis to a 5-cM region on chromosome 2q34. *Hum Genet* 1998;102:93–97.

102. Matsuo H, Kamakuro K, Saito M, et al. Familial paroxysmal dystonic choreoathetosis: clinical findings in a large Japanese family and genetic linkage to 2q. *Arch Neurol* 1999;56:721–726.

103. Su YR, Klanke CA, HousealTW, et al. Molecular cloning and physical and genetic mapping of the human anion exchanger isoform 3 (SLC2C) gene chromosome 2q36. *Genomics* 1994;22:605–609.

104. Plant GT, Williams AC, Marsden CD, et al. Familial paroxysmal dystonia induced by exercise. *J Neurol Neurosurg Psychiatry* 1984;47:275–279.

105. Kurlan R, Medved L, Shoulson I. Familial paroxysmal dystonic choreoathetosis: a family study. *Mov Disord* 1987;2:187–192.

106. Bathia KP, Soland VL, Marsden CD, et al. Paroxysmal exercise-induced dystonia: eight new sporadic cases and review of the literature. *Mov Disord* 1997;12 (6): 1007–1012.

107. Münchau A, Valente EM, Shahidi GA, et al. A new family with paroxysmal exercise-induced dystonia and migraine: a clinical and genetic study. *J Neurol Neurosurg Psychiatry* 2000;68:609–614.

108. Nardocci N, Lamperti E, Rumi V, et al. Typical and atypical forms of paroxysmal choreoathetosis. *Dev Med Child Neurol* 1989;31:670–674.

109. Wali GM. Paroxysmal hemidystonia induced by prolong exercise and cold. *J Neurol Neurosurg Psychiatry* 1992;55:236–237.

110. Guerrini R, Bonanni P, Nardocci N, et al. Autosomal recessive rolandic epilepsy with paroxysmal exercise-induced dystonia and writer's cramp: deliniation of the syndrome and gene mapping to chromosome 16p12-11.2. *Ann Neurol* 1999;45:344–352.

111. Neville BGR, Besag FMC, Marsden CD. Exercise-induced steroid dependent dystonia, ataxia, and alternating hemiplegia associated with epilepsy. *J Neurol Neurosurg Psychiatry* 1998;65:241–244.

112. Lugaressi E, Cirignotta F. Hypnogenic paroxysmal dystonia: epileptic seizure or a new syndrome? *Sleep* 1981;4:129–138.

113. Lugaressi E, Cirignotta F, Montagna P. Nocturnal paroxysmal dystonia. *J Neurol Neurosurg Psychiatry* 1986;49:375–380.

114. Lee BI, Lesser R, Pippenger CE, et al. Familial paroxysmal hypnogenic dystonia. *Neurology* 1985;35: 1357–1360.

115. Crowell JA, Anders TF. Hypnogenic paroxysmal dystonia. *J Am Acad Child Psychiatry* 1985;24:353–358.

116. Lehkuniek E, Micheli F, De Arbalaiz R, et al. Concurrent hypnogenic and reflex paroxysmal dystonia. *Mov Disord* 1988;3:290–294.

117. Tartara A, Manni R, Piccolo G. A long-lasting CBZ controlled case of hypnogenic paroxysmal dystonia. *Ital J Neurol Sci* 1988;9:73–76.

118. Godbout R, Montplaiser J, Rouleau I. Hypnogenic paroxysmal dystonia: epilepsy or sleep disorder? A case report. *Clin Electroencephal* 1985;16:136–142.

119. Biary N, Singh B, Bahau Y, et al. Posttraumatic paroxysmal nocturnal hemidystonia. *Mov Disord* 1994;9: 98–99.

120. Tinuper P, Cerullo A, Cirignotta F, et al. Nocturnal paroxysmal dystonia with short-lasting attacks: three cases with evidence for an epileptic frontal lobe origin of seizures. *Epilepsia* 1990;31:549–556.

121. de Saint-Martin A, Badinand N, Picard F, et al. Diurnal and nocturnal paroxysmal dyskinesia in young children: a new entity? *Rev Neurol* 1997;153(4):262–267.

122. Morley JB. Movement induced epilepsy: three case reports and comparison with a case of hemiballismus. *Proc Aust Assoc Neurol* 1970;7:19–24.

123. Oguni M, Oguni H, Kozasa M, et al. A case with nocturnal paroxysmal unilateral dystonia and interictal right frontal epileptic EEG focus: a lateralized variant of nocturnal paroxysmal dystonia. *Brain Dev* 1992; 14:412–416.

124. Meierkord H, Fish DR, Marsden CD, et al. Is nocturnal paroxysmal dystonia form of frontal lobe epilepsy? *Mov Disord* 1992;7:38–42.

125. Horner FH, Jackson LC. Familial paroxysmal choreoathetosis. In Barbeau A, Brunette JR, eds. *Progress in neuro-genetics*. Amsterdam: Excerpta Medica Foundation, 1969:745–751.

126. Fish DR, Marsden CD. Epilepsy masquerading as a movement disorder. In: Marsden CD, Fahn S, eds. *Movement disorders 3*. Oxford: Butterworth-Heinemann, 1994:346–358.

127. Scheffer IE, Bathia KP, Lopes-Cendes I, et al. Autosomal dominant nocturnal frontal lobe epilepsy: a distinctive clinical disorder. *Brain* 1995;118:61–73.

128. Scheffer IE, Bathia KP, Lopes-Cendes I, et al. Autosomal dominant nocturnal frontal lobe epilepsy misdiagnosed as a sleep disorder. *Lancet* 1994;343:515–517.

129. Philips HA, Scheffer IE, Berkovic SF, et al. Localization of a gene for autosomal dominant nocturnal frontal lobe epilepsy to chromosome 20q13.2. *Nat Genet* 1995;10:117–118.

130. Griggs RC, Moxley RT, Lafrance RA, et al. Hereditary paroxysmal ataxia: response to acetazolamide. *Neurology*1978;28:1259–1264.

131. Friedman J, Hollman PA. Acetazolamide responsive hereditary paroxysmal ataxia. *Mov Disord* 1987;2: 67–72.

132. Gancher ST, Nutt JC. Autosomal dominant episodic ataxia: a heterogeneous syndrome. *Mov Disord* 1986; 1:239–253.

133. Van Bogaert P, Van Nechel C, Goldman S, et al. Acetazolamide- responsive hereditary paroxysmal ataxia: report of a new family. *Acta Neurol Belg* 1993;93: 268–275.

134. Hawkes CH. Familial periodic ataxia: report of a family. *J Neurol Neurosurg Psychiatry* 1992;55:212–213.

135. Brunt ER, van Weerden TW. Familial paroxysmal kinesigenic ataxia and continuous myokymia. *Brain* 1990;113:1361–1382.

136. Griggs RC, Nutt JG. Episodic ataxias as channelopathies. *Ann Neurol* 1995;37:285–287.

137. Kramer P, Litt M, Browne D. Autosomal episodic ataxia represents at least two genetic disorders. *Ann Neurol* 1994;36:279.

138. Van Dyke DH, Griggs RC, Murphy MJ, et al. Hereditary myokymia and periodic ataxia. *J Neurol* 1975;25: 109–118.

139. Hanson PA, Martinez LB, Cassidy R. Contractures, continuous muscle discharge and titubation. *Ann Neurol* 1977;1:120–124.

140. Browne DL, Gancher ST, Nutt JG, et al. Episodic ataxia/myokymia syndrome is associated with point mutations in the human potassium channel gene, KCNA1. *Nat Genet* 1994;8:136–140.

141. Litt M, Kramer P, Browne D, et al. A gene for episodic ataxia/myokymia maps to chromosome 12p13. *Am J Hum Genet* 1994;55:702–709.

142. Adelman JP, Bond CT, Pessia M, et al. Episodic ataxia results from voltage-dependent potassium channels with altered functions. *Neuron* 1995;15:1449–1454.

143. Zerr P, Adelman JP, Maylie J. Episodic ataxia mutations in Kv1.1 alter potassium channel function by dominant negative effects or haploinsufficiency. *J Neurosci* 1998;18:2842–2848.

144. Zerr P, Adelman JP, Maylie J. Characterization of three episodic ataxia mutations in the human Kv1.1 potassium channel. *FEBS Lett* 1998;431:461–464.

145. Zuberi SM, Eunson LH, Spauschus A, et al. A novel mutation in the human voltage-gated potassium channel gene (*Kv1.1*) associates with episodic ataxia type 1 and sometimes with partial epilepsy. *Brain* 1999;122: 817–825.

146. Scheffer H, Brunt ER, Mol GJ, et al. Three novel KCNA1 mutations in episodic ataxia type I families. *Hum Genet* 1998;102:464–466.

147. Boland LM, Price DL, Jackson KA. Episodic ataxia/myokymia mutations functionally expressed in the Shaker potassium channel. *Neuroscience* 1999;91(4): 1557–1564.

148. Noebels JL. Targeting epilepsy genes. *Neuron* 1996; 16:241–244.

149. Browne DL, Brunt ER, Griggs RC, et al. Identification of two new KCNA1 mutations in episodic ataxia/myokymia families. *Hum Mol Genet* 1995;4:1671–1672.

150. Lubbers WJ, Brunt ERP, Scheffer H, et al. Hereditary myokymia and paroxysmal ataxia linked to chromosome 12 is responsive to acetazolamide. *J Neurol Neurosurg Psychiatry*1995;59:400–405.

151. Comu S, Giuliani M, Narayanan V. Episodic ataxia and myokymia syndrome: a new mutation of potassium channel gene Kv1.1. *Ann Neurol* 1996;40:684–687.

152. Vaamonde J, Artieda J, Obeso JA. Hereditary paroxysmal ataxia with neuromyotonia. *Mov Disord* 1991;6: 180–227.

153. Bulman DE. Phenotype variation and newcomers in ion channel disorders. *Hum Mol Genet* 1997;6:1679–1685.

154. Eunson LH, Rea R, Zuberi SM, et al. Clinical, genetic, and expression studies of mutations in the potassium channel gene KCNA1 reveal new phenotypic variability. *Ann Neurol* 2000;48:647–656.

155. Vahedi K, Joutel A, Van Bogaert P, et al. A gene for hereditary paroxysmal cerebellar ataxia maps to chromosome 19p. *Ann Neurol* 1995;37:289–293.

156. Joutel A, Bousser MG, Biousse V, et al. A gene for familial hemiplegic migraine maps to chromosome 19. *Nat Genet* 1993;5:40–45.

157. Kramer PL, Smith E, Carrero-Valenzuela R, et al. A gene for nystagmus associated episodic ataxia maps to chromosome 19p (abstract). *Am J Hum Genet* 1994;55 (suppl):A191.

158. Ophoff RA, Terwindt GM, Vergouwe MN, et al. Familial hemiplegic migraine and episodic ataxia type 2 are caused by mutations in the Ca(2+) channel gene CACNL1A4. *Cell* 1996;87:543–552.

159. Calandriello L, Veneziano L, Francia A, et al. Acetazolamide-responsive episodic ataxia in an Italian family refines gene mapping on chromosome 19p13. *Brain* 1997;120:805–812.

160. Baloh RW, Yue Q, Furman JM, et al. Familial episodic ataxia: clinical heterogeneity in four families linked to chromosome 19p. *Ann Neurol* 1997;41:8–16.

161. Yue Q, Jen JC, Thwe MM, et al. De nova mutation in CACNA1A caused acetazolamide-responsive episodic ataxia. *Am J Med Genet* 1998;77:298–301.

162. Yue Q, Jen JC, Nelson SF, et al. Progressive ataxia due to a missense mutation in a calcium-channel gene. *Am J Hum Genet* 1997;61:1078–1087.

163. Denier C, Ducros A, Vahedi K, et al. High prevalence of CACNA1A truncations and broader clinical spectrum in episodic ataxia type 2. *Neurology* 1999;52: 1816–1821.

164. Battistini S, Stenirri S, Piatti M, et al. A new CACNA1A gene mutation in acetazolamide-responsive familial hemiplegic migraine and ataxia. *Neurology* 1999;53:38–43.

165. Carrera P, Piatti M, Stenirri S, et al. Genetic heterogeneity in Italian families with familial hemiplegic migraine. *Neurology* 1999;53:26–33.

166. Jen J, Yue Q, Nelson SF, et al. A novel nonsense mutation in CACNA1A causes episodic ataxia and hemiplegia. *Neurology* 1999;53:34–37.

167. Tournier-Lasserve E. CACNA1A mutations: hemiplegic migraine, episodic ataxia type 2, and the others. *Neurology* 1999;53:3–4.

168. Baron DN, Dent CE, Harris H. Hereditary pellagra-like skin rash with temporary cerebellar ataxia, constant renal amino-aciduria and other bizarre biochemical features. *Lancet* 1956;2:421–428.

169. Dancis J, Hutzler J, Rokkones T. Intermittent branched-chain ketonuria: variant of maple-syrup-urine disease. *N Engl J Med* 1967;276:84–96.

170. Blass JP, Avigan J, Uhlendorf BV. A defect in pyruvate decarboxylase in a child with an intermittent movement disorder. *J Clin Invest* 1970;49:423–432.

171. Mayeux R, Fahn S. Paroxysmal dystonic choreoathetosis in a patient with familial ataxia. *Neurology* 1982;32:1184–1186.

172. Bathia K, Griggs RC, Ptacek LJ. Episodic movement disorders as channelopathies. *Mov Disord* 2000;15: 429–433.

173. Lennox WG, Lennox MA. *Epilepsy and related disorders. Vol 1.* Boston: Little, Brown, 1960.

174. Singh R, Macdonell RA, Scheffer IE, et al. Epilepsy and paroxysmal movement disorders in families: evidence for shared mechanisms. *Epileptic Disord* 1999;1 (2):93–99.

175. Kim MO, Im JH, Choi CG, et al. Proton MR spectroscopic findings in paroxysmal kinesigenic dyskinesia. *Mov Disord* 1998;13:570–575.

176. Wahnschaffe U, Fredow G, Heintz P, et al. Neuropathological studies in a mutant hamster model of paroxysmal dystonia. *Mov Disord* 1990;5:286–293.

Myoclonus and Paroxysmal Dyskinesias,
Advances in Neurology, Vol. 89,
edited by S. Fahn, et al.
Published by Lippincott Williams & Wilkins, Philadelphia, 2002.

36

Secondary Causes of Paroxysmal Dyskinesia

Jaishri Blakeley and Joseph Jankovic

Department of Neurology, Parkinson's Disease Center and Movement Disorders Clinic,
Baylor College of Medicine, Houston, Texas

Paroxysmal dyskinesias (PxD) are rare movement disorders that are involuntary, episodic, and sudden in onset. Movements may include any combination of dystonia, chorea, athetosis, or ballism. There are four major types of PxD that are differentiated by the event that precipitates the paroxysmal movement (see Chapter 35). PxD precipitated by sudden voluntary movements are termed kinesigenic (paroxysmal kinesigenic dyskinesia: PKD). PxD that occurs spontaneously at rest are termed non-kinesigenic (paroxysmal non-kinesigenic dyskinesia: PNKD). The two less common types of PxD are precipitated by exertion (paroxysmal exertion-induced dyskinesia: PED) or occur in the setting of sleep (paroxysmal hypnogenic dyskinesia: PHD) (1).

The pathophysiology of PxD is unknown; hence the distinction between PKD and PNKD is based chiefly on key clinical features. PKD occurs after a sudden voluntary movement and the episode is generally shorter in duration (seconds) and more frequent (multiple per day) than PNKD (1–4). PKD is also more responsive to pharmacotherapy, particularly anticonvulsant medications, than PNKD (5–7). In PNKD, more so than PKD, a wide range of factors including stress, temperature changes, fatigue, caffeine, and alcohol may exacerbate symptoms. Early reports attempted to describe the movement as choreic, athetotic, dystonic, or other. More recent reviews, however, suggest that the general term "dyskinesia" is more appropriate because the movements are often complex and in many cases are not witnessed by the diagnosing physician (1,2,7). Because PxD symptoms are episodic, sudden in onset and in some cases sensitive to anticonvulsant therapy, there is a long-standing controversy about whether the paroxysmal symptoms are due to movement versus epileptic disorders. Indeed, the early descriptions of PxD in the literature had titles such as "seizures induced by movement" (8,9) and "tonic seizures" (10). However, the rarity of abnormal electroencephalograms (EEG), the failure to document change in consciousness during or after episodes, and the similarity of PxD movements to those seen in other movement disorders argues against an cortical epileptic disorder, although paroxysmal events arising in subcortical (basal ganglia) structures has been postulated as a possible mechanism for this group of neurologic disorders.

In the majority of patients with PxD, there is evidence of familial inheritance (usually in an autosomal dominant pattern) or no specific etiology can be identified for their PxD. However, there are several cases in which there is a recognizable etiology associated with the PxD. Although there have been multiple case reports of secondary PxD, there has not been a large case series evaluating the characteristics, likely etiologies and response to treatment of secondary PxDs. We present a series of 20 patients in whom we identified an etiology for their PxD other than genetic or psychogenic and a review 130 cases of secondary PxD reported in the literature.

METHODS

Ninety-two patients diagnosed with PxD were identified from the Baylor College of Medicine Parkinson's Disease Center and Movement Disorders Clinic database of 12,063 patients evaluated between 1981 and 2000. Of those, 16 patients had incomplete records and were excluded from the study. Hence, 76 charts were reviewed for confirmation of the diagnosis of PxD and evidence of secondary etiologies. Inclusion criteria were (a) evidence of PxD by examination, review of videotape, and/or history; and (b) evidence of temporally and/or structurally related neurologic insult or disease. Exclusion criteria were (a) diagnosis of familial PxD, (b) positive family or personal history of dyskinesia or seizure disorder, and (c) evidence of a psychogenic etiology. Patients were diagnosed with psychogenic PxD if they had relief of symptoms with placebo, inconsistent neurologic examinations, false sensory examinations, or obvious psychiatric diagnoses (1,11).

All patients underwent thorough clinical evaluation at the Parkinson's Disease Center and Movement Disorders Clinic. PKD was diagnosed if sudden voluntary movements precipitated the involuntary movements. PNKD was diagnosed if the involuntary movements occurred spontaneously at rest. PHD was diagnosed when patients had episodic involuntary movements only during or emerging from sleep and PED was diagnosed when the involuntary movements followed prolonged physical exertion (1). None of the patients had changes in consciousness during or after the episodes, incontinence, or any other symptoms of seizure activity.

Charts were reviewed for demographics and the following clinical data: diagnosis, etiology, age at onset, temporal relationship between event and symptom onset, type and location of movement and injury, frequency and duration of symptoms, precipitants, exacer-

bating factors, progression of symptoms, presence of auras or pain, and treatment. Movements were categorized as dystonic, choreic, athetotic, or ballistic by the examining physician when possible, or in a few cases according to patient and witness reports. The predominant movement type was reported. However, in general the term dyskinesia was used to more accurately describe all of the patients with PxD, including those who had complex movements. Every effort was made to review all cases of secondary PxD previously published; however, there may be additional reports that were missed. Articles were included in the review if the symptoms described indicated that the movement was consistent with a paroxysmal dyskinesia (sudden onset, episodic, abnormal, involuntary movement without change in consciousness, or other evidence of seizure activity).

RESULTS

Of the 76 patients with PxD, 56 were excluded from analysis due to diagnosis of: familial PxD (31 patients), psychogenic PxD (21 patients), or alternative diagnoses (four patients). Twenty of the 76 patients had the diagnosis of secondary PxD (26%). Etiologies included peripheral trauma (six patients), vascular lesions (four patients), central traumatic lesions (four patients), kernicterus (two patients), and one patient each with multiple sclerosis (MS), cytomegalovirus (CMV) encephalitis, meningovascular syphilis, and migraine. There were ten men (mean age at onset: 41.4 years) and ten women (mean age at onset: 36.5 years). Although the range of age at onset varied widely from 2.5 to 79 years, vascular etiologies presented at older ages (mean 65) and trauma presented at younger ages (mean 33) (Table 36.1).

Ten patients were diagnosed with PNKD, three with PKD, and one with PHD according to the Demirkiran and Jankovic classification (1). Six patients had symptoms compatible with both PKD and PNKD, making classification difficult. These patients were referred to as "mixed" (Table 36.1).

TABLE 36.1. *Clinical features of secondary paroxysmal dyskinesias in 20 patients by suspected etiology*

Etiology	Age at onset	Gender	Diagnosis	Duration	Frequency	Precipitant	Exacerbating	Aura	Pain
Stroke	56	M	PNKD	1–2 hr	5/d		Fatigue	No	No
	68	M	PNKD	15–45 sec	1–2 min		Worse at night	No	No
	58	M	PNHD	<5 min	1/night			No	No
Peripheral trauma	79	F	Mixed	<5 min	1/mo → 1/wk	Stretching/yawning		No	No
	58	M	PKD	1 min	1–3/d	Rapid movement/rest		No	Yes
	17	F	PKD	<30 sec	5/wk → 5/d	Finger flexion		No	No
	29	F	PKD	Sec–min	1/hr	Rapid leg movement	Stress	Disorientation	No
	49	F	PNKD	30 min	6–8/d	Writing, walking		No	No
	39	F	Mixed	15–20 min	1 to 3/d → 5/day	Hand movements/light touch to arm/rest	Stress	No	No
	53	F	Mixed	2–12 hr	6–7/mo	Talking/rest	Stress/anxiety	"Pouf" sound	No
Central trauma	53	M	Mixed	1–45 min	1–5/d	Grasping, writing	Cold, fatigue	Left-hand tension	Yes
	17	M	PNKD	30 sec–2 min	3–6/d		Onset of headache	No	Yes
Kernicterus	7	M	PNKD	10–15 d	4/yr		Worse at night	No	Yes
	9	M	Mixed	5–10 min	1 to 30–40 min	Rapid movement/rest	Stress/anxiety	"Dizziness"	No
	2.5	F	PNKD	10 sec–2 min	0–20/d		Excitement activity	No	Yes
	18	M	PNKD	1–2 hr	Multiple/day			No	Yes
Meningiovascular syphilis	70	M	Mixed	10–15 min	3/d	Purposeful movements/rest		No	No
CMV encephalitis	7	F	PNKD	20–30 min	2/wk → 2/d		Stress/anxiety	Sweating, "gets quiet"	No
Multiple sclerosis	44	F	PNKD	10–15 sec	0–20/d		Heat	Right-face tension	No
Migraine	46	F	PNKD	5 min	2–3/wk	Occurs with migraine aura symptoms		No	No

PNKD, paroxysmal nonkinesigenic dyskinesia; PKD, paroxysmal kinesigenic dyskinesia; PHD, paroxysmal hypnogenic dyskinesia; *arrow* indicates that symptoms progressed to increased frequency.

The mean latency from the initial insult to the onset of PxD was 3 years, ranging from days (trauma) to 18 years (kernicterus). All three of the patients with PKD presented within 6 months of peripheral trauma. The patient with PHD suffered a stroke 6 years prior to the onset of PxD. In this case, the PxD symptoms were in the distribution of his resolved hemiparesis. In three cases, the underlying etiology was not identified until the workup for PxD was initiated, hence the temporal relationship between insult and onset of symptoms could not be determined. These cases had anatomically related lesions on MRI. Latency could not be accurately calculated in two additional patients in whom PxD symptoms developed on a background of chronic neurologic deficits (the patients with MS and history of multiple neurosurgeries, hydrocephalus and Arnold-Chiari malformation, respectively) (Table 36.2).

Dystonia was the most common primary movement (19 of 20 patients). When present, chorea, ballism, athetosis, and various hyperkinesias occurred concurrently with dystonia in all but one case. The patient with meningovascular syphilis had chorea without dystonia. There was no relationship between the type or location of the neurologic insult and the predominant type of movement. Consistent with previous reports (7,12,13), the majority of patients in this series (12 patients) had unilateral, axial distribution of the involuntary movement (seven right, five left). Three patients had bilateral dyskinesias and five had primary face and neck involvement. Nine patients had progression of their symptoms from one area of the body to another. One patient progressed from unilateral to bilateral involvement and one progressed from bilateral lower to bilateral upper extremities (Table 36.2).

All three PKD patients had short duration episodes (< 5 minutes) that occurred several times per day consistent with classic descriptions (1,4,12). There was pronounced variability in both frequency and duration of symptoms in the PNKD and mixed groups. PNKD patients had symptom durations rang-

ing from 10 seconds to 15 days. Five had short duration episodes (seconds to minutes), four had durations of 30 minutes to 2 hours, and one had episodes lasting 10 to 15 days. Seven of the PNKD patients had multiple episodes per day, two had weekly symptoms, and the patient with episodes lasting 15 days had symptoms four times a year. In the mixed group, four patients had symptom durations of 5 to 20 minutes, one had episodes lasting 1 to 45 minutes, and one had symptoms for up to 12 hours. Three patients with mixed had daily symptoms and three had symptoms weekly or monthly. There was no relationship between duration and frequency of symptoms in the PNKD and Mixed groups (Table 36.1).

Patients with kinesigenic symptoms (in both the PKD and mixed groups) reported rapid movements such as jumping up from a seated position, writing, flossing teeth, or purposeful hand movements as precipitants. Patients with PNKD were more likely to report exacerbating factors (seven patients) such as fatigue, anxiety, stress, and temperature changes than were patients with PKD (one patient) or mixed (four patients). One patient with mixed PKD/PNKD secondary to peripheral trauma had episodes at rest, with sudden movements and with tactile stimulation to the involved area (Table 36.1).

Six patients identified an aura before the paroxysmal episode. Of those, four had dyskinesias secondary to trauma (one PKD and three mixed). The patient with multiple sclerosis (MS) and the patient with cytomegalovirus (CMV) encephalitis also reported auras preceding the onset of dyskinesia (both PNKD). The dystonia was painful in five patients: four cases were secondary to trauma (one PKD, two PNKD and one mixed). The final case was PNKD secondary to kernicterus. There was no relationship between type of PxD and presence of aura or pain (Table 36.1).

There was no consistent pattern of response to therapies based on either the type or etiology of the PxD. However, anticonvulsants (four patients), clonazepam (three patients), and botulinum toxin injections into the ago-

TABLE 36.2. *Location and type of insult, location of symptoms, and latency between insult and symptom onset*

Suspected etiology	Location of insult	Location of PxD symptoms	Latency of onset
Stroke	L posterior frontal subcortical infarction	Neck and jaw contraction, orobuccal stereotypy	3 yr
	L cerebral peduncle and brainstem, R cerebellum and periventricular white matter infarcts on MRI	R wrist and MCP flexion → R toe flexion; foot inversion	3 yr
	R frontopartietal infarct on CT	L hand and elbow flexion → L leg flexion	6 yr
	R globus pallidus infarct, diffuse subcortical white matter infarcts on MRI	Bilateral MCP, PIP, DIP flexion	Unknown
Peripheral trauma	C6-7 disk herniation on MRI after fall	R wrist, 1st and 2nd PIP flexion	1 d
	Blunt trauma to R leg with residual nerve damage on EMG	R foot inversion → R hand → face	4 mo
	Neck trauma after MVA, nl. MRI of brain and neck	R knee extension and foot inversion → R arm ballism	1 wk
	C3-4 and C4-5 disk herniation after MVA	Laryngospasm	1 yr
	Fracture of L hand requiring multiple surgeries	L shoulder adduction, hand and elbow flexion → L foot inversion	6 mo
	R temporomandibular joint repair, nl. brain MRI	R masseter, temporalis, and submental contraction	1 mo
Central trauma	Repaired neural tube defect, chronic hydrocephalus, ventricular shunting and 6 shunt revisions, two tethered cord repairs, and posterior fossa decompression for Arnold-Chiari defect	L 1st–3rd digits extension and adduction → R hand and arm extension and occasionally → bilateral legs	2 yr after last surgery
	Repeat closed head injury with loss of consciousness, last injury with C1-4 subluxation	R foot inversion and leg extension	2 yr
	Perinatal anoxic brain injury, grade I intraventricular hemorrhage	L arm abduction, elbow flexion and pronation, L wrist and finger flexion	3 yr
	L midbrain and cerebral peduncle static lesions	R foot inversion, toe and hand flexion, and face contraction	Unknown
Kernicterus	Prolonged neonatal jaundice treated only with sun exposure, normal MRI of brain	L face contraction with L elbow flexion and athetosis of fingers → truncal dystonia and left leg extension	11 mo
	Neonatal jaundice, Rh incompatibility hemolysis requiring multiple blood transfusions, normal MRI	R hand extension with chorea; posterior neck extension	18 yr
Meningiovascular syphilis	Brainstem infarcts and R posterior parietal encephalomalacia, + CSF VDRL & MHA-TP	L arm and R leg	Unknown
CMV encephalitis	Small poorly defined lesion in L temporal area on MRI, positive CSF viral culture	Bilateral knee extension, ankle and toe flexion and foot inversion → L MCP and arm flexion, R hip flexion, hand athetosis and facial contraction	1 mo after diagnosis of encephalitis
Multiple sclerosis	Periventricular plaques, oligoclonal bands in CSF, classic history for MS	R blethorospasm, face contraction and neck contraction → left arm extension	13 yr (1st MS sx.), 4 mo R third nerve palsy
Migraine	Migraine headaches with aura, nl. MRI of brain	L face contraction with dysarthria	6-yr history of migraines

L, left; R, right; CT, computed tomography; MRI, magnetic resonance imaging; MCP, metacarpophalangeal; PIP, proximal interphalangeal; DIP, distal interphalangeal; MVA, motor vehicle accident; EMG, electromyelogram; CSF, cerebral spinal fluid; MS, multiple sclerosis; sx., symptom; nl., normal; *arrow* indicates progression of symptoms; VDRL, Venereal Disease Research Laboratories; MHA-TP, micronemagglutination-*Treponema pallidum* test.

nist muscle (two patients) were the most frequently effective monotherapies. Twelve of the 20 patients (60%) required only one therapy. All three patients with PKD had symptom relief with a single agent. In contrast, 50% of patients with PNKD (five patients) and 66% of patients with mixed PKD/PNKD (four patients) had symptom control with a single agent. Two patients with PNKD had symptom control with tetrabenazine and trihexyphenidyl, respectively, after failing trials with multiple conventional agents. Baclofen was effective in conjunction with clonazepam for the patient with PNKD secondary to MS and as a monotherapy for the patient with PHD secondary to stroke. Treatment of the underlying etiology relieved symptoms in two patients. The patient with meningovascular

TABLE 36.3. *Effective and ineffective therapies for secondary paroxysmal dyskinesia sorted by suspected etiology*

Etiology	Effective	Ineffective
Stroke	Clonazepam and botulinum toxin	Bromazepam, madopar
	Tetrabenazine	Phenytoin, carbamazepine, gabapentin, clonazepam, trihexyphenidyl, carbidopa/levodopa, botulinum toxin
	Baclofen	—
	Botulinum toxin and carbidopa/levodopa	—
Peripheral trauma	Botulinum toxin	—
	Carbamazepine	—
	Carbamazepine	Scopolamine
	Clonazepam	Phenytoin, acetazolamide
	Carbamazepine	—
	Botulinum toxin (IV diazepam and diphenhydramine for acute episodes)	Gabapentin, trazodone
Central trauma	Clonazepam	—
		—
	Clonazepam	Diazepam, baclofen, gabapentin, botulinum toxin
	Gabapentin and carbamazepine	Phenytoin, felbamate, clonazepam, carbidopa/levodopa
Kernicterus	None	Carbamazepine, clonazepam
	Trihexyphenidyl (IV diazepam and diphenhydramine for acute episodes)	Diphenhydramine, alprazolam, diazepam, carbamazepine, baclofen, cyclobenzaprine
Meningiovascular syphilis	IV Penicillin for neurosyphilis and carbidopa/levodopa	—
CMV encephalitis	Phenobarbitol	Clonazepam, trihexyphenidyl, carbamazepine, gabapentin, valproic acid
Multiple sclerosis	Clonazepam and baclofen	—
Migraine	Migraine prophylaxis (amitriptyline)	—

IV, intravenous.

syphilis responded well to intravenous penicillin and carbidopa-levodopa and the patient with PNKD associated with migraines had relief with migraine prophylaxis. As mentioned, carbidopa-levodopa was occasionally effective. In particular it alleviated symptoms in two patients with Mixed PKD/PNKD secondary to vascular lesions accompanied by vascular parkinsonism (Table 36.3).

ILLUSTRATIVE CASES

Case 1

Mixed PKDPKND Secondary to Multiple Neurosurgeries, Chronic Hydrocephalus, and Arnold-Chiari Malformation: A 54-year-old right-handed male presented with a 1-year history of episodic contraction of his left hand. The contractions begin in the left hand, progress to the right hand and in some in-

stances, to bilateral lower extremities. The episodes occur one to five times per day, last from 1 minute to 45 minutes, and are painful. All episodes are preceded by a sense of tightening in his left hand. There is no change in consciousness during or after the attacks. Attacks are precipitated by voluntary movements of his hands such as picking up a fork. Over time the symptoms progressed so that they also occur at rest when his hand is held in certain positions. He has no episodes during sleep. Cold and fatigue worsen the symptoms. Between episodes, he has long-standing problems with bowel and bladder control, limited bilateral eye abduction, scissoring gate, mild left arm weakness, and some sensory loss on the left arm. His extensive neurologic history includes myelomeningocele repaired by the obstetrician at the time of birth, chronic hydrocephalus requiring a ventriculoperitoneal shunt and six subsequent shunt revisions, two surgeries for repair of tethered cord, and posterior fossa decompression and repair of an Arnold-Chiari malformation. Despite this significant history, he had been stable and doing well at the time the paroxysmal movements began. The symptoms began 2 years after his last shunt revision surgery, but were diagnosed at the postoperative examination for the second tethered cord procedure. The patient is the only surviving child of ten siblings, all of whom died secondary to neural tube defects (presumably secondary to extensive radiation exposure in the patient's mother). He has no other family history and has two healthy adult sons. On examination, he had normal strength except 4/5 strength in bilateral iliopsoas and hamstring muscles and in the left distal upper extremity. He also had 3+ reflexes throughout and a scissoring gait. Dystonia characterized by extension of the fingers on bilateral hands and adduction and flexion of the thumbs was elicited by asking the patient to grasp a fork. Full laboratory analysis was negative except for an elevated creatinine phosphokinase level at 217. Magnetic resonance imaging (MRI) of the brain showed postoperative changes, atrophic dilatation of the lateral and third ventricles, and small chronic subdural fluid collections overlying both hemispheres. MRI of the cervical spine and EEGs were normal, as was a full genetic analysis. He was diagnosed with paroxysmal kinesigenic dyskinesia secondary to central trauma and started on clonazepam 1 mg three times a day. Within 1 week, the frequency and severity of symptoms significantly diminished.

Case 2

Paroxysmal Non-Kinesigenic Dyskinesia Secondary to Kernicterus: A 24-month-old right-handed girl presented with a history of episodic left facial spasms since 11 months of age. These progressed to involve left arm flexion and writhing movements of the fingers as well as dystonic contractions of the trunk and the left leg. The attacks last from 10 seconds to a few minutes, occur as many as 20 times

per day at rest and are increased in severity and frequency by excitement, crying and increased activity. She has no change in consciousness during or after the attacks. There is no loss of bowel or bladder control or abnormal eye movements. There is no aura or pain associated with the episodes and they do not occur during sleep. She had numerous waking and sleep EEGs and an MRI and CT of the brain that were all normal. Complete laboratory evaluation, neuro-ophthalmologic evaluation and 6-hour EEG monitoring were all normal. Medical history is significant for untreated perinatal jaundice (laboratory values were not available) and excessive drooling since infancy. There is a family history of "abnormal thumb movements" in a maternal grandfather and great grandfather after stroke and a history of "nerve tumors" in a maternal grandmother and uncle. General examination was normal except for significantly increased drooling. Neurologic examination was normal with the exception of extension of the left leg when walking and episodic flexion of the left arm with athetotic movements of the fingers and inversion of the left foot. She was diagnosed with paroxysmal non-kinesigenic hemidystonia and choreoathetosis secondary to kernicterus and treated with clonazepam one tablet three times a day. There was no improvement with clonazepam. She is currently undergoing a trial of phenytoin. A previous trial of carbamazepine was ineffective.

DISCUSSION

Paroxysmal dyskinesias (PxD) are rare, episodic and hyperkinetic movement disorders that are usually idiopathic (primary) or familial (genetic). We present 20 patients with secondary PxD and a review of 130 cases of secondary PxD reported in the literature. Reports of patients with secondary PxD differed from reports of patients with primary PxD chiefly in the wide range of age of onset (frequently related to the associated etiology), the variability of symptom duration, and the presence of both kinesigenic and non-kinesigenic symptoms in six patients. Unlike primary

PxD, many of the patients in this series had some abnormality on neurologic examination between episodes or developed PxD symptoms in areas where other neurologic symptoms had resolved. However, there were several similarities between secondary and primary PxD. Namely, our patients with secondary PKD had short duration, frequent episodes as seen in primary PKD (3,4). Dystonia was the most common movement (2,7), and patients with PNKD reported exacerbating factors with the highest frequency (1,4).

It is difficult to draw conclusions about treatments in secondary PxD because patients in this series were not started on uniform medications, doses or schedules, and assessments were subjective. However, we did find that, as in primary PxD, our patients responded well to anticonvulsant therapy and clonazepam; in many cases requiring only one agent for symptom control. Also similar to primary PxD, it was more difficult to control symptoms in PNKD and mixed disease than in PKD. Nonetheless, 50% of the PNKD group and 66% of the mixed group had symptom relief with a single agent. Unique to secondary PxD, treatment of the underlying etiology relieved symptoms in two cases. The relatively novel therapy of botulinum toxin injections into the agonist muscle was also observed to be effective in patients who had focal paroxysmal dystonia.

Several classification schemes have been proposed for PxD (1,4,14,15). These schemes briefly address secondary causes, but are primarily concerned with the more common idiopathic or familial forms of PxD. The classifications are organized according to clinical features such as duration of symptoms, type of movement, precipitating factors (kinesigenic or non-kinesigenic), and etiology (familial or acquired) (1,4,14,15). Many cases of secondary PxD fail to meet criteria for these classifications because they have marked variability in duration and frequency of symptoms. Moreover, the classifications do not address sensory precipitants. There are several reports of secondary PxD precipitated by sensory stimulation in the literature (16–19); we

had one such patient in this series. The most notable limitation of these classification schemes, however, is the inability to incorporate cases with features of both kinesigenic and non-kinesigenic dyskinesia. In the present series, this group accounted for 30% of all patients with secondary PxD. Awareness of this limitation will assist in identification and diagnosis of cases of secondary PxD that fail to meet criteria of the classifications.

The most frequent causes of secondary PxD identified from our series and from review of literature (total of 150 cases) are MS (37 cases, 25%), transient cerebral ischemia with or without orthostatic hypotension (32 cases, 21%), trauma (19 cases, 13%), stroke (13 cases, 9%), hypoglycemia or hyperglycemia (16 cases, 10%), central nervous system (CNS) infections (11 cases, 7%), anoxic brain injuries (six cases, 4%), and hypocalcemia secondary to hypoparathyroidism (five cases, 3%) (Fig. 36.1). These six causes accounted for 93% of the cases presented. Less common causes in this series and the literature include thyrotoxicosis (20); structural lesions such as ciatrix (8), Arnold-chiari malformation with syringomyelia (21), and parasagittal meningioma (22); systemic lupus erythematous (23); migraine; methylphenidate therapy (24); progressive supranuclear palsy (25); kernicterus; cystinuria (26); spinal cord lesion (19,27); AIDS (28,29); and a case in which masturbation by a young child was misdiagnosed as PxD (30) (Table 36.4).

Our case series includes many of the causes previously reported; however, there are some notable differences. For example, MS was the most commonly cited cause of secondary PxD in the literature, but was noted in only one of our patients. Similarly, we had no cases secondary to metabolic disorders although it is a common etiology of secondary PxD in the literature (Table 36.4). As mentioned, despite all efforts it is unlikely we included every reported case of secondary PxD. Hence, because of referral bias and the limitations of the literature review, we cannot determine the true prevalence of the various etiologies associated with secondary PxD.

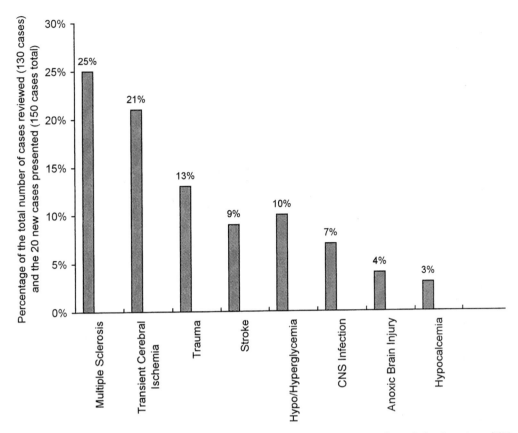

FIG. 36.1. The most common etiologies of secondary PxD based on review of the literature (130 cases) and the 20 cases from this series.

Despite these limitations, this series and review of literature demonstrates that there are a large variety of neurological lesions can lead to secondary PxD. The primary aim of this report and the following discussion is to draw attention to the characteristics of this movement disorder and to enhance the recognition of disease states capable of causing secondary PxD.

Multiple Sclerosis

PxD is a well-recognized manifestation of MS. In fact, it may be the presenting symptom of MS (31,32). Tranchant and associates (33) noted approximately 83 cases of PxD secondary to MS in the literature prompting him to describe PxD as "the most frequent move-

ment disorder described in MS." Shibasaki and colleagues (18) found 17% of the patients with MS they surveyed had paroxysmal dyskinesia, or what they termed "painful tonic seizures." Osterman and Westerberg (34) found that "tonic seizures" were second in frequency only to dysarthria and ataxia in their series on paroxysmal attacks in MS. Similarly, MS is the most frequently cited cause of secondary PxD in the literature (18, 19,31–39). The features of PxD in MS can be summarized as painful, predominantly dystonic movements precipitated by voluntary movement or sensory stimulation. The episodes are generally preceded by an aura (commonly paresthesias), are short in duration and occur many times per day (18, 31–34).

TABLE 36.4. *Published reports of secondary paroxysmal dyskinesias*

Etiology (Reference)	Cases	Location and type of movement	Category	Duration	Frequency	Lesion	Treatment
Vascular lesions							
Margolin and Marsden, 1982 (41)	4	Arm and leg: ballism and chorea	PNKD	1 min–1 h	Not reported	Carotid artery stenosis, cardiac aneurysm, HTN	Surgical revascularization and anticoagulation
Sunohara et al., 1984 (48)	1	Left arm and leg: dystonia	PKD	Duration of precipitating movement	—	Right posterolateral thalamus, left medial thalamus, and putamen	5-HTT and clonazepam
Baquis et al., 1985 (45)	8	Arm and leg: "shaking," "flailing," "flapping," "jerking," "twitching"	PKD, PNKD and positional	4 sec–5 min	Variable	Carotid artery stenosis; nl. head CT in 5 of 8 cases	Surgical revascularization
Yanagihara et al., 1985 (43)	12	Arm and leg: "rhythmic shaking," "jerking," "swinging"	Positional	Sec to min (sitting aborts)	4/wk–10/d	Carotid artery stenosis	Surgical revascularization
Merchut and Brumlik, 1986 (49)	1	Right hand, arm, and leg: painful dystonia	Mixed PKD & PNKD	30–60 sec	12–15/d	Left putaminal infarct, secondary to SLE with lupus anticoagulant	Carbamazepine
Bressman et al., 1988 (22)	1	Right: dystonia	PNKD	1 d to weeks	Daily to 1/yr	Ischemia	Not reported
Bennett and Fox, 1989 (40)	1	Left leg: dystonia and choreoathetosis	Positional	Whenever standing	4–5/d	Multiple small infarcts on CT of head	Aspirin
Tatemichi et al., 1990 (42)	1	Left leg: "twitching"	Positional	10 sec–2 min	6/d	Bilateral carotid artery stenosis	Carotid endarterectomy
Camac et al., 1990 (51)	1	Left hand progressing to arm, face, and leg: dystonia and choreoathetosis	PKD	<1 min	24/d	Right thalamic nuclei	Phenytoin
Fuh et al., 1991 (52)	1	Bilateral arms and legs, face: dystonia	PNKD	8–12 sec	5–15/h (in clusters)	Left frontoparietal and right parietooccipital perfusion deficit	Diazepam
Nijssen and Tijssen, 1992 (16)	1	Right leg and arm: dystonia, ballism, jerks, stereotypies	PKD (+ sensory stimulation)	<1 min	Variable	Left posterolateral thalamic infarct	Clonazepam, pinozide (unsuccessful)
Riley, 1996 (50)	1	Pharynx, larynx, and tongue	PKD	10–30 sec	6–20/d	Medullary hemorrhage	Phenytoin
Leira et al., 1997 (46)	1	Right arm >leg: dystonia, athetosis, myoclonus, "wandering limb"	Positional	1 min	10–15/d	Carotid artery stenosis	Modification of antihypertensive therapy
Baumgartner and Baumgartner, 1998 (47)	5	Arm and leg: "shaking" and "trembling"	Positional	Sec to min	Variable	Carotid artery stenosis; nl. head CT in 2 of 4 patients	Conservative and surgical revascularization
Uterga et al., 1999 (21)	1	Right arm: dystonia	PNKD	1 min	1–2/d	Left internal capsule and lenticular nucleus	
Zaidat et al., 1999 (44)	1	Left arm and hand: "shaking," "tremor-like"	PNKD	20 sec	6/d	Right cerebral hemisphere, right internal carotid artery occlusion	Right carotid endarterectomy
Posttraumatic							
Lance, 1963 (10)	1	Right arm, leg, and face: "painful tonic spasm"	PNKD, PNHD	10–30 sec (nocturnal-2 h)	6/d	Fall on right side; history of hemichoreoathetosis since 12 mo	Phenytoin and primidone
Osterman and Westerberg, 1975 (34)	1	Bilateral legs: painful dystonia	PKD	1 min	10–15/d	Fracture of odontoid after fall, cervical lesion	Carbamazepine
Robin, 1977 (56)	1	Left hand and arm: dystonia and choreoathetosis	PKD	5–10 sec	Several/day	Severe head injury s/p ejection from a plane	Phenobarbital

Reference	N	Clinical features	Type	Duration	Frequency	Lesion/etiology	Treatment
Perlmutter and Raichle, 1984 (58)	1	Right hand, arm, leg, face, and neck: dystonia	PNKD	Seconds	Every few minutes	Head and neck trauma: abnormal basal ganglia O_2 metabolism on PET	Phenytoin and trihexyphenidyl
Drake et al., 1986 (60)	3	Right hand, arm, and leg: "clonic jerking," athetosis, dystonia	PKD	1–2 min	Not reported	Closed head injury, coma, bilateral epidural hematomas, and s/p MVA	Phenobarbitone
		Right arm: dystonia, athetosis, "clonic jerking"	PKD	Several minutes	Not reported	Closed head injury, coma s/p fall from high height	Lorazepam
		Right arm and leg: ballism, dystonia, and "clonic jerks"	PNKD	Several minutes	Not reported	Closed head injury s/p moped accident	Phenobarbitone
Richardson et al., 1987 (57)	1	Left hemidystonia and hemichoreoathetosis	PKD	10 sec–3 min	<2/wk	Right frontal depressed skull fracture, contusion, and coma s/p MVA	Phenytoin
George et al., 1990 (17)	1	Right arm, leg, neck, and face: painful dystonia	PNKD (+ sensory stimulation)	5–30 sec	30/d	Cervical sprain s/p MVA	Diazepam
Biary et al., 1994 (59)	1	Right hemidystonia and athetosis of fingers	PNHD	3–12 min	2–5/night	Head injury and coma; left posterior putamen lesion s/p MVA	Acetazolamide
Multiple sclerosis							
Joynt and Green, 1962 (35)	4	Left arm, leg, and face: dystonia	PNKD	1–2 min	500–1000/ 6 mo	Not reported	Phenytoin, spontaneous remission
		Right arm and leg: painful dystonia	PNKD	60–90 sec	1–5/d	Not reported	Phenytoin
		Left hand and arm: dystonia	PNKD	5–10 sec	30/d	Not reported	Spontaneous remission
		Right arm and leg: dystonia	PNHD	1 min	Not reported	Not reported	Phenytoin
Lance, 1963 (10)	1	Left arm and leg: dystonia	PNKD	5 min	Not reported	Not reported	Not reported
Shibasaki and Kuroiwa, 1974 (18)	11	Right, left, or bilateral legs >arms and trunk; painful dystonia, jerking	9 PKD, (5 + sensory) 2PNKD	20 sec–2 min	1/h–1 every 5 min	Spinal cord, brainstem, cerebral, and cerebellar lesions	Carbamazepine and Phenytoin
Osterman and Westerberg, 1975 (34)	6	Not reported	Not reported	Not reported	Not reported	Not reported	Not reported
Berger et al., 1984 (31)	8	Right or left unilateral arm, leg, face, head, and neck dystonia, painful in 4	3 PKD 4 PNKD 1 PNHD?	15 sec–10 min	4–12/d	Not reported	Prednisone, phenytoin (3), carbamazepine (2), clorazepate (1)
Burguera et al., 1991 (36)	1	Right: hemidystonia	PKD	15–30 sec	10–20/d	Left thalamic lesion	Methylprednisone and carbamazepine
Roos et al., 1991 (37)	1	Right foot progressing to arm and head: dystonia	PKD	5–50 sec	5–10/h	Bilateral globus pallidus and putamen lesions	Phenytoin
Lugaresi et al., 1993 (38)	1	Left hand and foot, progressed to face: dystonia	PKD	3–30 min	1/d–1 every 10 d	Bilateral basal ganglia lesions	Not reported
Gatto et al., 1996 (39)	1	Bilateral: dystonia	PNKD	15–30 sec	15–30/d	Medulla oblongata	Carbamazepine
Cosentino et al., 1996 (19)	1	Right, left, and bilateral arm and leg: painful dystonia	Mixed PKD & PNKD (+ nociceptive stimulus)	10–20 sec	8–10/d	C2-7 intramedullary lesion	Valproate and acetazolamide
de Seze et al., 2000 (32)	1	Left arm: dystonia and choreoathetosis	PKD	30 sec–1 min	10/d	Right thalamus, internal pallidus, and posterior internal capsule lesions	Methylprednisone

Continued on next page

TABLE 36.4. *(Continued)*

Etiology (Reference)	Cases	Location and type of movement	Category	Duration	Frequency	Lesion	Treatment
Static brain lesions							
Falconer et al., 1963 (8)	1	Right leg, arm, and trunk: dystonia	Mixed PKD and PNKD	10–20 sec	8–40/d	Cortical scar: superior left hemisphere, near rolandic fissure	Surgical resection
Rosen, 1964 (98)	1	Bilateral arms, trunk: dystonia, face athetosis, oculogyria, and retrocollis	Mixed PKD and PNKD	15–60 sec	5–20/d	Perinatal hypoxic encephalopathy	Belladonna and diphenhydramine
Bressman et al., 1988 (22)	4	Trunk, neck, and limbs: dystonia	PNKD	10 sec–2 wk	1/d–1/mo	Anoxia (3 birth, 1 drug overdose)	Carbamazepine, trihexyphenidyl, clonazepam
Uterga et al., 1999 (21)	1	Left arm: dystonia	PNKD	15 min	1/mo	Arnold-Chiari malformation; cervical syringomyelia	—
Endocrine disorders							
Tabaee-Zadeh et al., 1972 (79)	1	Right arm, leg, and head: dystonia and choreoathetosis	?PED	30 sec	Several/wk	Hypocalcemia, idiopathic hypoparathyroidism, and basal ganglia calcifications	Calcium
Soffer et al., 1977 (78)	1	Right arm and leg, face: choreoathetosis, dystonia	PNKD	Min to hours	Not reported	Hypocalcemia, idiopathic hypoparathyroidism	Vitamin D and calcium
Fischbeck & Layzer, 1979 (20)	1	Bilateral arms and legs (L>R), face: dystonia and chorea	PKD	1–2 min	1–4 d	Thyrotoxicosis	Propylthiouracil, propranolol and potassium iodide
Newman and Kinkel, 1984 (70)	1	Bilateral limbs: choreoathetosis; opisthotonus	PNKD	Not reported	Not reported	Hypoglycemia due to insulinoma	Dextrose, reduction in insulin
Kato et al., 1987 (82)	1	Bilateral limbs, face: dystonia, choreoathetosis, and ballism	Mixed PKD and PNKD	15 sec	20/d	Hypocalcemia, basal ganglia calcification, familial idiopathic hypoparathyroidism	Vitamin D and phenytoin
Yamamoto and Kawazawa, 1987 (81)	1	Right shoulder, progressed to whole body: dystonia and chorea	PNKD	1–3 h	1–3/d	Hypocalcemia, basal ganglia calcification: pseudoidiopathic hypoparathyroidism	Vitamin D and calcium
Barabas and Tucker, 1988 (80)	1	Right hand, arm, and face: dystonia	PKD	15–30 sec	20/d	Hypocalcemia, basal ganglia calcification, hypoparathyroidism	Calcium
Haan et al., 1989 (75)	1	Bilateral arms, legs: choreoathetosis, buccolingual dyskinesia, and blepharospasm	PNKD	20 min	2–3 h after meals	Hyper- and hypoglycemia: presenting symptom of diabetes mellitus	Control of blood sugar
Morres and Dire 1989 (77)	2	Right arm, leg: "shaking"	PKD and PNKD	20 sec–10 min	Variable	Hyperglycemia	Control of blood sugar
Winer et al., 1990 (73)	1	Bilateral arms and legs: dystonia	PNKD	15 min–4 h	2–3/d	Hypoglycemia secondary to an islet cell tumor	Surgical resection

Study	N	Body involvement	Type	Duration	Dozens/day	Etiology	Treatment
Hennis et al., 1992 (76)	7	Unilateral right or left hand, arm, neck	"Focal seizures": PNKD (4) and PKD (3)	40 sec–5 min		Nonketotic hyperglycemia	Control of blood sugar (no response to antiepileptic medications)
Schmidt and Pillay, 1993 (71)	2	Bilateral arm, leg, neck, and face: chorea and dystonia	PNKD	2–15 min	10–15/y	Hypoglycemia secondary to an insulinoma	Glucose load
		Bilateral arms: choreoathetosis	PNKD	1–2 h	Not reported	Hypoglycemia secondary to insulin replacement	Glucose load
Clark et al., 1995 (74)	1	Right hand and arm: painful dystonia and choreoathetosis	PKD	3–5 min	8–10/d	Hyperglycemia, old left parietal infarct	Control of blood sugar
Shaw et al., 1996 (72)	1	Bilateral limbs and trunk: choreoathetosis and dystonia	PED and PNKD	30 min	Not reported	Hypoglycemia secondary to an insulinoma	Surgical resection

Miscellaneous etiologies

Study	N	Body involvement	Type	Duration	Dozens/day	Etiology	Treatment
Cavanagh et al., 1974 (26)	1	Bilateral limbs: painful dystonia, torticollis	PNKD	Several hours–several days	Several/week–monthly	Heterozygous cystinuria with mental retardation	Diazepam
Hutchinson and Bresnihan, 1983 (23)	1	Bilateral limbs: dystonia, pseudoathetosis	PKD	30 sec	20/d	Systemic lupus erythematosus	Azathioprine and prednisolone
Micheli et al., 1987 (83)	1	Right hand, arm, and leg: dystonia and choreoathetosis	PNKD	10 min–4 h	1–4/mo	Bilateral calcifications of the globus pallidus	Clonazepam
Nath et al., 1987 (29)	1	Dystonia	Not reported	Not reported	Not reported	AIDS, lesion in the left frontal region	Not reported
Bressman et al., 1988 (22)	1	Right leg: dystonia	PNKD	<5 min	2–12/yr	Parasagital meningioma	Clonazepam
	1	Right arm, neck, jaw, and tongue: dystonia	PNKD	2–5 min	1–6/d	Encephalitis	Clonazepam
Gay and Ryan et al., 1994 (24)	1	Bilateral limbs: dystonia and right or left head deviation	PKD	15–30 sec	1–5/d	Methylphenidate therapy	Carbamazepine (attacks persisted with discontinuation of methylphenidate)
Mink and Neil, 1995 (30)	1	Right limbs: dystonia, shaking in right foot	PNKD	<5 min–hours	5–6/d	Masturbation in a young child	None
Mirsattari et al., 1999 (28)	6	Unilateral (3) and bilateral limbs (3), neck and face (4): choreoathetosis, myoclonus, dysarthria, and postural tremor	PKD (2) and PNKD (4)	Min to days	Variable	HIV: toxoplasmosis encephalitis (1), herpes zoster (1), Kaposi sarcoma (1)	Antivirals, clonazepam (2), oxazepam (1), no response in 2 patients

AIDS, acquired immunodeficiency syndrome; CT, computed tomography; HIV, human immunodeficiency virus; HTN, hypertension; 5-HTT, ; MVA, motor vehicle accident; nl, normal; PED, paroxysmal exertion-induced dyskinesia; PET, positron emission tomography; PNHD, ; PNKD, paroxysmal nonkinesigenic dyskinesia; PKD, paroxysmal kinesigenic dyskinesia; SLE, systemic lupus erythematosus; s/p, status post.

The mechanism of PxD in MS is unknown; however, one widely accepted theory proposed by Osterman and Westerberg (34) is that there is ephaptic excitation and abnormal transmission in axons with damaged myelin resulting in paroxysmal movements. Lesions in the spinal cord are commonly cited in cases of PxD secondary to MS (18,19) and Osterman and Westerberg (34) focused their attention here. However, lesions throughout the CNS have been associated with PxD in MS including lesions in the cortex, basal ganglia, thalamus, and medulla (32,36,38,39). It is possible that the "transversely spreading activation of damaged axons" suggested by Osterman and Westerberg to be occurring in the spinal cord, is occurring throughout the CNS. Hence, demyelinating lesions anywhere along motor pathways (from cortex to the basal ganglia to the spinal cord) may result in PxD. Depending on the location of the lesion and the proximity of other tracts, ephaptic excitation may explain associated paresthesias, auras, and sensory precipitants.

Transient Ischemic Paroxysmal Dyskinesia

There are several reports of patients with paroxysmal movements associated with orthostasis or transient cerebral ischemia (40–47). These cases are distinct from other cases of PxD secondary to vascular lesions in that they occur with a change in posture, are frequently associated with presyncopal symptoms, are clinically similar to transient ischemia attacks (TIAs) and are reversible with interventions that increase cerebral perfusion. In several cases, anticoagulation or revascularization reversed the PxD (40,43,45,46). Yanagihara and associates (43) studied 12 patients with carotid occlusive disease who had repetitive involuntary movements (RIMs) precipitated by standing, walking, or neck extension. Of the 11 patients who underwent revascularization, seven had "excellent" outcomes, three had "fair-good" outcomes, and one died postoperatively of an unrelated disease. The median time from onset of the RIMs to revascularization was 6 months, suggesting early

intervention may have reversed the RIMs. The recognition of this particular PxD is crucial as early intervention to increase cerebral perfusion may prevent permanent movement disorders or future devastating infarctions.

Stroke

Stroke was present in four cases in this series and is a frequently cited cause of secondary PxD in the literature (16,21,22, 48–52). In this series and in many reported cases, the PxD symptoms develop in the same distribution of the stroke-related deficits and may occur after the immediate neurologic sequelae of the stroke has resolved. In several cases there is a direct link between vascular lesions in the thalamus, putamen and medulla and the development of PxD (16,48–51). These cases provide the most convincing evidence for a causal relationship between a focal neurological insult and the development of PxD. Moreover, they support the argument that PxD is a movement disorder rather than an epileptic disorder as the loss of key areas involved in the modulation of movement result in PxD symptoms.

Central and Peripheral Trauma

Trauma was the most common etiology for PxD in our series and it was the third most frequently cited cause of secondary PxD in our literature review (Table 36.4). That brain injury can result in movement disorders has been well established (53–55), and there are several reports of brain injury specifically associated with PxD (17,56–60). In some cases the PxD is related to a focal insult in an anatomically related area (58,59). In other cases focal PxD is associated with diffuse trauma to the CNS (59,60). Moreover, posttraumatic PxD has been reported in patients with seemingly minor injuries to the CNS (17). Similar to other post-traumatic movement disorders (61), there may be long intervals between the injury and the onset of the PxD. Perhaps general responses to injury such as inflammation and synaptic reorganization are involved in the generation of post-traumatic PxD. These processes occur over an unpredictable amount of time, and may account for the observed variability in the interval from injury to symptom onset.

Although the relationship between brain injury and resultant movement disorders is widely accepted, the notion that peripheral injury may also result in pathologic movements has only recently been recognized and remains highly controversial (62–67). Criticism of the concept of peripherally induced movement disorders focuses on the difficulty in defining the population that has peripheral injuries but never develops pathological movements (the "denominator problem") and inadequate diagnostic criteria (67). As the underlying mechanisms of PxD become better understood, these concerns may be addressed. Although the evidence is certainly incomplete, the noted temporal and anatomic relationships between the injuries and the subsequent movement disorders argue strongly for an association.

Although the mechanism underlying peripherally induced PxD is unknown, emerging evidence suggests that peripheral lesions may result in cortical and spinal reorganization (68,69). Aberrant reorganization of motor or sensory pathways may explain the observation that peripherally induced movement disorders have a propensity to progress from one body area to another. Three of our six patients with PxD secondary to peripheral trauma had progression to other body parts. Aberrant motor and sensory reorganization may also explain the precipitation of PxD symptoms by sensory stimulation in some patients with PxD secondary to trauma.

Metabolic Abnormalities

Several cases of hypoglycemia (70–73) and hyperglycemia (74–77) presenting with PxD have been reported. These cases are notable for the rapid and absolute reversal of symptoms with appropriate treatment of the underlying glucose abnormality and return of the symptoms with loss of glycemic control. The mechanism underlying both hypoglycemia and hyperglycemia is probably temporary cerebral hypoxia, because both hypoglycemia and hyperglycemia can cause focal reduction in blood flow. Although the pyramidal neurons of the cortex are known to be susceptible to hypoxia and may be contributing to the symptoms of PxD, it is unclear if the extrapyramidal motor circuits are particularly susceptible to glycemia-induced hypoxia. In addition, it is curious that although all people who experience symptomatic hypoglycemia or hyperglycemia presumably have some degree of neuronal hypoxia, only the rare patient develops PxD. Hennis and associates (76) suggested that the increased metabolism of gamma amino n-butyric acid (GABA) during hyperglycemia may allow for a decreased excitatory threshold, resulting in PxD. This is a plausible hypothesis since decreased GABA activity has been postulated to play a role in several disorders of the basal ganglia as a result of disinhibition of the pallido-thalamo-cortical-spinal circuit. Again, it is unclear why this would cause PxD exceptionally rarely although symptomatic hypoglycemia or hyperglycemia is common.

Like PxD secondary to glucose dysregulation, symptoms in patients with PxD secondary to hypocalcemia rapidly resolve with treatment of the underlying imbalance (78–81). There are frequently calcifications in the basal ganglia in patients with PxD secondary to hypocalcemia (79–82). Tabaee-Zadeh and associates (79) suggested that it is not the lesions to the basal ganglia alone that lead to PxD, but rather hypocalcemia causing hyperexcitability in susceptible basal ganglia neurons previously damaged by calcium deposits. This is supported by the fact that correction of the calcium reverses PxD symptoms even though the basal ganglia calcifications are unchanged (79–82). However, in another report, PxD was attributed to bilateral calcifications of the globus pallidus without any accompanying laboratory abnormalities (83). Once again, it is unclear why these neurons are particularly vulnerable in some patients.

Miscellaneous Central Nervous System Results

In addition to the numerous case reports of relatively unusual etiologies resulting in PxD (Table 36.4), we had several patients with diverse CNS insults including kernicterus, meningovascular syphilis, and CMV encephalitis. We also had a patient who had PxD associated with the aura of migraine headaches. In their series on PxD, Houser and associates (7) noted a patient with a history of migraine headaches, but they did not consider migraine as a cause. In our patient, the PxD symptoms occurred only prior to the onset of headache, were frequently accompanied by other auras such as visual disturbances, and were significantly relieved with migraine prophylaxis suggesting that migraine is the cause of the PxD symptoms. To our knowledge this is the first report of migraine as a cause of PxD, although migraine has long been considered one of the paroxysmal neurologic disorders.

Pathophysiology of Paroxysmal Dyskinesias

PxD is considered to be a disorder of the basal ganglia based on the following observations: (a) the movements seen in PxD are similar in nature to those seen in other basal ganglia disorders and resolve during sleep (84), (b) radiographic or structural abnormalities are frequently identified in the basal ganglia or its connections in patients with PxD (54, 58,85–87), (c) there is a distinct absence of epileptiform activity, (d) there is no loss of consciousness during episodes, and (e) there are no postictal changes in patients with PxD. In addition, Bhatia and colleagues (86) reported reversal of symptoms in a patient with PED after pallidotomy. This was the first report of structural manipulation within the basal ganglia leading to an improvement of PxD symptoms, strongly implicating the basal ganglia, or its connections, as the focal point of dysfunction in PxD. Furthermore, reviews of non-paroxysmal secondary dystonia have presented notable neuroimaging and neu-

ropathology data implicating structural involvement of the caudate, putamen, globus pallidus, and thalamus (88–90). However, controversy remains as to the exact pathophysiologic mechanisms and some investigators view PxD as a form of reflex epilepsy with subcortical seizure activity (8,91). This is supported by the paroxysmal nature of the movements and the positive response to antiepileptic medication. The notion of reflex epilepsy is further supported by the observation that sensory stimuli can produce a similar response in both reflex epilepsy and some cases of PxD. The presence of auras also supports the seizure hypothesis, as auras are classically associated with focal epileptiform activity. Nijssen and Tijssen (16) described a patient with PxD secondary to a infarction of the posterolateral thalamus and posterior arm of the internal capsule in which both voluntary movements and sensory stimulation induced dyskinesia. The lesion in the thalamus and the absence of epileptiform activity argues against epileptic origin for the movement disorder. Still, subcortical seizure activity within the basal ganglia cannot be excluded and indeed, the true pathophysiology may involve a combination of both mechanisms.

The observation that diverse causes such as symptomatic cerebral hypoperfusion, infarctions, hemorrhages, demyelinating lesions, trauma, and a host of other insults and metabolic abnormalities result in PxD suggests that PxD is the symptomatic expression of a variety of insults to the neuronal circuits modulating movement. Potentially, all of the implicated insults cause some degree of direct tissue damage, neurotransmitter dysregulation, hypoxia, and inflammatory responses associated with production of free radicals and excitatory neurotransmitters.

There are two general mechanisms that can adequately explain the symptoms observed in PxD. Because the episodes consist of hyperkinetic phenomenon, they likely represent either a state of primary hyperexcitability or loss of inhibition. While clearly an oversimplification, there is support for this hypothesis from several lines of evidence. Rehders and colleagues (92) showed that dopaminergic overactivity in the striatum was largely responsible for the severity of paroxysmal dystonia in mutant dystonic hamsters. Dystonic symptoms were worsened by injection of D2 agonist and amphetamine and alleviated by co-injections of D2 and D1 antagonists. This is supported by Gay and Ryan's (24) case report in which PxD was induced by methylphenidate in a previously healthy child. Methylphenidate is structurally related to amphetamine and is a powerful dopaminergic agonist. Fischbeck and Layzer (20) proposed hyperthyroidism similarly caused "thyroxine-induced hypersensitivity to dopamine," resulting in dopamine overactivity and PxD. While dopaminergic overactivity may account for some cases of secondary PxD, there are some cases of PxD in which dopamine replacement relieves symptoms (93). In fact, in the present series two patients responded well to carbidopa/levodopa.

Another possible cause of neuronal hyperexcitability is hypoxia through the accumulation of free radicals and excitatory amino acids such as glutamate and aspartate. There are cases of PxD secondary to cerebral vascular insufficiency in which there were no structural abnormalities on CT or MRI, but PET scanning revealed decreased oxygen metabolism. This, in turn, may contribute to increased production of excitatory amino acids (52,58).

There are some similarities between PxD and tardive dyskinesias (TD), an involuntary hyperkinetic movement disorder caused by exposure to dopamine receptor blocking drugs. Although the movements in TD are frequently persistent rather than paroxysmal, tardive involuntary ocular deviations, in particular, are commonly episodic and are frequently seen with facial dyskinesias similar to several of the cases described here (94,95). Micheli and associates (96) reported a patient with paroxysmal dystonic choreoathetosis with a history of mental retardation and a 15-year history of neuroleptic therapy. They suggested his symptoms represented a drug-induced

paroxysmal dystonia, directly linking PxD and TD. The similarities between PxD and TD suggest involvement of the dopaminergic system in at least some cases of PxD. The pathophysiology of TD remains unknown, however, it has long been hypothesized that TD is due to a compensatory increase in dopamine activity in response to receptor blockade, resulting in an imbalance in the dopaminergic-cholinergic pathways. Many patients with TD have symptom relief with anticholinergic medications. Indeed, the patient presented by Micheli and associates (96) had complete abatement of symptoms with trihexyphenidyl. There have been additional reports of PxD symptom abatement with anticholinergic therapy (97,98). It remains unclear why some cases of PxD respond to dopamine supplementation and some are worsened by increased dopamine, but respond to anticholinergic agents. However, the implication is that there is dopamine dysregulation within the basal ganglia in PxD.

There is significant clinical similarity between PxD and several paroxysmal disorders such as episodic ataxias, paramyotonia congenita, hyperekplexia, and hypokalemic periodic paralysis, which have been linked to ion channel disorders (99–101). This raises the possibility that PxD is also secondary to a channelopathy. Ion channels serve to maintain the functional integrity of the neuronal membranes and hence, directly impact neuronal excitability.

Several familial epilepsies have also been linked to ion channel dysfunction (99,100). Swoboda and colleagues (101) evaluated 11 families with histories of both nonfebrile infantile convulsions (IC) and PKD and confirmed linkage of the IC/PKD phenotype to the pericentric region of chromosome 16. This association further supports a channelopathy as a potential cause for PxD as there is genetic linkage of a known channelopathy (infantile convulsions) with a PxD phenotype.

Although the theory of channelopathy as the mechanism for PxD has been applied primarily to familial PxD, both idiopathic and secondary forms of PxD respond to medications such as acetazolamide and a variety of antiepileptic medications that stabilize neuronal membranes (1,2,102,103). Conceivably, the various etiologies implicated in secondary PxD ultimately result in ion channel dysfunction. The phenomenologic overlap between paroxysmal disorders such as epilepsy, migraine, PxD and periodic paralyses may be related to a shared ion channel defect (100). The emergence of data linking PxD to channelopathies may ultimately resolve the long-held controversy about whether PxD is a basal ganglia disorder or a form of epilepsy. It is quite possible that it is both: a disorder of ion channels within the circuits regulating movement.

SUMMARY

PxD are sudden, episodic, involuntary movement disorders that may include any combination of dystonia, chorea, athetosis, or ballism. The majority of reported cases are familial or idiopathic; however, there have been several reports of secondary PxD. We report 20 new cases of secondary, non-psychogenic PxD, and review 130 cases reported in the literature. The results suggest that although PxD is a rare disorder, secondary forms may be more common than previously recognized, accounting for 26% of all cases in our series. Secondary cases are notable for their variability in age of onset, the presence of both kinesigenic and non-kinesigenic symptoms in some patients, the prevalence of sensory precipitants, and most importantly, the reversal of symptoms when the underlying etiology is treated in some patients. In addition to MS, other causes to be considered in patients presenting with PxD include cerebral vascular insufficiency and stroke, trauma, metabolic abnormalities, and CNS infections. Awareness of the association of these etiologies with secondary PxD will permit prompt diagnoses and appropriate interventions. Potential pathophysiologic mechanisms including loss of inhibition or primary neuronal hyperactivity are discussed. In addition, recent hypotheses regarding channelopathies in relation to PxD are presented.

REFERENCES

1. Demirkiran M, Jankovic J. Paroxysmal dyskinesias: clinical features and classification. *Ann Neurol* 1995; 38:571–579.
2. Sethi KD. Paroxysmal dyskinesias. *Neurologist* 2000; 6:177–185.
3. Marsden CD. Paroxysmal choreoathetosis. In: Luders HO ed. *Advances in Neurology, Vol.70. Supplementary Sensorimotor Area.* Philadelphia: Lippincott-Raven, 1996:467–470.
4. Fahn S. The paroxysmal dyskinesias. In: Marsden CD, Fahn S, eds. *Movement disorders 3.* Oxford: Butterworth-Heinemann, 1994:310–345.
5. Demirkiran M, Jankovic J. Paroxysmal dyskinesias. *Curr Neurol* 1996;16:213–251.
6. Bhatia KP. The paroxysmal dyskinesias. *J Neurol* 1999;246:149–155.
7. Houser MK, Soland VL, Bhatia KP, et al. Paroxysmal kinesigenic choreoathetosis: a report of 26 patients. *J Neurol* 1999;246:120–126.
8. Falconer MA, Driver MV, Serafetinides EA. Seizures induced by movement: report of a case relieved by an operation. *J Neurol Neurosurg Psychiatry* 1963;26: 300–307.
9. Lishman WA, Symonds CP, Whitty CW, et al. Seizures induced by movement. *Brain* 1962;85:93–108.
10. Lance JW. Sporadic and familial varieties of tonic seizures. *J Neurol Neurosurg Psychiatry* 1963;26: 51–59.
11. Fahn S, Williams DT. Psychogenic dystonia. In: Fahn S, Marsden CD, Calne DB, eds. *Advances in neurology,Vol. 50. Dystonia 2.* New York: Raven Press, 1988: 431–455.
12. Kertesz A. Paroxysmal kinesigenic choreoathetosis. An entity within the paroxysmal choreoathetosis syndrome. Description of 10 cases, including 1 autopsied. *Neurology* 1967;17:680–690.
13. Plant G. Focal paroxysmal kinesigenic choreoathetosis. *J Neurol Neurosurg Psychiatry* 1983;46:345–348.
14. Lance JW. Familial paroxysmal dystonic choreoathetosis and its differentiation from related syndromes. *Ann Neurol* 1977;2:285–293.
15. Goodenough DJ, Fariello RG, Annis BL, et al. Familial and acquired paroxysmal dyskinesias. A proposed classification with delineation of clinical features. *Arch Neurol* 1978;35:827–831.
16. Nijssen PCG, Tijssen CC. Stimulus-sensitive paroxysmal dyskinesias associated with a thalamic infarct. *Mov Disord* 1992;7:364–366.
17. George MS, Pickett JB, Kohli H, et al. Paroxysmal dystonic reflex choreoathetosis after minor closed injury. *Lancet* 1990;336:1134–1135.
18. Shibasaki H, Kuroiwa Y. Painful tonic seizures in multiple sclerosis. *Arch Neurol* 1974;30:47–51.
19. Cosentino C, Torres L, Flores M, et al. Paroxysmal kinesigenic dystonia and spinal cord lesion. *Mov Disord* 1996;11:453–455.
20. Fishbeck KH, Layzer RB. Paroxysmal choreoathetosis associated with thyrotoxicosis. *Ann Neurol* 1979;6: 453–454.

21. Uterga JM, Portillo MF, Iriondo I, et al. Symptomatic paroxysmal dystonia (non-kinesigenic forms): two new cases. *Neurologia* 1999;14:190–192.

22. Bressman SB, Fahn S, Burke RE. Paroxysmal non-kinesigenic dystonia. In: Fahn S, Marsden CD, Calne DB, eds. *Advances in neurology, Vol. 50. Dystonia 2.* New York: Raven Press, 1988:403–413.

23. Hutchinson M, Bresnihan B. Neurological lupus erythematosus with tonic seizures simulating multiple sclerosis. *J Neurol Neurosurg Psychiatry* 1983;46:583–585.

24. Gay CT, Ryan SG. Paroxysmal kinesigenic dystonia after methylphenidate administration. *J Child Neurol* 1994;9:45–46.

25. Adam AM, Orinda DO. Focal paroxysmal kinesigenic choreoathetosis preceding the development of Steele-Richardson-Olszewski syndrome. *J Neurol Neurosurg Psychiatry* 1986;49:957–959.

26. Cavanagh NP, Bicknell J, Howard F. Cystinuria with mental retardation and paroxysmal dyskinesia in 2 brothers. *Arch Dis Child* 1974;49:662–664.

27. Previdi P, Buzi P. Paroxysmal dystonia due to a lesion of the cervical spinal cord: case report. *Ital J Neurol Sci* 1992;13:521–523.

28. Mirsattari SM, Roke Berry ME, Holden JK, et al. Paroxysmal dyskinesias in patients with HIV infection. *Neurology* 1999;52:110–114.

29. Nath A, Jankovic J, Pettigrew LC. Movement disorders and AIDS. *Neurology* 1987;37:37–41.

30. Mink JW, Neil JJ. Masturbation mimicking paroxysmal dystonia or dyskinesia in a young girl. *Mov Disord* 1995;10:518–520.

31. Berger JR, Sheremata WA, Melamed E. Paroxysmal dystonia as the initial manifestation of multiple sclerosis. *Arch Neurol* 1984;41:747–750.

32. DeSeze J, Stojkovic T, Destee M, et al. Parozysmal kinesigenic choreoathetosis as a presenting symptom of multiple sclerosis. *J Neurol* 2000;247:478–480.

33. Tranchant C, Bhatia KP, Marsden CD. Movement disorders in multiple sclerosis. *Mov Disord* 1995;10:418–423.

34. Osterman PO, Westerberg C-E. Paroxysmal attacks in multiple sclerosis. *Brain* 1975;98:189–202.

35. Joynt RJ, Green D. Tonic seizures as a manifestation in multiple sclerosis. *Arch Neurol* 1962;6:293–299.

36. Burguera JA, Catala J, Casanova B. Thalamic demyelination and paroxysmal dystonia in multiple sclerosis. *Mov Disord* 1991;6:379–381.

37. Roos RAC, Wintzen AR, Vielvoye G, et al. Paroxysmal choreoathetosis as presenting symptom of multiple sclerosis. *J Neurol Neurosurg Psychiatry* 1991;54:657–658.

38. Lugaresi A, Uncini A, Gambi D. Basal ganglia involvement in multiple sclerosis with alternating side paroxysmal dystonia. *J Neurol* 1993;240:257–258.

39. Gatto EM, Zurru MC, Rugilo C. Medullary lesions and unusual bilateral paroxysmal dystonia in multiple sclerosis. *Neurology* 1996;46:847–848.

40. Bennett DA, Fox JH. Paroxysmal dyskinesia secondary to cerebral vascular disease-reversal with aspirin. *Clin Neuropharmacol* 1989;12:215–216.

41. Margolin DI, Marsden CD. Episodic dyskinesias and transient cerebral ischemia. *Neurology* 1982;32:1379–1380.

42. Tatemichi TK, Young WL, Prohovnik I, et al. Perfusion insufficiency in limb-shaking transient ischemic attacks. *Stroke* 1990;21:341–347.

43. Yanagihara T, Piepgras DG, Klass DW. Repetitive involuntary movement associated with episodic cerebral ischemia. *Ann Neurol* 1985;18:244–250.

44. Zaidat OO, Werz MA, Landis DMD, et al. Orthostatic limb shaking from carotid hypoperfusion. *Neurology* 1999;53;650–651.

45. Baquis GD, Pessin MS, Scott RM. Limb shaking – A carotid TIA. *Stroke* 1985;16:444–448.

46. Leira EC, Ajax T, Adams HP. Limb-shaking carotid transient ischemic attacks successfully treated with modification of the antihypertensive regimen. *Arch Neurol* 1997;54:904–905.

47. Baumgartner RW, Baumgartner I. Vasomotor reactivity is exhausted in transient ischemic attacks with limb shaking. *J Neurol Neurosurg Psychiatry* 1998;65:561–564.

48. Sunohara N, Mukoyama M, Mano Y, et al. Action-induced rhythmic dystonia: an autopsy case. *Neurology* 1984;34:321–327.

49. Merchut MP, Brumlik J. Painful tonic spasms caused by putaminal infarction. *Stroke* 1986;17:1319–1321.

50. Riley DE. Paroxysmal kinesigenic dystonia associated with a medullary lesion. *Mov Disord* 1996;11:738–740.

51. Camac A, Greene P, Khandji A. Paroxysmal kinesigenic dystonic choreoathetosis associated with a thalamic infarct. *Mov Disord* 1990;5:235–238.

52. Fuh JL, Chang DB, Wang SJ, et al. Painful tonic spasms: an interesting phenomenon in cerebral ischemia. *Acta Neurol Scand* 1991;84:534–536.

53. Krauss JK, Trankle R, Kopp, KH. Post-traumatic movement disorders in survivors of severe head injury. *Neurology* 1996;47:1488–1492.

54. Marsden CD, Obeso JA, Zarranz JJ, et al. The anatomical basis of symptomatic hemidystonia. *Brain* 1985;108:463–483.

55. Jankovic J. Post-traumatic movement disorders: central and peripheral mechanisms. *Neurology* 1994;44:2006–2014.

56. Robin JJ. Paroxysmal choreoathetosis following head injury. *Ann Neurol* 1977;2:447–448.

57. Richardson JC, Howes JL, Celinski MJ, et al. Kinesigenic choreoathetosis due to brain injury. *Can J Neurol Sci* 1987;14:626–628.

58. Perlmutter JS, Raichle ME. Pure hemidystonia with basal ganglion abnormalities on positron emission tomography. *Ann Neurol* 1984;15:228–233.

59. Biary N, Singh B, Bahou Y, et al. Posttraumatic paroxysmal nocturnal hemidystonia. *Mov Disord* 1994;9:98–99.

60. Drake ME, Jackson RD, Miller CA. Paroxysmal choreoathetosis after head injury. *J Neurol Neurosurg Psychiatry* 1986;49:837–838.

61. Scott BL, Jankovic J. Delayed-onset progressive movement disorders after static brain lesions. *Neurology* 1996;46:68–74.

62. Jankovic, J, Van der Linden C. Dystonia and tremor induced by peripheral trauma: predisposing factors. *J Neurol Neurosurg Psychiatry* 1988;51:1512–1519.

63. Schott GD. Induction of involuntary movements by peripheral trauma. An analogy with causalgia. *Lancet* 1986;2:712–716.

64. Cardoso F, Jankovic J. Peripherally induced tremor and parkinsonism. *Arch Neurol* 1995;52:263–270.

65. Jankovic J. Can peripheral trauma induce dystonia and

other movement disorders? Yes! *Mov Disord* 2001; 16:7–12.

66. Sankhla C, Lai EC, Jankovic J. Peripherally induced oromandibular dystonia. *J Neurol Neurosurg Psychiatry* 1998;65:722–728.

67. Weiner WJ. Can peripheral trauma induce dystonia? No! *Mov Disord* 2001;16:13–22.

68. Cohen LG, Bandinelli S, Findley TW, et al. Motor reorganization after upper limb amputation in man. A study with focal magnetic stimulation. *Brain* 1991; 114:615–627.

69. Braune S, Schady W. Changes in sensation after nerve injury or amputation: the role of central factors. *J Neurol Neurosurg Psychiatry* 1993;56:393–399.

70. Newman RP, Kinkel WR. Paroxysmal choreoathetosis due to hypoglycemia. *Arch Neurol* 1984;41:341–342.

71. Schmidt BJ, Pillay N. Paroxysmal dyskinesia associated with hypoglycemia. *Can J Neurol Sci* 1993;20: 151–153.

72. Shaw C, Haas L, Miller D, et al. A case report of paroxysmal dystonic choreoathetosis due to hypoglycaemia induced by an insulinoma. *J Neurol Neurosurg Psychiatry* 1996;61:194–195.

73. Winer JB, Fish DR, Marsden CD, et al. A movement disorder as a presenting feature of recurrent hypoglycaemia. *Mov Disorder* 1990;5:176–177.

74. Clark JD, Pahwa R, Koller WC, et al. Diabetes mellitus presenting as paroxysmal kinesigenic dystonic choreoathetosis. *Mov Disord* 1995;10:353–355.

75. Haan J, Kremer HPH, Padberg G. Paroxysmal choreoathetosis as presenting symptom of diabetes mellitus. *J Neurol Neurosurg Psychiatry* 1989;52:133.

76. Hennis A, Corbin D, Fraser H. Focal seizures and nonketotic hyperglycaemia.. *J Neurol Neurosurg Psychiatry* 1992;55:195–197.

77. Morres CA, Dire DJ. Movement disorders as a manifestation of nonketotic hyperglycemia. *J Emerg Med* 1989;7:359–364.

78. Soffer D, Licht A, Yaar I, et al. Paroxysmal choreoathetosis as a presenting symptom in idiopathic hypoparathyroidism. *J Neurol Neurosurg Psychiatry* 1977; 40:692–694.

79. Tabaee-Zadeh MJ, Frame B, Kapphahn K. Kinesiogenic choreoathetosis and idiopathic hypoparathyroidism. *New Engl J Med* 1972;286:762–763.

80. Barabas G, Tucker SM. Idiopathic hypoparathyroidism and paroxysmal dystonic choreoathetosis. *Ann Neurol* 1988;24:585.

81. Yamamoto K, Kawazawa S. Basal ganglion calcifications in paroxysmal dystonic choreoathetosis. *Ann Neurol* 1987;22:556.

82. Kato H, Kobayashi K, Kohari S, et al. Paroxysmal kinesigenic choreoathetosis and paroxysmal dystonic choreoathetosis in a patient with familial idiopathic hypoparathyroidism. *Tohoku J Exp Med* 1987;151: 233–239.

83. Micheli F, Frenandez Pardal M, Casas Parera I, et al. Sporadic paroxysmal dystonic choreoathetosis associated with basal ganglia calcifications. *Ann Neurol* 1986;20:750.

84. Mount LA, Reback S. Familial paroxysmal choreoathetosis. Preliminary report on a hitherto undescribed

85. Hart YM, Tampieri D, Andermann E, Andermann F, Connolly M, Farrell K. Alternating paroxysmal dystonia and hemiplegia in childhood as a symptom of basal ganglia disease. *J Neurol Neurosurg Psychiatry* 1995; 59:453–454.

86. Bhatia KP, Marsden CD, Thomas DGT. Posteroventral pallidotomy can ameliorate attacks of paroxysmal dystonia induced by exercise. *J Neurol Neurosurg Psychiatry* 1998;65:604–605.

87. Lee MS, Marsden CD. Movement disorders following lesions of the thalamus or subthalamic region. *Mov Disord* 1994;9:493–507.

88. Hartmann A, Pogarell O, Oertel WH. Secondary dystonias. *J Neurol* 1998;245:511–518.

89. Obeso JA, Gimenez-Roldan. Clinicopathological correlation in symptomatic dystonia. In: Fahn S, Marsden CD, Calne DB, eds. *Advances in neurology, Vol. 50. Dystonia 2.* New York: Raven Press, 1988:113–122.

90. Janvas JL, Aminoff MJ. Dystonia and chorea in acquired systemic disorders. *J Neurol Neurosurg Psychiatry* 1998;65:436–445.

91. Stevens H. Paroxysmal Choreo-athetosis. A form of reflex epilepsy. *Arch Neurol* 1966;14:415–420.

92. Rehders JH, Loscher W, Richter A. Evidence for striatal dopaminergic overactivity in paroxysmal dystonia indicated by microinjections in a genetic rodent model. *Neuroscience* 2000;97:267–277.

93. Loong SC, Ong YY. Paroxysmal kinesigenic choreoathetosis: report of a case relieved by L-dopa. *J Neurol Neurosurg Psychiatry* 1973;36:921–924.

94. FitzGerald PM, Jankovic J. Tardive oculogyric crises. *Neurology* 1989;39:1434–1437.

95. Sachdev P. Tardive and chronically recurrent oculogyric crises. *Mov Disord* 1993;8:93–97.

96. Micheli F, Frenandez Pardal M, de Arbelaiz R, et al. Parozysmal dystonia responsive to anticholinergic drugs. *Clin Neuropharmacol* 1987;10:365–369.

97. Mushet GR, Dreifuss FE. Paroxysmal dyskinesia. A case responsive to benztropine mesylate. *Arch Dis Child* 1967;42,654–656.

98. Rosen JA. Paroxysmal choreoathetosis. Associated with perinatal hypoxic encephalopathy. *Arch Neurol* 1964;11:385–387.

99. Berkovic SF. Paroxysmal movement disorders and epilepsy. Links across the channel. *Neurology* 2000; 55:169–170.

100. Bhatia KP, Griggs RC, Ptácek LJ. Episodic movement disorders as channelopathies. *Mov Disord* 2000;15: 429–433.

101. Swoboda KJ, Soong B-W, McKenna C, et al. Paroxysmal kinesigenic dyskinesia and infantile convulsions. Clinical and linkage studies. *Neurology* 2000;55: 224–230.

102. Pereira AC, Loo WJ, Bamford M, et al. Use of lamotrigine to treat paroxysmal kinesigenic choreoathetosis. *J Neurol Neurosurg Psychiatry* 2000;68: 796–797.

103. Sethi KD, Hess DC, Huffnagle VH, et al. Acetazolamide treatment of paroxysmal dystonia in central demyelinating disease. *Neurology* 1992;42:919–921.

Myoclonus and Paroxysmal Dyskinesias,
Advances in Neurology, Vol. 89,
edited by S. Fahn, et al.
Published by Lippincott Williams & Wilkins, Philadelphia, 2002.

37

Transient Ischemic Attacks and Paroxysmal Dyskinesias: An Under-Recognized Association

*Néstor Gálvez-Jiménez, †Maurice R. Hanson, †Melanie J. Hargreave, and *Perla Peirut

*Department of Neurology, The Cleveland Clinic Florida, Weston, Florida;
†Department of Neurology, The Cleveland Clinic Florida, Naples, Florida

The paroxysmal dyskinesias may be classified as idiopathic or familial and secondary (symptomatic) (Tables 37.1, 37.2). Idiopathic or "familial" paroxysmal dyskinesias are a heterogeneous group of movement disorders (MDS) classified into four main categories as proposed by Demirkiran and Jankovic (1) and modified by Bhatia (2). These are paroxysmal kinesigenic dyskinesia (PKD), paroxysmal non-kinesigenic dyskinesia (PKND), paroxysmal exercise-induced dyskinesia (PED), and hypnogenic paroxysmal dyskinesia (HPD). Secondary or symptomatic paroxysmal dyskinesias resulting from transient ischemic attacks (TIA) have rarely been reported. In reviewing the literature, few reported cases of acute or paroxysmal dyskinesias associated with TIA have been reported (3). Most reported cases of vascular origin results in delayed symptoms and are usually due to focal cerebral lesions (4–21). Most of these reports are based on patients' descriptions of the abnormal movements as most were poorly witnessed by the treating physician, and predated the era of current neuroimaging and ultrasonographic techniques.

In recent years, we encountered five patients presenting to our institution for evaluation of transient ischemic episodes who had as their initial clinical presentation paroxysmal or acute hyperkinetic movement disorders. These episodes were quickly followed by focal neurologic deficits. The relation of the TIA as the cause of their symptoms was suspected based on the demographics of the patients such as age, risk factors for cerebrovascular athero-occlusive disease, clinical features, and phenomenology of the paroxysmal dyskinesias in association with focal neurologic symptoms. All episodes were wit-

TABLE 37.1. *Classification and causes of paroxysmal dyskinesias*

I. Idiopathic or familial paroxysmal dyskinesias
  a. Paroxysmal kinesigenic dyskinesias (PKD)
  b. Paroxysmal nonkinesigenic dyskinesias (PNKD)
  c. Exercise-induced dyskinesias (PED)
  d. Hypnogenic paroxysmal dyskinesias (HPD)
II. Secondary or symptomatic dyskinesias
  a. Vascular
    1. Vertebrobasilar transient ischemic attacks
    2. Generalized hemispheric hypoperfusion (carotid artery disease)
    3. Cerebral infarctions (thalamic, basal ganglia, internal capsule, parietal, frontal lobes)
  b. Basal ganglia calcifications
    1. Idiopathic or familial
    2. Hypoparathyroidism
  c. Metabolic
    1. Hypoglycemia
    2. Hypocalcemia
  d. Endocrine
    1. Hypoparathyroidism
  e. Infectious
    1. HIV disease
  f. Tumors
    1. Lymphoma

TABLE 37.2. *Types of movement disorders presenting as or associated with paroxysmal dyskinesias*

Hyperkinetic[a]
  Paroxysmal tremor (postural, resting, rubral, action induced)
  Chorea/ballism
  Dystonia
  Stereotypies
  Myoclonus
  Asterixis (negative myoclonus)
Akinetic/hypokinetic–rigid syndrome
  Parkinsonism[b]

[a]See text for references.
[b]This report.

nessed or induced by the examining physician and complete neurological evaluation and neuroimaging procedures led to the understanding of the pathogenesis of their symptoms in relation to transient ischemic episodes. Patients seen at our institution with paroxysmal dyskinesias due to metabolic, endocrine, infectious, or neoplastic causes were excluded.

CASE REPORTS

Patient 1

This 67-year-old woman presented to the emergency department of the Cleveland Clinic Florida Hospital (CCH) complaining of two episodes of sudden shaking of the right hand unaccompanied by warning signs. They lasted for approximately 2 minutes. During one of these episodes she had slurred speech. While in the emergency department she had an attack of sudden right hand and forearm tremor consisting predominantly of a fast frequency flexion/extension of the hand superimposed on a stiff trembling forearm, at the elbow. Slurred speech and weakness of the right upper and lower limb quickly followed. Her reflexes were normal, but a plantar extensor response was noted on the right. No dystaxia on heel to shin testing was present but mild clumsiness and past pointing on finger to nose testing was noted on the right upper extremity interpreted as due to limb weakness rather than ataxia. The rest of the neurologic

assessment was unremarkable. Computed axial (CT) tomography scan of the brain was unremarkable. Dupplex ultrasonography examination revealed a high-grade left carotid stenosis (75% to 95%). Transcranial Doppler ultrasonography (TCD) was normal except for a mild decrease in left middle and anterior cerebral flow velocities consistent with low pressures due to left internal carotid stenosis. Brain magnetic resonance imaging (MRI) demonstrated mild periventricular white matter changes consistent with ischemic leukomalacia. Magnetic resonance angiography (MRA) of the carotid arteries confirmed a 90% stenosis of the left internal carotid artery (Fig. 37.1). Cardiovascular evaluation was un-

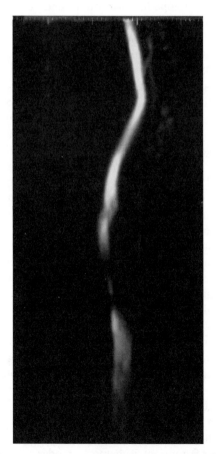

FIG. 37.1. MRA demonstrating a high-grade stenosis of the left internal carotid artery in patient 1.

remarkable. She underwent a left carotid endarterectomy followed by 325 mg of aspirin daily. The patient's attacks ceased.

Patient 2

A 72-year-old man presented with an 18-month history of short-lived episodes of sudden gait instability, slurred speech, and loss of manual dexterity during heat, fatigue, or stress. During an office evaluation and after 20 minutes of physical exercise, limb and gait ataxia with right hand tremor, micrographia with rigidity, and dysarthria developed. He also had upbeat nystagmus. The whole episodes lasted approximately 20 minutes. Carotid artery ultrasonography was unremarkable but a TCD demonstrated dampened flow of the basilar artery. Cardiovascular evaluation was unremarkable. A brain MRI demonstrated diffuse bilateral periventricular white matter ischemic lesions. Magnetic resonance angiography of the posterior circulation (Fig. 37.2) showed a severe high-grade steno-

sis of the right vertebral artery and a hypoplastic left vertebral artery. Cerebral angiography confirmed all MRA findings (greater than 80%, 1.5-cm stenotic segment of the right vertebral artery with a hypoplastic left vertebral artery). There was also a previously undiagnosed 70% left cavernous carotid artery tandem stenosis. Despite warfarin therapy, the attacks continued. He underwent a right vertebral artery balloon angioplasty resulting in a 50% residual stenosis. The attacks ceased.

Patient 3

A 70-year-old woman presented to the emergency room with two episodes of acute right hand shaking. During an attack, examination revealed intact cognition, dysarthria, and right limb dystaxia. Her right hand demonstrated a dystonic hand posturing while outstretched with "forced" abduction and extension of the fingers, ulnar hand deviation at the wrist, scooping of the hand, and slight op-

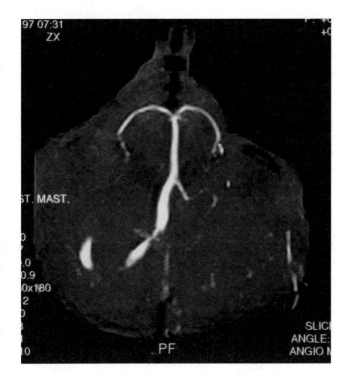

FIG. 37.2. Intracranial MRA demonstrating a high-grade stenosis of the right vertebral artery and a hypoplastic left vertebral artery in patient 2.

position of the fifth finger. A coarse, fast frequency flexion/extension rest hand tremor with tremorous handwriting was also present. All symptoms disappeared in approximately 30 minutes without residua. Carotid artery ultrasound, TCD, and cardiovascular assessments were normal. Electroencephalography (EEG) was normal. An emergency brain CT scan showed diffuse centrum semiovale ischemic periventricular white matter lesions with bilateral old lacunar infarcts in the striatum and left thalamus. No acute hemorrhages were noted. On follow-up brain MRI, no new lesions were observed 72 hours after admission. She began treatment with 325 mg of aspirin daily and had no further episodes.

Patient 4

A 73-year-old man who had an extracranial-intracranial (ECIC) bypass surgery presented with episodes of paroxysmal gait ataxia despite standard aspirin and ticlopidine therapy. Examination between attacks was normal. Brain MRI demonstrated an old left watershed ACA/MCA territory infarction and bilateral cerebellar lacunar strokes. Due to concerns about ECIC bypass reocclusion, a cerebral angiogram was performed. After a four-vessel cerebral angiogram, expressive aphasia with right hemiparesis ensued for approximately 1 hour. The angiogram demonstrated the prior findings of complete occlusion of both carotid arteries, a hypoplastic right vertebral artery, and a patent left ECIC bypass. The remaining of the anterior circulation and right MCA were fed through a dominant left vertebral and basilar artery system. The patient was kept in hospital for observation. Twelve hours before discharge, a paroxysmal arrhythmic and repetitive coarse jerky dystonic/myoclonic movement involving the left face, neck, shoulder, and proximal upper limb developed. Mini-mental status examination was normal with no corticospinal tract signs. His coordination was normal except for difficulty in performing finger-to-nose testing on the left due to interference from his adventitious movements. During this time, the movements disappeared during sleep, reappearing on awakening. The whole episode terminated abruptly after approximately 18 hours. Repeated brain CT scan was normal and three sequential EEG recordings during the attacks were normal, without evidence of periodic lateralizing epileptiform discharges. He was treated with warfarin. No further attacks have been reported.

Patient 5

A 76-year-old man was admitted to CCH because of an episode of a shaking leg lasting approximately 2 minutes followed by right leg weakness. He thought that a right hand tremor was also present during the attack. He denied slurred speech, diplopia, visual phenomena or phosphenes, dysphagia, sensory disturbances, clumsy hands, or gait difficulties. On admission, brain CT scan demonstrated an old lacunar infarct in the posterior limb of the right internal capsule. Carotid ultrasound and TCD studies were normal. Cardiovascular assessment was normal. While in hospital he had an episode of a rather coarse wide amplitude and jerky irregular alternating flexion/extension tremor affecting predominantly the hip joint accompanied by slight flexion/extension of the leg at the knee and a dystonic dorsiflexion of the foot and extension of the toes. His reflexes appeared to be increased during the attack. Slurred speech developed. This episode lasted approximately 3 minutes and was quickly followed by hemiparesis affecting the leg more than the arm. No tremor of the right upper limb was noted. His sensory examination was normal. A brain CT scan demonstrated no intraaxial or extraaxial lesions, hemorrhage, nor the presence of the hyperacute MCA sign. The patient did not receive recombinant tissue plasminogen activator as the episode resolved without residua 1 hour after onset of symptoms. Electroencephalography obtained immediately after the episode had neither epileptiform discharges nor focal slowing. Holter monitoring showed no arrhythmia and an MRA of the intracranial vasculature was unremarkable. He was placed on 325 mg of aspiring daily and heparin was discontinued. No further episodes have been reported.

DISCUSSION

Our patients comprise three women and two men with a mean age of 70 years (67 to 73 years). These episodes (all witness) lasted 10 to 30 minutes except in patient 4 in whom the abnormal movements began 12 hours after a four-vessel cerebral angiogram and lasted for approximately 18 hours. All patients had known risk factors for cerebrovascular athero-occlusive disease such as hypertension, smoking history, hyperlipidemia, peripheral vascular disease, and coronary artery disease (Table 37.3). The most common paroxysmal movement disorders observed in our patients were tremor in three patients, paroxysmal ataxia in two, acute limb dystonia in two, and an arrhythmic repetitive coarse, jerky movement affecting predominantly the left face, neck, shoulder, and proximal upper extremity with dystonic/myoclonic characteristics in one. In addition one patient had transient parkinsonism featured by micrographia and bradykinesia with limb tremor.

In cases 1,4, and 5, the associated symptoms were in keeping with distribution of the anterior circulation, and global bilateral cortical and subcortical hypoperfusion in case four. In these patients, involvement of the striatum via the lenticulostriatal (MCA) perforators and hypoperfusion of the head of the caudate via the recurrent artery of Heubner (ACA), in addition to the cortex, cannot be completely excluded (Figs. 37.3, 37.4). We may assume that the generation of these abnormal movements was a result of the greater involvement of the subcortical structures and associated connections and, to a lesser extent the cortical mantle. The lack of paroxysmal EEG abnormalities in these patients supports a subcortical origin of these abnormal movements. Cases 1 and 4 are similar to the earlier observations made by Miller-Fisher (22), Russell and Page (23), Yanagihara and associates (24), and Baquis and associates (25) where transient abnormal involuntary movements, predominantly "limb shaking," are manifestations of severe carotid artery athero-occlusive disease. Michel and colleagues (26) reported "shaking limbs" or tremor in the setting of severe carotid and basilar stenosis. Tatemichi and associates (27) demonstrated alterations of resting cerebral blood flow velocities using xenon-133 in a 63-year-old man with limb shaking and leg buckling associated with severe bilateral internal carotid artery disease. Baumgartner and Baumgartner (28), using CO_2 reactivity studies, demonstrated cerebral hemodynamic failure in five patients presenting with TIA and contralateral limb shaking. Differing from earlier case reports, our patients had, in addition to limb tremor, transient ataxia, myoclonic jerks, and dystonic limb posturing. In addition, patient 4 developed rhythmical facial, neck, and shoulder movements after angiography. Transient alteration or "irritation'" of a presumed brainstem generator resulting in a brainstem reticular origin of the movements is possible. These movements were akin to the brainstem reticular myoclonus described by Hallet and associates (29). Gordon and Lendon (30) reported a pathologically confirmed case of vertebrobasilar thrombosis and involuntary movement of the trunk, neck, and occasional twitching of the legs. Lai and Siegel (31) demonstrated brainstem-mediated locomotion and myoclonic jerks in 40 decerebrated cats. Histologic analysis showed hemorrhagic lesions in the retrorubral nucleus and ventral mesopontine junction. Hanna and Frank (32) described a patient with involuntary "pedaling alternating leg movements" as a release sign from uncal herniation giving further support for a brainstem generator. Similar hypotheses have been suggested to explain some of the abnormal movements seen in patients with restless legs syndrome and nocturnal myoclonus or periodic leg movement of sleep (33–35). Furthermore, EEG recordings did not support a cortical origin of his movements. Somatosensory evoked responses were unobtainable due to movement artifacts.

Baquis' (25) case descriptions emphasized the phenomenology of the abnormal limb

TABLE 37.3. Summary of patient clinical data

Patient number	Risk factors	Examination (during attack)	PHMD description	CT/MRI/ Angiography	Ultrasonography and other tests	Misc./ treatment
1	CAD, PVD, HTN, R carotid endart.	R arm and leg weakness, dysarthria	Coarse, moderate amplitude R arm tremor	MRA: 90% stenosis L ICA. L SCA 3 mm aneurysm	Carotid US: 70%–90% stenosis	Left carotid endart Aspirin 325 mg/d
2	CAD, ↑ chol, + smoker	Dysarthria, micrographia, stiffness, no limb weakness	Limb and gait-ataxia, R hand tremor	Diffuse bilateral white matter lesions High grade (tight) stenosis R vertebral artery (>80% 1.5 cm)	Carotid US: WNL TCD: low-flow basilar artery	Hemodinamic-dependent PHMD Angioplasty with residual 50% stenosis Rx: warfarin Rx: aspirin
3	HTN, DM, CAD, + smoker	Dysarthria, no limb weakness	R limb ataxia, dystonia, resting coarse, fast frequency flexion/ extension hand tremor for 30 min	Diffuse bilateral centrum semiovale lesions (CT scan) Lacunar infarcts bilateral striatum and L thalamus	Carotid US: WNL TCD: WNL Cardiac echo: WNL	
4	Bilateral EC/IC bypass	Gait ataxia, expressive aphasia and R hemiparesis	Arrythmic/repetitive, coarse, jerky, dystonic/myoclonic	MRI: L watershed infarction, cerebellar lacunar strokes Angiogram: complete occlusion both carotids, hypoplastic R vertebral artery, patent EC/IC bypass	EEG: WNL	Rx: warfarin
5	HTN, CAD, PVD, ↑ chol, + smoker	R leg weakness	R jerky leg movement followed by leg weakness	Lacunar infarct, posterior limb, R internal capsule	Carotid US: WNL TCD: WNL	Holter monitor: WNL Rx: aspirin

Endart, endarterectomy; HTN, hypertension; DM, diabetes mellitus; CAD, coronary artery disease; chol, cholesterol; SCA, superior cerebellar artery; ICA, internal carotid artery; Rx, treatment; PVD, peripheral vascular disease; PHMD, paroxysmal dyskinesia movement disorder; CT, computed tomography; MRA, magnetic resonance angiography; MRI, magnetic resonance imaging; EC/IC, external carotid/internal carotid; US, ultrasonography; WNL, within normal limits; TCD, transcranial Doppler ultrasonography; echo, echocardiography; EEG, electroencephalography; R, right; L, left.

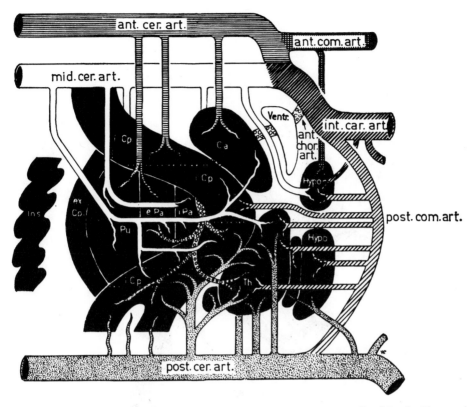

FIG. 37.3. Diagram demonstrating the vascularization of the basal ganglia. (Used with permission from Krayenbuhl HA, Yasargil MG. Cerebral angiography, 2d ed. Philadelphia: Lippincott, 1968.)

movements as shaking, trembling, twitching, flapping, or wavering lasting seconds to few minutes. All patients in Baquis' series had symptoms attributable to low perfusion pressures of the anterior circulation due to unilateral or bilateral carotid artery occlusion or high-grade stenosis. Patients 2, 4, 5, 6, and 8 had resolution of their symptoms after ECIC bypass surgery. Patients 3 and 7 were treated with platelet anti-aggregant agents and patient 1 had a carotid endarterectomy with complete control of symptoms. Miller-Fisher (22) who used terms such as twisting, shaking, or drawing made similar earlier observations, to describe the transient limb movements present in his patients. He further emphasized that seizures are rare in cases of carotid artery disease and that "limb shaking" was related to severe contralateral carotid artery disease.

In Yanagihara's (24) case series, five patients had limb shaking, six patients had limb jerks, and one patient had swinging of an arm. Only case 7 was described as having concomitant ataxia, but it is not clear if the ataxia was paroxysmal in nature. Electroencephalography failed to document epileptiform discharges in all patients. In five patients the EEG was normal and in seven, focal or generalized slowing was noted. Severe carotid artery stenosis or occlusion was present in all patients with resolution of symptoms after ECIC bypass or carotid endarterectomy.

Margolin and Marsden (36) were the first to use the term episodic dyskinesias when describing the paroxysmal movement disorders seen in patients in whom transient ischemic attacks were present. In their series of four patients, carotid artery disease was present in

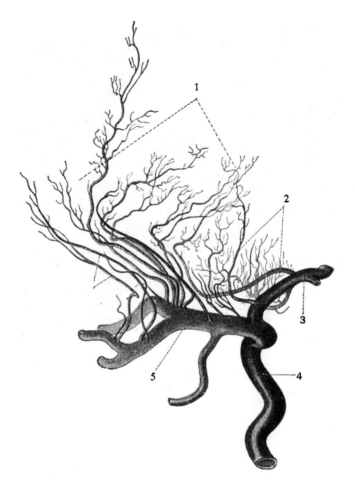

FIG. 37.4. The above drawing demonstrates the (*1*) striatolenticularis arteries, (*2*) the recurrent artery of Heubner also known as the anterior striatal artery, (*3*) anterior cerebral artery, (*4*) internal carotid artery, and (*5*) medial cerebral artery. (Used with permission from Krayenbuhl HA, Yasargil MG. Cerebral angiography, 2d ed. Philadelphia: Lippincott, 1968.)

two, hypertension in three, and a cardiac source of embolism was documented in one. Carotid endarterectomy, platelet anti-aggregant agents or anticoagulation resulted in symptom control in all patients. Athetosis or ballism was the predominant dyskinesias. They were described as writhing, snakelike, or wild gyrations. In a related letter to the editor, Stark (37) described a 53-year-old woman with systemic lupus erythematosus who had episodes of paroxysmal choreoathetosis associated with contralateral high-grade carotid artery stenosis. Symptoms improved after carotid endarterectomy.

Prick and Korten (38) described acute hemichorea/hemiballism or choreoathetosis in nine patients who had high-grade carotid artery stenosis. Four had symptoms on the side contralateral to the stenosis, four had both ipsilateral or bilateral carotid artery disease, and one had subclavian steal syndrome with left dyskinesias. One patient underwent a carotid endarterectomy with resolution of symptoms, another was treated with warfarin, one received no treatment, and the remaining six died. Two of their cases (cases 1 and 6) had some similarities to patient four of our series who had symptoms for a prolonged time (approximately 18 hours) affecting predominantly the face, neck, shoulder, and arm. Case 1 of Prick's series had symptoms lasting approximately 72 hours associated with complete occlusion of the right internal carotid artery. Case 6 had symptoms in both the face and platysma and a high-grade stenosis of the right internal carotid artery. As with our patient, neither case 1 nor 6 had loss of consciousness, or EEG demonstration of focal contralateral epileptiform discharges.

Other reports (39,40) linked Moya Moya disease with paroxysmal stimulus sensitive dyskinesia characterized by wrist extension, pronation, and athetosis. Thalamic infarctions may result in brief attacks of paroxysmal kinesigenic dystonic choreoathetosis (41), acute transient pseudo-choreoathetosis associated with proprioceptive sensory loss (42), and other transient dyskinesias (43). Attacks of paroxysmal, brief, painful, limb spasms (44) and hemichorea/hemiballism (45) have been associated with putaminal infarctions. Transient abrupt onset asterixis may result after midbrain (46) and thalamic infarctions (47). Kimber and Thompson (48) reported symptomatic hyperexplexia as a result of pontine infarction. Brainstem ischemia resulting in episodic undulating hyperkinesis of the tongue was reported by Postert and associates (49). Riley (50) described a 69-year-old man with paroxysmal kinesigenic dystonia affecting his throat and tongue from a medullary hemorrhage. Orthostatic limb shaking (51) and focal seizures (52) has also been reported with cerebral global hypoperfusion.

An interesting observation was the occurrence of paroxysmal or transient acute-onset parkinsonism in patient 2 manifest as micrographia, paroxysmal tremor and rigidity in addition to transient acute-onset ataxia, dysarthria, horizontal and vertical nystagmus after 20 minutes of physical exercise. All symptoms disappeared after 20 minutes of rest. This patient had compromised his posterior circulation with hemodynamically significant high-grade stenosis of the right vertebral artery and a hypoplastic left vertebral artery. In addition, he had a tandem high-grade stenosis of the left cavernous carotid artery. His symptoms disappear after vertebral artery angioplasty. Patient 3 in our series also had symptoms attributable to the posterior circulation. His symptoms consisted of dysarthria, and ataxia accompanying a coarse rapid flexion/extension rest tremor and dystonia. These patient's symptoms may be explained by direct involvement of the substantia nigra, red nucleus and nigrostriatal, cerebellofugal and thalamofugal projections in the area of Forel as well as the thalamus. Support for this assumption comes from our observation of distal low perfusion pressures in the vertebral, basilar, and posterior cerebral arteries as demonstrated using transcranial Doppler ultrasonography in patient 2. These structures depend on intact perfusion via the paramedian or lateral perforators branches of the basilar artery, the posterior choroidal artery and thalamoperforators, which are branches of the posterior cerebral and posterior communicating arteries (Fig. 37.5). Matsumoto and associates (53) demonstrated increased midbrain susceptibility to ischemia, followed by the thalamus and cerebral cortex using CO_2 reactivity in an experimental model of localized brainstem infarction. Patient 3 had a normal carotid ultrasound and transcranial doppler ultrasonography of the posterior circulation but brain MRI scan showed diffuse bilateral centrum semiovale white matter lesions, lacunar infarcts in the striatum and left thalamus consistent with small vessel arteriopathy. Furthermore, his symptoms improved with platelet anti-aggregant therapy.

Patients 3 and 5 of our series differ from those described in the literature, as their symptoms did not result from hemodynamically dependent large vessel athero-occlusive disease such as patients 1,2, and 4 but more likely due to small vessel athero-occlusive arteriopathy.

In conclusion, when strokes result in abnormal involuntary movements, they are delayed consisting of chorea/ballism, dystonia, tremor (cortical or thalamic), myoclonus, stereotypies, and generalized chorea due to bilateral basal ganglia strokes. Transient is-

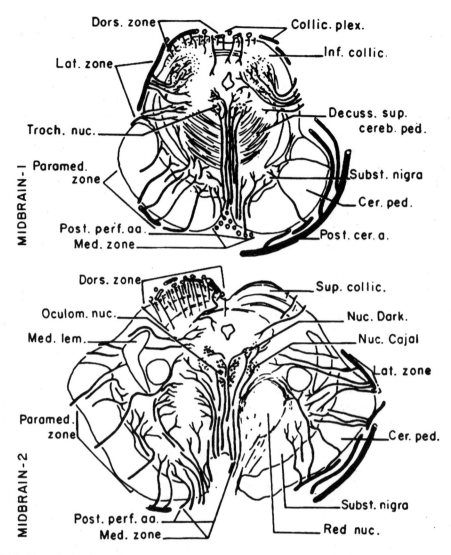

FIG. 37.5. Vascularization of the midbrain. (Modified and used with permission from Gillilan LA. Anatomy and embryology of the arterial system of the brain stem and cerebellum. In: Vinken PJ, Bruyn GW, eds. *Handbook of clinical neurology. Vol. 11.* New York: Elsevier, 1972.)

chemic attacks presenting as paroxysmal dyskinesias are rare. When patients present with paroxysmal dyskinesias, and have risk factors for cerebrovascular disease, transient ischemic attacks should be seriously considered and appropriately evaluated. These paroxysmal dyskinesias may be an accompaniment or the sole presentation of TIA and may complicate cerebral angiography. In addition to a "shaking limb" or tremor; dystonia, myoclonic jerks, myorrythmic-like movements, and transient parkinsonism may all be seen during a TIA. Treatment of the underlying cause for the TIA will be rewarding in most patients.

REFERENCES

1. Demirkiran M, Jankovic J. Paroxysmal dyskinesias: clinical features and classification. *Ann Neurol* 1995;38 (4):571–579.
2. Bhatia K. Idiopathic (familial) paroxysmal dyskinesias. *Semin Neurol* 2001;21(1):69–74.

3. Ghika-Schmid F, Ghika J, Regli F, et al. Hyperkinetic movement disorders during and after acute stroke: the Lausanne Stroke Registry. *J Neurol Sci* 1997;146: 109–116.

4. Marsden CD, Obeso J, Zarranz JJ, et al. The anatomical basis of symptomatic hemidystonia. *Brain* 1985;108: 463–483.

5. Burke RE, Stanley F, Gold AP. Delayed onset dystonia in patients with static encephalopathy. *J Neurol Neurosurg Psychiatry* 1980;43:789–797.

6. Demierre B, Rondot P. Dystonia caused by putamino-capsulo-caudate vascular lesions. *J Neurol Neurosurg Psychiatry* 1983;46:404–409.

7. Burton K, Farrel K, Li D, et al. Lesions of the putamen in dystonia: CT and magnetic resonance imaging. *Neurology* 1984;34:962–965.

8. Donat JR. Unilateral asterixis due to thalamic hemorrhage. *Neurology* 1980;30:83–84.

9. Ghika J, Bogousslavsky, Henderson J, et al. The jerky dystonic unsteady hand, a delayed complex hyperkinetic syndrome in posterior thalamic infarcts. *J Neurol* 1994; 241:537–542.

10. Dewey RR, Jankovic J. Hemiballism-hemichorea. Clinical and pharmacological findings in 21 patients. *Arch Neurol* 1989; 46:862–867.

11. Grimes JD, Hassan MN, Quarrington AH, et al. Delayed onset post hemiplegic dystonia. CT demonstration of basal ganglia pathology. *Neurology* 1982;32:1033–1035.

12. Bogousslavsky J, Regli F, Uske A. Thalamic infarcts: clinical syndromes, etiology and prognosis. *Neurology* 1988;38:837–848.

13. Goldblatt D, Markesbery W, Reeves AG. Recurrent hemichorea following striatal lesions. *Arch Neurol* 1974;31:51–54.

14. Klawans HL, Moses H, Nausieda PA, et al. Treatment and prognosis of hemiballism. *N Engl J Med* 1976;295: 1348–1350.

15. Donnan GA, Bladin PE, Berkovick SF, et al. The stroke syndrome of striatocapsular infarction. *Brain* 1991;114: 51–70.

16. Croisile B, Tourniaire D, Confavreux C, et al. Bilateral damage to the head of the caudate nuclei. *Ann Neurol* 1989;25:313–314.

17. Richetfield EK, Twyman R, Berent S. Neurological syndromes following bilateral damage to the head of the caudate nuclei. *Ann Neurol*1987;22:768–771.

18. Feve AP, Fenelon G, Remy P, et al. Axial motor disturbances after hypoxic lesion of the globus pallidus. *Mov Disord* 1993;8:321–326.

19. Maraganore DI, Less AJ, Marsden CD. Complex stereotypies after right putaminal infarction: a case report. *Mov Disord* 1991;6:358–361.

20. Lee MS, Lee SA, Heo JH, et al. A patient with resting tremor and a lacunar infarction at the border between the thalamus and the internal capsule. *Mov Disord* 1993;8:244–246.

21. Sethi KD, Nicholar FT, Yaghmai F. Chorea due to basal ganglia lacunar infarcts. *Mov Disord* 1987;2:61–66.

22. Fisher CM. Concerning recurrent transient cerebral ischemic attacks. *Can Med J* 1962;86:1091–1099.

23. Ross Russell W, Page GR. Critical Perfusion of brain and retina. *Brain* 1983;106:419–434.

24. Yanagihara T, Piepgrass DG, Klass DW. Repetitive involuntary movement associated with episodic cerebral ischemia. *Ann Neurol* 1985; 18: 244–250.

25. Baquis GD, Michael MD, Pessin S, et al. Limb shaking-A carotid TIA. *Stroke* 1985;16(3):444–448.

26. Michel B, Lemarquis P, Nicoli F, et al. Abnormal postural movements: carotid transient ischemic episodes? *Rev Neurol (Paris)* 1989;145(12):853–855.

27. Tatemichi TK, Young WL, Prohovnik I, et al. Perfusion insufficiency in limb-shaking transient ischemic attacks. *Stroke* 1990;21:341–347.

28. Baumgartner RW, Baumgartner I. Vasomotor reactivity is exhausted in transient ischemic attacks with limb shaking. *J Neurol Neurosurg Psychiatry* 1998;65: 561–564.

29. Hallet M, Chadwick D, Marsden CD, et al. Reticular reflex myoclonus: a physiological type of human posthypoxic myoclonus. *J Neurol Neurosurg Psychiatry* 1979; 42:52–55.

30. Gordon N, Lendon M. Vertebro-basilar thrombosis and involuntary movements. *Dev Med Child Neurol* 1985; 27:664–667.

31. Lai YY, Siegel JM. Brainstem-mediated locomotion and myoclonic jerks. I. Neural substrates. *Brain Res* 1997; 745:257–264.

32. Hanna JP, Frank JI. Automatic stepping in the pontomedullary stage of central herniation. *Neurology* 1995;45:985–986.

33. Lugaresi E, Cirignotta F, Coccagna G, et al. Nocturnal myoclonus and restless syndrome. *Adv Neurol* 1986;43: 295–307.

34. Sachdev P. *Akathisia and restless legs*. Cambridge, UK: Cambridge University Press, 1995.

35. Galvez-Jimenez N, Khan T. Ropinirole and restless legs syndrome. *Mov Disord* 1999;14(5):890–892.

36. Margolin DI, Marsden CD. Episodic dyskinesias and transient cerebral ischemia. *Neurology* 1982;32:1379–1380.

37. Stark SR. Transient dyskinesias and cerebral ischemia. *Neurology*1985;35:445.

38. Prick JJW, Korten JJ. Unilateral involuntary movements of acute onset in the adult, nine case reports and an alternative pathophysiological hypothesis. *Clin Neurol Neurosurg* 1988;90(4):321-327.

39. Nijssen PCG, Tijssen CC. Stimulus-sensitive paroxysmal dyskinesias associated with a thalamic infarct. *Mov Disord* 1992;7(4):364–366.

40. Suzuki J, Kodama N. Moyamoya disease-a review. *Stroke* 1983;14:104–109.

41. Camac A, Green P, Khandji A. Paroxysmal kinesigenic dystonic choreoathetosis associated with a thalamic infarct. *Mov Disord* 1990;5(3):235–238.

42. Lee MS, Kim YD, Kim JT, et al. Abrupt onset of transient pseudochoreoathetosis associated with propioceptive sensory loss as a result of a thalamic infarction. *Mov Disord* 1998;13:184–186.

43. Milandre L, Brosset C, Gabriel B, et al. Transient dyskinesias associated with thalamic infarcts. Report of five cases. *Rev Neurol (Paris)* 1993;149:402–406.

44. Merchut MP, Barumlik J. Painful tonic spasms caused by putaminal infarction. *Stroke* 1986;17:1319–1321.

45. Kase CS, Gilbert MD, Maulsby MD, et al. Hemichorea-hemiballism and lacunar infarction in the basal ganglia. *Neurology*1981;31:452–455.

46. Bril V, Sharpe JA, Ashby P. Midbrain asterixis. *Ann Neurol*1979;6:362–364.

47. Wayne-Massey E, Clay Goodman J, Stewart C, et al. Unilateral asterixis: motor integrative dysfunction in focal vascular disease. *Neurology* 1979;29:1188–1190.

48. Kimber TE, Thompson PD. Symptomatic hyperekplexia occurring as a result of pontine infarction. *Mov Disord* 1997;12:814–815.
49. Postert T, Amoiridis G, Pohlau D, et al. Episodic undulating hyperkinesias of the tongue associated with brainstem ischemia. *Mov Disord.* 1997;12:619–621.
50. Riley D. Paroxysmal kinesigenic dystonia associated with a medullary lesion. *Mov Disord* 1996;11: 738–740.
51. Zaidat OO, Werz MA, Landis DM, et al. Orthostatic limb shaking from carotid hypoperfusion. *Neurology* 1999;53(2):650–651.
52. Riley TL, Friedman JM. Stroke, orthostatic hypotension, and focal seizures. *JAMA* 1981;245:1243–1244.
53. Matsumoto S, Kuwubara S, Moritake K. Effects of cerebrovascular autoregulation and C02 reactivity in experimental localized brainstem infarction. *Neurol Res* 2000;22(2):197–203.
54. Krayenbuhl HA, Yasargil MG. *Cerebral angiography*, 2d ed. Philadelphia: Lippincott, 1968.
55. Gillilan LA. Anatomy and embryology of the arterial system of the brain stem and cerebellum. In: Vinken PJ, Bruyn GW, eds. *Handbook of clinical neurology. Vol. 11.* New York: Elsevier, 1972.

Myoclonus and Paroxysmal Dyskinesias,
Advances in Neurology, Vol. 89,
edited by S. Fahn, et al.
Published by Lippincott Williams & Wilkins, Philadelphia, 2002.

38

Epilepsy and Paroxysmal Dyskinesia: Co–occurrence and Differential Diagnosis

Renzo Guerrini, Lucio Parmeggiani, and *Giorgio Casari

*Neurosciences Unit, Institute of Child Health and Great Ormond Street Hospital For Children, The Wolfson Centre, London, United Kingdom; *Human Molecular Genetics Unit, Stem Cell Research Institute, IRCCS San Raffaele Hospital, Milan, Italy*

Epilepsy and paroxysmal dyskinesia (PD) may be difficult to differentiate clinically. Although in the past it has been hypothesized that episodes of PD could represent a form of epilepsy (1–3), the current understanding is that the two disorders are distinct (4).

However, there are several recent reports of families in which some individuals presented either or both paroxysmal disorders, with different age-related expression. Co-occurrence makes it likely that a common, genetically determined, pathophysiologic abnormality is variably expressed in the cerebral cortex and in basal ganglia.

A rather homogeneous syndrome of autosomal dominant infantile convulsions and paroxysmal (dystonic) choreoathetosis (ICCA) was described in 20 families from France, China, Japan, and the United States (5–9). Linkage analysis allowed the mapping of the disease gene to partially overlapping loci in the pericentromeric region of chromosome 16.

Additional autosomal dominant pedigrees are on record, from Australia and Italy, in which epilepsy was variably associated with paroxysmal kinesigenic or exercise-induced dystonia (10,11).

A pedigree in which three members in the same generation were affected by rolandic epilepsy (RE), paroxysmal exercise-induced dystonia (PED), and writer's cramp (WC) was reported from Italy (7). Linkage analysis showed a common homozygous haplotype in a critical region spanning 6 cM and entirely included within the critical region described in the French families (5), partially overlapping with the critical region assigned to the North American families (8) and distinct but contiguous to the critical region described in the Japanese families (9). Clinical analogies and linkage findings suggest that the same gene could be responsible for these clinically overlapping syndromes, with specific mutations accounting for each of these mendelian disorders.

In fact, chromosome 16 could harbor a family of genes that give rise to paroxysmal disorders, as suggested by the linkage to partially overlapping markers spanning from the pericentromeric region to 16q22.1 of two large pedigrees of Indian and African American origin with autosomal dominant paroxysmal dyskinesia.

Ion channel genes are potentially interesting candidates for syndromes featuring both these paroxysmal neurologic disorders.

Ion channel gene defects have been demonstrated in some genetic forms of epilepsies (12–14), of paroxysmal movement disorders (15–17), and of other neurologic disorders associating different paroxysmal manifestations

(18–20), with considerable clinical variability. Different mutations in the same ion channel gene (CACNL 1A4) cause two different paroxysmal nonepileptic disorders in humans (episodic ataxia type 1 [19]; and familial hemiplegic migraine [20]) and absence seizures in the mouse mutant (21,22). It is, therefore, highly probable that ion channel gene disorders could provide the pathophysiological link for co-occurrence of epilepsy and PD. Increased awareness of the possible co-occurrence of these two paroxysmal neurologic disorders will certainly increase the number of observations in the next few years.

In the present chapter we analyze the clinical elements that support the differential diagnosis between epilepsy and paroxysmal dyskinesia and review the syndromic association of idiopathic epilepsy and paroxysmal dyskinesia.

PAROXYSMAL DYSKINESIA AND EPILEPSY: DIFFERENTIAL DIAGNOSIS

Dermirkiran and Jankovich (23) classified their patients with PD into three main categories: (a) kinesigenic PDs (with attacks usually lasting less than 5 minutes); (b) exercise-induced PDs (with attacks usually lasting more than 5 minutes), and (c) nonkinesigenic PDs (with attacks usually lasting hours).

Most sporadic and all familial cases of PD are idiopathic. The familial (dominant) form of non-kinesigenic PD is linked to chromosome 2q (24–26). Putaminal or thalamic lesions have been demonstrated using neuroimaging in some patients with sporadic PD (27–29). Causes of symptomatic PD, accounting for a minority of sporadic cases include infarctions (27,28), multiple sclerosis (29,30), hypoxic encephalopathy (31); thyrotoxicosis (32), hypoparathyroidism (33), and diabetes mellitus (34). Carbamazepine and phenytoin are often effective in controlling attacks at dosages producing the same plasma levels effective in epilepsy or at lower levels (4,35). Sodium valproate seems to be less effective (35).

It has been argued that PDs, either kinesigenic or nonkinesigenic, may represent one expression of epilepsy (36–38), because of the paroxysmal character, the possible presence of prodromic aura-like symptoms, the short duration of the attacks and their response to antiepileptic drugs. Most of the cases described as movement-induced epileptic seizures by Lishman and associates (1), presented with childhood-onset episodes of focal or generalized stiffening followed by choreoathetotic movements, with preserved consciousness. While some of these patients could have had paroxysmal kinesigenic choreoathetosis, others had epileptiform EEG abnormalities and possibly a form of reflex epilepsy akin to startle epilepsy. This is also possible for the patients with spontaneous or movement-induced paroxysmal dyskinetic attacks that appeared following brain injury (39,40). In general, the presence of sustained twisting, athetosic or choreic movements, lack of EEG abnormalities during attacks, lack of episodes of unresponsiveness, which would mean spread of seizure activity outside the frontal lobes, all indicate a nonepileptic origin (4).

On the other hand, some ictal manifestations that are typical of frontal lobe seizures have often been misdiagnosed as due to idiopathic PD (for review see Fish and Marsden [41]), because of their semiology (42) and of their frequent occurrence in patients without any brain lesion and without any accompanying ictal EEG changes (43). Lugaresi and Cirignotta (44) introduced the term nocturnal PD when describing a group of patients with frequent brief, sleep-related attacks characterized by predominantly dystonic movements. Lack of any ictal or interictal scalp EEG abnormality has added to the difficulty in correctly diagnosing the nature of such episodes, as confirmed by several subsequent reports (45–48). Although it took 10 years from the first description by Lugaresi and Cirignotta (44) before the paroxysmal dystonic-like nocturnal episodes were found to be accompanied by ictal scalp EEG activity in a few patients (49), previous studies with depth electrodes had demonstrated that similar attacks were actually the expression of seizure activity in the mesial frontal lobe (46,50). Absence of ictal EEG changes in the surface EEG is not surprising considering the mesial and deep location of the area of seizure origin in these patients. Using both subdural strips and depth electrodes, Lombroso (51) demonstrated that choreoathetosis-like seizures might be accompanied by ictal activity involving both the supplementary sensorimotor cortex and the homolateral caudate nucleus. Although such a spread might be particularly frequent due to the strong cortico-subcortical connections existing between the supplementary sensorimotor cortex and the basal ganglia (52–54), its actual frequency and the respective role of the cortical and subcortical structures in producing the dyskinetic-like seizure pattern have yet to be determined.

Dystonic posturing may also occur during seizures originating in the temporal lobe (55), during which it is usually accompanied by additional, often prominent ictal features such as unresponsiveness and automatisms, and it is secondary to the spread of the ictal discharge to the frontal and parietal cortex (56).

Startle-induced epileptic seizures may sometimes mimic paroxysmal dyskinetic attacks. A sudden stimulus, either acoustic or somatosensorial, may trigger sudden dystonic posturing or stiffening, which may involve a body segment, a hemibody, or be generalized, often without any obvious impairment of consciousness (57–59). Most patients with startle epilepsy have a brain lesion producing congenital hemiplegia and present, in addition, spontaneous seizures that may be similar or different from the reflex-induced attacks. Ictal scalp EEG activity may be difficult to recognize in those patients whose attacks are characterized by diffuse stiffening, which determines a great amount of scalp muscle activity obscuring the concomitant ictal discharge. In this type of seizure, depth electrode studies have demonstrated that seizure activity involves the supplementary motor area or the primary motor cortex (58). The following sequence has been hypothesized (60): surprise stimulation—startle reaction—afferent proprioceptive volley—epileptic seizure. The initial startle response and the subsequent motor seizure may produce a bizarre paroxysmal dystonic posturing.

TRUE ASSOCIATION OF EPILEPSY AND PAROXYSMAL DYSKINESIA

Co-occurrence of epilepsy and PD in the same individual or their familial aggregation is not infrequent (35,61–66). Both paroxysmal non-kinesigenic (or dystonic) choreoathetosis (37,61,63,64,66) and paroxysmal exercise-induced dystonia (PED) (62) have been described in patients also suffering from epilepsy. However, only recently it has become evident that epilepsy and PD can be associated within a definite syndrome with mendelian inheritance (Table 38.1). Szepetowski and associates (5) described four families from the north of France showing a homogeneous syndrome of familial infantile convulsions, expressed as an autosomal dominant trait, together with variably expressed paroxysmal (dystonic) choreoathetosis (ICCA) (5). Of the 29 affected members of the four families, 22 had infantile partial seizures, almost always with early motor signs and beginning between the fourth and tenth month of life; 12 of those with seizures as well as three others had dyskinetic attacks starting in childhood or early adolescence, which were exercise-induced in six. While epileptic seizures were limited to infancy, it remains to be clarified whether the dyskinetic attacks were likewise age-related. Linkage analysis performed under the assumption of an autosomal dominant pattern of inheritance with a penetration of 0.8, allowed the mapping of the disease gene to the pericentromeric region of chromosome 16, in a 10 cM interval, between D16S401 and D16S517. Lee and colleagues (45) confirmed both the syndrome and linkage to the same chromosomal region in a Chinese family in which nine members in three generations were affected. A different phenotypic expression of the disorder was represented in the Chinese pedigree

TABLE 38.1. *Syndromes in which epilepsy and paroxysmal dyskinesia co-occur or in which either disorder is associated with other paroxysmal neurologic manifestations*

Epilepsy and paroxysmal dyskinesia	Epilepsy and other paroxysmal neurologic manifestations	Paroxysmal dyskinesia with other paroxysmal neurologic manifestations
Autosomal dominant paroxysmal (dystonic) choreoathetosis and benign infantile convulsions (5,8,9,45) Linkage: chromosome 16, pericentromeric	Episodic ataxia type I and infantile convulsions (78) Gene: potassium channel KCNAI	Autosomal dominant paroxysmal choreoathetosis and episodic ataxia (68) Linkage: chromosome 1p
Autosomal recessive RE with PED and WC (7) Linkage: chromosome 16p12-11.2	Familial herniplegic migraine and seizures (79) Linkage: chromosome 1p31	Autosomal dominant paroxysmal dystonic choreoathetosis with classic migraine (26) Linkage: chromosome 2q
Autosomal dominant kinesigenic PD, migraine, hemiplegic migraine and generalized epilepsy with febrile seizures (11)	Familial hemiplegic migraine and benign infantile convulsions (80)	Autosomal dominant PED and migraine (81)
Autosomal dominant PED and epilepsy (10)	Benign infantile convulsions, idiopathic generalized epilepsy, episodic ataxia, migraine (11)	

PD, paroxysmal dyskinesia; PED, paroxysmal exercise-induced dystonia; RE, rolandic epilepsy; WC, writer's cramp.

by seizure recurrence at a later age, predominantly generalized rather than partial seizures, episodes of status epilepticus in some individuals, and by a very mild expression and duration of dyskinetic attacks. Phenytoin was reported to be effective in stopping both dyskinetic episodes and seizures, which, in any case, disappeared by the age of 20 to 30 years. Linkage analysis not only confirmed gene assignment to the pericentromeric region of chromosome 16 but also the finding that individuals carrying the disease haplotype in the critical region may be clinically unaffected (5).

Sadamatsu and associates (67) described a pedigree in which five members in three consecutive generations were affected by a form of paroxysmal kinesigenic choreoathetosis with attacks precipitated by sudden movement or exercise. Attacks had started during school age in all individuals and had disappeared or were greatly reduced in frequency in the three patients reaching adulthood. Four of the five affected patients had suffered generalized convulsions during infancy with no recurrence at a later age with or without treat-

ment in most of them. The authors stressed that video-EEG monitoring during dyskinetic attacks in two patients showed no EEG changes, consistently with nonepileptic origin, adding to the evidence that epilepsy and PD are distinct manifestations. To reinforce this observation, they ruled out genetic linkage with five known chromosomal regions previously linked to epilepsy or movement disorders (1p [68], 2q33-35 [24, 25], 6p21.2-11 [69] and I0q23.3-q24). They did not realize, however, that they were describing a syndrome identical to ICCA. However, Tomita and colleagues (9) subsequently linked to chromosome 16p 11.2-q 12.1 the same family and seven other families, five of which presented with paroxysmal kinesigenic choreoathetosis and infantile convulsions and two with paroxysmal kinesigenic choreoathetosis alone. This locus partially overlaps the ICCA critical region and is contiguous to but not overlapping with the RE-PED-WC locus (7).

A subsequent report from Swoboda and colleagues (8) confirmed the linkage to the pericentromeric chromosome 16 (from D16S3131 to D16S3396) of a syndrome of paroxysmal dyskinesia and infantile convulsions (PKD/IC), clinically similar to ICCA. The PKD/IC critical region partially overlaps with both the ICCA (from D16S3131 and D16S517) and RE-PED-WC (D16S3131) critical regions. These authors reported 11 families with different ethnic background in which 44 individuals were affected by PKD (42 patients), IC (37 patients) or both (18 patients). Episodes of IC were brief and spontaneous and remitted by age 3 years in the absence of treatment. Onset was between 3 and 18 months of age. Age at onset for PKD was around 11 years. Episodes were triggered by sudden movement in all cases. Three individuals also reported episodes during physical exertion such as running or swimming. PKD episodes lasted uniformly less than 5 minutes, the majority lasting only seconds. Most individuals remained symptomatic at the time of participation in the study; virtually all reported improvement with age over 25 years.

In addition to familial observations, two sporadic patients with clinical features and outcome identical to the ICCA syndrome are on record (70,71).

Singh and associates (11) described an Australian family of Anglo-Saxon origin in which nine members in three generations presented with epilepsy (febrile seizures and febrile seizures plus), kinesigenic PD, migraine and hemiplegic migraine, in various combinations (febrile seizures and kinesigenic PD co-occurred in two patients).

Perniola and associates (10) reported an Italian family with six affected individuals in three generations, exhibiting a syndrome characterized by long-duration PED attacks beginning between age 5 and 10 years and disappearing between age 18 and 30 years, accompanied by different seizure types: absences during school age in three patients; complex partial seizures in adolescence and adulthood in one patient; generalized tonic-clonic seizures beginning after 10 years and with uncertain evolution in two other patients. Additional findings were myotonic discharges in one patient and mild mental retardation in three.

A pedigree in which three members in the same generation were affected by rolandic epilepsy, PED, and writer's cramp was recently reported (7). Both the seizures and PD had a strong age-related expression that peaked during childhood, while the WC, also appearing in childhood, had been stable since diagnosis. Clonazepam had some efficacy in reducing PED attacks in one patient, while acetazolamide had no significant effect. Genome-wide linkage analysis carried out under the assumption of recessive inheritance identified a common homozygous haplotype in a critical region spanning 6 cM between markers D16S3133 and D16S3131 on chromosome 16, cosegregating with the affected phenotype and producing a multipoint (LOD) score value of 3.2. Although the RE-PED-WC syndrome has unique features, it presents striking analogies with the ICCA syndrome, linked to a 10 cM region between D16S401 and D16S517 that entirely includes the 6 cM of the RE-PED-WC critical region. The same gene could be responsible for both RE-PED-WC and ICCA, with specific mutations accounting for each of these mendelian disorders. A similar finding has been reported for the chloride channel 1 gene (CLCN1), whose mutations are found in Becker and Thomsen disease, both associated with generalized myotonia. Becker disease is transmitted through an autosomal recessive pattern of inheritance, whereas Thomsen disease is transmitted in an autosomal dominant fashion (70).

Bennett and associates (72) recently linked to chromosome 16p11.2-q11.2 an African American family with paroxysmal kinesigenic dyskinesia (PKD). The critical regions for PKD and for ICCA partially overlap by > 6 cM between D16S769 and D16S517 and those for PKD/IC and ICCA overlap by approximately 7.4 cM between D16S3131 and D16S517 (Fig. 38.1). Different mutations of the same gene or two distinct genes may underlie these disorders. PKD and RE-PED-WC critical regions are contiguous but non-overlapping since D16S3131 (representing the RE-PED-WC lower boundary) and D16S769 (the PKD upper boundary) map at no recom-

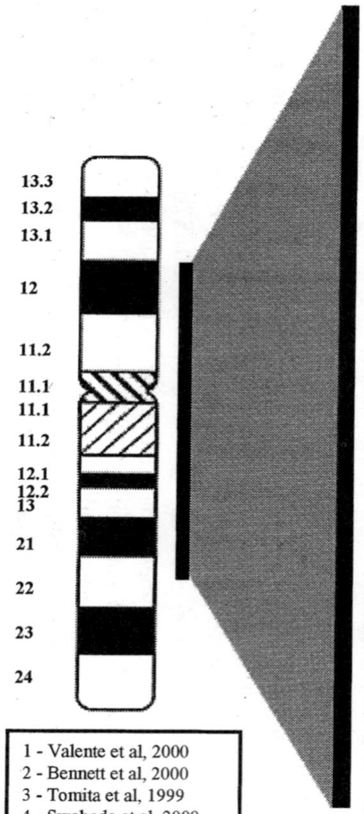

Locus	PKD[1]	PKD[2]	PKD/IC[3]	PKD/IC[4]	ICCA[5]	RE-PED-WC[6]	BFIC[7]
D16S401	D16S401	D16S401	D16S401	*D16S401*	D16S401	D16S401	*D16S401*
D16S3133	D16S3133	D16S3133	D16S3133	*D16S3133*	*D16S3133*	*D16S3133*	*D16S3133*
D16S3068	D16S3068	D16S3068	D16S3068	*D16S3068*	*D16S3068*	*D16S3068*	*D16S3068*
D16S3131	D16S3131	D16S3131	D16S3131	*D16S3131*	*D16S3131*	*D16S3131*	*D16S3131*
D16S769	D16S769	D16S769	*D16S769*	*D16S769*	D16S769	D16S769	D16S769
D16S3100	D16S3100	*D16S3100*	*D16S3100*	*D16S3100*	D16S3100	D16S3100	*D16S3100*
D16S3093	D16S3093	*D16S3093*	*D16S3093*	*D16S3093*	D16S3093	D16S3093	*D16S3093*
SPN	SPN	*SPN*	*SPN*	*SPN*	SPN	SPN	*SPN*
D16S517	D16S517	*D16S517*	*D16S517*	*D16S517*	*D16S517*	D16S517	*D16S517*
D16S3120	D16S3120	*D16S3120*	*D16S3120*	D16S3120	D16S3120	D16S3120	*D16S3120*
D16S261	D16S261	*D16S261*	*D16S261*	D16S261	D16S261	D16S261	*D16S261*
D16S753	D16S753	*D16S753*	*D16S753*	D16S753	D16S753	D16S753	*D16S753*
D16S3396	D16S3396	*D16S3396*	*D16S3396*	D16S3396	D16S3396	D16S3396	*D16S3396*
D16S416	D16S416	*D16S416*	*D16S416*	D16S416	D16S416	D16S416	*D16S416*
D16S685	*D16S685*	*D16S685*	D16S685	D16S685	D16S685	D16S685	*D16S685*
D16S419	*D16S419*	*D16S419*	D16S419	D16S419	D16S419	D16S419	*D16S419*
D16S771	*D16S771*	*D16S771*	D16S771	D16S771	D16S771	D16S771	*D16S771*
D16S415	*D16S415*	D16S415	D16S415	D16S415	D16S415	D16S415	*D16S415*
D16S503	*D16S503*	D16S503	D16S503	D16S503	D16S503	D16S503	D16S503

Chromosome 16 band positions: 13.3, 13.2, 13.1, 12, 11.2, 11.1, 11.1, 11.2, 12.1, 12.2, 13, 21, 22, 23, 24

1 - Valente et al, 2000
2 - Bennett et al, 2000
3 - Tomita et al, 1999
4 - Swoboda et al, 2000
5 - Szepetowski et al, 1997
6 - Guerrini et al, 1999
7 - Caraballo et al, 2001

FIG. 38.1. Schematic drawing showing loci (*italic bold*) where the different disorders featuring epilepsy and paroxysmal dyskinesia have been mapped on chromosome 16.

bination. These mapping data indicate the presence of more than one gene responsible for these two forms (73). An additional family with paroxysmal kinesigenic choreoathetosis (EKD2) has recently been linked to a slightly more telomeric region on chromosome 16, partially overlapping with the PKD locus (74). EKD2 spans between 16q13 and 16q22.1 (markers D16S685 to D16S503). The EKD2 region, however, does not overlap with those identified in any of the families featuring both epilepsy and paroxysmal dyskinesia. Finally Caraballo and co-workers (75) linked to chromosome 16p12-q12 seven families from Argentina and France in which 24 subjects presented with a pure form of benign familial infantile convulsions (BFIC) inherited as autosomal dominant trait. Although the critical region spans from D16S401 to D16S415, a maximum two-point LOD score was demonstrated for D16S3131 and SPN. These markers are completely included in the ICCA critical region, they appear contiguous to that of RE-PED-WC (7), and they partially overlap with those of two PKD/IC syndromes (8,9) and of one PKD syndrome (72) (Fig. 38.1). There is therefore evidence for two or more genes clustering to human chromosome 16 that cause epilepsy, paroxysmal dyskinesia or both.

Clinical and neurophysiologic abnormalities producing the epilepsy/PD syndromes are possibly caused by disturbances involving the motor cortex as well as the basal ganglia with epilepsy usually being manifested earlier than PD. It also appears that when defining the syndromic spectrum of genetically determined epilepsy and PD, as well as other paroxysmal neurologic disorders, one must make sure that general concepts of idiopathic/benign transient disorders be satisfied rather than expecting a strictly age-related expression. For example, variable phenotypic expressions of epilepsy were observed in association with mutation of the SCN1B gene (12) and variable age of onset of convulsions was present in the family with benign neonatal (extending to infancy) convulsions showing the KCNQ2 mutation (13). Different mutations of the disease gene, the existence of modifier genes and the influence of environmental factors may account for intrafamilial and interfamilial phenotypic variability. Ion channel genes are potential candidates for syndromes featuring both epilepsy and PD, as well as other syndromes in which either epilepsy or PD occur in association with other paroxysmal neurologic manifestations (Table 38.1). Different mutations of the same ion channel can produce different phenotypes, presumably via different functional effects. In families with epilepsy and PD the same mutation causes different age-related phenotypic manifestations. A possible explanation may relay on age-related expression of different subunits of the same ion channel (76). IC could be caused by a mutation in a channel causing cortical hyperexcitability in the first years of life, subsequently remitting when channel function is restored by other subunits. Peaking of functional expression of the mutated ion channel subunits at a later age in the basal ganglia would lead to later appearance of PKD (77).

The transient expression of both epilepsy and PD has certainly caused their association to be under-recognized. Only recently, due to a better knowledge of the two disorders and widespread use of video-EEG techniques, has their association been better assessed. Increased awareness of their possible co-occurrence in the same patient, either in the same period of life or at different ages, will certainly increase the number of observations in the next few years.

REFERENCES

1. Lishman WA, Symonds CP, Whitty CWM, C. Seizures induced by movement. *Brain* 1962;85:93–108.
2. Whitty CWM, Lishman WA, FitzGibbon JP. Seizures induced by movement: a form of reflex epilepsy. *Lancet* 1964;i:1403–1406.
3. Burger U, Lopez RI, Elliott FA. Tonic seizures induced by movement. *Neurology* 1972;22:656–659.
4. Fahn S. The paroxysmal dyskinesias. In: Marsden CD, Fahn S, eds. *Movement disorders 3*. Oxford: Butterworth-Heinemann, 1994:310–345.
5. Szepetowski P, Rochette J, Berquin J, et al. Familial infantile convulsions and paroxysmal choreoathetosis: a new neurological syndrome linked to pericentromeric

region of human chromosome 16. *Am J Hum Genet* 1997;61:889–898.

6. Lee BI, Lesser RP, Pippenger CE, et al. Familial paroxysmal hypnogenic dystonia. *Neurology* 1985;35:1357–1360.

7. Guerrini R, Bonanni P, Nardocci N, et al. Autosomal recessive rolandic epilepsy with paroxysmal exercise-induced dystonia and writer's cramp: delineation of the syndrome and gene mapping to chromosome 16p12-11.2. *Ann Neurol* 1999;45:344–352.

8. Swoboda KJ, Soong BW, McKenna C, et al. Paroxysmal kinesigenic dyskinesia and infantile convulsions. Clinical and linkage studies. *Neurology* 2000;55:224–230.

9. Tomita H, Nagamitsu S, Wakui K, et al. Paroxysmal kineisgenic choreoathetosis locus maps to chromosome 16p1 1.2-q12. 1. *Am J Hum Genet* 1999;65:1688–1697.

10. Perniola T, Margari MG, De laco MG, et al. Discinesia parossistica indotta dall'esercizio fisico ed epilessia: descrizione di una famiglia. *Bole Lega It. Epiessia* 1998;47:51–54.

11. Singh R, Macdonnel RAL, Sheffer LE, et al. Epilepsy and paroxysmal movement disorders in families: Evidence for shared mechanisms. *Epil Disord* 1999;1:93–99.

12. Wallace RH, Wang DW, Singh R, et al. Febrile seizures and generalized epilepsy associated with a mutation in the Na+-channel b1 subunit gene SCNIB. *Nat Genet* 1998;19:366–370.

13. Singh NA, Charlier C, Stauffer D, et al. A novel potassium channel gene, KCNQ2, is mutated in an inherited epilepsy of newborns. *Nat Genet* 1998;18:25–29.

14. Charlier C, Singh NA, Ryan SG, et al. A pore mutation in a novel KQT-like potassium channel gene in an idiopathic epilepsy family. *Nat Genet* 1998;18:53–55.

15. Browne DL, Gancher ST, Nutt JG, et al. Episodic ataxia/myokymia syndrome is associated with point mutations in the human potassium channel gene, KCNA I. *Nat Genet* 1994;8:136–140.

16. Litt M, Kramer P, Browne D, et al. A gene for episodic ataxia/myokymia maps to chromosome 12q13. *Am J Hum Genet* 1994;55:702–709.

17. Vahedi K, Joutel A, Van Bogaert P, et al. A gene for hereditary paroxysmal cerebellar ataxia maps to chromosome 19p. *Ann Neurol* 1995;37:289–293.

18. Ophoff RA, van Eijk R, Sandkuijl LA, et al. Genetic heterogeneity of familial herniplegic migraine. *Genomics* 1994;22:21–26.

19. Ophoff RA, Terwindt GM, Vergouwe MN, et al. Familial hemiplegic migraine and episodic ataxia type-2 are caused by mutations in the CA2+ channel gene CACNL 1A4. *Cell* 1996;87:543–552.

20. Joutel A, Ducros A, Vahedi K et al. Genetic heterogeneity of familial hemiplegic migraine. *Am J Hum Genet* 1994;55:1162–1172.

21. Fletcher CF, Lutz CM, O'Sullivan CM, et al. Absence epilepsy in tottering mutant mice is associated with calcium channel defects. *Cell* 1996;87:607–617.

22. Burgess DL, Jones JM, Meisler NM, et al. Mutations of the Ca $^{2+}$ channel β subunit gene Cchb4 is associated with ataxia and seizures in the lethargic (1h) mouse. *Cell* 1997;88:385–392.

23. Demirkiran M, Jankovic J. Paroxysmal dyskinesias: clinical features and classification. *Ann Neurol* 1995;38:571–579.

24. Fouad GT, Servidei S, Durcan S, et al. A gene for familial paroxysmal dyskinesia (FPD I) maps to chromosome 2q. *Am J Hum Genet* 1996;59:135–139.

25. Fink JK, Rainer S, Wilkowski J, et al. Paroxysmal dystonic choreoathetosis: tight linkage to chromosome 2q. *Am J Hum Genet* 1996;59:140–145.

26. Hofele K, Benecke R, Auburger G. Gene locus FPDI of the dystonic Mount-Reback type of autosomal dominant paroxysmal choreoathetosis. *Neurology* 1997;49:1252–1256.

27. Merchut MP, Brumlik J. Painful tonic spasms caused by putaminal infarction. *Stroke* 1986;17:1319–1321.

28. Camac A, Greene P, Khandiji A. Paroxysmal kinesigenic dystonic choreoathetosis associated with a thalamic infarct. *Mov Disord* 1990;5:235–238.

29. Burguera JA. Thalamic demyelination and paroxysmal dystonia in multiple sclerosis. *Mov Disord* 1991;6:379–381.

30. Miley CE, Forster FM. Paroxysmal signs and symptoms in multiple sclerosis. *Neurology* 1974;24:458–461.

31. Rosen JA. Paroxysmal choreoathetosis: associated with perinatal hypoxic encephalopathy. *Arch Neurol* 1964;11:385–387.

32. Fischbeck KH, Layzer RB. Paroxysmal choreoathetosis associated with thyrotoxicosis. *Ann Neurol* 1979;6:453–454.

33. Tabaee-Zadeh WJ, France B, Kapphahn K. Kinesigenic choreoathetosis and idiopathic hypoparathyroidism. *New Engl J Med* 1972;286:762–763.

34. Clark JD, Pahwa R, Koller WC, et al. Diabetes mellitus presenting as paroxysmal kinesigenic dystonic choreoathetosis. *Move Disord* 1995;10:353–355.

35. Hwang W-J, Lu C-S, Tsai J-J. Clinical manifestations of 20 Taiwanese. patients with paroxysmal kinesigenic dyskinesia. *Acta Neurol Scand* 1998;98:340–345.

36. Spiller WG. Subcortical epilepsy. *Brain* 1927;50:171–187.

37. Hudgins RL, Corbin KB. An uncommon seizure disorder: familial paroxysmal choreoathetosis. *Brain* 1966;89:199–204.

38. Stevens H. Paroxysmal choreoathetosis: a form of reflex epilepsy. *Arch Neurol* 1966;14:415–420.

39. Robin JJ. Paroxysmal choreoathetosis following head injury. *Ann Neurol* 1977;2:447–448.

40. Richardson JC, Howes JL, Celinski MJ, et al. Kinesigenic choreoathetosis due to brain injury. *Can J Neurol Sci* 1987;14:626–628.

41. Fish DR, Marsden CD. Epilepsy masquerading as a movement disorder. In: Marsden CD, Fash S, eds. *Movement Disorders 3.* Oxford: Butterworth-Heinemann, 1994:346–359.

42. Morris HH, Dinner DS, Luders H, et al. Supplementary motor seizures: clinical and electroencephalographic findings. *Neurology* 1988;38:1975–1982.

43. Scheffer IE, Bhatia KP, Lopes-Cendes I, et al. Autosomal dominant frontal epilepsy misdiagnosed as sleep disorder. *Lancet* 1994;343:515–517.

44. Lugaresi E, Cirignotta F. Hypnogenic paroxysmal dystonia: epileptic seizure or a new syndrome? *Sleep* 1981;4:129–138.

45. Lee WL, Tay A, Ong FIT, et al. Association of infantile convulsions with paroxysmal dyskinesias (ICCA syndrome): Confirmation of linkage to human chromosome 16p12-q12 in a Chinese family. *Hum Genet* 1998;103:608–612.

46. Rajna P, Kundra O, Halasz P. Vigilance level-dependent

tonic seizures—epilepsy or sleep disorder? A case report. *Epilepsia* 1983;24:725–733.

47. Godbout R, Montplaisir J, Rouleau L. Hypnogenic paroxysmal dystonia: epilepsy or sleep disorder? A case report. *Clin EEG* 1985;6:136.

48. Crowell JA, Anders TF. Hypnogenic paroxysmal dystonia. *J Am Acad Child Psychiatry* 1985;24:353–358.

49. Tinuper P, Cerullo A, Cirignotta F, et al. Nocturnal paroxysmal dystonia with short fasting attacks. Three cases with evidence for an epileptic frontal lobe origin of seizures. *Epilepsia* 1990;31:549–556.

50. Niedermyer E, Walker AE. Mesial frontal epilepsy. *Electroencephalography Clin Neurophysiol* 1971;31: 104–105.

51. Lombroso CT. Paroxysmal choreoathetosis: an epileptic or non-epileptic disorder? *Ital J Neurol Sci* 1995; 16:271–277.

52. Goldman PA, Nauta WJH. An intricately patterned prefronto-caudate projection. *J Comp Neurol* 1977;171: 369–386.

53. Selemon LD, Goldman-Rakic PS. Longitudinal topography and interdigitation of corticostriatal projections in the rhesus monkey. *J Neurosci* 1985;5:776–794.

54. Walker EA. Pre-frontal lobe epilepsy. *Int J Neurol* 1966; 5:422–429.

55. Kotagal P, Luders H, Morris HH, et al. Dystonic posturing in complex partial seizures of temporal lobe onset: a new lateralizing sign. *Neurology* 1989;39:196–201.

56. Bossi L, Munari C, Stoffels C, et al. Somatomotor manifestations in temporal lobe epilepsy. *Epilepsia* 1984; 25:70–76.

57. Gastaut H, Tassinari CA. Triggering mechanisms in epilepsy: the electroclinical point of view. *Epilepsia* 1966;7:86–138.

58. Bancaud J, Talairach J, Bonis A. Physiopathogenesis of reflex epilepsies. *Rev Neurol* 1967;117:441–453.

59. Guerrini R, Genton P, Bureau M, et al. Reflex seizures are frequent in patients with Down syndrome and epilepsy. *Epilepsia* 1990;31:406–417.

60. Bancaud J, Talairach J, Lamarche M, et al. Neurophysiopathological hypothesis on startle epilepsy in man. *Rev Neurol* 1975;131:559–571.

61. Lance JW. Familial paroxysmal dystonic choreoathetosis and its differentiation from related syndromes. *Ann Neurol* 1977;2:285–293.

62. Plant GT, Williams AC, Marsden CD, et al. Familial paroxysmal dystonia induced by exercise. *J Neurol Neurosurg Psychiatry* 1984;47:275–279.

63. Fukuyama Y, Okada R. Hereditary kinaesisthetic reflex epilepsy: report of five pedigrees with seizures induced by movements and review of literature. *Proc Aust Assist Neurol* 1968;5:583–587.

64. Pryles CV, Livingston S, Ford FR. Familial paroxysmal choreoathetosis of Mount and Reback: study of a second family in which this condition is found in association with epilepsy. *Pediatrics* 1952;9:44–47.

65. Bhatia KP, Soland VL, Marsden CD, et al. Paroxysmal exercise-induced dystonia: eight new sporadic cases and a review of the literature. *Mov Disord* 1997;12: 1007–1012.

66. Jung S, Chen KM, Brody JA. Paroxysmal choreoathetosis. *Neurology* 1973;23:749–755.

67. Sadamatsu M, Masui A, Sakai T, et al. Familial paroxysmal kinesigenic choreoathetosis: an electrophysiologic and genotypic analysis. *Epilepsia* 1999;40:942–949.

68. Auburger G, Ratzlaff T, Lunkes A, et al. A gene for autosomal dominant paroxysmal choreoathetosis/spasticity (CSE) maps to the vicinity of a potassium channel gene cluster on chromosome Ip, probably within 2 cM between DIS443 and DIS197. *Genomics* 1996;31: 90–94.

69. Liu AW, Delgado-Escueta AV, Serratosa JM, et al. Juvenile myoclonic epilepsy locus in chromosome 6p21.2-p11: linkage to convulsions and electroencephalography trait. *Am J Hum Genet* 1995;57:368–381.

70. Koch MC, Steinmeyer K, Lorenz C, et al. The skeletal muscle chloride channel in dominant and recessive human myotonia. *Science* 1992;257:797–800.

71. Echenne B, Rivier F, Humbert Claude V, et al. Benign familial infantile convulsions. *Arch Pediatr* 1999;6: 54–58.

72. Bennett LB, Roach ES, Bowcock AM. Locus for paroxysmal kinesigenic dyskinesia maps to human chromosome 16. *Neurology* 2000;54:125–130.

73. Guerrini R, Parmeggiani L, Bonanni P, et al. Locus for paroxysmal kinesigenic dyskinesia maps to human chromosome 16 [letter]. *Neurology* 2000;55:735.

74. Valente EM, Spacey SD, Wali GM, et al. A second paroxysmal kinesigenic choreoathetosis locus (EKD2) mapping on 16qI3-q22.1 indicates a family of genes which give rise to paroxysmal disorders on human chromosome 16. *Brain* 2000;123:2040–2045.

75. Caraballo R, Pavek S, Lemainque A, et al. Linkage of benign familial infantile convulsions to chromosome 16p 12-q 12 suggests allelism to the infantile convulsions and choreoathetosis syndrome. *Am J Hum Genet* 2001;68:788–794.

76. Tinel N, Lauritzen 1, Choabe C, Lazdunski M, et al. The KCNQ2 potassium channel: splice variants, functional and development expression. Brain localization and comparison with KCNQ3. *FEBS Lett* 1998;483:171–176.

77. Berkovic SF. Paroxysmal movement disorders and epilepsy. Links across the channel. *Neurology* 2000;55: 169–170.

78. Zuberi SM, Eunson LH, Spauschus A, et al. A novel mutation in the human voltagegated potassium channel gene (Kv 1. 1) associates with episodic ataxia type I and sometimes with partial epilepsy. *Brain,* 1999;122: 817–825.

79. Gardner K, Barmada M, Ptacek LJ, et al. A new locus for herniplegic migraine maps to chromosome lq3l. *Neurology* 1997;49:1231–1238.

80. Terwindt GM, Ophoff RA, Lindhout D, et al. Partial cosegregation of familial herniplegic migraine and a benign infantile epileptic s yndrome. *Epilepsia* 1997;38: 15–21.

81. Munchau A, Valente EM, Shahidi GA, et al. A new family with paroxysmal exercise induced dystonia and migraine: a clinical and genetic study. *J Neurol Neurosurg Psychiatry* 2000;68:609–614.

Myoclonus and Paroxysmal Dyskinesias,
Advances in Neurology, Vol. 89,
edited by S. Fahn, et al.
Published by Lippincott Williams & Wilkins, Philadelphia, 2002.

39

Animal Models of Paroxysmal Dystonia

Angelika Richter and Wolfgang Löscher

Department of Pharmacology, Toxicology and Pharmacy, School of Veterinary Medicine Hannover,
Hannover, Germany

Non-episodic dyskinesias can be experimentally induced by drugs or neurolesions in animals (1–3). Furthermore, several mutant rodents have been reported to exhibit permanent dystonic symptoms (2,3). A rare inherited (recessive) hyperkinetic disorder in dogs, the Scotty cramps in Scottish terriers, is characterized by episodes of generalized involuntary movements with co-contractions of flexors and extensors which are precipitated by exercise, fear, or excitement (4). This movement disorder possibly shares similarities to symptoms of paroxysmal dystonia in humans, but has not yet been extensively examined. Recently, a dystonic phenotype associated with a mutation of the neuronal sodium channel *SCN8a* has been described in mouse mutant *med^J* crossed with strain C3H (5). These mutant mice show muscle weakness and frequent movement-induced periods of tremor and twisting of the trunk. The episodes of abnormal postures of the limbs and trunk last 2 seconds to 1 minute. This phenotype, probably a consequence of low level *SCN8a* channel expression, occurs in the absence of any pathomorphologic changes within the CNS. Although the novel mutant mouse might represent a model of kinesogenic dystonia, there seems to be a need for further studies, such as electroencephalographic examinations (5). Clearly defined animal models of paroxysmal dyskinesias are, therefore, still restricted to the genetically dystonic hamster (3).

THE *DT^{SZ}* MUTANT HAMSTER

Clinical Signs in Genetically Dystonic Hamsters

In the *dt^{sz}* mutant hamster, an inbred line of Syrian hamsters, attacks of generalized dystonic and choreoathetotic movements occur in response to mild stress and sometimes also spontaneously. These hereditary motor impairments, which are transmitted by an autosomal recessive gene, were initially misdiagnosed as a reflex epilepsy (6). The original gene symbol was, therefore, *sz* (for seizures). Emphasizing the necessity for careful evaluation of animal models, more detailed examinations revealed that the attacks are not epileptic seizures (7), but show several features in common with paroxysmal non-kinesogenic dystonic choreoathetosis (PDC) in humans (3,8,9): (a) Episodes of twisting movements and abnormal postures last several hours in mutant hamsters and can be precipitated by stress and caffeine, while the progression of dystonic symptoms is often aborted by sleep. (b) The consciousness is not altered during attacks, e.g., the animals react to different external stimuli. (c) EEG recordings failed to disclose any ictal or interictal epileptogenic activities in cortical areas, hippocampus, basal ganglia nuclei (striatum, globus pallidus) or nucleus ruber. (d) Altered EMG patterns found in *dt^{sz}* hamsters are comparable to those determined in patients with dystonia. (e) As in patients with PDC, benzodiazepines and neuroleptics exerted beneficial effects, while classical antiepileptics such as phenytoin were not effective or even worsened dyskinesia in mutant hamsters. The comparable drug response suggests that the dt^{sz} hamster is suitable for preclinical drug testing. (f) By using standard techniques (e.g. silver staining), no morphologic abnormalities could be detected within the CNS of mutant hamsters. Neither signs of neurodegenerations nor a general retardation of brain development seems to be involved in the syndrome of mutant hamsters (10,11). In summary, the genetically dystonic hamster represents a valid animal model of idiopathic PDC (3,8).

A score system for rating severity of dystonic attacks in mutant hamsters (Fig. 39.1)

has been shown suitable to examine drug effects on the severity of dyskinesia (7). Among the wide range of drugs tested in dt^{sz} hamsters during the past years (3), most marked beneficial effects were observed after acute treatments with various GABA-potentiating drugs, antidopaminergic compounds and adenosine receptor agonists (3,12,13), while drugs which disturb GABAergic inhibition or compounds, known to cause a selective increase of the dopaminergic activity, as well as methylxanthines (caffeine, theophylline), which enhance the striatal dopaminergic activity by their adenosine antagonistic action (3,14), worsened the dystonic syndrome. A dramatic aggravation of dystonia in mutant hamsters was provoked by the sodium chan-

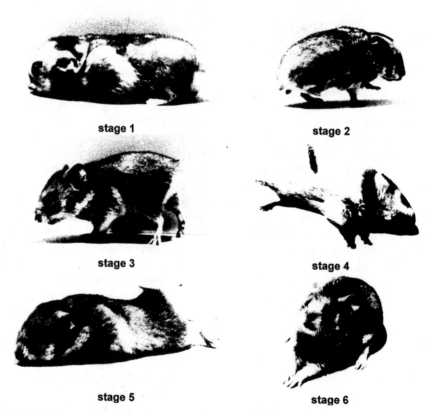

stage 1   stage 2

stage 3   stage 4

stage 5   stage 6

FIG. 39.1. Dystonic movements and postures in dt^{sz} hamsters (7). The dyskinetic syndrome in mutant hamsters consists of a sequence of motor disturbances. Therefore, the severity of dystonia can be rated according to a six-point score-system (for further explanations see section 1). Not all animals reach stage 6. The individual maximum stage is usually reached within 3 hours.

nel blockers lamotrigine and riluzole (15,16). Apart from preclinical drug testing, pharmacological examinations done in mutant hamsters are helpful for interpretations of neurochemical findings (see below).

The severity of dyskinetic symptoms shows an age-dependent time course with first occurrence of dystonic attacks on about day 16 of life, a maximum severity of the attacks at an age of 30 to 40 days of life and a complete remission of the stress-inducible movement disorder at an age of about 10 weeks. Nevertheless, paroxysmal dystonia in mutant hamsters is obviously not really transient because relapses of dystonia occur in females during late pregnancy (17) and the prodystonic drugs lamotrigine and riluzole can provoke severe attacks in male and female hamsters over 10 weeks of age (15,16). The vitality is normal in mutant hamsters, probably because of the paroxysmal nature of the dystonic syndrome, and the age-dependent time course of dystonia contributes to an unaltered fertility, although the onset of puberty was found to be retarded in male and female dt^{sz} hamsters (3,17).

Investigations of the Pathophysiology of Paroxysmal Dystonia in dt^{sz} Mutants

Over the past decade several studies have been done in the hamster model (and for comparisons in non-dystonic control hamsters) to identify the underlying mechanism of the dystonic syndrome (3). The paroxysmal nature of dyskinesias in dt^{sz} hamsters provides the possibility for a separation of changes that are secondary to abnormal motor patterns. Furthermore, the age dependence of paroxysmal dystonia proves the relevance of pathophysiologic changes for the occurrence of dystonia by ontogenetic studies; that is, alterations detected at an age of maximum severity should be reduced or disappeared in older animals after spontaneous remission of stress-inducible attacks. A disadvantage of the hamster model is that the genome of Syrian hamsters is not well characterized. Therefore, the gene defect has not yet been recognized, but current studies could at least exclude a DYT1 defect (A. Schneider and A. Richter, unpublished observations), supporting the findings in humans that the pathogenesis of dystonias is heterogenous (18). The main findings of pharmacologic and neurochemical studies of various neurotransmitter systems, such as inhibitory and excitatory amino acids or monoamines, and of neuromodulators as well as studies on neuronal activities are summarized in the following.

Neurochemical Alterations in dt^{sz} Mutants

By neurochemical examinations, which included 14 to over 100 brain regions and subregions, most changes were detected in the striatum and ventral thalamic nuclei of dt^{sz} hamsters (3). There is strong evidence that disturbed GABAergic inhibition and enhanced dopaminergic activity are critically involved in the dystonic syndrome of dt^{sz} hamsters.

Examinations of the Dopaminergic System: Measurements of levels of dopamine and its metabolites in tissue homogenates of different brain regions, examinations of tyrosine hydroxylase by immunhistochemistry and by in-situ hybridization as well as analyses of dopamine transporter binding (3,10,19) did not disclose any abnormalities in dystonic hamsters. Although the dopaminergic system is obviously intact in this animal model (unaltered density of dopaminergic neurons and of their terminals), autoradiographic analyses of dopamine receptor density revealed a reduced dopamine D_1 and D_2 receptor binding in the dorsal striatum (20). In view of pharmacologic observations, this has been interpreted as a receptor down-regulation; that is, as a consequence of an enhanced dopamine release (20), which may be temporary (e.g., induced by stress or caffeine), thereby not leading to changes detectable by the above mentioned examinations (21). Dopamine receptor antagonists, such as haloperidol and clozapine, exerted beneficial effects, while compounds that increase dopaminergic activity, such as the receptor agonist apomorphine or the uptake inhibitor GBR 12909, aggravated dystonia after systemic administrations in mutant hamsters (3,13,19). Recent pharmacologic manipulations of the dopaminergic system in the striatum of mutant hamsters clearly demonstrated that striatal dopaminergic overactivity plays a crucial role for the manifestation of paroxysmal dystonia (21). Striatal injections of the dopamine D_2 receptor agonist quinpirole significantly worsened the dystonic syndrome, while combined microinjections of D_1 and D_2 receptor antagonists exerted striking beneficial effects (21). Based on several more recent observations, the striatal dopaminergic overactivity could be secondary to impaired GABAergic inhibition.

Examinations of the GABAergic System: The GABA levels were found to be reduced in the striatum of dt^{sz} hamsters at an age of maximum severity but not after remission of paroxysmal dystonia (3). Furthermore, Burgunder and associates (10) detected a reduced expression of the GABA-synthesizing enzyme glutamic acid decarboxylase (GAD) in dystonic hamsters. Therefore, an increased affinity and density of benzodiazepine binding sites on the $GABA_A$ receptor in the striatum, determined in mutant hamsters at the age of most marked severity of paroxysmal dystonia, but not in older animals after the remission of stress-inducible dyskinesia (22), probably reflects an up-regulation of these sites. This interpretation referred to previous pharmacologic observations, which demonstrated that GABAmimetic drugs exerted marked antidystonic efficacy after systemic administrations (3).

The neurochemical alterations in the striatum and an increased basal activity of striatal projection neurons (see below) prompted us to determine the number and density of striatal aspiny GABAergic interneurons, which co-express the calcium-binding protein parvalbumin, in dt^{sz} hamsters by immunohistochemical investigations. These interneurons constitute only 3% to 5% of the cells in the rodent neostriatum but are the main inhibitory source in the striatum (23,24). By using a stereologic counting method in a blinded

fashion, the number of all striatal parvalbumin-immunoreactive GABAergic interneurons was determined. A significant reduction in the number (-41%; $p < 0.0001$) and density (-26%; $p=0.0006$) of interneurons was found within the whole neostriatum of dt^{sz} hamsters at the most sensitive age (32 days of life) in comparison to age- and sex-matched non-dystonic control hamsters (25). Most marked decreases of the number and density became evident in the anterior ($-48\%/-44\%$) and posterior ($-43\%/-29\%$) striatum, but a significant deficit was also detected in the subregions of the middle part of the striatum, that is, in the dorsomedial, dorsolateral, ventromedial, and ventrolateral striatum of mutant hamsters (number: 27% to 31%; density: 17% to 21%). Furthermore, the density of the fibers of GABAergic interneurons was lower in mutant animals, while the extent of parvalbumin-labeling in single neurons was similar in both animal groups (25). To examine the functional relevance of the reduction of these inhibitory interneurons, the effects of the $GABA_A$-receptor agonist muscimol on severity of dystonia were investigated after microinjections into the striatum and after systemic administrations. Muscimol improved the dystonic syndrome after striatal injections to a similar extent as after systemic treatment, supporting the importance of the deficiency of striatal GABAergic interneurons for the occurrence of dyskinesia in the hamster model (25,26). Recently, ontogenetic examinations revealed that the deficit of striatal GABAergic interneurons disappeared in older (>90 days) dt^{sz} hamsters after spontaneous remission of age-dependent dystonia (Richter and Hamann, unpublished observations). Thus, a retarded development of these interneurons obviously plays a critical role in the pathogenesis of paroxysmal dystonia. Quantitative determinations of the density of the fibers of GABAergic interneurons are under way to examine if the lowered density persists after age-depenent remission. This could explain the enhanced susceptibility to sodium channel blockers; that is, the drug-induced dystonic attacks in older dt^{sz} hamsters after remission of stress-inducible dyskinesia (15, 16), because GABAergic interneurons communicate through electrotonic coupling, which may be further disturbed by sodium channel blockers (24). The consequence of altered neuronal synchronization in the striatum, as indicated by previous quantitative electroencephalographic depth electrode recordings in *dt^sz* hamsters (27), may be also relevant for occurrence of motor disturbances in *med^J* mutant mice with lower sodium channel expression. First *in vitro* electrophysiologic experiments of striatal neurons did not reveal abnormalities of basal sodium currents in mutant hamsters (28).

The marked deficit of striatal GABAergic interneurons that cannot be detected by histological standard techniques, as used in previous neuropathologic investigations in mutant hamsters (11), possibly represents the primary defect in this animal model. Thereby several previous pharmacological, neurochemical and electrophysiologic findings in *dt^sz* hamsters (3) can be explained. This structural defect obviously leads by disinhibition of striatal projection neurons to an abnormal basal ganglia output (Fig. 39.2B, see below).

Examinations of Neuronal Activities in dt^sz *Mutants*

2-Deoxyglucose (2-DG)-uptake studies, undertaken in mutant hamsters during the manifestation of a dystonic attack, have shown an abnormal neuronal activity in discrete regions of the motor system (29). In comparison to non-dystonic control hamsters (treated in the same manner as *dt^sz* hamsters), the 2-DG-uptake, which reflects particularly synaptic activities, was significantly increased in the dorsomedial striatum, in the ventromedial, ventrolateral, ventral anterior nuclei of the thalamus, in the medial vestibular nucleus and was dramatically enhanced in the nucleus ruber, while a reduced uptake was found in the reticular thalamic nucleus and a more marked decrease was detected in the deep cerebellar nuclei. Although this study essentially contributed to the decision of

which nuclei could be involved in the manifestation of this movement disorder and should be therefore investigated in more detail, the strength of the 2-DG method is limited. Thus, by these examinations it cannot be decided which type of neurons shows altered activity and whether these changes are merely secondary to abnormal movements. Therefore, single unit recordings from striatal GABAergic projection neurons were carried out in anesthetized (fentanyl/gallamine) hamsters; that means, in the absence of dystonic attacks.

In accordance with the deficiency of striatal GABAergic interneurons (Fig. 39.2B), single unit recordings revealed an increased basal activity (+58.3%, $p < 0.01$) of striatal GABAergic projection neurons in *dt^sz* hamsters (30). As shown by recent experiments, the firing rate of GABAergic neurons was significantly decreased (−69.5%; $p < 0.001$) in the entopeduncular nucleus (the homologue of the internal segment of the globus pallidus, GPi, in primates) of mutant hamsters, probably due to an enhanced striatoentopeduncular inhibition (25). Furthermore, the firing patterns were found to be more irregular in the entopeduncular nucleus of dyskinetic animals (Bennay, Gernert, Löscher, Richter, unpublished observations). In line with an age-dependent normalization of striatal GABAergic interneurons, recent single unit recordings have shown that the basal entopeduncular activity in older *dt^sz* hamsters; (after remission of stress-inducible dystonia), reach comparable levels to those determined in age-matched control hamsters (31). In the globus pallidus (globus pallidus externus in primates) the neuronal activity only tended to be increased (+40%, with a wide range) and no significant changes of the discharge rates could be detected in the substantia nigra pars reticulata (±0%) of mutant hamsters at the most sensitive age of dystonia (25,32). Thus, in contrast to the direct, striato-entopeduncular pathway, the neuronal activity is obviously not significantly disturbed within the striatonigral and indirect (striato-pallidal) pathway, at least in the absence of dystonic attacks.

In view of the paroxysmal nature of dyskinesia in *dt^sz* hamsters, the permanent deficit of striatal GABAergic interneurons, resulting in an enhanced striato-entopeduncular activity, seems not to cause motor disturbances by itself. However, this structural defect may lead to a disinhibition of stress- (or caffeine) induced dopamine-release in the striatum and thereby to the manifestation of a dystonic attacks (Fig. 39.2C). This is indicated by the prevention of dystonic attacks after intrastriatal injections of D_1/D_2-receptor antagonists (21).

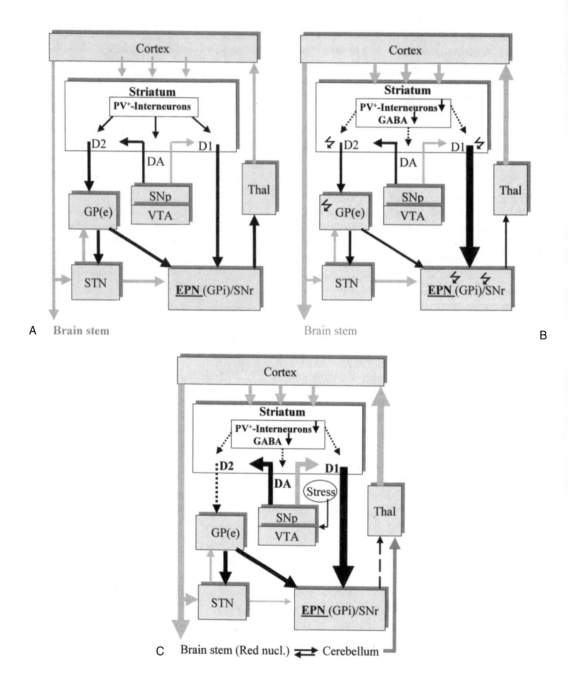

Activation of dopamine D_1 receptors, predominantly located on of the direct pathway, leads to a further inhibition of the entopeduncular nucleus. Because stimulation of dopamine D_2 receptors is known to inhibit the projection to the globus pallidus, the prodystonic effects of the D_2 receptor agonist quinpirole after microinjections into the striatum suggest that alterations within the indirect pathway contribute to the manifestation of dyskinesia in mutant hamsters (21). The consequence of stimulations of D_2 receptors on striatopallidal projection neurons would be (via disinhibition of GABAergic pallidal neurons) a decreased activity of subthalamic neurons, thereby a reduced excitation of the entopeduncular nucleus. An increased activity of inhibitory synapses and a reduced activity of excitatory synapses could explain the lack of 2-DG changes within the entopeduncular nucleus of mutant hamsters during the occurrence of dystonic attacks (29). The abnormal 2-DG uptake in brainstem and cerebellar nuclei could be secondary to reduced basal ganglia output or to disturbed motor patterns.

Furthermore, the reduced activity of entopeduncular GABAergic neurons leads to a disturbed innervation of the lateral habenula, as suggested by abnormal *c-fos* expression in the lateral habenula during dystonic attacks in dt^{sz} hamsters (33), and to a reduced thalamic inhibition. However, the 2-DG uptake was increased within the ventral thalamic nuclei during the manifestation of a dystonic attack (29). This could be caused by an enhanced excitatory input from deep cerebellar nuclei, because 2-DG uptake studies indicated a secondary disinhibition of these structures during dystonic attacks. A significantly increased binding of a ligand at the phencyclidine site in the ion channel of the *N*-methyl-D-aspartate receptor within the ventrolateral thalamic nucleus (34), at least partly, supports this explanation. Apart from considerations about the thalamo-cortical activity, which deserve further studies, the mechanisms that lead to the recovery from a dystonic attack remain to be explored. One explanation, which could be clarified by further microdialysis studies of extracellular dopamine levels in dt^{sz}

FIG. 39.2. Schematic diagram of the basal ganglia motor circuit in (**A**) normal animals (non-dystonic control hamsters) and in dt^{sz} mutant hamsters in the absence of dystonic attacks (**B**) and during a dystonic attack (**C**). Inhibitory connections are represented by black arrows and excitatory projections by gray arrows. Changes in neuronal activities are indicated by the thickness of the arrows. As shown by single unit recordings (*zigzag arrows*) in anaesthetized hamsters (fentanyl, gallamine), i.e., in the absence of dystonia (**B**), the activity of striatal GABAergic projection neurons was significantly increased, which is probably related to the deficit of striatal parvalbumin-reactive (PV+) inhibitory interneurons. The consequence is a dramatic decrease of the entopeduncular activity (EPN, globus pallidus internus (GPi) in primates), while no significant changes were found in the globus pallidus (GP, in primates the external [e] segment) or in the substantia nigra pars reticulata (SNr). An enhanced dopaminergic activity caused by triggers, such as stress and caffeine, seems to be essential for the manifestation of dystonic attacks in mutant hamsters (**C**), as indicated by striatal manipulations of the dopaminergic system, but is probably secondary to deficiencies of striatal GABAergic interneurons. An increased stimulation of dopamine D2 receptors, which are thought to be predominantly located on the striatopallidal neurons, resulting in a further decrease of the entopeduncular activity, aggravated dystonia in dt^{sz} hamsters. 2-DG studies have shown an increased uptake within the dorsomedial striatum, a subregion of altered dopamine receptor binding, which may be due to enhanced synaptic activity of dopaminergic and/or glutamatergic neurons. Further significant changes of 2-DG uptake in ventral nuclei and the reticular nucleus of the thalamus (Thal), in brain stem structures (dramatic increases in the red nucleus) and in the deep cerebellar nuclei during dystonic attacks suggest that altered activity in these motor areas contributes to the occurrence of dystonic attacks.

hamsters, is that an increased dopamine release results in an enhanced release of other neurotransmitters or neuromodulators (e.g., adenosine) which leads to a gradual decrease of striatal dopaminergic activity until the disappearance of a dystonic attack.

CONCLUSIONS

In summary, striatal dysfunctions, leading to an abnormal basal ganglia output, are critically involved in paroxysmal dyskinesia in the hamster model. In line with the findings in levodopa-induced dyskinesias of parkinsonian monkeys, which suggest that a decreased neuronal activity of the GPi plays an important role in this movement disorder (35), paroxysmal dystonia in dt^{sz} hamsters is related to a reduced discharge rate and an irregular firing pattern of entopeduncular neurons (25). These data substantiate the hypothesis of the pathophysiology of dyskinesias in humans (36,37). However, in contrast to considerations about the neurochemical basis of dystonias (38) the dopaminergic system seems not to be the culprit in paroxysmal dystonia of the hamster model. Striatal dopaminergic overactivity seems to be essential for the manifestation of dystonic attacks in the hamster model, but is probably secondary to GABAergic disinhibition. Although hyperkinetic movement disorders, such as symptomatic dystonia and choreoathetosis, are often associated with striatal lesions (39,40), parvalbumin-reactive GABAergic interneurons have not yet been examined in autopsy material from patients. The relation between losses of interneurons and projection neurons could be essential for the occurrence of dystonia, which could explain that striatal lesions do not always cause dystonic symptoms. The inborn deficit of striatal GABAergic interneurons in dt^{sz} hamsters indicates that the GABAergic system deserves attention in human dyskinesias, particularly in types in which GABA-potentiating drugs exert beneficial effects, such as in PDC (8,9).

ACKNOWLEDGMENTS

The examinations of genetically dystonic hamsters were funded by the Deutsche Forschungsgemeinschaft (Lo275/4-1-3, Ri 845/1-1) and in part by the Dystonia Medical Research Foundation.

REFERENCES

1. Jankovic J, Fahn S. Dystonic disorders. In: Jankovic J, Tolosa E, eds. *Parkinson's disease and movement disorders*. New York: Lippincott-Williams&Wilkins, 1998: 513–552.
2. Lorden JF.Animal models of dystonia. In: Tsui JKC, Calne DB, eds. *Handbook of dystonia*. New York: Marcel Dekker, 1995:5–42.
3. Richter A, Löscher W. Pathophysiology of idiopathic dystonia: findings from genetic animal models. *Prog Neurobiol* 1998;54:633–677.
4. Meyers KM, Padgett GA, Dickson WM. The genetic basis of a kinetic disorder in Scottish terrier dogs. *J Hered* 1970;61:189–192.
5. Sprunger LK, Escayg A, Tallaksen-Greene S, et al. Dystonia associated with mutation of the neuronal sodium channel *Scn8a* and identification of the modifier locus *Scnm1* on mouse chromosome 3. *Hum Mol Genet* 1999;8:471–479.
6. Yoon CH, Peterson JS, Corrow D. Spontaneous seizures: a new mutation in Syrian golden hamsters. *J Hered* 1976;67:115–116.
7. Löscher W, Fisher JE Jr, Schmidt D, et al. The *sz* mutant hamster: a genetic model of epilepsy or of paroxysmal dystonia? *Mov Disord* 1989;4:219–232.
8. Demirkiran M, Jankovic J. Paroxysmal diskinesias: clinical features and classification. *Ann Neurol* 1995;38:571–579.
9. Fahn S. The paroxysmal dyskinesias. In: Marsden CD, Fahn S, eds. *Movement disorders 3*. Oxford: Butterworth-Heinemann, 1994:311–345.
10. Burgunder J-M, Richter A, Löscher W. Expression of cholecystokinin, somatostatin, thyrotropin-releasing hormone, glutamic acid decarboxylase and tyrosine hydroxylase genes in the central nervous motor systems of the genetically dystonic hamster. *Exp Brain Res* 1999;129:114–120.
11. Wahnschaffe U, Fredow G, Heintz P, et al. Neuropathological studies in a mutant hamster model of paroxysmal dystonia. *Mov Disord* 1990;5:286–293.
12. Richter A, Hamann M, Bartling C. CGS 21680 exerts marked antidystonic effects in a genetic model of paroxysmal dyskinesia. *Eur J Pharmacol* 2000;404(3):299–302.
13. Richter A, Löscher W. The atypical neuroleptic clozapine exerts antidystonic activity in a mutant hamster model. Comparison with haloperidol. *Eur J Pharmacol* 1993;242:309–312.
14. Richter A, Hamann M. Effects of adenosine receptor agonists and antagonists in a genetic animal model of paroxysmal dystonia. *Primary Brit J Pharmacol* 2001;134:343–352.

15. Richter A, Gernert M, Löscher W. Prodystonic effects of riluzole in an animal model of idiopathic dystonia related to decreased total power in the red nucleus? *Eur J Pharmacol* 1997;332:133–142.
16. Richter A, Löschmann PA, Löscher W. The novel antiepileptic drug lamotrigine exerts prodystonic effects in a hamster model of paroxysmal dystonia. *Eur J Pharmacol* 1994;264:345–351.
17. Löscher W, Blanke T, Richter A, et al. Gonadal sex hormones and dystonia: experimental studies in genetically dystonic hamsters. *Mov Disord* 1995;10:92–102.
18. Fahn S, Bressman SB, Marsden CD. Classification of dystonia. In: Fahn S, Marsden CD, DeLong MR, eds. *Advances in neurology, Vol. 78. Dystonia 3*. New York: Lippincott-Raven, 1998:1–10.
19. Nobrega JN, Gernert M, Löscher W, et al. Tyrosine hydroxylase immunreactivity and [3H]WIN 35,428 binding to the dopamine transporter in a hamster model of idiopathic paroxysmal dystonia. *Neuroscience* 1999;92:211–217.
20. Nobrega JN, Richter A, Tozman N, et al. Quantitative autoradiography reveals regionally selective changes in dopamine D_1 and D_2 receptor binding in the genetically dystonic hamster. *Neuroscience* 1996;71:927–936.
21. Rehders JH, Löscher W, Richter A. Evidence for striatal dopaminergic overactivity in paroxysmal dystonia indicated by microinjections in a genetic rodent model. Neuroscience 2000;97:267–277.
22. Pratt DG, Möhler H, Richter A, et al. Regionally selective and age-dependent alterations in benzodiazepine receptor binding in the genetically dystonic hamsters. *J Neurochem* 1995;64:2153–2158.
23. Kawaguchi Y, Wilson CJ, Augood SJ, et al. Striatal interneurons: chemical, physiological and morphological characterization. *Trends Neurosci* 1995;18:527–535.
24. Koos T, Tepper JM. Inhibitory control of neostriatal projection neurons by GABAergic interneurons. *Nature Neurosci* 1999;2:467–472.
25. Gernert M, Hamann M, Bennay M, et al. Deficit of striatal parvalbumin-reactive GABAergic interneurons and decreased basal ganglia output in a genetic rodent model of idiopathic paroxysmal dystonia. J Neurosci 2000;20:7052–7058.
26. Hamann M, Löscher W, Richter A. Striatal dysfunctions of the GABAergic system in a genetic animal model of primary paroxysmal dystonia indicated by pharmacological examinations. *Eur J Neurosci* 2000;12(suppl 11):399.
27. Gernert M, Richter A, Rundfeldt C, et al. Quantitative EEG analysis of depth electrode recordings from several brain regions of mutant hamsters with paroxysmal dystonia discloses frequency changes in the basal ganglia. *Mov Disord* 1998;13:509–521.
28. Siep E, Richter A, Köhling R. Sodium currents in striatal neurons from dystonic dt^{sz} hamsters. *Soc Neurosci Abstr* 2000;26:1538.
29. Richter A, Brotchie JM, Crossman AR, et al. [^{3}H]-2-Deoxyglucose uptake study in mutant dystonic hamsters: abnormalities in discrete brain regions of the motor system. *Mov Disord* 1998;13:718–725.
30. Gernert M, Richter A, Löscher W. Alterations in spontaneous single unit activity of striatal subdivisions during ontogenesis in mutant dystonic hamsters. *Brain Res* 1999;821:277–285.
31. Bennay M, Gernert M, Richter A. Spontaneous remission of paroxysmal dystonia coincides with normalization of entopenduncular activity in dt^{sz} mutants. *J Neurosci* 2001;21:RC153(1–4).
32. Gernert M, Richter A, Löscher W. In vivo extracellular electrophysiology of pallidal neurons in dystonic and nondystonic hamsters. *J Neurosci Res* 1999;57:894–905.
33. Ebert U, Gernert M, Löscher W, et al. Abnormal expression of c-*fos* in the lateral habenula during dystonic attacks in mutant hamsters. *Brain Res* 1996;728:125–129.
34. Nobrega JN, Richter A, Jiwa D, et al. Autoradiographic analysis of NMDA receptor binding in dystonic hamster brains. *Brain Res* 1997;744:161–165.
35. Crossman AR, Brotchie JM. Pathophysiology of dystonia. In: Fahn S, Marsden CD, DeLong MR, eds. *Advances in neurology*. Vol. 78. *Dystonia 3*. New York: Lippincott-Raven, 1998:19–25.
36. Wichmann T, DeLong MR. Functional and pathophysiological models of the basal ganglia. *Curr Opin Neurobiol* 1996;6:751–758.
37. Vitek JL, Zhang J, Evatt M, et al. GPi pallidotomy for dystonia: Clinical outcome and neuronal activity. In: Fahn S, Marsden CD, DeLong MR, eds. *Advances in neurology*. Vol. 78. *Dystonia 3*. New York: Lippincott-Raven, 1998:211–219.
38. Todd RD, Perlmutter JS. Mutational and biochemical analysis of dopamine in dystonia. *Mol Neurobiol* 1998;16:135–147.
39. Bhatia KP, Marsden CD. The behavioural and motor consequences of focal lesions of the basal ganglia in man. *Brain* 1994;117:859–876.
40. Craver RD, Duncan MC, Nelson JS. Familial dystonia and choreoathetosis in three generations associated with bilateral striatal necrosis. *J Child Neurol* 1996;11:185–188.

Myoclonus and Paroxysmal Dyskinesias,
Advances in Neurology, Vol. 89,
edited by S. Fahn, et al.
Published by Lippincott Williams & Wilkins, Philadelphia, 2002.

40

Molecular Biology of Episodic Movement Disorders

Louis J. Ptáček and *Ying-Hui Fu

*Departments of Neurology And Human Genetics, *Departments of Neurobiology and Anatomy,
Howard Hughes Medical Institute, University of Utah, Salt Lake City, Utah*

Paroxysmal dyskinesias and episodic ataxias are a rare group of conditions manifesting as abnormal involuntary movements or ataxia lasting a brief duration. Interestingly, both these disorders share striking similarities with other episodic disorders of the nervous system. For example, episodic ataxia has some features similar to periodic paralysis and in one family was misdiagnosed as periodic paralysis. This mistake serendipitously led to acetazolamide, a drug helpful to many periodic paralysis patients, being discovered to be of benefit in preventing the episodes of ataxia (1).

The discovery of the molecular defects resulting in the periodic paralyses led to recognition of the role of ion channel mutants in episodic neurologic disease. This group of disorders, the channelopathies, has now grown to include not only muscle diseases, but also epilepsies, movement disorders, headache and cardiac dysrhythmias (Table 40.1). The examples are not limited to humans; several mouse epilepsies are included in this group. Once genes causing such disorders are identified, biologic function of the wild type and mutant proteins can be assayed to shed light on the pathophysiologic basis of the disorders. Physiologic characterization of sodium channel mutations has defined a number of alterations of channel function that can result in a myotonic or paralytic phenotype

(2–6). Study of naturally occurring mutations in ion channels will not only lead to better understanding of pathogenesis, but also to greater insights into structure-function relationships of ion channels.

All of these disorders can be confounded by phenocopies simulating the disease in a family but lacking recognized molecular defects (7). Understanding of the molecular and pathophysiologic basis of episodic disorders may lead to testable hypotheses regarding the pathophysiologic basis of episodic movement disorders for which the cause is not (as yet) known.

EPISODIC ATAXIA

The episodic ataxias are disorders of intermittent ataxia often with completely normal cerebellar function between attacks that usually segregate as autosomal dominant traits. There are two distinct forms. Episodic ataxia type 1 (EA1) is a disorder involving both the central nervous system and peripheral nervous system and manifest as episodic ataxia with myokymia. The attacks usually last from seconds to several minutes and may occur many times during the day. Myokymia, a muscle rippling resulting from motor nerve hyperexcitability is often seen in the muscles around the eyes and in small hand muscles. It can be demonstrated by electromyography.

TABLE 40.1. *Cloned genes and mapped loci for episodic disorders*

Disease	Chromosome	Gene	Ion Channel
Neuromuscular disorders			
Hyperkalemic periodic paralysis	17q24	*SCN4A* (32,33)	Sodium channel
Paramyotonia congenita	17q24	*SCN4A* (34,35)	Sodium channel
Potassium aggravated myotonia	17q24	*SCN4A* (36)	Sodium channel
Hypokalemic periodic paralysis 1	1q32	*CACNA1S* (37,38)	Calcium channel
Myotonia congenita	7q35	*CLCN1* (39–40)	Chloride channel
Myasthenic syndrome	2q	*CHRNA4*	Acetylcholine receptor
Myasthenic syndrome	17p	*CHRNB*	Acetylcholine receptor
Myasthenic syndrome	17	*CHRNE*	Acetylcholine receptor
Ataxic disorders			
Episodic ataxia with myokymia (type 1)	12p13	*KCNA1* (7)	Potassium channel
Episodic ataxia with nystagmus (type 2)	19p13	*CACNA1A* (23)	Calcium channel
Spinocerebellar ataxia type 6	19p13	*CACNA1A* (42)	Calcium channel
(Familial hemiplegic migraine)	19p13	*CACNA1A* (23)	Calcium channel
Paroxysmal dyskinesias			
Familial paroxysmal nonkinesigenic dyskinesia	2q33-35 (17,24)	?	?
Paroxysmal choreoathetosis/ spasticity	1p (53)	?	?
Infantile convulsions and paroxysmal choreoathetosis	16p12q-12 (25,26)	?	?
Familial paroxysmal kinesigenic dyskinesias	16p11.2-q12.1 (15)	?	?
Autosomal dominant nocturnal frontal lobe epilepsy	20q13	*CHRNA4* (28,29)	Nicotinic acetylcholine receptor
Autosomal dominant nocturnal frontal lobe epilepsy	15q24	*CHRNA4* (30)	Nicotinic acetylcholine receptor
Hereditary hyperekplexia	5q32	*GLRA1* (31)	Glycine receptor
Epilepsy			
Benign familial neonatal convulsions (type 1)	20q33-35	*KCNQ2* (43)	Potassium channel
Benign familial neonatal convulsions (type 2)	8q24	*KCNQ3* (44)	Potassium channel
Experimental mouse epilepsy disorders[a]	Various	Various	Various
Long QT syndromes[b]	Various	Various	Various

[a]Mouse epilepsy models: *tottering* and *learner* mice; *CACA1A* (45); calcium channel; *lethargic mouse*; *CCNB4*, calcium channel (46); *stargazer* mouse; *CACNG2*, calcium channel (47); *slow wave epilepsy*; *SLC9A1*, Na/H transporter (48); *Frings* (49); unknown gene defect.
[b]Long QT intervals syndromes, potassium or sodium channels on different genes (50–52).

These patients occasionally benefit from acetazolomide or from anticonvulsants such as phenytoin or valproic acid (1).

Episodic ataxia type 2 is a similar disorder and is also transmitted as an autosomal dominant trait. Attacks in patients with EA2 occur with episodes of markedly impaired truncal ataxia. Interictal nystagmus is frequently seen. These patients almost invariably benefit from acetazolomide (8). Unlike EA1, patients with this disorder often develop persistent cerebellar signs that accompany cerebellar atrophy demonstrated by magnetic resonance imaging.

FAMILIAL PAROXYSMAL DYSKINESIA

The paroxysmal dyskinesias include a clinically heterogeneous group of disorders that have shared features of episodic hyperkinetic movement disorder. These conditions can be either hereditary or acquired. Among the hereditary forms of paroxysmal dyskinesia, there are four main types.

Paroxysmal Kinesigenic Dyskinesia

The kinesigenic form occurs in early childhood and attack frequency frequently decreases in adult life. The hyperkinetic movements are initiated by movements or change in velocity. The attacks in these patients frequently manifest as choreoathetosis induced by a sudden change in position classically from a sitting to standing position. Even changes in velocity (going from walking slowly to walking more quickly) can initiate the episode. Attacks commonly involve the hemibody, in some almost always the same side or alternating sides. Patients with PKD frequently have dozens of attacks per day and respond dramatically to low doses of carbamazepine (9,10). We have recently demonstrated infantile convulsions as part of the phenotypic spectrum of this disorder in many such families. PKD can be seen in patients with episodic ataxia type 1 resulting from mutations in a voltage-gated potassium channel (7).

Paroxysmal Non-Kinesigenic Dyskinesia

PNKD is characterized by spontaneous attacks that tend to be more dystonic in nature. Attacks are frequently precipitated by alcohol, caffeine, stress, or fatigue, last sometimes up to 6 to 8 hours and are infrequent compared to PKD. Attacks in these patients do not benefit from antiepileptics such as carbamazepine, and recent reports (11) and personal experience suggest some patients may respond to levodopa.

Paroxysmal Exercise-Induced Dyskinesia

PED is distinct from the kinesigenic form in that the attacks occur after 10 or 15 minutes of continuing exercise rather than at the initiation of movement. The attacks are usually dystonic and appear in the body part involved in the exercise most commonly the legs after prolonged walking or running (12).

Paroxysmal Hypnogenic Dyskinesia

Paroxysmal hypnogenic dyskinesia (PHD) occurs at night during sleep and is often initially erroneously suspected to represent night terrors or other forms of sleep disorders (13). In a large proportion (if not all) of these cases especially the familial variety, these nocturnal dyskinesias are due to mesial frontal lobe seizures that are often difficult to pick up on surface EEG recordings. The eponym autosomal dominant nocturnal frontal lobe epilepsy (ADNFLE) (14) has recently been given to describe this condition in six families in whom affected members had typical PHD attacks.

Although these disorders are quite distinct in the most classical forms, study of a large number of families is revealing in that there is a significant amount of overlap among all of the paroxysmal dyskinesias among families that map to the known genetic loci (15).

ALTERNATING HEMIPLEGIA OF CHILDHOOD

Alternating hemiplegia of childhood (AHC) is a clinical disorder of unknown origin, first described in 1971 (16). The clinical manifestations typically occur before 1 year of age, but there are cases with onset later in childhood. In AHC, episodes of intermittent neurologic dysfunction usually manifest as hemiplegia. A single attack generally affects only one side but can be bilateral. Over time, the attacks can alternate from side to side. These features, along with the onset in early childhood, are the hallmarks for which this disorder was named. The rarity and severity of this disorder has made elucidation of the pathophysiologic basis difficult. Clues that there may be a hereditary basis to AHC exist.

Furthermore, AHC shares overlapping features with a large group of episodic neurologic diseases.

EPISODIC DISORDERS OF THE NERVOUS SYSTEM SHARE MANY CLINICAL FEATURES

All of the episodic movement disorders mentioned here as well as the periodic paralyses and various migraine and epilepsy syndromes share the common feature of having episodic attacks on a normal background, at least at the onset of the disease. In many of these disorders, attacks are frequently precipitated by stress and fatigue. Other precipitating factors that overlap many of these disorders include altered serum potassium levels and certain foods. Similarly, most are amenable to treatment. Moreover, there is overlap of these disorders with regard to therapeutic response to various agents. For example, carbamazepine is effective in preventing seizures in many epilepsy patients and also dramatically reduces incidence of attacks in patients with familial kinesigenic dyskinesia (17). Mexilitene, an antiarrhythmic agent, is also very effective in treating myotonia in some patients with periodic paralysis (18). Acetazolamide and other carbonic anhydrase inhibitors are beneficial to patients with periodic paralysis, myotonias, episodic ataxia (1,18), and also some paroxysmal dyskinesias (12). These similarities suggest common pathophysiologic bases that are shared among some or all of these disorders. In addition, there are syndromes that include features of multiple episodic disorders. For example, Andersen's syndrome is a rare disorder in which patients have both periodic paralysis and cardiac dysrhythmia (19,20). In some forms of episodic ataxia, additional attacks of paroxysmal dyskinesia can be seen (21). Migraine and epilepsy appear to occur at higher than expected rates in families with paroxysmal dyskinesias (17,22, and Ptacek, unpublished results).

PATHOPHYSIOLOGIC SIMILARITIES ARE PRESENT IN EPISODIC DISORDERS

The similarities shared by episodic movement disorders, periodic paralysis, and some forms of epilepsy suggest that insights into the pathogenesis of such disorders may shed light on understanding of the pathophysiology of episodic movement disorders. The first episodic movement disorder gene to be identified was KCNA1, the gene causing EA1 (7). It was not surprising that this disorder, which has many similarities with the periodic paralyses, results from mutations in a voltage-gated potassium channel gene that is evolutionarily related to the sodium and calcium channel genes now known to cause the periodic paralyses. Subsequently, the gene for episodic ataxia type 2 (EA2) has been cloned and is another related gene encoding a P/Q type calcium channel in the central nervous system (23). Different mutations in that same gene also result in a separate phenotype, familial hemiplegic (23). The gene causing paroxysmal non-kinesigenic dyskinesia has been mapped to chromosome 2q; although the gene has not yet been identified, it is thought to be in the vicinity of different ion channel genes (17,24). Recently, two articles describing families with infantile convulsions and paroxysmal choreoathetosis (called the ICCA syndrome) have been linked to chromosome 16p12-q12 (25,26). Attacks in the affected members in both these papers were very brief, frequent, and induced by sudden exertion and therefore similar to PKD (26). A recent report localized eight Japanese families with PKD to this same region (27). Although the gene is not known again this area is in the vicinity of ion channel genes. ADNFLE is genetically heterogenous and two different mutations in two families in the alpha 4 subunit of the neuronal acetylcholine receptor (CHRNA4) on 20q13.2 have been found (28,29). Recently another family with ADNFLE has been also been linked to CHRNA4 which is not at chromosome 20q but on chromosome 15q24 (30).

Pharmacologic studies of the two *CHRNA4* mutations have shown different effects *in vitro*, although both mutations appear to impair calcium entry into cells (29,30).

The list of genes that, when mutated, can result in episodic neurologic phenotypes is growing rapidly (Table 40.1). We should know soon whether the paroxysmal dyskinesias and other episodic movement disorders are the result of ion channel mutations. If not, these disorders could result from mutations in genes that encode proteins that modulate ion channel function.

Given the recognition of many familial episodic movement disorders and the powerful tools of genetics, we will continue to see an explosion of information regarding the pathophysiology of these interesting and mysterious disorders. Such insights will lead to better diagnosis and disease classification and will provide well-characterized patient population for therapeutic trials. Ultimately, these discoveries will lead not only to new insights about pathophysiology but also treatment of paroxysmal movement disorders.

REFERENCES

1. Griggs RC, Moxley RT, Lafrance RA, et al. Hereditary paroxysmal ataxia: response to acetazolamide. *Neurology* 1978;28:1259–1264.
2. Cummins TR, Zhou J, Sigworth FJ, et al. Functional consequences of a Na+ channel mutation causing hyperkalemic periodic paralysis. *Neuron* 1993;10: 667–678.
3. Cannon SC, Strittmatter SM. Functional expression of sodium channel mutations identified in families with periodic paralysis. *Neuron* 1993;10:317–326.
4. Yang N, Ji S, Zhou M, et al. Sodium channel mutations in paramyotonia congenita exhibit similar biophysical phenotypes *in vitro. Proc Natl Acad Sci USA* 1994;91: 12785–12789.
5. Ptáček LJ, Griggs RC. Familial periodic paralyses. In: Andreoli T, ed. *The molecular biology of membrane transport disorders. 3rd ed.* New York: Plenum, 1996.
6. Cannon SC. From mutation to myotonia in sodium channel disorders. *Neuromusc Disord*1997;7:241–249.
7. Browne DL, Gancher ST, Nutt JG, et al. Episodic ataxia/myokymia syndrome is associated with point mutations in the human potassium channel gene, KCNA1. *Nat Genet* 1994;8:136–140.
8. Lubbers WJ, Brunt ER, Scheffer H, et al. Hereditary myokymia and paroxysmal ataxia linked to chromo-

some 12 is responsive to acetazolamide. *J Neurol Neurosurg Psychiatry* 1995;59:400–405.
9. Houser MK, Soland VL, Bhatia KP, et al. Paroxysmal kinesigenic choreoathetosis: a report of 26 cases. *J Neurol* 1999;246:120–126.
10. Demirkirin M, Jankovic J. Paroxysmal dyskinesias: clinical features and classification. *Ann Neurol* 1995;4: 571–579.
11. Fink JK, Hedera P, Mathay JG, et al. Paroxysmal dystonic choreoathetosis linked to chromosome 2q:clinical analysis and proposed pathophysiology. *Neurology* 1997;49:177–183.
12. Bhatia KP, Soland VL, Marsden CD, et al. Paroxysmal exercise induced dystonia:eight new cases and a review of the literature. *Mov Disord* 1997;12:1007–1012.
13. Scheffer IE, Bhatia KP, Lopes-Cendes I, et al. Autosomal dominant frontal lobe epilepsy misdiagnosed as a sleep disorder. *Lancet* 1994;343:515–517.
14. Scheffer IE, Bhatia KP, Lopes Cendes I, et al. Autosomal dominant nocturnal frontal lobe epilepsy. A distinctive clinical disorder. *Brain*1995;118:61–73.
15. Swoboda KJ, McKenna C, Soong B-W, et al. Paroxysmal kinesigenic dyskinesia and infantile convulsions: clinical and linkage data in eleven families. *Neurology* 2000;55:224–230.
16. Verret S, Steele JC. Alternating hemiplegia in childhood: a report of eight patients with complicated migraine beginning in infancy. *Pediatrics* 1971;47: 675–680.
17. Fouad GT, Servidei S, Durcan S, et al. A gene for familial paroxysmal dyskinesia (FPD1) maps to chromosome 2q. *Am J Hum Genet* 1996;59:135–139.
18. Ptáček LJ, Johnson KJ, Griggs RC. Genetics and physiology of the myotonic muscle disorders. *N Engl J Med* 1993;328:482–489.
19. Tawil R, Ptáček LJ, Pavlakis SG, et al. Andersen's syndrome: potassium-sensitive periodic paralysis, ventricular ectopy, and dysmorphic features. *Ann Neurol* 1994; 35:326–330.
20. Sansone V, Griggs RC, Meola G, et al. Andersen's syndrome: a distinct periodic paralysis. *Ann Neurol* 1997; 42:305–312.
21. Griggs RC, Nutt JG. Episodic ataxias as channelopathies [editorial; comment]. *Ann Neurol* 1995;37: 285–287.
22. Munchau A, Valente EM, Shahidi GA, et al. A new family with paroxysmal exercise-induced dystonia and migraine: a clinical and genetic study. *J Neurol Neurosurg Psychiatry* (in press).
23. Ophoff RA, Vergouwe MN, van Eijk R, et al. Familial hemiplegic migraine and episodic ataxia type-2 are caused by mutations in the Ca2+ gene CACNL1A4. *Cell* 1996;87:543–552.
24. Fink JK, Rainier S, Wilkowski J, et al. Paroxysmal dystonic choreoathetosis: tight linkage to chromosome 2q. *Am J Hum Genet* 1996;59:140–145.
25. Szepetowski P, Rochette J, Berquin P, et al. Familial infantile convulsions and paroxysmal choreoathetosis: a new neurological syndrome linked to the pericentromic region of human chromosome 16. *Am J Hum Genet* 1997;61:889–898.
26. Lee WL, Tay A, Ong HT, et al. Association of infantile convulsions with paroxysmal dyskinesias (ICCA syn-

drome): confirmation of linkage to human chromosome 16p12-q12 in a Chinese family. *Hum Genet* 1998;103: 608–612.

27. Tomita H, Nagamitsu S, Wakui K, et al. Paroxysmal kinesigenic choreoathetosis locus maps to chromosome 16p11.2-q12.1. *Am J Hum Genet* 1999;65:1688-1697.

28. Steinlein OK, Mulley JC, Propping P, et al. A missense mutation in the neuronal nicotinic acetylcholine receptor alpha4 subunit is associated with autosomal dominant nocturnal frontal lobe epilepsy. *Nat Genet* 1995;11:201–202.

29. Steinlein OK, Magnusson A, Stoodt J, et al. An insertion mutation of the CHRNA4 gene in a family with autosomal dominant nocturnal frontal lobe epilepsy. *Hum Mol Genet* 1997;6:943–947.

30. Phillips HA, Scheffer IE, Crossland KM, et al. Autosomal dominant nocturnal frontal-lobe epilepsy: genetic heterogeneity and evidence for a second locus at 15q24. *Am J Hum Genet* 1998;63:1108–1116.

31. Shiang R, Ryan SG, Zhu YZ, et al. Mutations in the alpha 1 subunit of the inhibitory glycine receptor cause the dominant neurologic disorder, hyperplexia. *Nat Genet* 1993;5:351–358.

32. Ptáček LJ, George AL Jr, Griggs RC, et al. Identification of a mutation in the gene causing hyperkalemic periodic paralysis. *Cell* 1991;67:1021–1027.

33. Rojas CV, Wang JZ, Schwartz LS, et al. A Met-to-Val mutation in the skeletal muscle Na+ channel alpha-subunit in hyperkalemic periodic paralysis. *Nature* 1991;354:387–389.

34. Ptáček LJ, George AL, Jr., Barchi RL, et al. Mutations in an S4 segment of the adult skeletal muscle sodium channel cause paramyotonia congenita. *Neuron* 1992;8: 891–897.

35. McClatchey AI, Van den Bergh P, Pericak Vance MA, et al. Temperature-sensitive mutations in the III-IV cytoplasmic loop region of the skeletal muscle sodium channel gene in paramyotonia congenita. *Cell* 1992;68: 769–774.

36. Ptáček LJ, Tawil R, Griggs RC, et al. Sodium channel mutations in acetazolamide-responsive myotonia congenita, paramyotonia congenita, and hyperkalemic periodic paralysis. *Neurology* 1994;44:1500–1503.

37. Ptáček LJ, Tawil R, Griggs RC, et al. Dihydropyridine receptor mutations cause hypokalemic periodic paralysis. *Cell* 1994;77:863–868.

38. Fontaine B, Vale Santos J, Jurkat Rott K, et al. Mapping of the hypokalemic periodic paralysis (HypoPP) locus to chromosome 1q31-32 in three European families. *Nat Genet* 1994;6:267–272.

39. Koch MC, Steinmeyer K, Lorenz C, et al. The skeletal muscle chloride channel in dominant and recessive human myotonia. *Science* 1992;257:797–800.

40. George AL Jr, Crackower MA, Abdalla JA, et al. Molecular basis of Thomsen's disease (autosomal dominant myotonia congenita). *Nat Genet* 1993;3:305–310.

41. Zhang J, George AL Jr, Griggs RC, et al. Mutations in the human skeletal muscle chloride channel gene (CLCN1) associated with dominant and recessive myotonia congenita. *Neurology* 1996;47:993–998.

42. Zhuchenko O, Bailey J, Bonnen P, et al. Autosomal dominant cerebellar ataxia (SCA6) associated with small polyglutamine expansions in the alpha 1A-voltage-dependent calcium channel. *Nat Genet* 1997;15: 62–69.

43. Singh NA, Charlier C, Stauffer D, et al. A novel potassium channel gene, KCNQ2, is mutated in an inherited epilepsy of newborns. *Nat Genet* 1998;18:25–29.

44. Charlier C, Singh NA, Ryan SG, et al. A pore mutation in a novel KQT-like potassium channel gene in an idiopathic epilepsy family [see comments]. *Nat Genet* 1998;18:53–55.

45. Doyle J, Ren X, Lennon G, et al. Mutations in the Cacnl1a4 calcium channel gene are associated with seizures, cerebellar degeneration, and ataxia in tottering and leaner mutant mice. *Mam Genome* 1997;8: 113–120.

46. Burgess DL, Jones JM, Meisler MH, et al. Mutation of the Ca2+ channel beta subunit gene Cchb4 is associated with ataxia and seizures in the lethargic (lh) mouse. *Cell* 1997;88:385–392.

47. Letts VA, Felix R, Biddlecome GH, et al. The mouse stargazer gene encodes a neuronal Ca2+-channel gamma subunit [see comments]. *Nat Genet* 1998;19: 340–347.

48. Cox GA, Lutz CM, Yang CL, et al. Sodium/hydrogen exchanger gene defect in slow-wave epilepsy mutant mice. *Cell* 1997;91:139–148.

49. Skradski SL, White HS, Ptáček LJ. Genetic mapping of a locus (mass1) causing audiogenic seizures in mice. *Genomics* 1998;49:188–192.

50. Wang Q, Curran ME, Splawski I, et al. Positional cloning of a novel potassium channel gene: KVLQT1 mutations cause cardiac arrhythmias. *Nat Genet* 1996; 12:17–23.

51. Wang Q, Shen J, Splawski I, et al. SCN5A mutations associated with an inherited cardiac arrhythmia, long QT syndrome. *Cell* 1995;80:805–811.

52. Splawski I, Tristani-Firouzi M, Lehmann MH, et al. Mutations in the hminK gene cause long QT syndrome and suppress IKs function. *Nat Genet* 1997;17:338–340.

53. Auburger G, Ratzlaff t, Lunkes A, et al. A gene for autosomal dominant paroxysmal choreoathetosis/spasticity (CSE) maps to the vicinity of a potassium channel gene cluster on chromosome 1p, probable within 2 cM between D1S443 and D1S197. *Genomics* 1996;31:90–94.

Myoclonus and Paroxysmal Dyskinesias,
Advances in Neurology, Vol. 89,
edited by S. Fahn, et al.
Published by Lippincott Williams & Wilkins, Philadelphia, 2002.

41

Genetics of Episodic Ataxia

Joanna C. Jen and *Robert W. Baloh

Department of Neurology, UCLA School of Medicine, Los Angeles, California;
*Department of Neurology and Surgery, UCLA Medical School, Neurotology Laboratory,
UCLA Medical Center, Los Angeles, California

Episodic ataxia syndromes are rare, usually dominantly inherited disorders with incomplete penetrance characterized by attacks of clumsiness and imbalance triggered by stress or fatigue and often dramatically responsive to acetazolamide. Like other paroxysmal neurologic disorders responsive to acetazolamide, episodic ataxias had long been hypothesized to be channelopathies, neuromuscular disorders caused by mutations in ion channel genes. Indeed, point mutations in genes encoding neuronal ion channels cause two different subtypes of episodic ataxia.

Episodic ataxia syndromes are clinically and genetically heterogeneous. Episodic ataxia type 1 (EA1; MIM 176260) is characterized by episodes of imbalance with persistent myokymia, fine twitching or rippling, which may be difficult to see except in small muscles of the hand and face but is detectable by electromyography (EMG) (1,2). The onset is usually in infancy, with spontaneous resolution during the teens. Exercise, fatigue, hormonal changes, or startle can trigger ataxic attacks. Each episode may last from seconds to minutes and recur many times a day. Linkage analysis in large pedigrees with EA1 established that the locus for this disorder resided on chromosome 12p13, where there was a cluster of potassium channel-encoding genes (3). Point mutations were subsequently identified in *KCNA1* encoding the Kv1.1 subunit, a human homologue of *Shaker* delayed rectifier

voltage-gated potassium channel (4). Each subunit contains six putative transmembrane segments S1-S6. S4 with positively charged amino acid residues at every third position is thought to be the voltage sensor. S5, S6, and the p-loop connecting S5-S6 likely form the channel pore, as is the case in a bacterial potassium channel, the structure of which was recently solved by x-ray crystallography (5). Four such subunits assemble to form a functional channel complex. Found in synaptic zones of axons of cerebellar basket cells and paranodal regions along axons of motor neurons, Kv1.1 is important in neuronal excitability, action potential generation, impulse conduction, and neurotransmission (6). This distribution also correlates well with clinical manifestations of cerebellar and peripheral nerve dysfunction in EA1. Functional studies of heterologously expressed mutant channels have demonstrated altered channel properties (7–13). Kv1.1 null mice exhibited generalized seizures and abnormal neurotransmission at the neuromuscular junction, but there was no evidence of ataxia (14).

Episodic ataxia type 2 (EA2; MIM 601011) is characterized by episodes of slurring of speech and gait imbalance lasting hours to days with interictal gaze-evoked or rebound nystagmus. The age of onset ranges from infancy to early childhood. The attacks may occur spontaneously or may be triggered by physical exertion, fatigue, emotional stress, or excitement. Many experienced their first attacks while playing sports or performing activities associated with emotional excitement. There is usually little neurologic impairment at baseline, but progressive ataxia with cerebellar atrophy develops in some patients. Linkage analysis in large pedigrees with EA2 mapped the disease locus to chromosome 19p13, where familial hemiplegic migraine (another rare, dominantly inherited, paroxysmal neurologic disorder) had previously been mapped. Of the known genes in this chromosomal region of interest, *CACNA1A*, a gene encoding a neuronal calcium channel subunit, was considered a likely candidate. EA2 and FHM were indeed allelic disorders. In unrelated families with EA2 or FHM, point mutations were subsequently identified in *CACNA1A* encoding the $Ca_v2.1$ subunit of the neuronal P/Q type voltage-gated calcium channel (15–23), which is prominently expressed in cerebellar Purkinje and granule cells and at the neuromuscular junction. Later, modest expansions in polyglutamine-encoding CAG repeats in several splice variants of *CACNA1A* were found to cause spinocerebellar ataxia type 6 (SCA6), which is a dominant ataxic syndrome of late onset (24) with acetazolamide-responsive episodic features in some patients (25,26). The $Ca_v2.1$ subunit has four homologous domains, each with six transmembrane segments, similar to the voltage-gated potassium channel subunits. The $Ca_v2.1$ subunit assemble with several auxiliary subunits to form a functional channel complex. Electrophysiologic studies of EA2/FHM mutant channels expressed in cell lines demonstrated altered biophysical properties (23,27,29), in contrast to barely detectable changes in mutant channels harboring polyglutamine expansions (30,31). *In vitro* studies in our laboratory of EA2 mutant channels showed marked reductions in calcium conductance. Prompted by the complaint of fluctuating weakness and previous diagnosis of myasthenia in some patients with EA2, we performed EMG and single-fiber EMG *in vivo* to examine neuromuscular transmission, which is coupled to the pre-

synaptically located P/Q type voltage-gated calcium channels. That these channels are the target of autoantibodies in paraneoplastic Eaton Lambert myasthenic syndrome further emphasizes the importance of these channels in neurotransmission at the neuromuscular junction (32). SFEMG demonstrated jittering and blocking, which is indicative of abnormal synaptic transmission. Abnormal channel function may contribute to impaired neurotransmission at the neuromuscular junction, which could reflect similarly abnormal neurotransmission in the cerebellum. Spontaneous recessive mouse mutants *tottering*, *rolling-Nagoya*, and *leaner* with mutations in the mouse homollog of *CACNA1A* suffer from ataxia and/or seizures, with marked cerebellar atrophy (33,34). Null mice also exhibit cerebellar atrophy, while there was no apparent pathology in heterozygotes (35,36).

How mutation in *KCNA1* and *CACNA1A* cause episodic ataxia with progressive features remains poorly understood. These rare channelopathies are instructive models to study the important roles of ion channels in neuronal function and behavior. Of note, reminiscent of the mouse mutants, coexistence of episodic ataxia and epilepsy has been observed in human, thus suggesting shared mechanisms between paroxysmal movement disorders and seizures.

REFERENCES

1. VanDyke DH, Griggs RC, Murphy MJ, et al. Hereditary myokymia and periodic ataxia. *J Neurol Sci* 1975;25 (1):109–118.
2. Brunt ER, van Weerden TW. Familial paroxysmal kinesigenic ataxia and continuous myokymia. *Brain* 1990; 113(pt 5):1361–1382.
3. Litt M, Kramer P, Browne D, et al. A gene for episodic ataxia/myokymia maps to chromosome 12p13. *Am J Hum Genet* 1994;55(4):702–709.
4. Browne DL, Gancher ST, Nutt JG, et al. Episodic ataxia/myokymia syndrome is associated with point mutations in the human potassium channel gene, KCNA1. *Nat Genet* 1994;8(2):136–140.
5. Doyle DA, Morais Cabral J, Pfuetzner RA, et al. The structure of the potassium channel: molecular basis of K+ conduction and selectivity. *Science* 1998;280 (5360):69–77.
6. Wang H, Kunkel DD, Martin TM, et al. Heteromultimeric K+ channels in terminal and juuxtaparanodal regions of neurons. *Nature* 1993;365(6441):75–79.

7. Adelman JP, Bond CT, Pessia M, et al. Episodic ataxia resultsfrom voltage dependent potassium channels with altered functions. *Neuron* 1995;15(6):1449–1454.

8. D'Adamo MC, Liu Z, Adelman JP, et al. Episodic ataxia type-1 mutations in the hKv1.1 cytoplasmic pore region alter the gating properties of the channel. *Embo J* 1998;17(5):1200–1207.

9. Zerr P, Adelman JP, Maylie J. Characterization of three episodic ataxia mutations in the human Kv1.1 potassium channel. *FEBS Lett* 1998;431(3):461–464.

10. Zerr P, Adelman JP, Maylie J. Episodic ataxia mutations in Kv1.1 alter potassium channel function by dominant negative effects or haploinsufficiency. *J Neurosci* 1998; 18(8):2842–2848.

11. Boland LM, Price DL, Jackson KA. Episodic ataxia/ myokymia mutations functionally expressed in the Shaker potassium channel. *Neuroscience* 1999;91(4): 1557–1564.

12. Bretschneider F, Wrisch A, Lehmann-Horn F, et al. Expression in mammalian cells and electrophysiological characterization of two mutant Kv1.1 channels causing episodic ataxia type 1 (EA-1). *Eur J Neurosci* 1999; 11(7):2403–2412.

13. Spauschus A, Eunson L, Hanna MG, et al. Functional characterization of a novel mutation in KCNA1 in episodic ataxia type 1 associated with epilepsy. *Ann NY Acad Sci*1999;868:442–446.

14. Smart SL, Lopantsev V, Zhang CL, et al. Deletion of the K(V)1.1 potassium channel causes epilepsy in mice. *Neuron* 1998;20(4):809–819.

15. Ophoff RA, Terwindt GM, Vergouwe MN, et al. Familial hemiplegic migraine and episodic ataxia type-2 are caused by mutations in the Ca2+ channel gene CACNL1A4. *Cell* 1996;87(3):543–552.

16. Yue Q, Jen JC, Nelson SF, et al. Progressive ataxia due to a missense mutation in a calcium-channel gene. *Am J Hum Genet* 1997;61(5):1078–1087.

17. Yue Q, Jen JC, Thwe MM, et al. De novo mutation in CACNA1A caused acetazolamide-responsive episodic ataxia. *Am J Med Genet* 1998;77(4):298–301.

18. Battistini S, Stenirri S, Piatti M, et al. A new CACNA1A gene mutation in acetazolamide-responsive familial hemiplegic migraine and ataxia [see comments]. *Neurology*1999;53(1):38–43.

19. Carrera P, Piatti M, Stenirri S, et al. Genetic heterogeneity in Italian families with familial hemiplegic migraine [see comments]. *Neurology* 1999;53(1): 26–33.

20. Denier C, Ducros A, Vahedi K, et al. High prevalence of CACNA1A truncations and broader cliinical spectrum in episodic ataxia type 2. *Neurology* 1999;52(9): 1816–1821.

21. Friend KL, Crimmins D, Phan TG, et al. Detection of a novel missense mutation and second recurrent mutation in the CACNA1Agene in individuals with EA-2 and FHM. *Hum Genet* 1999;105(3):261–265.

22. Jen J, Yue Q, Nelson SF, et al. A novel nonsense mutation in CACNA1A causes episodic ataxia and hemiplegia [see comments]. *Neurology* 1999;53(1):34–37.

23. Guida S, Trettel F, Pagnutti S, et al. Complete loss of p/q calcium channel activity caused by a cacna1a missense mutation carried by patients with episodic ataxia type 2. *Am J Hum Genet* 2001;68(3):759–764.

24. Zhuchenko O, Bailey J, Bonnen P, et al. Autosomal dominant cerebellar ataxia (SCA6) associated with small polyglutamine expansions in the alpha 1A voltage dependent calcium channel. *Nat Genet* 2001;15(1):62–69.

25. Jodice C, Mantuano E, Veneziano L, et al. Episodic ataxia type 2 (EA2) and spinocerebellar ataxia type 6 (SCA6) due to CAG repeat expansion in the CACNA1A gene on chromosome 19p. *Hum Mol Genet* 1997;6 (11):1973–1978.

26. Jen JC, Yue Q, Karrim J, et al. Spinocerebellar ataxia type 6 withh positional vertigo and acetazolamide responsive episodic ataxia. *J Neurol Neurosurg Psychiatry* 1998;65(4):565–568.

27. Kraus RL, Sinnegger MJ, Glossmann H, et al. Familial hemiplegic migraine mutations change alpha1A Ca2+ channel kinetics. *J Biol Chem*1998;273(10):5586–5590.

28. Hans M, Luvisetto S, Williams ME, et al. Functional consequences of mutations in the human alpha1A calcium channel subunit linked to familial hemiplegic migraine. *J Neurosci*1999;19(5):1610–1619.

29. Kraus RL, Sinnegger MJ, Koschak A, et al. Three new familial hemiplegic migraine mutants affect P/Q-type Ca(2+) channel kinetics. *J Biol Chem* 2000;27(13): 9239–9243.

30. Matsuyama ZMW, Mori Y, Kawakami H, et al. Direct alteration of the P/Q-type Ca2+ channel property by polyglutamine expansion in spinocerebellar ataxia 6. *J Neurosci* 1999;19.

31. Restituito S, Thompson RM, Eliet J, et al. The polyglutamine expansion in spinocerebellar ataxia type 6 causes a beta subunit-specific enhanced activation of P/Q-type calcium channels in Xenopus oocytes. *J Neurosci* 2000;20(17):6394–6403.

32. Kim YI, Neher E. IgG from patients with Lambert-Eaton syndrome blocks voltage-dependent calcium channels. *Science*1988;239(4838):405–408.

33. Fletcher CF, Lutz CM, O'Sullivan TN, et al. Absence epilepsy in tottering mutant mice is associated with calcium channel defects. *Cell* 1996;87(4):607–617.

34. Mori Y, Wakamori M, Oda S, et al. Reduced voltage sensitivity of activation of P/Q-type Ca2+ channels is associated with the ataxic mouse mutation rolling Nagoya (tg(rol)). *J Neurosci* 2000;20(15):5654–5662.

35. Jun K, Piedras-Renteria ES, Smith SM, et al. Ablation of P/Q-type Ca(2+) channel currents, altered synaptic transmission, and progressive ataxia in mice lacking the alpha(1A)-subunit. *Proc Natl Acad Sci USA* 1999;96 (26):15245–15250.

36. Fletcher CF, Tottene A, Lennon VA, et al. Dystonia and cerebellar atrophy in Cacna1a null mice lacking P/Q calcium channel activity. *Faseb J* 2001;5:5.

Myoclonus and Paroxysmal Dyskinesias,
Advances in Neurology, Vol. 89,
edited by S. Fahn, et al.
Published by Lippincott Williams & Wilkins, Philadelphia, 2002.

42

Autosomal Dominant Nocturnal Frontal Lobe Epilepsy

*Gholam K. Motamedi and †Ronald P. Lesser

*Epilepsy Center; Department of Neurology, Georgetown University School of Medicine and Hospital;
†Department of Neurology, Johns Hopkins University School of Medicine, Baltimore, Maryland

Approximately 30,000 genes, of the total human genome of 100,000, are expressed specifically in the nervous system. The gene products for a few thousands of them are known. Dysfunction of at least 1,000 genes can cause neurologic disorders. However, the responsible genes for only a small number of inherited neurologic diseases have been identified, and only a few of them are related to epilepsy. Thus the study of genetic diseases of the nervous system, epilepsy in particular, is still in its infancy (1).

Epilepsies with a presumed genetic etiology (idiopathic epilepsies) are predominantly of generalized type and have complex or multifactorial rather than monogenic mode of inheritance. This group represents 39% to 59% of all epilepsies and includes primarily the generalized epilepsies, such as epilepsy with generalized tonic-clonic seizures only, childhood and juvenile absence epilepsy, and juvenile myoclonic epilepsy (JME) (2), although there is controversy regarding the mode of inheritance of JME (3–13).

There are over 200, mostly rare, symptomatic epilepsies known to be inherited as single-gene disorders but only a few of them carry chromosomal assignments (14). The genes for most of this group have been discovered over the past few years starting with the discovery of the genetic defect in AD-NFLE, the first genetic defect described in an idiopathic epilepsy (15).

The monogenic epilepsy syndromes for which the genetic defects have been discovered include autosomal dominant nocturnal frontal lobe epilepsy (ADNFLE) linked to chromosomes 20q and 15q (15–18), benign familial neonatal convulsions (BFNCs) genetically linked to chromosome regions 20q and 8q (19–23), generalized epilepsy with febrile seizures plus (GEFS+1) and benign familial infantile convulsions (BFIC) linked to 19q13 (24), GEFS+2 linked to 2q24 (25–28), progressive myoclonic epilepsy of Unverricht-Lundborg type (EPM1) linked to 21q (29–33), progressive myoclonus epilepsy of Lafora type (EPM2) linked to 6q (2,34), and neuronal ceroid lipofuscinoses linked to 1p, 11p, 13q, 15q, 16p (35,36). ADNFLE is the only one of these epilepsy types causing partial seizures. The recessively inherited generalized epilepsy syndrome of childhood progressive epilepsy with mental retardation (northern epilepsy syndrome) maps to chromosome 8p23 and has recently been described as a form of neuronal ceroid-lipofuscinosis with an exceptionally protracted course (37–39).

Recently three other autosomal dominant partial epilepsy syndromes have been described. Familial temporal lobe epilepsy has been reported to be linked to chromosome 10q but its genetic defect is still unknown (40–43). Autosomal dominant partial epilepsy with variable foci (FPEVF) has been mapped to chromosome 22q (44). Autosomal dominant rolandic epilepsy and speech dyspraxia remain to be studied further (45).

EPILEPSY AS A CHANNELOPATHY

The products of gene mutations in AD-NFLE, BFNCs, GEFS+, and possibly JME (4–12) are associated with ion channels (Table 42.1).

Increasing evidence from animal studies suggest that dysfunctional ion channels are responsible for epilepsy (46). Some types of epilepsy are caused by abnormalities in potassium channels. Mice lacking the voltage-gated Shaker-like potassium channel Kv1.1 α-subunit develop frequent spontaneous seizures (47). Point mutation in the human potassium channel gene KCNA1 (the human homologue of Kv1.1) was recently reported in patients with episodic ataxia type 1 (EA1) and partial epilepsy. The mutation results in substitution of arginine for threonine in a highly conserved position in the second transmembrane segment of the channel (48).

Mutations in another set of human potassium channel genes KCNQ2 and KCNQ3

identified through positional cloning were found in families with benign familial neonatal convulsions (BFNC). These two along with two other genes, KVLQT1 and nKQT, now form a new family of voltage-gated potassium channel genes known as the long QT family. KVLQT1 (KCNQ1) is responsible for the inherited form of long QT syndrome (49). Mutations in the Drosophilae seizure (sei) locus cause temperature-induced hyperactivity, followed by paralysis. The product of this mutation is the Drosophilae homologue of HERG, which encodes an inwardly rectifying potassium channel. This channel is mutated in one form of hereditary long QT syndrome in humans (50).

Generalized epilepsy with febrile seizures plus (GEFS+1), a generalized epilepsy with a complex inheritance pattern, has been linked to chromosome region 19q13.1 with identification of a mutation in the voltage-gated sodium channel β1 subunit gene (SCN1B). The mutation changes a conserved cysteine residue. Co-expressing the mutant β-1 subunit with a brain Na^+-channel α-subunit in *Xenopus* oocytes, the investigators have shown that the mutation interfered with the ability of the subunit to modulate channel-gating kinetics, consistent with a loss-of-function allele (27,28). GEFS+2 has been linked to 2q24 with identification of a muta-

TABLE 42.1. *Genetic epilepsy syndromes with monogenic mode of inheritance associated with ion channel mutations*

Epilepsy syndrome	Gene (chromosome)	Gene product
Autosomal dominant nocturnal frontal lobe epilepsy	CHRNA4 (20q, 15q)	Mutation in the second transmembrane region of the α4 subunit of the neuronal nicotinic acetylcholine receptor (nAChR)
Benign familial neonatal convulsions	KCNQ2, KCNQ3 (20q, 8q)	Mutation in the pore-forming region of the voltage-gated potassium channel
Generalized epilepsy with febrile seizures plus	SCN1B (19q)	Mutation in the β1-subunit of voltage-gated sodium channel
Generalized epilepsy with febrile seizures plus	SCN1A (2q)	Mutation in the α subunit of voltage-gated sodium channel
Benign familial infantile convulsions	SCN1B (19q)	Mutation in the β1-subunit of voltage-gated sodium channel
Juvenile myoclonic epilepsy[a]	CHRNA7 (6p, 15q)	Mutation in the α7 subunit of the nicotinic cholinergic receptor

[a]There is controversy regarding the inheritance of juvenile myoclonic epilepsy.

tion in SCN1A, the gene coding the α-subunit of voltage-gated sodium channel (25,26).

Benign familial infantile convulsions (BFIC), also a rare autosomal dominant epilepsy syndrome has been recently mapped to chromosomes 19q. These patients present with partial, then generalized, seizures, with onset at age 3 months. Usually the seizures cease spontaneously after 1 year without treatment, leaving no neurologic abnormalities. Given the phenotypical similarity between BFIC and GEFS+, SCN1B is a candidate gene for BFIC (24).

There is controversy regarding the evidence in favor of JME being a single-gene disorder linked to chromosomes 6p and 15q. Interestingly, a candidate gene region on chromosome 15q is located near the region containing CHRNA7, a gene encoding the α7 subunit of the nicotinic cholinergic receptor (6–8,10).

Linkage analysis has confirmed a pericentromeric locus on chromosome 16 as a major locus in 11 families with paroxysmal kinesigenic dyskinesia (PKD) and infantile convulsions (51). PKD is considered a reasonable candidate for an ion channel disorder, as it has been observed in patients with episodic ataxia type 1 due to mutations in the potassium channel gene KCNA1 (12p) (52).

The gene for ADNFLE has been found to be a mutation in the neuronal acetylcholine receptor (nAChR) α4-subunit gene (CHRNA4) on chromosome region 20q13.2-q13.3, associated with a Ser248Phe or Ser252Leu amino acid exchange, or 776ins3 in the gate-forming second transmembrane domain (TM2). This was the first discovered genetic defect in an idiopathic human epilepsy syndrome that happens to be a localization-related epilepsy (15,17,18,53) (Figs. 42.1, 42.2).

HISTORICAL BACKGROUND AND CLINICAL PRESENTATION

The description of ADNFLE as a distinct epilepsy syndrome in 1994 (54,55), was preceded by conflicting data over three decades, of a complex of "abnormal nocturnal motor and behavioral phenomena" described as a series of conditions including paroxysmal nightmares (56), episodic nocturnal wandering (ENW) (57,58), paroxysmal awakenings (59), nocturnal paroxysmal dystonia (NPD) (60,61), paroxysmal arousals during sleep (PAS) (62), and paroxysmal periodic motor attacks during sleep (63).

These case reports described mostly young patients typically in their second or third decade of life who presented with a history of frequent episodes of brief, nocturnal, stereotyped awakening from non-REM sleep followed by screaming, violent limb movements, unintelligible vocalizations, and ambulation. The frequency ranged from two or three per year to several per night, in some cases with a periodic repetition every 20 to 60 seconds and a tendency to occur in the early morning hours. Some had a history or family history of parasomnias. Some patients appeared to have a disorder with an autosomal dominant inheritance (64). Patients were responsive to antiepileptic drugs, carbamazepine in particular. Their interictal electroencephalogram (EEG) occasionally revealed epileptiform discharges but remained normal during the recorded episodes.

The possibility that the entity now called ADNFLE might be a new epileptic syndrome was suggested approximately 25 years ago (57,59), and it was later suggested to possibly be of frontal lobe origin (63). Frontal lobe epilepsy *per se* had been well described before (65–69), and later reports even further characterized it (70–77). More recently, video-EEG monitoring and polysomnography distinguished the EEG and semiologic characteristics of the new syndrome and emphasized the epileptic and possibly frontal lobe origin of the episodes. Despite the inevitable terminologic ambiguities that resulted in describing the disorder as consisting of "short attacks" of NPD, ENW, or PAS, the authors were moving toward recognizing the syndrome as a new diagnostic entity (61–63, 78–84). Moreover, comparison between NPD, daytime frontal lobe seizures, and nocturnal motor attacks of known epileptic origin did

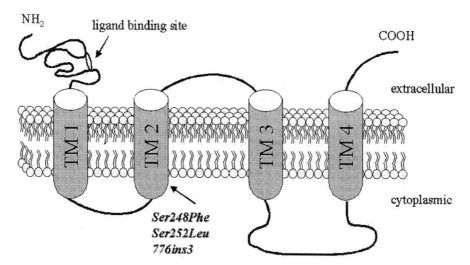

FIG. 42.1. Schematic representation of the α-4 subunit of the neuronal nicotinic acetylcholine receptor (nAChR), encoded by the gene CHRNA4, and composed of four hydrophobic transmembrane domains (TM1-4). TM2 contributes to the pore of the ion channel, where the three ADNFLE mutations occur (*arrow*). (Modified with permission from Steinlein OK. New insights into the molecular and genetic mechanisms underlying idiopathic epilepsies. *Clin Genet* 1998;54(3):169–175.)

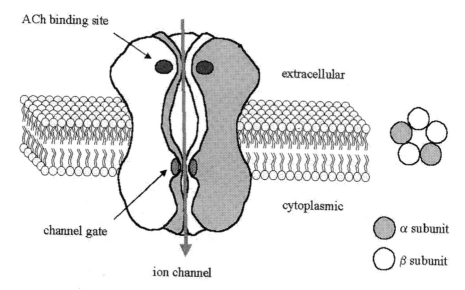

FIG. 42. 2. The neuronal nicotinic acetylcholine receptor (nAChR) is a heteropentameric ligand-gated ion channel consisting of five α2β3 subunits. A horizontal view is shown on the *left* and a cross-sectional view (i.e., from above) is shown on the *right*. (Used with permission from Bate L, Gardiner M. Molecular genetics of human epilepsies. *Expert reviews in molecular medicine.* Cambridge: University Press, 1999.)

not support the idea that NPD was a separate diagnostic entity (86).

Eventually Scheffer and associates reported a nocturnal frontal lobe epilepsy syndrome of clear autosomal dominant inheritance (ADNFLE) in 47 individuals spanning six generations from five unrelated families in Australia, Britain, and Canada (54,55). These families presented a homogeneous clinical epilepsy syndrome. Many of these patients had been misdiagnosed as having non-epileptic disorders. One patient had only infrequent stress-related "nightmares" and never sought medical care. Mildly affected cases were recognized only because of a diagnosed parent. The penetrance was 69%. The authors emphasized that the autosomal dominant nature of this condition had been previously unrecognized because of under-reporting or misdiagnosis and also because of the stigma attached to epilepsy (55,87).

There was a direct relationship between the severity and frequency of seizures and the age of onset; the earlier the onset the more severe the disease. The average age of onset varied from 2 months to 52 years (mean, 11.7 years). The clusters consisted of typically four to 11, but as high as 72, episodes of brief nocturnal motor seizures per night. Most of the episodes originated in light sleep, usually early, but occurred in early morning as well. Mean duration of the recorded episodes was 20 seconds (range, 5 seconds to 5 minutes). Seventy percent of the patients reported an aura that included a wide variety of sensory, somatosensory, and psychic phenomena. The episodes started with vocalization or a gasp followed by eye opening and staring. The motor activity included thrashing, hyperkinetic activity, tonic stiffening, clonic jerking, grabbing, crawling, sitting up during the episode, forced hyperextension, and flinging out of bed. Although the majority of the patients believed that they remained conscious during the attack, most of them reported tongue biting or incontinence. Postictal periods were brief. In more than half of the patients, seizures secondarily generalized. Seizures persisted through adult life, becoming less severe beyond the fifth decade. Intellect and neurologic examination were normal, and neuroimaging was unremarkable (54,55).

One third of the patients were taking antiepileptic medications at the time of diagnosis. Carbamazepine at the average dose of 690 mg per day was highly effective and its discontinuation in adult life was associated with seizure recurrence. Phenytoin was effective as well but valproate was not. Interictal EEG was normal in the majority of patients (84%), while the rest showed bilateral or unilateral activity with frontal or anterior quadrant predominance. Ictal EEG did not record any epileptiform activity in the majority of patients, while in others it showed bilateral frontal sharp and slow activity with extension to the central and parietal areas (55).

MOLECULAR GENETICS

Genetic mapping of ADNFLE in a large Australian kindred, to chromosome 20q13.2-q13.3 (16), paved the way for the identification of Ser248Phe mutation in exon 5 of CHRNA4, the gene encoding the α4 subunit of the neuronal nicotinic acetylcholine receptor (nAChR), located in the same region (15). This missense mutation induced by a C to T transition replaces neutral serine by the complex aromatic phenylalanine in the sixth amino acid position (homologous to Ser248 of the Torpedo (α subunit), a highly conserved amino acid residue in the second transmembrane, channel lining domain (TM2). Most of the other subunits of the human nAChR conserve Ser248 except for α7 and α8. Charged amino acids line the channel pore and selectively let through the ions that can pass into the cell (Figs. 42.1, 42.2) (15). Neuronal nAChRs are involved in cognition, learning, memory, arousal, anxiety, depression, cerebral blood flow and metabolism, and an increasing number of disorders including ADNFLE, Alzheimer's disease, Parkinson's disease, and schizophrenia (88).

The neuronal nAChR is a pentameric ligand-gated ion channel composed of various combinations (homomeric or heteromeric) of various complements of membrane spanning α or β subunits (α2-9 and β2-4). It has a 2α3β stoichiometry with the possibility of more than one α subunit subtype within a pentamer. The encoding gene (CHRNA4) is expressed in all layers of the frontal cortex. The multiplicity of the subunits provides the basis for the heterogeneity observed in the structure and function of nAChR. Each subunit of the nAChR, about 500 amino acid in length, consists of an extracellular ligand-binding N-terminal domain, four hydrophobic membrane spanning domains (TM1-4), and several loops connecting TM1-4 (15,88–90). Upon binding to nicotine, nAChR undergoes a conformational change, opening the channel. According to one model, serine 248 is located beneath a tight hydrophobic ring at the most constricted part of the closed channel pore (88,91).

Electrophysiologic investigation of the mutated channel (Ser248Phe) coexpressed with the wild type in *Xenopus* oocytes demonstrated faster desensitization (reduced response to a transmitter during repeated or prolonged application) of the mutated channel upon activation by acetylcholine, and slower recovery from the desensitized state to a conducting state. This possibly indicates a destabilization of the ion channel open configuration. The mutant receptor also showed a sevenfold decrease in apparent affinity to acetylcholine, and desensitization in response to agonist concentrations 3,000 times lower than that in controls (89,92).

Two further mutations in the TM2 domain of CHRNA4 gene have been reported in families with ADNFLE. These include an insertion mutation (776ins3), and a missense mutation (Ser252Leu), in separate Norwegian and Japanese families, respectively (18,93–95). Independent Ser248Phe mutations have been reported in families from northern Norway and Spain (the latter was named Ser252Phe, according to different numbering) (53,96). Insertion of three nucleotides (GCT) at the nucleotide position 776 in the coding region for the C-terminal end of TM2 domain, results in an extra leucine. Electrophysiologic investi-

gation of the changes induced by this mutation in *Xenopus* oocytes revealed a significant reduction of the channel permeability of calcium, while a tenfold increase in the apparent affinity for acetylcholine was observed. Despite looking dissimilar in their electrophysiologic properties, both mutations, Ser248Phe and 776ins3, result in loss of function by inducing receptor hypoactivity and decreased calcium influx. The common end result of both mutations is consistent with the phenotypic similarity observed in patients with different genotypes (18,96).

But how do mutations that induce fast desensitization, decrease calcium influx, and therefore render the neuronal nAChR hypoactive, cause seizures? It has been shown that neuronal nAChR is involved in the modulation of other neurotransmitter release, in fast synaptic transmission, and acts as a modifier of neuronal excitability (89,97–100). Bertrand and associates and Weiland and colleagues have suggested that accumulation of ACh in the synaptic cleft induces desensitization of receptors containing mutant subunits. The resultant neuronal nAChR hypoactivity may disturb the balance between the excitatory and inhibitory synaptic transmission by affecting the inhibitory regulating pathways such as those regulated by $GABA_A$ receptor, leading to abnormal fast spike discharges (89, 92,97,99).

Cholinergic projections to the frontal lobes may play an important role in sleep, as evidenced by their role in synchronization of spindles in stage 2 sleep. It is possible that abnormalities in this same cholinergic input result in the increased seizure frequency seen in stage 2 sleep in some patients with ADNFLE (101).

And why should a Mendelian disorder present as a localization-related rather than generalized seizure? Variability in neuronal nAChR subunit composition in different parts or layers of the frontal cortex (even within a given patient) may alter the way in which a disorder such as ADNFLE is expressed (15). Variability in unrelated factors could modify the way in which nAChR receptor changes affect cerebral function. This in turn would mean that the presence of ADNFLE would not necessarily, by itself, predict all aspects of the clinical expression of the disorder, as demonstrated by criteria such as ictal semiology, scalp EEG, and ictal SPECT. Second, it is possible that more than one disorder could express itself clinically as ADNFLE. For example, Picard and associates report a member of a family diagnosed on clinical grounds to have ADNFLE but in whom they could not definitely establish linkage to chromosomal regions thought specific for ADNFLE. This patient's seizures appeared clinically and on scalp EEG to originate in the left frontal lobe. Intracerebral recording revealed a primary focus in the opercular-insular cortex. (40,102).

The genetic heterogeneity of ADNFLE has been further explored. Phillips and colleagues reported families in which ADNFLE is unlinked to the CHRNA4 region on chromosome 20q13.2, and sporadic cases in which no evidence of defective CHRNA4 was found. Interestingly one of the families showed evidence of linkage to 15q24, in a region close to the CHRNA3/CHRNA5/CHRNB4 cluster encoding $\alpha3/\alpha5/\beta4$ subunits of neuronal nAChR, respectively (17). Picard and colleagues did not find the CHRNA4 mutation in any of eight European families clinically diagnosed with ADNFLE, nor did Oldani and his colleagues among 38 patients in 28 Italian pedigrees, or Provini and associates in their 21 patients with ADNFLE. These authors suggest the locations of other neuronal nAChR subunits as candidate regions for further linkage studies in such ADNFLE families (40,103,104).

RELATIONSHIP BETWEEN CLINICAL PRESENTATION AND GENETIC MECHANISMS

As further insight was provided by molecular genetics to the nature of the disease, the latest comprehensive clinical-genetic studies have contributed to better delineation of ADNFLE as an independent clinical and genetic entity, and older descriptive terms such as episodic nocturnal wandering, paroxysmal

awakenings, and nocturnal paroxysmal dystonia have been abandoned (40,81,83,84,94–96, 102–108).

The clinical presentation of ADNFLE as described by Scheffer and associates in their original kindred remains the standard (55). This phenotype, in independent families with similar genetic mutations, has not shown significant differences in symptoms, although there is some intrafamilial and interfamilial variability (40,102). More noticeable clinical heterogeneity is seen when comparing families with different genetic mutations. Three Japanese families with ADNFLE, with a novel mutation (Ser252Leu), did not have auras and were not aware of their episodes (55,94,95). All three children in these families had behavioral problems such as hyperactivity and two of them also had mild mental retardation. Co-occurrence of ADNFLE and mental retardation was thought coincidental in a family reported from Germany (108).

There are more phenotypic differences between families with ADNFLE caused by mutations in neuronal nAChR $\alpha4$ subunit on chromosome 20q, and those not linked to chromosome 20q. Age of onset, nocturnal clusters of hyperkinetic and dystonic movements, and favorable response to carbamazepine are among the common features in the group with 20q linkage, but enuresis, diurnal attacks, tiredness on awakening, and daytime somnolence were seen only in those without this linkage (53,55,102,103). The phenotypic similarity between the independent Norwegian families, the Spanish family, and the original Australian kindred, all with different genetic backgrounds, suggests that the Ser248Phe mutation is the major factor determining the phenotype rather than other background genes (96).

Seizures of patients with ADNFLE generally respond well to carbamazepine and also have responded to phenytoin. It's possible that these seizures would also respond to oxcarbazepine, because it is similar to carbamazepine. Valproic acid is often used for seizures of frontal lobe origin, but doesn't appear to be effective for ADNFLE.

The genetic heterogeneity and clinical variability of the different autosomal dominant partial epilepsy syndromes continue to challenge those interested in the genetics of epilepsy (55,105,109). Of particular interest is the variability of expression, even among members of the same family who have the same genetic defect. This emphasizes the likelihood that, even when we can define the single genetic defect responsible for the occurrence of ADNFLE in a patient, we still need to understand the multiple influences responsible for the clinical expression of the disorder in that individual.

REFERENCES

1. Hall ZW. Molecular approaches to diseases of the nervous system. An introduction to molecular neurobiology. Sinauer Assoc., 1992.
2. Seratossa JM. Idiopathic epilepsies with a complex mode of inheritance. *Epilepsia* 1999;40(suppl 3): 12–16.
3. Steinlein OK. Idiopathic epilepsies with a monogenic mode of inheritance. *Epilepsia*1999;40(suppl 3):9–11.
4. Liu AW, Delgado-Escueta AV, Serratosa JM, et al. Juvenile myoclonic epilepsy locus in chromosome 6p21.2-p11: linkage to convulsions and electroencephalography trait. *Am J Hum Genet* 1995;57(2): 368–381.
5. Liu AW, Delgado-Escueta AV, Gee MN, et al. Juvenile myoclonic epilepsy in chromosome 6p12-p11:locus heterogeneity and recombinations. *Am J Med Genet* 1996;63(3):438–446.
6. Sander T, Bockenkamp B, Hildmann T, et al. Refined mapping of the epilepsy susceptibility locus EJMI on chromosome 6. *Neurology* 1997;49(3):842–847.
7. Sander T, Kretz R, Williamson MP, et al. Linkage analysis between idiopathic generalized epilepsies and the GABA(A) receptor alpha5, beta3, and gamma3 subunit cluster on chromosome 15. *Acta Neurol Scand* 1997;96(1):1–7.
8. Sander T, Schultz H, Vieira-Saeker AM, et al. Evaluation of a putative major susceptibility locus for juvenile myoclonic epilepsy on chromosome 15q14. *Am J Med Genet* 1999;88(2):182–187.
9. Elmslie FV, Williamson MP, Rees M, et al. Linkage analysis of juvenile myoclonic epilepsy and microsatellite loci spanning 61 cM of chromosome 6p in 19 nuclear pedigrees provides no evidence for susceptibility locus in this region. *Am J Hum Genet* 1996;59 (3):653–663.
10. Elmslie FV, Rees M, WIlliamson MP, et al. Genetic mapping of a major susceptibility locus for juvenile myoclonic epilepsy on chromosome. *Hum Mol Genet* 1997;6(8):1329–1334.
11. Guipponi M, Thomas P, Girard-Reydet C, et al. Lack of association between juvenile myoclonic epilepsy and GABRA5 and GABRB3 genes. *Am J Med Genet* 1997;74(2):150–153.
12. Delgado-Esccueta AV, Medina MT, Serratosa JM, et al. Mapping and positional cloning of common idiopathic generalized epilepsies: juvenile myoclonus epilepsy and childhood absence epilepsy. *Adv Neurol* 1999; 79:351–374.
13. Goodwin H, Chioza B, McCormic D, et al. Positive association found between the α7 nicotinic acetylcholine receptor subunit gene and idiopathic generalized epilepsy. *Neurology* 2000;54(7):A356.
14. Berkovic SF, Scheffer IE. Epilepsies with single gene inheritance. *Brain Dev* 1997;19(1):13–18.
15. Steinlein OK, Mulley JC, Propping P, et al. A missense mutation in the neuronal nicotinic acetylcholine receptor alpha4 subunit is associated with autosomal dominant nocturnal frontal lobe epilepsy. *Nat Genet* 1995; 11(2):201–203.
16. Phillips HA, Scheffer IE, Berkovic SF, et al. Localization of a gene for autosomal dominant nocturnal frontal lobe epilepsy to chromosome 20q 13.2. *Nat Genet* 1995;10(1):117–118.
17. Phillips HA, Scheffer IE, Crossland KM, et al. Autosomal dominant nocturnal frontal-lobe epilepsy: genetic hetrogeneity and evidence for a second locus at 15q24. *Am J Hum Genet* 1998;63(4):1108–1116.
18. Steinlein OK, Magnusson A, Stoodt J, et al. An insertion mutation of the CHRNA4 gene in a family with autosomal dominant nocturnal frontal lobe epilepsy. *Hum Mol Genet* 1997;6(6):943–947.
19. Leppert M, Anderson VE, Quattlebaum T, et al. Benign neonatal convulsions linked to genetic markers on chromosome 20. *Nature* 1989;337:647–648.
20. Lewis TB, Leach RG, Ward K, et al. Genetic heterogeneity in benign familial neonatal convulsions: Identification of a new locus on chromosome 8q. *Hum Genet* 1993;53:670–675.
21. Biervert C, Schroeder BC, Kubisch C, et al. A potassium channel mutation in neonatal human epilepsy. *Science* 1998;279:403–406.
22. Singh NA, Charlier C, Stauffer D, et al. A novel potassium channel gene, KCNQ2, is mutated in an inherited epilepsy of newborns. *Nat Genet* 1998;18:25–29.
23. Charlier C, Singh NA, Ryan SG, et al. A pore mutation in a novel KQT-like potassium channel gene in an idiopathic epilepsy family. *Nat Genet* 1998;18:53–55.
24. Moulard B, Buresi C, Malafosse A. Study of the voltage-gated sodium channel beta 1 subunit gene (SCN1B) in the benign familial infantile convulsions syndrome (BFIC). *Hum Mutat* 2000;16:139–142.
25. Escayg A, MacDonald B, Meisler M, et al. Mutations of SCN1A, encoding a neuronal sodium channel, in two families with GEFS+2. *Nat Genet* 2000;24: 343–345.
26. Moulard B, Guipponi M, Chaigne D, et al. Identification of a new locus for generalized epilepsy with febrile seizures plus (GEFS+) on chromosome 2q24-q33. *Am J Hum Genet* 1999;65:1396–1400.
27. Wallace RH, Wang DW, Singh R, et al. Febrile seizures and generalized epilepsy associated with a mutation in the Na+ channel beta1 subunit gene SCN1B. *Nat Genet* 1998;19(4):366–370.
28. Scheffer IE, Berkovic SF. Generalized epilepsy with febrile seizures plus. A genetic disorder with heterogeneous clinical phenotypes. *Brain* 1997;120(pt 3): 479–490.
29. Lehesjoki AE, Koskimiemi M, Sistonen P, et al. Local-

ization of a gene for progressive myoclonus epilepsy to chromosome 21q22. *Proc Natl Acad Sci USA* 1991; 88:3696–3699.

30. Lehesjoki AE, Koskimiemi M. Progressive myoclonus epilepsy of Unverricht-Lundborg type. *Epilepsia* 1999; 40(suppl 3):23–28.

31. Pennacchio LA, Lehesjoki AE, Stone NE, et al. Mutations in the gene encoding cystatin B in progressive myoclonus epilepsy. *Science* 1996;271(5256):1731–1734.

32. Virtaneva K, Paulin L, Krahe R, de la Chapelle A, et al. The minisatellite expansion mutation in EPMI: resolution of an initial discrepancy. Mutations in brief No. 186. Online. *Hum Mutat* 1998;12(3):218.

33. Bate L, Gardiner M. Molecular genetics of human epilepsies. *Expert reviews in molecular medicine.* Cambridge: University Press, 1999.

34. Minassian BA, Sainz J, Serratosa JM, et al. Genetic locus heterogeneity in Lafora's progressive myoclonus epilepsy. *Ann Neurol* 1999;45(2):262–265.

35. Mole S, Gardiner M. Molecular genetics of the neuronal ceroid lipofuscinoses. *Epilepsia* 1999;40(suppl 3):29–32.

36. Wheeler RB, Sharp JD, Mitchell WA, et al. A new locus for variant late infantile neuronal ceroid lipofuscinosis-CLN7. *Mol Genet Metab* 1999;66(4):337–338.

37. Hirvasniemi A, Lang H, Lehesjoki AE, et al. Northern epilepsy syndrome: an inherited childhood onset epilepsy with associated mental deterioration. *J Med Genet* 1994;31(3):177–182.

38. Tahvanainen E, Ranta S, Hirvasniemi A, et al. A gene for a recessively inherited human childhood progressive epilepsy with mental retardation maps to the distal short arm of chromosome 8. *Proc Natl Acad Sci USA* 1994;91(15):7267–7270.

39. Herva R, Tyynela J, Hirvasniemi A, et al. Northern epilepsy: a novel form of neuronal ceroid-lipofuscinosis. *Brain Pathol* 2000;10:215–222.

40. Picard F, Baulac S, Kahane P, et al. Dominant partial epilepsies: a clinical, electrophysiological and genetic study of 19 european families. *Brain* 2000;123(pt 6): 1247–1262.

41. Gambardella A, Messina D, Le Piane E, et al. Familial temporal lobe epilepsy autosomal dominant inheritance in a large pedigree from southern Italy. *Epilepsy Res* 2000;38(2-3):127–132.

42. Cendes F, Lopes-Cendes I, Andermann E, et al. Familial temporal lobe epilepsy: a clinically heterogeneous syndrome. *Neurology* 1998;50(2):554–557.

43. Berkovic SF. Epilepsy genes and the genetics of epilepsy syndromes: the promise of new therapies based on genetic knowledge. *Epilepsia* 1997;38(suppl 9):S32–S36.

44. Xiong L, Labuda M, Li DS, et al. Mapping of a gene determining familial partial epilepsy with variable foci to chromosome 22q11-q12. *Am J Hum Genet* 1999; 65(6):1698–1710.

45. Scheffer IE, Jones L, Pozzebon M, et al. Autosomal dominant rolandic epilepsy and speech dyspraxia: A new syndrome with anticipation. *Ann Neurol* 1995; 38 (4):633–642.

46. Noebels JL. Targeting epilepsy genes. *Neuron* 1996; 16(2):241–244.

47. Smart SL, Lopantsev V, Zhang CL, et al. Deletion of the K(V)1.1 potassium channel causes epilepsy in mice. *Neuron* 1998;20(4):809–819.

48. Zuberi SM, Eunson LH, Spauschus A, et al. A novel mutation in the human voltage-gated potassium channel gene (Kv1.1) associates with episodic ataxia type 1 and sometimes with partial epilepsy. *Brain* 1999; 122(pt 5):817–825.

49. Leppert M, Singh N. Benign familial neonatoral epilepsy with mutations in two potassium channel genes. *Curr Opin Neurol* 1999;12(2):143–147.

50. Wang XJ, Reynolds ER, Deak P, et al. The seizure locus encodes the Drosophila homolog of the HERG potassium channel. *J Neurosci* 1997;17(3):882–890.

51. Swoboda KJ, Soong B, McKenna C, et al. Paroxysmal kinesigenic dyskinesia and infantile convulsions: clinical and linkage studies. *Neurology* 2000;55(2): 224–230.

52. Griggs RC, Nutt JG. Episodic ataxias as channel-opathies. *Ann Neurol* 1995;37:285–287.

53. Saenz A, Galan J, Caloustian C, et al. Autosomal dominant nocturnal frontal lobe epilepsy in a Spanish family with a Ser252Phe mutation in the CHRNA4 gene. *Arch Neurol* 1999;56(8):1004–1009.

54. Scheffer IE, Bhatia KP, Lopes-Cendes I, et al. Autosomal dominant frontal epilepsy misdiagnosed as sleep disorder. *Lancet* 1994;343(8896):515–517.

55. Scheffer IE, Bhatia KP, Lopes-Cendes I, et al. Autosomal dominant nocturnal frontal lobe epilepsy. A distinctive clinical disorder. *Brain* 1995;118 (pt 1):61–73.

56. Boller F, Wright DG, Cavalieri R, et al. Paroxysmal "nightmares". Sequel of a stroke responsive to diphenylhydantoin. *Neurology* 1975;25(11): 1026–1028.

57. Pedley TA, Guilleminault C. Episodic nocturnal wanderings responsive to anticonvulsant drug therapy. *Ann Neurol* 1977;2(1):30–35.

58. Maselli RA, Rosenberg RS, Spire JP. Episodic nocturnal wanderings in non-epileptic young patients. *Sleep* 1988;11(2):156–161.

59. Peled R, Lavie P. Paroxysmal awakenings from sleep associated with excessive daytime somnolence: a form of nocturnal epilepsy. *Neurology* 1986;36(1):95–98.

60. Lugaresi E, Cirignotta F. Hypnogenic paroxysmal dystonia: epileptic seizure or a new syndrome? *Sleep* 1981;4(2):129–138.

61. Tinuper P, Cerullo A, Cirignotta F, et al. Nocturnal paroxysmal dystonia with short-lasting attacks: three cases with evidence for an epileptic frontal lobe origin of seizures. *Epilepsia* 1990;31:549–556.

62. Montagna P, Sforza E, Tinuper P, et al. Paroxysmal arousals during sleep. *Neurology* 1990;40:1063–1066.

63. Sforza E, Montagna P, Rinaldi R, et al. Paroxysmal periodic motor attacks during sleep: clinical and polygraphic features. *Electroencephalogr Clin Neurophysiol* 1993;86(3):161–166.

64. Lee BI, Lesser RP, Pippenger CE, et al. Familial paroxysmal hypnogenic dystonia. *Neurology* 1985;35: 1357–1360.

65. Tharp BR. Orbital frontal seizures. An unique electroencephalographic and clinical syndrome. *Epilepsia* 1972;13(5):627–642.

66. Geier S, Bancaud J, Talairach J, et al. The seizures of frontal lobe epilepsy. A study of clinical manifestations. *Neurology* 1977;27:951–958.

67. Rasmussen T. Characteristics of a pure culture of frontal lobe epilepsy. *Epilepsia* 1983;24(4):482–493.

68. Williamson PD, Spencer DD, Spencer SS, et al. Complex partial seizures of frontal lobe origin. *Ann Neurol* 1985;18:497–504.

69. Waterman K, Purves SJ, Kosaka B, et al. An epileptic syndrome caused by mesial frontal lobe seizure foci. *Neurology* 1987;37:577–582.

70. Chang C-N, Ojemann LM, Ojemann GA, et al. Seizures of fronto-orbital origin: a proven case. *Epilepsia* 1991;32:487–491.

71. Stores G, Zaiwalla Z, Bergel N. Frontal lobe complex partial seizures in children: a form of epilepsy at particular risk of misdiagnosis. *Dev Med Child Neurol* 1991;33:998–1009.

72. Ajmone-Marsan C. Preoperative electroencephalographic localization of large epileptogenic zones in the frontal and temporal lobes. *Can J Neurol Sci* 1991; 18(suppl 4):564–565.

73. Quesney LF. Preoperative electroencephalographic investigation in frontal lobe epilepsy: electroencephalographic and electrocorticographic recordings. *Can J Neurol Sci* 1991;18(suppl 4):559–563.

74. Henry TR, Mazziotta JC, Engel J Jr. The functional anatomy of frontal lobe epilepsy studied with PET. *Adv Neurol* 1992;57:449–463.

75. Saygi S, Katz A, Marks DA, et al. Frontal lobe partial seizures and psychogenic seizures: Comparison of clinical and ictal characteristics. *Neurology* 1992;42: 1274–1277.

76. Salanova V, Morris HH, Van Ness PC, et al. Comparison of scalp electroencephalogram with subdural electrocorticogram recordings and functional mapping in frontal lobe epilepsy. *Arch Neurol* 1993;50:294–299.

77. Salanova V, Morris HH, van Ness P, et al. Frontal lobe seizures: electroclinical syndromes. *Epilepsia* 1995;36: 16–24.

78. Montagna P. Nocturnal paroxysmal dystonia and nocturnal wandering. *Neurology* 1992;42(suppl 6):61–67.

79. Oguni M, Oguni H, Kozasa M, et al. A case with nocturnal paroxysmal unilateral dystonia and interictal right frontal epileptic EEG focus: a lateralized variant of nocturnal paroxysmal dystonia? *Brain Dev* 1992; 14(6):412–416.

80. Hirsch E, Sellal F, Maton B, et al. Nocturnal paroxysmal dystonia: a clinical form of focal epilepsy. *Neurophysiol Clin* 1994;24(3):207–217.

81. Plazzi G, Montagna P, Tinuper P, et al. Autosomal dominant nocturnal frontal lobe epilepsy. *Epilepsia* 1997;38(6):738; discussion 739–740.

82. Plazzi G, Tinuper P, Montagna P, et al. Epileptic nocturnal wanderings. *Sleep* 1995;18(9):749–756.

83. Ambrosetto G. Autosomal dominant nocturnal frontal lobe epilepsy. *Epilepsia* 1997;38(6):739–740.

84. Oldani A, Zucconi M, Ferini-Strambi L, et al. Autosomal dominant nocturnal frontal lobe epilepsy: electroclinical picture. *Epilepsia* 1996;37(10):964–976.

85. Meierkord H, Fish DR, Marsden CD, et al. Is nocturnal paroxysmal dystonia a form of frontal lobe epilepsy? *Mov Disord* 1992;7:38–42.

86. Meierkord H. Epilepsy and sleep. *Curr Opin Neurol* 1994;7(2):107–112.

87. Thomas P, Picard F, Hirsch E, et al. Autosomal dominant nocturnal frontal lobe epilepsy. *Rev Neurol (Paris)* 1998;154(3):228–235.

88. Paterson D, Nordberg A. Neuronal nicotinic receptors in the human brain. *Prog Neurobiol* 2000;61(1): 75–111.

89. Bertrand S, Weiland S, Berkovic SF, et al. Properties of neuronal nicotinic acetylcholine receptor mutants from humans suffering from autosomal dominant nocturnal frontal lobe epilepsy. *Br J Pharmacol* 1998;125 (4):751–760.

90. Wevers A, Jeske A, Lobron C, et al. Cellular distribution of nicotinic acetylcholine receptor subunit mRNAs in the human cerebral cortex as revealed by nonisotopic in situ hybridization. *Brain Res* 1994;25 (1-2):122–128.

91. Steinlein OK. New insights into the molecular and genetic mechanisms underlying idiopathic epilepsies. *Clin Genet* 1998;54(3):169–175.

92. Weiland S, Witzemann V, Villarroel A, et al. An amino acid exchange in the second transmembrane segment of a neuronal nicotinic receptor causes partial epilepsy by altering its desensitization kinetics. *FEBS Lett* 1996;398(1):91–96.

93. Magnusson A, Nakken KO, Brubakk E. Autosomal dominant frontal epilepsy. *Lancet* 1996;347:1191–1192.

94. Ito M, Kobayashi K, Fujii T, et al. Electroclinical picture of autosomal dominant nocturnal frontal lobe epilepsy in a Japanese family. *Epilepsia* 2000;41(1): 52–58.

95. Hirose S, Iwata H, Akiyoshi H, et al. A novel mutation of CHRNA4 responsible for autosomal dominant nocturnal frontal lobe epilepsy. *Neurology* 1999;53(8): 1749–1753.

96. Steinlein OK, Stoodt J, Mulley J, et al. Independent occurrence of the CHRNA4 Ser248Phe mutation in a Norwegian family with nocturnal frontal lobe epilepsy. *Epilepsia* 2000;41(5):529–535.

97. Lena C, Changeux JP, Mulle C. Evidence for "preterminal" nicotinic receptors on GABAergic axons in the rat interpeduncular nucleus. *J Neurosci* 1993;13(6): 2680–2688.

98. Dani JA. Properties underlying the influence of nicotinic receptors on neuronal excitability and epilepsy. *Epilepsia* 2000;41:1063–1065.

99. McGehee DS, Heath MJ, Gelber S, et al. Nicotine enhancement of fast excitatory synaptic transmission in CNS by presynaptic receptors. *Science* 1995;269 (5231):1692–1696.

100. Gray R, Rajan AS, Radcliffe KA, et al. Hippocampal synaptic transmission enhanced by low concentrations of nicotine. *Nature* 1996;383(6602):713–716.

101. Scheffer IE. Autosomal dominant nocturnal frontal lobe epilepsy. *Epilepsia* 2000;41(8):1059–1060.

102. Hayman M, Scheffer IE, Chinvarun Y, et al. Autosomal dominant nocturnal frontal lobe epilepsy: demonstration of focal frontal onset and intrafamilial variation. *Neurology* 1997;49(4):969–975.

103. Oldani A, Zucconi M, Asselta R, et al. Autosomal dominant nocturnal frontal lobe epilepsy. A video-polysomnographic and genetic appraisal of 40 patients and delineation of the epileptic brain. *Brain* 1998; 121(pt 2):205–223.

104. Provini F, Plazzi G, Tinuper P, et al. Nocturnal frontal lobe epilepsy. A clinical and polygraphic overview of 100 consecutive cases. *Brain* 1999;122(pt 6):1017–1031.

105. Picard F, Bertrand S, Steinlein OK, et al. Mutated nicotinic receptors responsible for autosomal dominant nocturnal frontal lobe epilepsy are more sensitive to carbamazepine. *Epilepsia* 1999;40(9):1198–1209.

106. Nakken KO, Magnusson A, Steinlein OK. Autosomal

dominant nocturnal frontal lobe epilepsy: an electro-clinical study of a Norwegian family with ten affected members. *Epilepsia* 1999;40(1):88–92.

107. Zucconi M, Oldani A, Smirne S, et al. The macrostructure and microstructure of sleep in patients with autosomal dominant nocturnal frontal lobe epilepsy. *J Clin Neurophysiol* 2000;17(1):77–86.

108. Khatami R, Neumann M, Schulz H, et al. A family with autosomal dominant nocturnal frontal lobe epilepsy and mental retardation. *J Neurol* 1998;245(12):809–810.

109. Ferini-Strambi L, Bozzali M, Cercignani M, et al. Magnetization transfer and diffusion-weighted imaging in nocturnal frontal lobe epilepsy. *Neurology* 2000; 54(12):2331–2333.

Myoclonus and Paroxysmal Dyskinesias,
Advances in Neurology, Vol. 89,
edited by S. Fahn and S. J. Frucht.
Lippincott Williams & Wilkins, Philadelphia © 2002.

43

Clinical Spectrum and Genetics of Rolandic Epilepsy

*Bernd A. Neubauer, †Andreas Hahn, †Ulrich Stephani, and †Hermann Doose

*Division of Neuropediatrics, Justus-Liebig-University, Giessen, Germany; †Department
of Neuropediatrics, University of Kiel, Kiel, Germany

ELECTRO-CLINICAL SPECTRUM

Rolandic epilepsy (RE) or benign epilepsy of childhood with centrotemporal spikes belongs to the idiopathic partial epilepsies also including benign psychomotor epilepsy and benign occipital epilepsy (1).

The first description of RE as an unique electroclinical syndrome can be credited to Nayrac and Beaussart in 1957 (2). The epilepsy accounts for approximately one sixth of all childhood epilepsies, and has a prevalence of greater than 1/1000 (3,4). A slight, but consistent predominance of males has been documented. Age at onset varies from 3 to 13 years of age; in the majority of cases, epilepsy manifests not before school age (5). Clinical and electroencephalographic remission of epilepsy without intellectual deficit before 15 to 16 years of age is the rule (1,6). Clinically, RE is characterized by brief, simple, partial, hemifacial motor seizures, frequently having associated somatosensory symptoms. These partial seizures have a tendency to evolve into generalized tonic clonic seizures. Both seizure types are often related to sleep. Characteristic features are: (a) somatosensory onset with unilateral paresthesias involving the tongue, lips, gums, and inner cheeks; (b) unilateral, tonic, clonic or tonic-clonic convulsions involving the face, lips, tongue, as well as the pharyngeal and laryngeal muscles, causing (c) speech arrest

and drooling due to sialorrhea and saliva pooling. At this stage the seizure may end, or it may develop into a generalized major convulsion. Nocturnal seizures, the most frequent variant of this syndrome, frequently become generalized. Generalized tonic-clonic seizures are by a wide margin the most frequently observed seizure type. Nonfacial partial motor and unilateral seizures have also been reported (1). Complex partial seizures are not observed (5). Seizure frequency is low with many patients suffering only one seizure during the course of disease. Recently, a placebo-controlled trial has demonstrated that sulthiame is highly effective and well tolerated in patients with RE (7).

The electroencephalographic hallmark of RE are blunt high-voltage characteristically shaped epileptic discharges predominantly of centrotemporal location (Fig. 43.1). The most prominent element of this specific waveform is a negative spike or sharp wave that is preceded by a well-defined, short duration prepositivity, and often followed by a prominent positive wave whose amplitude is frequently up to 50% that of the preceding spike or sharp wave (5). These centrotemporal spike or sharp slow waves (CTS) are activated by sleep and tend to spread from side to side, frequently with the features of a horizontal dipole (8). At younger age, children with RE also tend to show spike or sharp slow waves in the posterior temporal or occipital regions

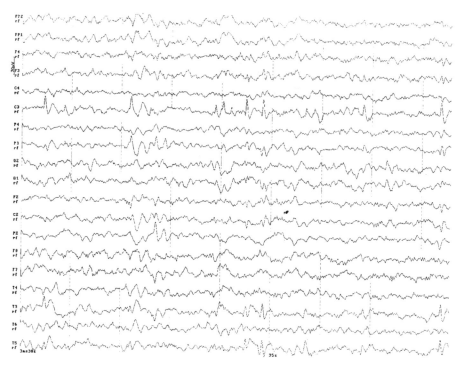

FIG. 43.1. EEG of a 7-year-old girl with RE. Centrotemporal left-sided spikes at rest.

that with maturation can be replaced by, or occur simultaneously with spike or sharp slow waves in the centrotemporal area (1,9).

A normal intelligence and a normal neurologic status are considered a prerequisite for diagnosis of RE (6). However, it is hard to conceive that RE should protect against other types of neurologic disorders. One would rather expect to find it equally distributed in all groups of the population (9). Doose investigated the clinical symptoms of 41 probands with familial CTS. Besides subjects displaying the characteristic clinical features of RE, he also observed children with largely divergent clinical symptoms (e.g., atypical absences, febrile convulsions, complex-partial seizures and mental retardation without seizures) (10). He concluded that CTS are the symptom of a widespread genetic liability responsible not only for RE, but for a broad spectrum of epileptic and non-epileptic disorders (10). In a unifying pathogenic concept of idiopathic partial epilepsies the responsible

basic mechanism has been termed hereditary impairment of brain maturation (HIBM) (11).

In 1982, Aicardi and Chevrie (12) first reported seven patients who fulfilled the main criteria for RE, but who also suffered from secondarily generalized minor seizures. Because of the overall good prognosis, they coined the term atypical benign partial epilepsy (ABPE). Recently, Hahn and co-workers investigated the clinical and electroencephalographic spectrum of ABPE, which is by far less prevalent than RE because they doubted the good prognosis with respect to mental development (13). Criteria for diagnosis of ABPE consisted of detection of focal sharp or spike slow waves indiscernible from those in RE with activation by sleep in at least one EEG, and occurrence of generalized minor seizures of focal origin (i.e., myoclonic, atonic-astatic seizures and atypical absences). In the 43 children studied, mental development prior to onset of epilepsy was retarded in 26%. In addition to generalized minor

TABLE 43.1. *Seizure symptomatology in 43 subjects with atypical benign partial epilepsy*

Seizure symptomatology	Number (%)
Generalized minor seizures	**43 (100)**
Atonic-astatic seizures	31 (72)
Atypical absences	30 (70)
Myoclonic seizures	10 (23)
Status of minor seizures	17 (40)
Focal seizures	**27 (63)**
Simple partial seizures involving other areas than the orofacial region	19 (44)
Unilateral seizures	9 (21)
Simple partial seizures involving the orofacial region	6 (14)
Versive seizures	5 (12)
Focal atonic seizures	4 (9)
Complex partial seizures	1 (2)
Generalized tonic-clonic seizures (GTCS)	**19 (44)**
GTCS without focal symptoms	19 (44)
GTCS with focal symptoms not involving the orofacial region	13 (30)
GTCS with focal symptoms involving the orofacial region	8 (19)
Others	**18 (42)**
Questionable seizures	8 (19)
Unclassifiable seizures	7 (18)
Febrile convulsions	5 (12)
Neonatal seizures	2 (6)

From Hahn A, Pistohl J, Neubauer BA, et al. Atypical "benign" partial epilepsy or pseudo-Lennox-syndrome. Part I: symptomatology and long-term prognosis. *Neuropediatrics* 2001;32:1–8, with permission.

seizures of focal origin, 28% of patients suffered from Rolandic, 44% from generalized tonic-clonic, 21% from unilateral, 44% from partial motor, 12% from versiv (12%), 9% from focal atonic, and 2% from complex-partial seizures (Table 43.1). Despite an exceptionally pronounced activation of epileptic discharges during sleep resulting in a bioelectrical status in 51% of patients and a temporarily often therapy-resistant course, 84% of patients reached clinical remission and all subjects older than age 15 became seizure-free. However, 56% of patients were left with persistent mental deficits (13). Based on these findings, the authors concluded that there are significant clinical overlaps particularly with RE, but also with electrical status epilepticus during sleep and Landau-Kleffner syndrome.

GENETICS

In 1964, Bray and Wiser (14) reported that CTS, the associated EEG trait of RE, follow an autosomal dominant mode of inheritance with high but incomplete penetrance. In 1975, Heijbel and colleagues tested this hypothesis in the families of 19 children with RE. In the siblings of these children who were investigated by wake and sleep recordings they found that 11 of 32 (34%) showed Rolandic discharges. Based on these findings, they came to the identical conclusion as did Bray and Wiser (15). Ottman questioned this conclusion for a possible ascertainment bias was not taken into account (16). In both series only approximately 10% of trait carriers had seizures, which corresponds roughly to the ratio of prevalences of RE (1/500 to 1/1000) and the EEG trait (approximately 2%). Only a small minority of CTS carriers suffer from seizures. In those who do, additional generalized genetic EEG traits (e.g., 3-Hz generalized spikes and waves, photosensitivity) might contribute to the manifestation of epilepsy (9). More recently, Doose and associates studied 188 siblings of epileptic children with CTS and observed CTS in 14% of siblings (17).

Although the exact mode of inheritance remains equivocal, the previously mentioned studies demonstrate that the CTS trait, the electroencephalographic hallmark of RE, is genetically determined. Therefore, EEG investigations at the age of expression can be conducted and multiplex families with several affected relatives (siblings) can be ascertained. This should allow delineating the symptoms associated with the neurobiologic marker as defined by its EEG morphology and its familial occurrence. As previously stated, the clinical symptoms associated with the CTS trait seem not to be limited to what is defined as classic RE. EEG analysis of the relatives of subjects with ABPE disclosed sharp or spike slow waves as characteristic of RE in 40% of siblings in whom EEGs were performed at the age of maximum penetrance (3–10 years) (13,18). This number is by far higher than the rate found in siblings of patients with RE by a comparable method (17). From these data, the authors concluded that ABPE and RE may have a common underlying genetic etiology, and that the high rate of sharp waves in ABPE siblings, the polymorphous seizure symptoms and the massive extent of epileptic discharges point to a very strong expressivity of the underlying genetic disturbance. However genetic heterogeneity has to be expected (13,18).

Recently, in several handicapped children with de novo deletions of 1q43 and 7q seizures and EEG findings (similar to those found in benign rolandic epilepsy) were reported (19,20). Several linkage studies have been applied to families with RE or CTS, respectively. Reese and associates (21), Whitehouse and colleagues (22), and Neubauer and associates (23) excluded 6p21 (EJM1), the fragile X site, 20q13 (EBN1), and 8q24 (EBN2) by linkage analysis. First positive evidence for linkage in RE was found on chromosome 15q14. It was concluded that either the alpha 7 AChR subunit gene (which is located there) or another closely linked gene are implicated in pedigrees with RE and that the trait is genetically heterogeneous (24). Recently, Mount and co-workers showed that the gene of a cation chloride cotransporter (KCC4) is also located within this region (25).

Further research will have to elucidate the relevance of these findings for the under-standing for the most common idiopathic epilepsy syndrome of childhood.

REFERENCES

1. Dalla Bernardina B, Chiamenti C, Capovilla G, et al. Benign partial epilepsies in childhood. In: Roger J, Buneau M, Dravet CH, et al. *Epileptic syndromes in infancy, childhood and adolescence*. London: John Libbey and Co., 1985;137–149.
2. Nayrac P, Beaussart M. Les pointes-ondes prérolandiques: expression EEG trés particulière. Etude électroclinique de 21 cas. *Rev Neurol* 1957;99:201–206.
3. Hejbel J, Blom S, Bergfors PG. Benign epilepsy of children with centrotemporal EEG foci in childhood. A study of incidence rate on outpatient care. *Epilepsia* 1975;16:657–664.
4. Cavazutti GBL, Capella L, Nalin A. Longitudinal study of epileptiform EEG patterns in normal children. *Epilepsia* 1980;21:43–55.
5. Lüders H, Lesser RP, Dinner DS, et al. Benign focal epilepsy of childhood. In: Lüders H, Lesser RP, eds. *Epilepsy-electroclinical syndromes*. London: Springer-Verlag, 1987:303–346.
6. Commission on classification and terminology of the international league against epilepsy. Proposal for revised classification of epilepsies and epileptic syndromes. *Epilepsia* 1989;30:389–399.
7. Rating D, Wolf C, Bast T. Sulthiame as monotherapy in children with benign childhood epilepsy with centrotemporal spikes: a 6-month randomized, double-blind, placebo-controlled study. Sulthiame study group. *Epilepsia* 2000;41:1284–1288.
8. Gutierrez AR, Brick JF, Bodensteiner J. Dipole reversal: an ictal feature of benign partial epilepsy with centrotemporal spikes. *Epilepsia* 1990;31:544–548.
9. Doose H, Neubauer B, Carlsson G. Children with benign focal sharp waves in the EEG—developmental disorders and epilepsy. *Neuropediatrics* 1996;27:1–15.
10. Doose H. Symptomatology in children with focal sharp waves of genetic origin. *Eur J Pediatr* 1989;149:210–215.
11. Doose H, Baier WK. Benign partial epilepsies and related conditions: multifactorial pathogenesis with hereditary impairment of brain maturation. *Eur J Pediatr* 1989;149:152–158.
12. Aicardi J, Chevrie JJ. Atypical benign partial epilepsy of childhood. *Dev Med Child Neurol* 1982;24:281–292.
13. Hahn A, Neubauer BA, Stephani U, et al. Atypical "benign" partial epilepsy or pseudo-Lennox-syndrome. I. Symptomatology and long-term prognosis. *Neuropediatrics* 2001;32:1–8.
14. Bray PF, Wiser WC. Evidence for a genetic etiology of temporal-central abnormalities in focal epilepsy. *New Engl J Med* 1964;271:926–933.
15. Hejbel J, Blom S, Rasmuson M. Benign epilepsy of childhood with centrotemporal EEG foci. A genetic study. *Epilepsia* 1975;16:285–293.
16. Ottman R. Genetics of the partial epilepsies: a review. *Epilepsia* 1989;30:107–111.
17. Doose H, Brigger-Heuer B, Neubauer BA. Children with focal sharp waves: clinical and genetic aspects. *Epilepsia* 1997;38:788–796.
18. Doose H, Hahn A, Neubauer BA, et al. Atypical "be-

nign" partial epilepsy or pseudo-Lennox-syndrome. II. Genetic study. *Neuropediatrics* 2001;32(1):9-13.

19. Vaughn BV, Greenwood RS, Aylsworth AS, et al. Similarities of EEG and seizures in del(1q) and benign rolandic epilepsy. *Pediatr Neurol* 1996;15:261–264.

20. Burke MS, Carroll JE, Burket RC. Benign rolandic epilepsy and chromosome 7q deletion. *J Child Neurol* 1997;12:148–149.

21. Reese M, Diebold U, Doose H, et al. Benign childhood epilepsy with centrotemporal spikes and the focal sharp wave trait is not linked to the fragile X region. *Neuropediatrics* 1993;24:211–213.

22. Whitehouse W, Diebold U, Parker K, et al. Exclusion of linkage of genetic focal shar waves of the HLA region on chromosome 6p in families with benign partial epilepsy with centrotemporal sharp waves. *Neuropediatrics* 1993;24:208–210.

23. Neubauer B, Moises HW, Läβker U, et al. Benign childhood epilepsy with centrotemporal spikes and electroencephalography trait are not linked to EBN1 and EBN2 of benign neonatal familial convulsions. *Epilepsia* 1997;38:782–787.

24. Neubauer BA, Fiedler B, Himmelein B, et al. Centrotemporal spikes in families with Rolandic epilepsy. Linkage to chromosome 15q14. *Neurology* 1998;51:1608–1612.

25. Mount DB, Mercado A, Song L, et al. Cloning and characterization of KCC3 and KCC4, new members of the cation-chloride cotransporter gene family. *J Biol Chem* 1999;274:16355–16362.

Subject Index

Page numbers followed by f indicate figures; page numbers followed by t indicate tables

A

Acetazolamide
  in blocking synchronous motor activity in
      animal model, 277, 278f
  for episodic disorders of nervous system, 382,
      383, 394, 453, 454, 456
  mechanism of action, 275–276
Acetylcholine receptors, in autosomal dominant
      nocturnal frontal lobe epilepsy, 465, 466f,
      467–469
Action myoclonus, 13–14, 15
  electrophysiology, 31
  in multiple system atrophy, 81
  in posthypoxic myoclonus, 85–86
Acyclovir, 70
Alcohol use/abuse, myoclonic dystonia and, 5,
      188, 190, 190t
Aldolase C
  after global brain ischemia
      distribution, 338f, 339–341, 340f, 347–348,
          348f, 349f
      Purkinje cell loss, 342, 347, 348, 355–357
  function, 357
  measurement, 335
Alexander disease, 115
Alkalosis, 61
Aluminum toxicity, 54–55
Alzheimer's disease
  electrophysioly, 32–33
  genetics, 177
  myoclonus features in, 32–33
  myoclonus incidence in, 20, 22
Amantadine
  myoclonus induced by, 63, 78–79
  serotonin syndrome induced by, 65–66
2-(Amino-methyl) phenylacetic acid (AMPA),
      333
AMPA. *See* (Amino-methyl) phenylacetic acid
Amphetamine, 65
Amyloidosis, 147
Analgesic drugs, 68
Andersen disease, 205, 207
Anesthetic agent-induced myoclonus, 61
Animal studies, 9–10
Antibiotic drugs, adverse effects, 69–70

Anticonvulsant drugs, 64–65
Antidepressant drugs, adverse effects, 66–67
Antihelminthic drugs, 70
Antihistamine drugs, 64
Arnold-Chiari malformation, paroxysmal
      dyskinesia secondary to, 404, 406–407,
      408
Arsenic toxicity, 55
Arteriovenous malformation, spinal myoclonus
      caused by, 138
Assessment, 15–16
  pallido-pontal-nigral degeneration, 36
  periodic limb movements, 146
  posthypoxic myoclonus, 87
  restless leg syndrome, 146
  startle responses, 153, 153t
  toxin- and drug-induced myoclonus, 49
  Truong-Fahn scale, 361
  unified rating scale
      clinical application, 362–363
      components, 362
      equipment and procedures, 363–364
      evaluation of myoclonus at rest, 367–368f
      evaluation of myoclonus with action,
          369–372f
      functional tests, 373–374f
      goals, 361–362
      historical development, 361
      patient questionnaire, 365–366f
      scoring, 363, 375–376f
      stimulus sensitivity evaluation, 369f
      validity, 362
      videotape protocol, 364t
Asterixis, 15
  classification, 103
  as complication of Parkinson disease treatment,
      78
  definition, 49
  focal central nervous system lesion in, 112
  in metabolic/toxic encephalopathy, 112
  in toxin- and drug-induced myoclonus, 49–53
Ataxia, episodic. *See* Episodic ataxia
Ataxia, progressive myoclonic, 15
  associated metabolic disorders, 31, 32t
  Ramsay Hunt syndrome and, 5–6